D0959353

A WORD BOOK

IN PATHOLOGY & LABORATORY MEDICINE

SHEILA B. SLOANE

Formerly President, Medi-Phone, Inc.
Author, The Medical Word Book

JOHN L. DUSSEAU, M.A.

Vice President and Editor-in-Chief, Retired
W.B. Saunders Company

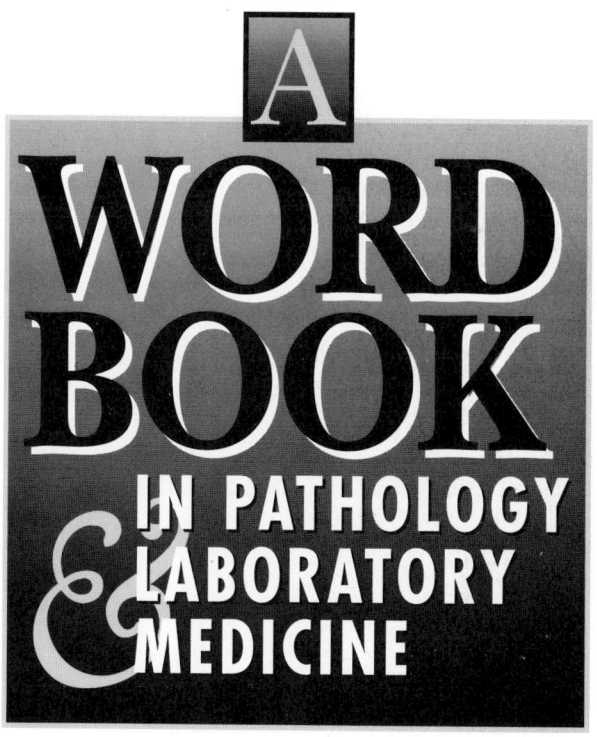

A WORD BOOK IN PATHOLOGY & LABORATORY MEDICINE

2ND

EDITION

W.B. SAUNDERS COMPANY

A Division of Harcourt Brace & Company

Philadelphia   London   Toronto   Montreal   Sydney   Tokyo

W.B. SAUNDERS COMPANY
A Division of Harcourt Brace & Company

The Curtis Center
Independence Square West
Philadelphia, Pennsylvania 19106

Library of Congress Cataloging-in-Publication Data

Sloane, Sheila B.
  A word book in pathology and laboratory medicine / Sheila B.
Sloane, John L. Dusseau. — 2nd ed.
      p.   cm.
  Includes bibliographical references.
  ISBN 0–7216–4040–0
  1. Pathology—Terminology.   2. Medical laboratory technology—
Terminology.   I. Dusseau, John L.   II. Title.
  [DNLM: 1. Pathology—terminology.   2. Diagnosis Laboratory—
terminology.   QZ 15 S634w 1995]
  RB115.S56   1995
  616.07′014—dc20
  DNLM/DLC   94–30881

A WORD BOOK IN PATHOLOGY AND LABORATORY
MEDICINE, Second Edition   ISBN   0–7216–4040–0

Copyright © 1995, 1984 by W.B. Saunders Company.

All rights reserved. No part of this publication may be reproduced or transmitted in any
form or by any means, electronic or mechanical, including photocopy, recording, or any
information storage and retrieval system, without permission in writing from the
publisher.

Printed in the United States of America

Last digit is the print number: 9   8   7   6   5   4

Dedicated
to
All those who enforce
the necessary accuracy of medicine

Preface

In its first edition *A Word Book in Pathology and Laboratory Medicine* met a distinct need in medical transcription, its six hundred pages providing a careful listing of the language of two comprehensive specialties of medicine. One might then suppose that revision would require updating of terms and slight deletion of what had become obsolete. But this proved not to be so for a reason simply put but not so simply resolved: The vocabulary of pathology and laboratory medicine comprises all the terms of the separate disciplines of bioscience and all the terms of medicine and surgery and their separate specialties, so that selection of new words and phrases required discrimination lest the work attain a cumbersome size beyond its needs. Even so, some fifteen thousand new words, phrases, and abbreviations have been added to this second edition, and all entries of more than one word have been consistently cross-referenced. We hope that we have been able to achieve a happy course midway between superfluity and insufficiency.

Nowhere was the question of proper detail more troublesome than in the issue of how anatomy was to be treated. From Morgagni on, pathology has had its foundation in knowledge of human structure, so we make no apology for an abundance of anatomical terms, both in the Latin of the *Nomina Anatomica* and in their English equivalents. Further, we have not hesitated to include relatively simple terms whose spelling poses no problem to anyone, because such words round out the dimensions and define the scope of our subject. Similarly, the pages to follow are generously seasoned with abbreviations and eponyms, because the former are an international language of medicine and the latter are a puzzle in orthography.

As before, we have been guided by our belief that the complex and difficult vocabulary of pathology and laboratory medicine needs an accurate and comprehensive listing for use by transcriptionists, medical secretaries, record librarians, and laboratory technologists, who often need to find a word and its proper spelling in the context of its relation to other or similar technical terms or to whole phrases. This is why there are, on the pages to follow, many general headings under which are listed appropriate subentries, so that the user, familiar with only part of a complex phrase, will find entry points to its complete form. Logophilia is not a syndrome listed in this book; but it is a common condition in medicine—the love of words, especially new and polysyllabic ones. Hence, perhaps even the working pathologist or laboratory physician may find this workaday vocabulary useful, for medical terms (and their ingenious abbreviations) are almost beyond computation in number and often beyond comprehension in their Greek and Latin roots. For the latter we have added plurals to those entries whose plural is often more singular than its singular form.

The words themselves must be both accurate and in current use, and, to this purpose, we have had recourse to contemporary reference sources and journals of medicine and investigation; but we have not hesitated to include now obsolete species names and other terms that appear frequently in the older literature. It is not to gainsay the accuracy of our sources to note that they sometimes differ in details of terminology. Thus, we have needed help not only from the W.B. Saunders Company editorial staff but from our diligent typists and proofreaders as well. None could have been more helpful, careful, and perceptive in their task than Donna Ciccotelli, Michaelina Lombardi, Roy Foster, and Wynette Kommer. If errors remain, they are those of our own commission. Whatever their number, it would have been significantly greater without the help we herewith gratefully acknowledge. We also appreciate the role of the American Association for Medical Transcription, whose seminars and publications have been valuable to us and whose leaders and members have done so much to ensure high standards of proficiency in a demanding and difficult profession.

We conclude by hoping that this new edition will serve its purpose and its users well, that its place on the desktop may be secure, and that readers will make known to us their corrections and suggestions. We have tried to be judicious in selection of terms and wakeful in reading of proof, but no book has more significant criticism than that arising from its daily use.

Sheila B. Sloane

John L. Dusseau

Contents

PART I

THE VOCABULARY

A — absolute temperature
absorbance
acetum
ampere
A amyloid
Ångström unit
anode
anterior
artery
atropine
axial
mass number
total acidity
A. — *Actinomyces*
Anopheles
a_1 — antichymotrypsin
A_2 — aortic second sound
a or A — ampere
anode
area
asymmetric
total acidity
α — alpha (q.v.)
a/A ratio
AA — acetic acid
alveolar-arterial
aminoacetone
amyloid associated
arachidonic acid
ascending aorta
atomic absorption
aa — arteries
AA or aa — of each (ana)
AA protein
AAA — abdominal aortic aneurysm
androgenic anabolic agent
AAAF — albumin autoagglutinating
factor
AAAS — American Association for
the Advancement of
Science
AABB — American Association of
Blood Banks
AAC — antibiotic-associated pseudomembranous colitis
AACC — American Association for
Clinical Chemistry
AACIA — American Association for
Clinical Immunology
and Allergy

AAI — American Association of Im-
munologists
AAM — American Academy of Mi-
crobiology
AAMI — Association for the Ad-
vancement of Medical In-
strumentation
AAN — American Association of
Neuropathologists
AAP — American Association of Pathologists
AAPA — American Association of
Pathologist Assistants
AAPB — American Association of
Pathologists and Bacteri-
ologists
AAR — antigen–antiglobulin reaction
AAS — aortic arch syndrome
atomic absorption spectrophotometry
AAT — alpha-antitrypsin
AAV — adeno-associated virus
AB —abnormal
abortion
alcian blue
asbestos body
asthmatic bronchitis
axiobuccal
A/B — acid–base ratio
Ab — antibody
ABA — antibacterial activity
abacterial thrombotic
endocarditis
A band
abarticular gout
abasia
a. astasia
a. atactica
choreic a.
paralytic a.
paroxysmal trepidant a.
spastic a.
a. trepidans
abatement
Abbé's
condenser
test plate
Abbé-Estlander flap

Abbé-Zeiss
    apparatus
    counting chamber
Abbott-Rawson tube
Abbott's Stain for Spores
ABC — absolute basophil count
        American Blood Commis-
            sion
        antigen-binding capacity
        aspiration biopsy cytology
        axiobuccocervical
ABD, abd, or abd — abdomen
                        abdominal
ABDOM, Abdom, or
    abdom — abdomen
                abdominal
abdomen
abdominal
    a. aneurysm
    a. aorta
    a. aortic aneurysm
    a. dropsy
    a. esophagus
    a. fibromatosis
    a. fistula
    a. heart
    a. inguinal ring
    a. kidney
    a. lymph node
    a. muscle deficiency syn-
        drome
    a. reflex
    a. viscera
    a. watersheds
abdominopelvic
abdominoperineal
abducens
    a. nerve
    a. nucleus
abducent nerve
abductor
    a. digiti minimi muscle
    a. longi and extensor brevis
        pollicis muscles
    a. pollicis muscle
ABE — acute bacterial endocarditis
Abel expert system
Abell-Kendall method
Abell's method
Abelson's
    murine leukemia virus
    oncogene

Abernethy's sarcoma
aberrant
    a. duct
    a. ductule
    a. goiter
    a. hemoglobin
    a. pancreas
    a. renal vessels
    a. rest
    a. tissue
aberration
    chromatic a.
    chromosomal a.
    dioptric a.
    distantial a.
    heterosomal a.
    homosomal a.
    interchromosomal a.
    intrachromosomal a.
    karyotype a.
    meridional a.
    newtonian a.
    penta-X chromosomal a.
    spherical a.
    tetra-X chromosomal a.
    triple-X chromosomal a.
abetalipoproteinemia
    familial recessive a.
ABG — axiobuccogingival
        arterial blood gases
abietic acid
abiotrophy
ABL — abetalipoproteinemia
        axiobuccolingual
ablastin
ablate
ablatio
    a. placentae
    a. retinae
ablation
    pituitary a.
    radioiodine a.
ABLB — alternate binaural loudness
            balance
ablepharon
ABMA — anti–basement membrane
            antibody
ABN, Abn, or abn — abnormal
abnormal
    a. chorion
    a. chorionic villi
    a. endochondral ossification

a. flow
a. glucose tolerance test
a. mucopolysacchariduria
a. shortening
abnormality
    bone marrow a.
    chromosomal a.
    chromosome a.
    cytologic a.
    fetal a.
    morphologic a.
    nonspecific hepatocellular a.
    traumatic a.
ABO
    agglutinins
    antibodies
    antigens
    blood group
    compatibility
    erythroblastosis
    hemolytic disease of newborn
    incompatibility
    typing
ABO-RH typing
aborted ectopic pregnancy
abortion
    afebrile a.
    ampullar a.
    artificial a.
    complete a.
    contagious a.
    criminal a.
    habitual a.
    imminent a.
    incomplete a.
    induced a.
    inevitable a.
    infected a.
    justifiable a.
    missed a.
    septic a.
    spontaneous a.
    therapeutic a.
    threatened a.
    tubal a.
abortive
    a. infection
    a. neurofibromatosis
    a. viral disease
abortus fever
ABP — arterial blood pressure
abraded wound

Abraham's protocol
Abrams' test
abrasion
Abrikosov's (Abrikossoff's) tumor
abrin
abruptio placentae
Abrus
ABS — alkylbenzene sulfonate
abscess
    acute a.
    a. aerobic culture
    alveolar a.
    amebic a.
    amebic a. of liver
    apical a.
    appendiceal a.
    Bartholin's a.
    Bezold's a.
    bicameral a.
    bone a.
    brain a.
    breast
    Brodie's a.
    bursal a.
    cerebral a.
    cerebral epidural a.
    chronic a.
    cold a.
    collar-button a.
    crypt a.
    diffuse a.
    Douglas's a.
    dry a.
    Dubois's a.
    embolic a.
    epidural a.
    fecal a.
    follicular a.
    gas a.
    gravitation a.
    gummatous a.
    hematogenous a.
    hepatic a.
    hot a.
    hypostatic a.
    ischiorectal a.
    kidney a.
    Kogoj's a.
    lacunar a.
    lung a.
    lymph node a.
    mastoid a.

metastatic a.
migrating a.
miliary a.
Munro's a.
mycotic a.
nocardial a.
orbital a.
otic a.
pancreatic a.
parafrenal a.
parametric a.
parametritic a.
paranephric a.
parotid a.
Pautrier's a.
pelvic a.
perforating a.
periappendiceal a.
periarticular a.
perinephric a.
perirectal a.
peritonsillar a.
periureteral a.
periurethral a.
phlegmonous a.
Pott's a.
premammary a.
psoas a.
pulmonary a.
pyemic a.
renal cortical a.
residual a.
retrobulbar a.
retrocecal a.
retropharyngeal a.
satellite a.
septicemic a.
shirt-stud a.
stellate a.
stercoral a.
sterile a.
stitch a.
subacute a.
subdiaphragmatic a.
subepidermal a.
subhepatic a.
subperiosteal a.
subphrenic a.
subungual a.
sudoriparous a.
syphilitic a.
thecal a.

thymic a.
Tornwaldt's (Thornwaldt's) a.
tropical a.
tuberculous a.
tubo-ovarian a.
verminous a.
wandering a.
worm a.
abscissa
abscopal
absence
    acquired a.
    congenital a.
Absidia
    A. *corymbifera*
    A. *ramosa*
absolute
    a. alcohol
    atmosphere a.
    a. cell increase
    a. eosinophil count
    a. iodine uptake
    a. leukocytosis
    a. polycythemia
    a. retention time
    a. scale
    a. system of units
    a. temperature
    a. temperature scale
    a. unit
    a. value
    a. viscosity
    a. zero
absorb
absorbance
absorbed dose
absorbefacient
absorbency index
absorbent
    carbon dioxide a.
    a. gland
absorber
absorption
    a. atelectasis
    atomic a.
    a. cavities
    a. cell
    a. coefficient
    a. constant
    disjunctive a.
    a.-equivalent thickness

a. of erythrocyte anti-
bodies
fat a.
iron a.
a. spectrum
absorptive
a. cell
a. lipemia
absorptivity
molar a.
specific a.
abstinence
alimentary a.
ABV — Adriamycin, bleomycin, and
vinblastine
AC — acromioclavicular
adrenal cortex
air conduction
anodal closure
anterior chamber
anticoagulant
anticomplementary
anti-inflammatory corticoid
aortic closure
atriocarotid
auriculocarotid
axiocervical
Ac — actinium
ac — acute
ACA — adenocarcinoma
acacia
"academy rash"
Academy of Clinical Laboratory Physicians and Scientists
acalculous cholecystitis
acanthamebiasis
acanthamebic keratitis
Acanthamoeba
A. *castellani*
A. *hartmannella*
A. *keratitis*
acanthella
acanthion
Acanthobdella
Acanthocephala
Acanthocheilonema
A. *perstans*
A. *streptocerca*
acanthocyte
acanthocytosis
acanthoid cell
acantholysis

acantholytic dysplasia
acanthoma
a. adenoides cysticum
basal cell a.
clear cell a.
Degos's a.
pilar sheath a.
a. verrucosa seborrheica
acanthomatous
a. ameloblastoma
a. ameloblastomic fibroma
acanthor
acanthorrhexis
acanthosis
glycogen a.
a. nigricans
penile a.
acanthotic
acanthrocyte
acanthrocytosis
acapnia
acapnial alkalosis
acarbia
acardia
acardiacus
acardius
acariasis
acaricide
Acaridae
Acarus
A. *folliculorum*
A. *gallinae*
A. *hordei*
A. *rhyzoglypticus hyacinthi*
A. *scabiei*
A. *siro*
acaryote
acatalasemia
acatalasia
acatamathesia
acataphasia
acathectic
acathexia
Acaulium
ACC — adenoid cystic carcinoma
anodal closure contrac-
tion
accelerant
accelerated
a. idioventricular rhythm
a. silicosis

acceleration
>growth a.
>negative a.

accelerator
>a. factor
>a. globulin
>proserum prothrombin conversion a.
>prothrombin a.
>serum a.
>serum prothrombin conversion a.
>serum thrombotic a.
>a. urinae

accelerin

accentuator

acceptor
>hydrogen a.
>oxygen a.
>proton a.

access
>exit a.
>multiple a.
>sequential a.
>a. time

accessory
>a. adrenal cortex
>a. atrium
>a. breast
>a. cells
>a. chromosome
>a. gland
>a. nasal sinus
>a. nerve
>a. nucleus cuneatus
>a. obturator nerve
>a. organ
>a. pancreas
>a. pancreatic duct
>a. paraflocculus
>a. parotid gland
>a. saphenous vein
>a. scrotum
>a. sinus
>a. sinus mucus
>a. spleen
>a. structure

access time

accident
>cardiovascular a.
>cerebral vascular a.
>cerebrovascular a.

accidental
>a. host
>a. parasite

ACCL — anodal closure clonus

acclimation

accommodation

account
>dose a.

accrementition

accreta
>placenta a.

accretion

accumulation
>a. of carbohydrates
>a. of complex lipids
>galactocerebroside a.
>a. of glycogen
>intracellular a.
>a. of pigments
>a. of protein

accumulator

accuracy
>photometric a.
>wavelength a.

ACD — absolute cardiac dullness
>acid-citrate-dextrose
>anterior chest diameter

ACE — adrenocortical extract
>angiotensin converting enzyme

A cell

acellular

acenocoumarin

acentric

acephalous

acephalus
>a. dibrachius
>a. dipus
>a. monobrachius
>a. monopus
>a. paracephalus
>a. sympus

acervuline

acervulus (pl., acervuli)

acestoma

acetabulectomy

acetabulum (pl., acetabula)

acetal

acetaldehyde

acetaldehydrase

acetamide

acetaminophen
    a. assay
    a. hepatic toxicity
acetanilid
acetarsone
acetate
    betamethasone a.
    cellulose a.
    deoxycorticosterone a.
    ethyl a.
    isoamyl a.
    mercuric a.
    methyl a.
    a. replacement factor
    a. trestolone
acetazolamide
Acetest
acetic
    a. acid
    a. acid and potassium ferrocya-
      nide test
    a. acid-alcohol-formalin
    a. aldehyde
    a. anhydride–acetic acid–sul-
      furic acid reagent
    a. naphthalene
    a. orcein
acetoacetate
acetoacetic acid aciduria
acetoacetyl-coenzyme A
    a.-CoA reductase
    a.-CoA thiolase
acetoacetylglutathione hydrolase
acetoacetylhydrolipoate hydrolase
acetoarsenite
Acetobacter
    A. aceti
    A. melanogenus
    A. oxydans
    A. rancens
    A. roseus
    A. suboxydans
    A. xylinum
acetocarmine
acetohexamide
acetoin
    a. dehydrogenase
    a. test
acetol kinase
acetolysis
acetone
    a. body

a. compound
a. fixative
a.-insoluble antigen
isopropyl a.
a. test
acetonemia
acetonemic
acetonitrile
acetonuria
aceto-orcein stain
acetophenazine
acetophenetidin
acetrizoate
aceturate
    diminazene a.
acetyl
    a. chloride
    a. glycerol ether phospho-
      choline
    a. peroxide
    a. sulfisoxazole
acetylaminodeoxyglucosephosphate
    isomerase
acetylaminodeoxyglucose phospho-
    mutase
β-acetylaminodeoxyglucosidase
acetylaminofluorene
acetylaspartic acid; *N*-acetylaspartic
    acid
acetylated hemoglobin
acetylation
acetylcarbromal
acetylcholine
    a. channel
    a. receptor
acetylcholinesterase assay
acetyl-coenzyme A
    a.-CoA acetyltransferase
    a.-CoA acyltransferase
    a.-CoA carboxylase
    a.-CoA hydrolase
    a.-CoA synthetase
N-acetyl-L-cysteine
acetyldigitoxin
acetylene
    a. dichloride
    a. tetrachloride
    a. trichloride
acetylesterase
N-acetyl-D-galactosamine
acetylgalactosaminidase
N-acetylglucosamine

N-acetyl-β-D-glucosaminidase
N-acetylhexosamine
N-acetylmannosamine
acetylmethadol
acetylmethylcarbinol
acetyl-β-methylcholine
N-acetylmuramate
N-acetylmuramic acid
N-acetylneuraminate
N-acetylprocainamide
acetylsalicylic acid
acetylserotonin methyltransferase
acetylsulfadiazine crystals
acetylsulfamethoxazole crystals
acetyltransferase
 acetyl-CoA a.
ACG — apexcardiogram
AcG — accelerator globulin
ACH — adrenocortical hormone
ACh — acetylcholine
achalasia
 biliary a.
 esophageal a.
 pelvirectal a.
 sphincteral a.
 ureteral a.
AChE — acetylcholinesterase
Achillea
Achilles
 bursa
 reflex
 tendon
achillodynia
achlorhydria
achlorhydric
 a. anemia
 a. pepsia
Acholeplasma laidlawii
Acholeplasmataceae
acholic
acholuria
acholuric jaundice
achondrogenesis
achondroplasia
 homozygous a.
achondroplastic dwarfism
achondroplasty
Achorion
 A. schoenleini
 A. violaceum
achrestic anemia
achroacyte

achroacytosis
achrodextrin; achroodextrin
achromacyte
achromasia
achromate
achromatic
 a. lens
 a. net
 a. objective
 a. spindle
achromatin
achromatism
achromatocyte
achromatolysis
achromatophil
achromatophilia
achromatosis
achromatous
achromaturia
achromia
 congenital a.
 cortical a.
 a. parasitica
 a. unguium
achromic
 a. erythrocyte
 a. nevus
Achromobacter
Achromobacteraceae
achromocyte
achromophil
achromophilic
achromophilous
achroodextrin; achrodextrin
Achucárro's stain
achylia
achylic anemia
acid
 abietic a.
 acetic a.
 acetoacetic a.
 N-acetylaspartic a.
 N-acetylmuramic a.
 acetylsalicylic a.
 N-acylneuraminic a.
 adenylic a.
 a. agglutination
 a. alcohol
 aldaric a.
 aldonic a.
 alginic a.
 aliphatic a.

allantoic a.
alpha amino a.
amino a.
aminoacetic a.
α-aminoadipic a.
aminobenzoic a.
γ-aminobutyric a.
aminocaproic a.
aminoglutaric a.
aminohippuric a.
aminohydroxybenzoic a.
aminoisobutyric a.
aminolevulinic a.
aminopenicillanic a.
6-aminopenicillanic a.
aminosuccinic a.
a. anhydride
a. anhydride method
anthranilic a.
arachidonic a.
argininosuccinic a.
aromatic a.
ascorbic a.
asparagic a.
asparaginic a.
aspartic a.
aurin tricarboxylic a.
behnic a.
1,2-benzenedicarboxylic a.
benzoic a.
benzoylaminoacetic a.
binary a.
bisphosphoglyceric a.
boric a.
Brönsted-Lowry a.
butanoic a.
butyric a.
cacodylic a.
caffeic a.
canavaninosuccinic a.
capric a.
caproic a.
caprylic a.
carbolic a.
carbonic a.
γ-carboxyglutamic a.
carminic a.
catechinic a.
catechuric a.
cerebronic a.
a. challenge test
chenodeoxycholic a.

chloranilic a.
chloric a.
chloroacetic a.
chlorophenoxyacetic a.
chlorotoloxyacetic a.
cholic a.
chromic a.
chromium-51-
    ethylenediaminetetra-
    acetic a.
chromonucleic a.
a. citrate dextrose
citric a.
complementary deoxyribonu-
    cleic a.
conjugate a.
cytidylic a.
decanoic a.
dehydroascorbic a.
deoxyadenylic a.
deoxycholic a.
deoxycytidylic a.
deoxyguanylic a.
deoxyribonucleic a.
deoxyuridic a.
diacetic a.
dibasic a.
dicarboxylic a.
2,4-dichlorophenoxy acetic a.
diethylbarbituric a.
diethylene-
    triaminepentaacetic a.
dihydrofolic a.
dihydroxymandelic a.
dihydroxyphenylacetic a.
3,5-dinitrobenzoic a.
dipicolinic a.
docosahexaenoic a.
a. dye
edetic a.
eicosapentaenoic a.
eicosatrienoic a.
elaidic a.
a. elution slide test
epsilon a.
epsilon-aminocaproic a.
essential fatty a.
ethacrynic a.
ethanoic a.
ethylenediaminetetraacetic a.
a. fast
a.-fast bacilli

fatty a.
folic a.
folinic a.
a. formaldehyde hematin
formic a.
formiminoglutamic a.
free a.
a. fuchsin
fumaric a.
gamma-carboxyglutamic a.
gastric a.
glacial acetic a.
D-glucaric a.
glucuronic a.
glutamic a.
glutaric a.
glyceroboric a.
glycochenodeoxycholic a.
glycocholic a.
glycodeoxycholic a.
glycolithocholic a.
a. glycoprotein
guanidino-aminovaleric a.
guanylic a.
a. halide
a. hematin
a. hemolysin test
heptanoic a.
hexadecanoic a.
hexanoic a.
hexuronic a.
hippuric a.
homogentisic a.
homovanillic a.
hyaluronic a.
hydrochloric a.
hydrocyanic a.
hydrofluoric a.
a. hydrolase
hydroperoxyeicosatetraenoic a.
hydroxy a.
hydroxyanthranilic a.
p-hydroxybenzoic a.
hydroxybutyric a.
hydroxyeicosatetraenoic a.
hydroxyethanesulfonic a.
hydroxyheptadecatrienoic a.
5-hydroxyindoleacetic a.
O-hydroxyphenylacetic a.
p-hydroxyphenyllactic a.
p-hydroxyphenylpyruvic a.
ibotenic a.

iduronic a.
imidazolepyruvic a.
imino a.
indolaceturic a.
indoleacetic a.
indollactic a.
inorganic a.
inosinic a.
a. intoxication
iodic a.
iodoalphionic a.
a. ionization constant
isobutyric a.
isocitric a.
isovaleric a.
keto a.
ketoadipate a.
ketoadipic a.
ketoglutaric a.
kojic a.
lactic a.
lauric a.
leukocyte ascorbic a.
Lewis a.
lignoceric a.
linoleic a.
linolenic a.
lipoic a.
lithic a.
lithocholic a.
long-chain fatty a.
a. magenta
malic a.
malonic a.
medium-chain fatty a.
mercaptoacetic a.
metaphosphoric a.
3-methoxy-4-
    hydroxymandelic a.
methylacetic a.
α-methylacetoacetic a.
methylmalonic a.
monoaminodicarboxylic a.
monoaminomonocarboxylic a.
monobasic a.
monocarboxylic a.
morrhuic a.
a. mucopolysaccharide
muramic a.
mycolic a.
myristic a.
nalidixic a.

nitrilotriacetic a.
nucleic a.
a. number
octadecanoic a.
octanoic a.
oleic a.
organic a.
orotic a.
orotidylic a.
orthophosphoric a.
oxalic a.
oxaloacetic a.
oxo a.
3-oxobutyric a.
2-oxoglutaric a.
oxolinic a.
oxybutyric a.
palmitic a.
palmitoleic a.
p-aminohippuric a.
pantothenic a.
para-aminobenzoic a.
para-aminohippuric a.
para-aminosalicylic a.
paracetic a.
pentetic a.
perchloric a.
performic a.
a. perfusion test
phenaceturic a.
phenyllactic a.
phenylpyruvic a.
a. phosphatase
a. phosphate
phosphatidic a.
6-phosphogluconic a.
phosphoglyceric a.
5-phosphomevalonic a.
phosphomolybdic a.
phosphonic a.
phosphonoacetic a.
phosphoric a.
phthalic a.
phytanic a.
phytic a.
picric a.
polyadenylic a.
polybasic a.
polyenoic a.
polyglutamic folic a.
polyphosphoric a.
polyunsaturated fatty a.

polyuridylic a.
pristanic a.
propanoic a.
prostanoic a.
prussic a.
pteroic a.
pteroylglutamic a.
pteroylmonoglutamic a.
4-pyridoxic a.
pyrophosphoric a.
pyruvic a.
quinolinic a.
quisqualic a.
a. radical
radioiodinated fatty a.
a. reaction
retinoic a.
ribonucleic a.
ribothymidylic a.
ricinoleic a.
saccharic a.
salicylic a.
salicylsalicylic a.
salicylsulfonic a.
saturated fatty a.
a. seromucoid
serum uric a.
sialic a.
a. sialomucin
silicic a.
soluble ribonucleic a.
a. stain
stearic a.
succinic a.
sugar a.
sulfanilic a.
sulfinic a.
sulfonic a.
sulfuric a.
sulfurous a.
tannic a.
tartaric a.
taurochenodeoxycholic a.
taurocholic a.
taurodeoxycholic a.
taurolithocholic a.
teichoic a.
ternary a.
n-tetracosanoic a.
tetrahydrofolic a.
thio a.
thioctic a.

thioglycolic a.
thiolaminopropionic a.
thymidylic a.
titratable a.
toluic a.
total fatty a's
tranexamic a.
tribasic a.
tricarboxylic a.
trichloroacetic a.
2,4,5-trichlorophenoxy
    acetic a.
tuberculostearic a.
tungstic a.
UDP-glucuronic a.
UDP-iduronic a.
undecylenic a.
uric a.
uridine diphosphoglucuronic a.
uridylic a.
a. urine
urobenzoic a.
urocanic a.
uronic a.
ursodeoxycholic a.
vaccenic a.
valeric a.
valproic a.
a. value
vanillactic a.
vanillic a.
vanillylmandelic a.
vinegar a.
xanthurenic a.
xanthylic a.
y-carboxyglutamic a.
acid-alcohol-formalin
    acetic a.-a.-f.
Acidaminococcus fermentans
acidaminuria
acid-base
    a.-b. balance
    a.-b. indicator
    a.-b. nomogram
    a.-b. ratio
acidemia
    argininosuccinic a.
    metabolic a.
    methylmalonic a.
    organic a.
    propionic a.

acid-fast
    a.-f. bacilli
    a.-f. bacterium
    a.-f. stain
    a.-f. staining methods
α_1-acid glycoprotein
acidic dye
acidifiable
acidified
    a. ethanol
    a. serum tests
acidifier
acidify
acidimetry
acidity
    a. reduction test
    titratable a.
    total a.
acid-lability test
acidocyte
acidocytopenia
acidocytosis
acidogenic
acidophil; acidophile
    a. adenoma
    alpha a.
    a. body
    a. cell
    epsilon a.
    a. granule
acidophilic
    a. adenome
    a. body
    a. erythroblast
    a. index
    a. leukocyte
    a. normoblast
acidosis
    carbon dioxide a.
    compensated a.
    diabetic a.
    hypercapnic a.
    hyperchloremic a.
    lactic a.
    metabolic a.
    orotic a.
    potassium a.
    renal tubular a.
    respiratory a.
    a. test
    uncompensated a.
    uremic a.

acidotic
acid phosphatase
    a. p. assays
    cupric ion-inhibited a. p.
    prostatic a. p.
    a. p. staining
    tartrate-inhibited a. p.
    a. p. test
acid-Schiff stain
acid-secretion rate
aciduria
    acetoacetic a.
    beta-aminoisobutyric a.
    argininosuccinic a.
    glycolic a.
    methylmalonic a.
    organic a.
    orotic a.
    paroxysmal a.
    propionic a.
    pyroglutamic a.
    xanthurenic a.
aciduric
acinar
    a. cell carcinoma
    a. cell tumor
    a. development
    a. gland
Acinetobacter
    A. *anitratus*
    A. *calcoaceticus*
    A. *calcoaceticus anitratus*
    A. *calcoaceticus lwoffi*
    A. *parapertussis*
    A. *lwoffi*
acinic
    a. cell adenocarcinoma
    a. cell carcinoma
    a. cell tumor
    a. cell tumor of salivary
      gland
aciniform
acinitis
acinose carcinoma
acinotubular gland
acinous
    a. adenocarcinoma
    a. carcinoma
    a. gland
acinus (pl., acini)
    hyperplastic a.
    liver a.

    neoplastic a.
    prostatic a.
acivicin
ACl — aspiryl chloride
ACLA — American Clinical Laboratory Association
aclacinomycin A
Acladium
aclasis
    diaphyseal a.; diaphysial a.
    tarsoepiphyseal a.
ACLPS — Academy of Clinical Laboratory Physicians and Scientists
ACM — albumin-calcium-magnesium
acne
    a. atrophica
    a. conglobata
    a. fulminans
    a. rosacea
    a. rosacea keratitis
    a. vulgaris
acneiform
acolumellate
aconitase
cis-aconitate hydratase
aconitine
aconitrate dehydrogenase
Aconitum
acoustic
    a. coupler
    a. labyrinth
    a. nerve
    a. neurilemoma
    a. neuroma
    a. radiation
    a. schwannoma
ACP — acid phosphatase
    acyl-carrier protein
    American College of Pathologists
    American College of Physicians
    anodal-closing picture
    aspirin, caffeine, phenacetin
acquired
    a. agammaglobulinemia
    a. antigen
    a. atrophy
    a. character
    a. C1 inhibition deficiency
    a. defect

a. deformity
a. dysplasia
a. hemolytic anemia
a. hemolytic icterus
a. hypogammaglobulinemia
a. ichthyosis
a. idiopathic sideroblastic anemia
a. immune deficiency syndrome
a. immunodeficiency syndrome
a. leukoderma
a. leukopathia
a. megacolon
a. methemoglobinemia
a. nevus
a. sideroachrestic anemia
a. toxoplasmosis
acral lentiginous melanoma
acrania
acraturesis
Acrel's ganglion
Acremonialla
Acremonium
acridine
a. dye
a. hydrochloride
a. orange stain
tetramethyl a.
acridinylamino
acridinyl anisidide
acriflavine
acroanesthesia
acroasphyxia
acrobystitis
acrocentric chromosome
acrocephalosyndactyly
acrocephaly
acrochordon
acrocyanosis
acrodermatitis
a. chronica atrophicans
a. continua
a. enteropathica
a. perstans
acrodolichomelia
acrodynia
acroedema
acrofacial
a. dysostosis
a. syndrome

acrokeratoelastoidosis
acrokeratosis
paraneoplastic a.
a. verruciformis
acrolein phenylhydrazine
acromegalia
acromegalic giantism
acromegalogigantism
acromegaloidism
acromegaly
acromelia
acromelic dwarfism
acromicria
acromioclavicular joint
acromion
acronarcotic poison
acronine
acro-osteolysis
acropachy
acropachyderma
acroparesthesia
acropathy
acroposthitis
acroscleroderma
acrosclerosis
acrosomal
a. granule
a. vesicle
acrosome reaction
acrospiroma
eccrine a.
acrostealgia
Acrotheca pedrosoi
Acrothesium floccosum
acrotrophoneurosis
acrylamide gel electrophoresis
acrylonitrile
ACS — American Cancer Society
American Chemical Society
American College of Surgeons
American Society of Cytology
anodal-closing sound
antireticular cytotoxic serum
Association of Clinical Scientists
ACSV — aortocoronary saphenous vein
ACT — activated coagulation time
anticoagulant therapy

Actaea
ACTe — anodal-closure tetanus
ACTH — adrenocorticotropic
       hormone
ACTH-endorphin precursor
ACTH-RF — adrenocorticotropic hor-
       mone–releasing
       factor
ACTH-secreting adenoma
ACTH stimulation test
actin
      a. binding protein
      a. filament
      a. isoform
actinic
      a. dermatitis
      a. keratosis
      a. porokeratosis
      a. reticuloid
actinide
α-actinin
actinium
Actinobacillus
      A. *actinomycetemcomitans*
      A. *equuli*
      A. *lignieresii*
      A. *mallei*
      A. *pseudomallei*
      A. *suis*
actinochemistry
Actinomadura
      A. *madurae*
      A. *pelletierii*
Actinomyces
      A. *bovis*
      A. *congolensis*
      A. *eriksonii*
      A. *gonidiaformis*
      A. *israelii*
      A. *muris*
      A. *muris-ratti*
      A. *naeslundii*
      A. *necrophorus*
      A. *odontolyticus*
      A. *pseudonecrophorus*
      A. *rhusiopathiae*
      A. *vinaceus*
      A. *viscosus*
actinomyces
Actinomycetaceae
Actinomycetales

actinomycete
      nocardioform a.
      thermophilic a.
actinomycetic infection
actinomycetoma
actinomycin
actinomycosis
      cervicofacial a.
      thoracic a.
actinomycotic
      a. appendicitis
      a. mycetoma
actinomyoma
actinophage
actinophytosis
Actinoplanaceae
Actinoplanes teichomyceticus
Actinopoda
action
      ball-valve a.
      buffer a.
      calorigenic a.
      capillary a.
      cumulative a.
      diastasic a.
      diastatic a.
      law of mass a.
      opsonic a.
      reflex a.
      specific dynamic a.
      tampon a.
      thermogenic a.
      trigger a.
      vitaminoid a.
action potential
      biphasic a. p.
      cardiac a. p.
      compound muscle a. p.
      compound nerve a. p.
      monophasic a. p.
      muscle a. p.
      polyphasic a. p.
      serrated a. p.
activated
      a. charcoal
      a. coagulation time
      a. complex
      a. lymphocyte
      a. macrophage
      a. partial prothrombin time
      a. partial thromboplastin substi-
        tution test

a. partial thromboplastin time
a. protein C inhibitor

activating
a. agent
a. enzyme

activation
allosteric a.
a. analysis
complement a.
contact a.
cross a.
latency of a.
lymphocyte a.
ovum a.
photometrazol a.
plasma a.
a. unit

activator
plasminogen a.
polyclonal a.
prothrombin a.
single-chain urokinase-like plasminogen a.

active
a. chronic hepatitis
a. chronic inflammation
a, electrode
a. rosette test
a. sensitization
a. transport
a. zone

activity
blood granulocyte-specific a.
chemotactic a.
colony-stimulating a.
a. determination
erythroid-potentiating a.
estrogenic hormone a.
general gonadotropic a.
insulin-like a.
multiplication-stimulating a.
nonsuppressible insulin-like a.
optical a.
plasma insulin a.
plasma renin a.
postheparin lipolytic a.
a. ratio
relative specific a.
renal vein renin a.
rheumatoid factor–like a.
thyroxine-specific a.
tissue plasminogen a.

total antitryptic a.
tryptic a.

activity ratio
cumulated a. r.

actomyosin
platelet a.

Actonia

ACTP — adrenocorticotropic polypeptide

actuate

Acuaria

acusector

acute
a. abscess
a. anterior poliomyelitis
a. appendicitis
a. bacterial endocarditis
a. bronchial cerebellar ataxia
a. bronchitis
a. bronchopneumonia
a. cardiovascular disease
a. cellular rejection
a. cerebellar ataxia
a. cholecystitis
a. compression triad
a. crescentic glomerulonephritis
a. diffuse peritonitis
a. disseminated encephalomyelitis
a. disseminated myositis
a. disseminated lupus erythematosus
a. epidemic infectious adenitis
a. erythroleukemia
a. exudative glomerulone-
phritis
a. febrile jaundice
a. fibrinous pleuritis
a. focal hepatitis
a. fulminating meningococcal
septicemia
a. gangrenous appendicitis
a. gastritis
a. gelatinous pneumonia
a. glomerulonephritis
a. goiter
a. granulocytic leukemia
a. hemolytic anemia
a. hemolytic transfusion reaction

a. hemorrhagic bronchopneumonia
a. hemorrhagic cholecystitis
a. hemorrhagic cystitis
a. hemorrhagic erosive gastritis
a. hemorrhagic glomerulonephritis
a. hemorrhagic inflammation
a. hemorrhagic leukoencephalitis
a. hemorrhagic pancreatitis
a. hemorrhagic ulceration
a. idiopathic polyneuritis
a. infarct
a. infectious disease
a. infective endocarditis
a. inflammation
a. inflammatory exudate
a. inflammatory infiltrate
a. inflammatory membrane
a. inflammatory necrosis
a. inflammatory transudate
a. intermittent porphyria
a. interstitial nephritides
a. interstitial nephritis
a. isolated myocarditis
a. lymphoblastic leukemia
a. lymphocytic leukemia
a. mastitis
a. megakaryoblastic leukemia
a. megakaryocytic leukemia
a. miliary tuberculosis
a. monarthritis
a. monocytic (monoblastic) leukemia
a. myeloblastic leukemia
a. myelocytic leukemia
a. myelogenous anemia
a. myelogenous leukemia
a. myeloid leukemia
a. myelomonocytic leukemia
a. myocardial infarction
a. necrotizing enterocolitis
a. nephritis
a. nephrosis
a. nonlymphoblastic leukemia
a. nonlymphocytic leukemia
a. nonspecific lymphadenitis
a. pancreatitis
a. parenchymatous hepatitis
a. paroxysmal myoglobinuria

a. pericarditis
a. phase protein
a. phase reactants
a. phase reaction
a. posthemorrhagic anemia
a. post-streptococcal glomerulonephritis
a. prelymphocytic leukemia
a. progranulocytic leukemia
a. promyelocytic leukemia
a. pseudomembranous candidiasis
a. pulmonary alveolitis
a. purulent otitis media
a. pyelonephritis
a. pyogenic membrane
a. recurrent rhabdomyolysis
a. renal failure
a. respiratory disease
a. respiratory distress syndrome
a. respiratory failure
a. rickets
a. salivary adenitis
a. serous synovitis
a. splenic tumor
a. splenitis
a. suppurative appendicitis
a. thyroiditis
a. tuberculosis
a. tubular necrosis
a. ulcerative colitis
a. undifferentiated leukemia
a. uric acid nephropathy
a. viral hepatitis
a. yellow atrophy
ACVD — acute cardiovascular disease
acycloguanosine
acyclovir
acyesis
acyl
a. carrier proteins
a. halide
a. peroxide
acylase
acylation
acylcarnitine
acylcholine acylhydrolase
acyl-coenzyme A
a.-CoA dehydrogenase
a.-CoA synthetase
acylglycerol

acylhydrolase
    triacylglycerol a.
N-acylneuraminic acid
acylphosphatase
acyl-plasminogen streptokinase activator complex
N-acylsphingosine deacylase
acyltransferase
    acetyl-CoA a.
    lecithin-cholesterol a.
    phosphatidylcholine-cholesterol a.
AD — anodal duration
    average deviation
    axiodistal
    axis deviation
A & D — ascending and descending
ADA — adenosine deaminase activity
    anterior descending artery
adactyly
adamantanamine
adamantine prisms
adamantinoma
    a. of long bones
    pituitary a.
    a. polycysticum
adamantoblast
adamantoblastoma
adamantoma
Adamkiewicz's test
adamsite
Adams-Stokes attack
Adansonia
adaptation
    cellular a.
    color a.
    dark a.
    enzymatic a.
    genetic a.
    light a.
    phenotypic a.
    photopic a.
    retinal a.
    scotopic a.
adaptive
    a. enzyme
    a. hormone
    a. hypertrophy
    a. radiation

ADC — anodal-duration contraction
    average daily census
    axiodistocervical
ADCC — antibody-dependent cell-mediated cytotoxicity
addict
addiction
    alcohol a.
    drug a.
Addis count
addisonian
    a. anemia
    a. crisis
addisonism
Addison's
    anemia
    keloid
addition
    binary a.
    a. polymer
    a. reaction
additive
addresin
adduct
adduction
adductor
    a. brevis muscle
    a. canal
    a. hallucis muscle
    a. longus muscle
    a. magnus muscle
    a. pollicis muscle
Adelomycetes
A delta fibers
ADEM — acute disseminated encephalomyelitis
adenalgia
adenasthenia
adendritic
adenectomy
adenectopia
adenia
adenine
    a. arabinoside
    a. deaminase
    a. diphosphate
    a. hypoxanthine
    a. nucleotide
    a. phosphoribosyltransferase deficiency
    a. sulfate
    a. triphosphate

adenitis
    acute epidemic infectious a.
    acute salivary a.
    cervical a.
    mesenteric a.
    phlegmonous a.
    a. tropicalis
adenocanthoma
adenoameloblastoma
adenoangiosarcoma
adenocarcinoma
    acinic cell a.
    acinous a.
    alveolar a.
    anaplastic a.
    axillary lymph node a.
    bronchioalveolar node a.
    bronchiolar a.
    bronchogenic a.
    clear cell a.
    colloid a.
    colorectal a.
    ductal a.
    endometrial a.
    follicular a.
    gastric a.
    gelatinous a.
    Gleason II a.
    Hürthle cell a.
    infiltrating duct a.
    inflammatory a.
    a. in situ
    lobular a.
    metastatic prostatic a.
    medullary a.
    mesonephric a.
    mucinous a.
    mucoid a.
    papillary a.
    polymorphous low-grade a.
    polypoid a.
    prostatic a.
    renal a.
    sebaceous a.
    signet ring a.
    sweat gland a.
    terminal duct a.
    testicular a.
    trabecular a.
    undifferentiated a.
    urachal a.
adenocele

adenocellulitis
adenochondroma
adenochondrosarcoma
adenocystic
    a. carcinoma
    a. ovary
adenocystoma
adenocyte
adenodiastasis
adenoepithelioma
adenofibroma edematodes
adenofibromyoma
adenofibrosis
adenogenous
adenohypophyseal hormone
adenohypophysis
adenoid
    a. cystic breast cancer
    a. cystic carcinoma
    a. facies
    a. squamous cell carcinoma
    a. tumor
adenoiditis
adenoleiomyofibroma
adenolipoma
adenolipomatosis
    symmetric a.
adenolymphocele
adenolymphoma
adenolysis
adenoma
    acidophilic a.
    acidophil stem cell a.
    ACTH-producing a.
    ACTH-secreting a.
    a. adamantium
    adnexal a.
    adrenal cortical a.
    adrenocortical a.
    aldosterone-producing a.
    aldosterone-secreting a.
    alpha subunit a.
    a. alveolare
    angioinvasive a.
    apocrine a.
    atypical a.
    basal cell a.
    basophilic a.
    bile duct a.
    black a.
    bronchial a.
    canalicular a.

carcinoma ex pleomorphic a.
C cell a.
ceruminous a.
chief cell a.
chromophilic a.
chromophobic a.
clear cell a.
colloid a.
corticotrope a.
corticotroph a.
corticotropin-producing a.
cortisol-producing a.
a. destruens
embryonal a.
endocrine active a.
endocrine inactive a.
a. endometrioides ovarii
eosinophilic a.
fetal a.
fibroid a.
a. fibrosum
follicular a.
Fuchs's a.
functional a.
gastric a.
gastrin-secreting a.
glucocorticoid-secreting a.
glycoprotein a.
gonadotrope a.
gonadotropin-producing a.
growth hormone–producing a.
hepatocellular a.
a. hidradenoides
Hürthle cell a.
hyalinizing trabecular a.
hyperfunctional a.
islet cell a.
lactating a.
lactotroph a.
langerhansian a.
Leydig cell a.
lipid-rich a.
lipid tubular a.
liver cell a.
macrofollicular a.
malignant a.
mammosomatotroph a.
mammosomatotropic a.
mesonephric a.
microfollicular a.
mineralocorticoid-secreting a.
mineral-secreting a.

mixed cell a.
mixed somatotroph-lactotroph
    a.
monomorphic a.
mucinous a.
multiple a.
nephrogenic a.
nonfunctional a.
nonsecreting a.
nonsecretory a.
null cell a.
oncocytic a.
ovarian tubular a.
a. ovarii testiculare
oxyphil a.
papillary a.
papillary cystic a.
paraganglioma-like a.
parathyroid a.
Pick's tubular a.
pigmented a.
pituitary a.
pleomorphic a.
plurihormonal a.
polypoid a.
prolactin-producing a.
prostatic a.
racemose a.
renal a.
renal cortical a.
sebaceous a.
a. sebaceum
signet-ring cell a.
somatotrope a.
somatotrophic a.
a. sudoriparum
sweat duct a.
testicular tubular a.
thyroid-stimulating hor-
    mone–secreting a.
thyrotrope a.
thyrotropin-producing a.
toxic a.
trabecular a.
trabecular-tubular a.
TSH-secreting a.
tubulovillous a.
tubular a.
undifferentiated cell a.
urachal a.
villous a.
virilizing a.

handwritten: not 2deryz, but iDXA

adenomalacia
adenomatoid
    a. nodule
    a. odontogenic tumor
    a. tumor
adenomatosis
    erosive a.
    familial endocrine a.
    fibrosing a.
    multiple endocrine a.
    pluriglandular a.
    polyendocrine a.
    pulmonary a.
adenomatous
    a. goiter
    a. hyperplasia
    a. hypertrophy
    a. nodule
    a. polyp
adenomegaly
adenomere
adenomyoepithelioma
adenomyofibroma
adenomyoma
adenomyomatosis
adenomyosarcoma
adenomyosis uteri
adenoncus
adenopathy
adenophlegmon
adenophthalmia
adenophyma
    a. psammopapillare
adenosalpingitis
adenosarcoma
    müllerian a.
adenosclerosis
adenosine
    a. arabinoside
    a. 3',5'-cyclic phosphate
    a. deaminase
    a. deaminase deficiency
    a. diphosphate
    a. kinase
    a. monophosphate
    a. phosphate
    a. phosphorylase
    a. triphosphatase
    a. triphosphatase, calcium-activated
    a. triphosphatase, magnesium-activated

    a. triphosphate
    a. triphosphate pyrophosphohydrolase
adenosinediphosphate deaminase
adenosinetriphosphatase
adenosis
    blunt duct a.
    fibrosing a.
    microglandular
    sclerosing a.
    vaginal a.
adenosquamous carcinoma
adenosyl
adenosylcobalamin deficiency
S-adenosyl-L-homocysteinase
S-adenosylhomocysteine
S-adenosylmethinone
adenosyltransferase
    methionine a.
adenoviral
    a. conjunctivitis
    a. pneumonia
adenovirus
    a. culture
    a. immunofluorescence
    oncogenic a.
adenyl
    a. cyclase
    a. kinase
adenylate
    a. cyclase
    a. kinase deficiency
adenylic acid
adenylosuccinase
adenylosuccinate lyase
adenylpyrophosphatase
adenylyl
adenylylation
adenylylsulfate kinase
adenylyltransferase
    nicotinamide mononucleotide a.
ADG — atrial diastolic gallop
    axiodistogingival
ADH — alcohol dehydrogenase
    antidiuretic hormone
ADH deficiency
adherence
    bacterial a.
    immune a.
adherens
    zonula a.

adherent
>   a. pericarditis
>   a. pericardium

adhesion
>   amniotic a.
>   fibrinous a.
>   fibrous a.
>   intestinal a.
>   a. molecule
>   sublabial a.

adhesive
>   a. capsulitis
>   a. chronic pachymeningitis
>   a. inflammation
>   a. mediastinopericarditis
>   a. pericarditis
>   a. peritonitis
>   a. phlebitis
>   a. pleurisy
>   a. vaginitis

ADI — axiodistoincisal
adiadochokinesia
Adiantum
adiaspiromycosis
adiasporosis
Adie's pupil
adiphenine hydrochloride
adipic
adipocele
adipoceratous
adipocere
adipocyte
adipokinesis
adipokinetic hormone
adipolysis
adipolytic
adiponecrosis
adipose
>   a. cell
>   a. degeneration
>   a. infiltration
>   a. tissue
>   a. tumor

adiposis
>   a. cardiaca
>   a. cerebralis
>   a. dolorosa
>   a. hepatica
>   a. orchica
>   a. tuberosa simplex
>   a. universalis

adiposity
>   hamartomatous a.

adiposogenital dystrophy
adiposuria
aditus (pl., aditi)
adjuvant
>   Freund's a.
>   mycobacterial a.
>   a. radiotherapy

adjuvanticity
Adler's test
adnexa
>   a. mastoidea
>   a. oculi
>   a. uteri

adnexal
>   a. adenoma
>   a. carcinoma
>   a. neoplasms
>   a. tumor

adnexitis
ADO — axiodisto-occlusal
adonidine
adoral
ADP — adenosine diphosphate
ADP/ATP — adenosine/adenosine tri-
>   phosphate ratio

ADR — Alzheimer's disease research
adrenal
>   a. amyloidosis
>   a. antibody
>   a. aplasia
>   a. apoplexy
>   a. atrophy
>   a. artery
>   a. ascorbic acid depletion test
>   a. capsule
>   a. cortex cyst
>   a. cortical adenoma
>   a. cortical carcinoma
>   a. cortical cell
>   a. cortical hyperplasia
>   a. crisis
>   a. cyst
>   a. cytomegaly
>   a. disease
>   a. ectopia
>   a. feminizing syndrome
>   a. function test
>   a. ganglioneuroma
>   a. gland
>   a. gland virilizing syndrome
>   a. heterotopia

a. hypoplasia
a. "incidentalomas"
a. insufficiency
a. leukodystrophy
Marchand's a's
a. mass
a. medulla
a. medullary hyperplasia
a. neoplasm
a. neuroblastoma
a. pheochromocytoma
a. pseudocyst
a. rest tumor
a. scan
a. steroidogenesis
a. tuberculosis
a. tumor
a. vein
a. virilism
a. virilization
a. weight factor
Adrenalin
adrenaline
adrenalitis
    autoimmune a.
adrenalopathy
adrenarche
    delayed a.
    precocious a.
adrenergic
a. blockade
a. blocking
a. neuron blockade
α-adrenergic blockade
β-adrenergic
    β-a. antagonist
    β-a. blockade
adrenochrome
adrenocortical
a. adenoma
a. antibody
a. cell
a. extract
a. hormone
a. inhibition test
a. insufficiency
a. rest
a. rest tumor
a. suppression
adrenocorticoid
adrenocorticosteroid

adrenocorticotropic
a. cell
a. hormone
a. hormone assay
a. hormone–releasing factor
a. hormone reserve
a. hormone stimulation test
a. hormone suppression test
a. polypeptide
adrenocorticotropin
adrenodoxin
adrenogenital syndrome
adrenoleukodystrophy
adrenomyeloneuropathy
adrenoreceptor
adrenomedullary
    a. hormone
    a. triad
adrenomegaly
adrenopathy
Adriamycin
ADS — antibody deficiency syndrome
        antidiuretic substance
Adson's maneuver
adsorb
adsorbate
adsorbed plasma
adsorbent
    gastrointestinal a.
adsorption
    agglutinin a.·
    chemical a.
    a. chromatography
    physical a.
ADT — adenoside triphosphate
adult
a. cystic teratoma
a. gonococcal conjunctivitis
a. hemoglobin
a. hemolytic-uremic syndrome
a. medulloepithelioma
a. polycystic disease
a. respiratory distress syndrome
a. T-cell leukemia
a. T-cell lymphoma
a. tuberculosis
adulteration
adulthood
adult-onset diabetes
adventitious
a. albuminuria
a. cell
a. cyst

adynamia
>hereditary a.

adynamic
>a. ileus
>a. ureter

AE — antitoxineinheit (antitoxin unit)

Aedes
>A. *aegypti*
>A. *albopictus*
>A. *cinereus*
>A. *flavescens*
>A. *leucocelaenus*
>A. *scutellaris pseudoscutellaris*
>A. *sollicitans*
>A. *spencerii*
>A. *taeniorhynchus*

AEF — allogenic effect factor
AEG — air encephalogram
AEM — analytical electron microscope
AEP — average evoked potential
AEq — age equivalent
aequorin
AER — aldosterone excretion rate
>auditory evoked response
>average evoked response

aerated
aeration
Aerobacter
>A. *aerogenes*
>A. *cloacae*
>A. *lipolyticus*
>A. *liquefaciens*
>A. *subgroup* A, B, C

aerobe
>obligate a.

aerobia
aerobian
aerobic
>a.-anaerobic infection
>a. bacterium
>a. blood culture
>a. diphtheroids
>a. metabolism
>a. respiration
>a. spore-forming bacilli

aerobiosis
aerobiotic
aerocele
Aerococcus viridans
aerodermectasia

aeroembolism
aerogen
aerogenesis
aerogenic
aerogenous
Aeromonas
>A. *hydrophila*
>A. *liquefaciens*
>A. *punctata*
>A. *salmonicida*
>A. *shigelloides*
>A. *sobria*

aeropathy
aerophagia
aerophil; aerophile
aerophilic
aerophilous
aeroplankton
aerosis
aerosol
aerosolized pentamidine
aerotaxis
aerotitis media
aerotolerant
aerotonometer
aerotropism
AET — absorption-equivalent thickness
AEV — avian erythroblastosis virus
AF — acid-fast
>aldehyde fuchsin
>amniotic fluid
>antibody-forming
>aortic flow
>atrial fibrillation
>atrial flutter

AFB — acid-fast bacilli
AFC — antibody-forming cells
afebrile abortion
affective
afferent
>a. arteriole
>a. lymph node
>a. neuron
>a. pathway

affinity
>chemical a.
>a. chromatography
>a. constant
>electron a.
>functional a.
>intrinsic a.

a. labeling
a. maturation
a. purification
testosterone-binding a.
AFIB — atrial fibrillation
afibrinogenemia
congenital a.
AFIP — Armed Forces Institute of Pathology
AFL — atrial flutter
aflatoxicosis
aflatoxin-producing fungus
AFP — alpha fetoprotein
anterior faucial pillar
African
histoplasmosis
lymphoma
sleeping sickness
tick-borne fever
trypanosomiasis
aftergilding
afterimage
negative a.
positive a.
afterload
AFX — atypical fibroxanthoma
AG — albumin-globulin
antiglobulin
atrial gallop
axiogingival
A/G — albumin/globulin ratio
Ag — antigen
silver
AGA — appropriate for gestational age
agammaglobulinemia
acquired a.
Bruton's a.
congenital a.
Swiss-type a.
transient a.
X-linked a.
Agamodistomum ophthalmobium
Agamomermis
Agamonema
Agamonematodum migrans
aganglionic megacolon
aganglionosis
agar
ascitic a.
bile-esculin a.
bile salt a.

bird seed a.
bismuth sulfite a.
blood a.
Bordet-Gengou a.
brain-heart infusion a.
brillant green a.
buffered charcoal yeast extract a.
casein a.
chocolate a.
Christensen's urea a.
citrate a.
colistin-nalidixic acid a.
Columbia blood a.
corn meal a.
cystine-tellurite blood a.
cystine trypticase a.
Czapek-Dox a.
deep a.
deoxycholate-citrate a.
deoxyribonuclease a.
dextrose a.
a. diffusion method
DNase a.
egg-yolk a.
Emmon's modification of Sabouraud's dextrose a.
eosin–methylene blue a.
glucose-cysteine a.
heart infusion a.
Hektoen a.
Hektoen enteric a.
inhibitory mold a.
Kliger iron a.
Löffler's a.
lysine iron a.
MacConkey a.
malt a.
Martin-Lester a.
Middlebrook's a.
Mueller-Hinton a.
mycobiotic a.
mycosel a.
niger seed a.
nitrate a.
nutrient a.
Pfeiffer's blood a.
phenylalanine a.
phenylethyl alcohol a.
phenylethyl alcohol blood a.
a. plate count
potato dextrose a.

rabbit blood a.
Regan-Lowe a.
Sabhi a.
Sabouraud's dextrose a.
Salmonella-Shigella a.
Schaedler blood a.
serum a.
sheep-blood a.
Simmon's citrate a.
soybean casein digest blood a.
Thayer-Martin a.
thistle seed a.
Trichophyton a.
triosulfate-citrate bile salts and
    sucrose a.
triple sugar iron a.
trypticase soy a.
tryptic soy a.
urea a.
Wilkins-Chilgren a.
xylose-lysine-deoxycholate a.

Agarbacterium
Agaricaceae
Agaricus
agarose gel electrophoresis
agenesis
bladder a.
cerebellar a.
gonadal a.
pure red cell a.
renal a.
testicular a.
thymic a.
thyroidal a.
vas deferens a.

agent
activating a.
adrenergic blocking a.
adrenergic neuron blocking a.
alkylating a.
androgenic anabolic a.
antibacterial a.
antifungal a.
bacteriostatic a.
biologic alkylating a.
caudalizing a.
chelating a.
cholinergic blocking a.
Eaton a.
embedding a.
etiologic a.
ganglionic blocking a.

gonadotropin-releasing a.
Gordon's a.
Hawaii a.
infectious a.
initiating a.
levigating a.
lysing a.
Marburg a.
Marcy a.
Norwalk a.
oxidizing a.
Pittsburgh pneumonia a.
progestational a.
reducing a.
surface-active a.
thrombolytic a.
transforming a.
vacuolating a.
virus-inactivating a.
wetting a.
Agent Orange
AGEPC — acetyl glyceryl ether phos-
            phocholine
AGG — agammaglobulinemia
agglutin
agglutinating antibody
agglutination
acid a.
bacterial a.
bacteriogenic a.
chick cell a.
cold a.
direct a.
false a.
H a.
indirect a.
intravascular a.
latex a.
macroscopic a.
mediate a.
microscopic a.
O a.
passive a.
platelet a.
reverse a.
salt a.
slide latex a.
spontaneous a.
T a.
a. test
a. titer
Treponema pallidum a.

tube a.
Vi a.
agglutinative thrombus
agglutinator
    rheumatoid a.
agglutinin
    ABO a's
    a. adsorption
    alpha a.
    anti-Rh a.
    beta a.
    blood group a's
    cold a.
    cross-reacting a.
    febrile a.
    flagellar a.
    group a.
    H a.
    Haupt-a.
    immune a.
    latex a.
    leukocyte a.
    Mg a.
    O a.
    platelet a.
    Rh a.
    saline a.
    Salmonella a.'s
    serum a.
    somatic a.
    warm a.
    wheat germ a.
agglutinogen
aggregate
    a. anaphylaxis
    cytoplasmic a.
    cytoplasmic crystalline a.
    cytoplasmic lipid a.
    cytoplasmic macromolec-
        ular a.
    nuclear a.
    nuclear crystalline a.
    nuclear lipid a.
aggregated
    a. albumin
    a. microspheres
aggregation
    platelet a.
aggregometer
    platelet a.
aggressive infantile fibromatosis
agitation

AGL — acute granulocytic leukemia
    aminoglutethimide
aglobulia
aglobuliosis
aglobulism
aglomerular
aglutition
aglycemia
aglycogenosis
aglycone
aglycosuria
aglycosuric
AGN — acute glomerulonephritis
agnathus
agnocobalamin
agnogenic myeloid metaplasia
agnosia
agonadal
agonadism
agonal
    a. leukocytosis
    a. thrombosis
    a. thrombus
agonist
    opioid a.
agoraphobia
AGR — Aniridia, genitourinary mal-
        formations, and mental re-
        tardation complex
agranular
    a. endoplasmic reticulum
    a. leukocyte
agranulocyte
agranulocytic angina
agranulocytosis
    Kostmann's infantile genetic a.
agranuloplasia
agranuloplastic
agraphia
A/G (albumin/globulin) ratio test
agretope
Agrobacterium
AGS — adrenogenital syndrome
AGT — antiglobulin test
AGTT — abnormal glucose toler-
        ance test
ague
AGV — aniline gentian violet
agyria
AH — acetohexamide
    amenorrhea and hirsutism
    aminohippurate

antihyaluronidase
arterial hypertension
hypermetropic astigmatism
AHA — acquired hemolytic anemia
autoimmune hemolytic
anemia
ahaptoglobinemia
AHD — arteriosclerotic heart disease
atherosclerotic heart disease
A hemoglobin
AHF — antihemophilic factor
AHG — antihemophilic globulin
antihuman globulin
AHH — arylhydrocarbon hydroxylase
alpha-hydrazine analogue of
histidine
AHLE — acute hemorrhagic leukoencephalitis
AHLS — antihuman lymphocyte
serum
AHP — air at high pressure
AHT — antihyaluronidase titer
augmented histamine test
AI — angiotensin I
aortic incompetence
aortic insufficiency
apical impulse
axioincisal
AIBA — aminoisobutyric acid
AIC — aminoimidazole carboxamide
AID — acute infectious disease
AIDS — acquired immune deficiency
syndrome
acquired immunodeficiency
syndrome
AIDS-related complex
AIDS-related syndrome
AIDS-related virus
AIDS serology
AIEP — amount of insulin extract-
able from the pancreas
AIH — artificial insemination, homol-
ogous
AIHA — autoimmune hemolytic
anemia
AII — angiotension II
AIII — angiotension III
AILD — angioimmunoblastic lymph-
adenopathy with dyspro-
teinemia
AIN — acute interstitial nephritides
acute interstitial nephritis

ainhum
AIO — amyloid of immunoglobulin
origin
AIP — acute intermittent porphyria
automated immunoprecipi-
tation
average intravascular pressure
air
alveolar a.
a. embolism
a. embolus
a. foil
liquid a.
a. monitor
a. pollution
residual a.
venous alveolar a.
air-borne infection
airway
a. conductance
nasal a.
oropharyngeal a.
a. resistance
AITT — arginine insulin tolerance test
AIU — absolute iodine uptake
AIVR — accelerated idioventricular
rhythm
AJCCS — American Joint Committee on Cancer Staging
Ajellomyces
A. *dermatitidis*
A. dermatitis
AK — adenylate kinase
akaryocyte
akathisia
akeratosis
Akeridae
akinesia
akinetic mutism
Akiyama's procedure
AKT1 virus
AKT8 retrovirus
AL — albumin
axiolingual
AL-721
AL protein
Al — aluminum
ALA — aminolevulinic acid
axiolabial
ALA dehydratase

ALA synthetase
ala (pl., alae)
    a. auris
    a. nasi
alactasia
ALAD — abnormal left axis deviation
              aminolevulinic acid dehydratase
ALAG — axiolabiogingival
ALAL — axiolabiolingual
alamecin
alanine
β-alanine
    β-a. aminotransferase
    β-a. aminotransferase assay
    β-a. dehydrogenase
    β-a.-glutamate transaminase
    β-a.-ketoacid aminotransferase
    β-a.-ketoglutarate transaminase
    β-a.-oxoglutarate aminotransferase
    β-a. transaminase
alaninemia
alaninuria
alanyl-RNA synthetase
alastrim
alb — albumin
Albarrán's gland
Albert-Linder bone sectioning
Albert's stain
albicans
albiduria
albinism
    ocular a.
    oculocutaneous a.
albino
albinuria
Albright's hereditary osteodystrophy
albukalin
albumin
    a. A
    acetosoluble a.
    acid a.
    aggregated a.
    alkali a.
    a. assay
    a. B
    Bence Jones a.
    blood a.
    bovine serum a.
    caseiniform a.

chromated serum a.
chromium 51–labeled a.
a. clearance
coagulated a.
crystalline egg a.
derived a.
a.-globulin ratio
hematin a.
human serum a.
iodinated human serum a.
iodinated I 125 serum a. (human)
iodinated I 131 serum a. (human)
iodinated marcoaggregated a.
iodinated serum a.
macroaggregated a.
a. Mexico
a. microspheres
a. Naskapi
native a.
normal human serum a.
Patein's a.
a. quotient
radioactive iodinated serum a.
radio-iodinated serum a.
serum a.
a. suspension test
a. tannate
technetium Tc 99m serum a.
a. test
thyroxine-binding a.
triphenyl a.
a. X
a. X_1
albuminaturia
albumin-calcium-magnesium
albuminemia
albumin-globulin ratio
albuminiferous
albuminiparous
albuminocholia
albuminocytological
albuminogenous
albuminoid degeneration
albuminoptysis
albuminorrhea
albuminous
    a. degeneration
    a. granules
albuminuria
    adventitious a.

Bamberger's a.
benign a.
cardiac a.
colliquative a.
cyclic a.
digestive a.
essential a.
febrile a.
functional a.
intermittent a.
lordotic a.
march a.
neuropathic a.
orthostatic a.
physiologic a.
postrenal a.
prerenal a.
regulatory a.
transient a.
albuminuric
albumose-free tuberculin
albumosuria
Bence Jones a.
Bradshaw's a.
enterogenic a.
pyogenic a.
ALC — approximate lethal concentration
axiolinguocervical
Alcaligenes
A. *bookeri*
A. *bronchosepticus*
A. *denitrificans*
A. *faecalis*
A. *marshallii*
A. *metalcaligenes*
A. *odorans*
A. *recti*
A. *viscolactis*
alcaptonuria
Alcian blue
alcohol
absolute a.
acid a.
aliphatic a.
alkyl a.
allyl a.
amyl a.
anhydrous a.
benzyl a.
blood a.
butyl a.

caprylic a.
dehydrated a.
a. dehydrogenase
diacetone a.
dihydric a.
ethyl a.
a. fixation
grain a.
isoamyl a.
isobutyl a.
isopropyl a.
methyl a.
monohydric a.
octyl a.
phenylethyl a.
a. poisoning
polyhydric a.
polyvinyl a.
propyl a.
a. radical
sugar a.
a. thermometer
wood a.
alcoholic
a. cardiomyopathy
a. cirrhosis
a. coma
a. formalin
a. hepatitis
a. hyalin
a. myopathy
a. steatosis
alcoholism
alcohol-soluble eosin
ALD — aldolase
aldaric acid
aldehyde
acetic a.
a. adduct
a. dehydrogenase
a. fixative
a. fuchsin
a. oxidase
Alder bodies
Alder-Reilly
anomaly
bodies
Alder's constitutional granulation
anomaly
aldicarb
aldimine

alditol
aldofuranose
aldohexose
aldolase
    a. deficiency
    allothreonine a.
    fructose a.
    fructose-bisphosphate a.
    fructose 1-phosphate a.
    a. test
aldonic acid
aldonolactonase
aldopentose
aldophosphamide
aldopyranose
aldose
    a. 1-epimerase
    a. mutarotase
    a. reductase
aldosterone
    a. excretion rate
    a.-producing adenoma
    a.-producing carcinoma
    a.-producing tumor
    a.-secreting carcinoma
    a.-secreting tumor
    a. secretion defect
    a. secretion rate
    a.-stimulating factor
    a. stimulation test
    a. suppression test
aldosteronism
aldosteronoma
aldotransferase
aldotriose
aldrin
Aletris
aleukemia
aleukemic
    a. granulocytic leukemia
    a. leukemia
    a. lymphadenosis
    a. lymphocytic leukemia
    a. monocytic leukemia
    a. myelosis
aleukemoid
aleukia hemorrhagica
aleukocytic
aleukocytosis
aleuriospore
alexia
    cortical a.

alexin
aleydigism
ALG — antilymphocyte globulin
       antithoracic duct lympho-
         cyte globulin
       axiolinguogingival
alga
algae
algesidystrophy
algid malaria
algin
alginate
alginic acid
Alginobacter
Alginomonas
algodystrophy
algoid cell
algorithm
algor mortis
algoscopy
ALH — anterior lobe hormone
       anterior lobe of the hy-
         pophysis
alicyclic hydrocarbon
alienia
aliesterase
alignment
alimentary
    a. diabetes
    a. glycosuria
    a. hypoglycemia
    a. lipemia
    a. osteopathy
    a. tract
    a. tract smear
alimentation
alimentotherapy
aliphatic
    a. acid
    a. alcohol
    a. hydrocarbon
    a. saturated hydrocarbon
    a. unsaturated hydrocarbon
aliquot
alizarin
    a. cyanin
    a. indicator
    a. purpurin
    a. red
    a. red S
    a. test
    a. yellow

alk — alkaline
alkalemia
alkalescence
alkalescens-dispar
alkali
    caustic a.
    a. denaturation test
    fixed a.
    a. metal
    a.-soluble nitrogen
    a. test
    a. tolerance test
    volatile a.
alkalimetry
    Engel's a.
alkaline
    a. earth metal
    a. intoxication
    a. phosphatase
    a. phosphotungstate
    a. reaction
    a. RNase
    a. tide
    a. toluidine
    a. tuberculin
    a. urine
    a. wave
alkaline phosphatase
    a.p. activity of granular leukocytes
    a.p. antialkaline phosphatase method
    a.p. isoenzyme electrophoresis
    leukocyte a.p.
    a.p. staining
    a.p. test
alkalinuria
alkaloid
    a. test
    vinca a's
alkalosis
    acapnial a.
    compensated a.
    hypokalemic a.
    metabolic a.
    nonrespiratory a.
    potassium a.
    respiratory a.
alkalotic
alkaluria
alkane

alkannin paper
alkapton bodies
alkaptonuria test
alkene
alkenyl
alkoxide ion
alkoxy
alkoxyaryl hydroxylase
alk phos — alkaline phosphatase
alkyl
    a. alcohol
    a. aryl ammonium bromide
    a. aryl ammonium chloride
    a. aryl polyether sulfate
    a. aryl polyether sulfonate
    a. dimethyl benzyl ammonium bromide
    a. dimethyl benzyl ammonium chloride
    a. dimethyl-3,4-dichlorobenzene ammonium chloride
    a. dimethyl ethyl ammonium bromide
    a. dimethyl ethyl ammonium chloride
    a. dimethyl ethylbenzyl ammonium bromide
    a. dimethyl ethylbenzyl ammonium chloride
    a. hydroxyethyl imidazolinium chloride
    a. mercuric chloride
    a. mercuric phosphate
    a. naphthyl methyl pyridium chloride
    a. peroxide
    a. phenol polyglycol ether
    a. quaternary ammonium bromide
    a. quaternary ammonium chloride
    a. sodium-N-methyltaurate
    a. sodium sulfate
    a. sodium sulfonate
    a. toluyl methyl trimethyl ammonium chloride
    a. trimethyl ammonium bromide
    a. trimethyl ammonium chloride

alkylate
alkylating agent
alkylation
alkylbenzene sulfonate
alkylhalidase
alkylnitrosamine
alkyne
ALL — acute lymphoblastic leukemia
        acute lymphocytic leukemia
allantoic
     a. acid
     a. cyst
     a. duct
allantoicase
allantoin
allantoinase
allantoinuria
allantois
allele
     multiple a's
     a.-specific oligonucleotide
     a.-specific oligonucleotide
       probes
allelic
     a. exclusion
     a. genes
allelocatalysis
allelotaxis
Allen-Doisy
     test
     unit
Allen's
     correction
     test
allergen
     atopic a.
allergenic protein preparations
allergen-specific IgE antibody
allergic
     a. asthma
     a. conjunctivitis
     a. dermatitis
     a. encephalitis
     a. encephalomyelitis
     a. gastroenteropathy
     a. granulomatosis
     a. granulomatous angiitis
     a. neuritis
     a. pneumonitis
     a. prostatitis
     a. purpura
     a. reaction

     a. rhinitis
     a. transfusion reaction
allergoid
allergy
     atopic a.
Allescheria boydii
allescheriosis
allesthesia
allethrin
alloagglutinin
alloalbuminemia
alloantibody
alloantigen
alloantigen-D antibody
allobarbital
allocation
     storage a.
allochezia
Allodermanyssus sanguineus
allogeneic; allogenic
     a. antigen
     a. effect factor
     a. graft
     a. inhibition
     a. lymphoma
     a. transplantation
allograft
allogroup
alloimmune
alloimmunization
allometric
allometry
allophanamide
allophenic
alloplasia
alloplasmatic
alloploidy
allopolyploidy
allopurinol
allosteric
     a. activation
     a. effector
     a. enzyme
     a. inhibition
allosterism
allostery
allothreonine aldolase
allotope
allotopia
allotoxin
allotrope
allotropic

allotropism
allotropy
allotype
    Am (alpha-marker) a.
    Gm (gamma-marker) a.
    Km (kappa-marker) a.
    latent a.
    nominal a.
    simple a.
    a. suppression
allotypic
    a. determinant
    a. marker
allotypy
alloxan-Schiff reaction
alloxuremia
alloxuria
alloy
allyl
    a. alcohol
    a. aldehyde
    a. isothiocyanate
    a. sulfide
    a. sulfocarbamide
    a. thiocarbamide
    a. tribromide
ALME — acetyl-lysine methyl ester
Almén's test for blood
ALMI — anterior lateral myocardial
        infarct
ALN — anterior lymph node
ALO — axiolinguo-occlusal
Alocinma
alogia
aloin
alopecia
    a. areata
    congenital sutural a.
    a. mucinosa
    a. universalis
ALP — alkaline phosphatase
    antilymphocyte plasma
alpha
    a. acid glycoprotein
    a. acidophil
    a.-adrenergic receptor
    a. agglutinin
    a. amino acid
    a. amino acid nitrogen
    a. amino nitrogen test
    a.-amylase
    a.-amylose

a. antichymotrypsin
a.-antiplasmin
a_1-antitrypsin
a. band
a.-beta variation
a. blockade
a. cells
a. chain disease
a. decay
a.-delta sleep pattern
a.-difluoromethylornithine
5-a.-dihydrotestosterone
a.-dinitrophenol
a.-estradiol
a.-fetoglobin
a.-fetoprotein
a. globulin antibodies
α_1 globulin
α_2 globulin
a.-1-4 glucosidase
a. granules
a. heavy chain disease
a. helix
a. hemolysin
a. hemolysis
a.-hypophamine
a. interferon
a.-ketoglutarate
a. lactalbumin
a.-lipoprotein
a. lobeline
a_2 macroglobulin
a. melanocyte-stimulating
  hormone
a. metachromasia
a.-methyldopa
a. motor neuron
a.-naphthol thiourea
a.-naphthyl acetate esterase reaction
a. particles
a. protease inhibitor
a. radiation
a. ray
a. receptors
5-a. reductase
a. rhythm
a. seromucoid
a. staphylolysin
a. streptococcus
a. substance
a.-thalassemia intermedia

a.-thalassemia trait
α_1 thymosin
a.-tocopherol
a.-trypsin
a. unit
a. variant rhythm
alpha$_1$-acid glycoprotein
alpha-adrenergic receptor
alpha$_2$-antiplasmin
alpha$_1$-antitrypsin
alpha$_1$-antitrypsin deficiency
alpha$_1$-fetoglobulin
alpha$_1$-fetoprotein
alpha$_1$-inhibitor
alpha$_2$-macroglobulin
alpha$_2$-macroglobulin inhibitor
alphameric
alphanumeric
alpha-particle detector
alpha$_1$-seromucoid
alphaprodine hydrochloride
alphavirus
alphazurine
alprazolam
ALS — amyotrophic lateral sclerosis
        antilymphatic serum
        antilymphocyte serum
alseroxylon
Alsever's solution
Alstonia
ALT — alanine aminotransferase
ALTEE — acetyl-L-tyrosine ethyl
                ester
alteration
        bone matrix a.
        cartilage matrix a.
        chromosome a.
        crystalline macromolecule a.
        cyclic tissue a.
        cytologic a.
        cytoplasmic a.
        cytoplasmic fiber a.
        cytoplasmic fibril a.
        cytoplasmic filament a.
        cytoplasmic lipid a.
        cytoplasmic matrix a.
        decidual a.
        extracellular fibril a.
        extracellular matrix a.
        fibrocartilaginous matrix a.
        Golgi's cavity a.
        Golgi's membrane a.

Golgi's vacuole a.
Golgi's vesicle a.
hematopoietic maturation a.
leukocytic maturation a.
mitochondria cristae a.
mitochondrial matrix a.
mitochondrial membrane a.
Nissl substance a.
nuclear-cytoplasmic ratio a.
nuclear membrane a.
nucleolar a.
pH a.
predecidual a.
syncytial a.
alternans
        electrical a.
        a. of the heart
        pulsus a.
Alternaria tenuis
alternating current
alternation
        cardiac a.
        a. of generations
alternative
        a. complement pathway
        a. hypothesis
        a. inheritance
altitude
        a. anoxia
        a. sickness
Altmann's
        aniline-acid fuchsin stain
        fixative
        granule
alum
        a. carmine
        chrome a.
        a.-precipitated pyridine
        a.-precipitated toxoid
alumina
        hydrated a.
aluminosis
aluminum
        a. acetate
        a. carbonate
        a. chloride
        a. compound
        a. dihydroxyaminoacetate
        a. hydroxide
        a. hydroxide gel
        a. oxide
        a. phosphate
        a. toxicity

ALV — avian leukosis virus
alveolar
    a. abscess
    a. adenocarcinoma
    a. air
    a. air equation
    a.-arterial carbon dioxide.
    a.-arterial oxygen
    a. asthma
    a. bronchiole
    a.-capillary block
    a. carcinoma
    a. cell
    a. cell carcinoma
    a. cell tumor
    a. cyst
    a. duct
    a. edema
    a. emphysema
    a. epithelium
    a. fenestra
    a. gland
    a. hydatid
    a. hydatid cyst
    a. macrophage
    a. mucosa
    a. nerve
    a. phagocyte
    a. pore
    a. proteinosis
    a. rhabdomyosarcoma
    a. sac
    a. sarcoma
    a. septa
    a. soft part sarcoma
    a. ventilation equation
alveolectomy
alveolitis
    acute pulmonary a.
    diffuse fibrosing a.
    extrinsic allergic a.
alveoloclasia
alveolus (alveoli)
    dental a.
    pulmonary a.
alveus
ALW — arch-loop-whorl
alymphia
alymphocytic
alymphocytosis
alymphoplasia
    Nezelof's typs of thymic a.
    thymic a.

Alzheimer's
    disease
    fibrillary degeneration
Am — alveolar macrophage
    ametropia
    amperemeter
    anovular menstruation
    axiomesial
    myopic astigmatism
AM antigens
Am — americium
Am (alpha marker) allotype
AMA — American Medical Association
amacrine cells
Amanita
    A. *muscaria*
    A. *pantherina*
    A. *phalloides*
    A. *rubescens*
    A. *verna*
    A. *virosa*
Amanitaceae
amanitine
amantadine hydrochloride
amaranth
amarillic typhus
amasacrine
amastia
amastigote
amaurosis
amaurotic familial idiocy
amazia
Ambard's
    constant
    laws
ambenonium chloride
amber mutation
ambient
    a. air
    a. temperature
    a. temperature and pressure, saturated
ambiguous external genitalia
Amblyomma
amblyopic neuropathy
amboceptor
    bacteriolytic a.
    Bordet's a.
    hemolytic a.
ambomycin

Ambrosia
ambutonium
ambutoxate
Ambystoma tigrinum
AMC — axiomesiocervical
AMD — alpha-methyldopa
    axiomesiodistal
ameba (amebae)
    coprozoic a.
    intestinal a.
    nonpathogenic a.
amebiasis
amebic
    a. abscess
    a. abscess of liver
    a. colitis
    a. cyst
    a. cystitis
    a. diarrhea
    a. dysentery
    a. encephalitis
    a. granuloma
    a. hepatitis
    a. meningitis
    a. meningoencephalitis
    a. peritonitis
    a. prevalence rate
    a. ulcer
amebocyte
ameboflagellate
ameboid movement
ameboma
ameburia
amegakaryocytic thrombocytopenia
amelanotic
    a. melanoma
    a. nevus
amelia
ameloblast
ameloblastic
    a. adenomatoid tumor
    a. carcinoma
    a. fibroma
    a. fibro-odontoma
    a. fibrosarcoma
    a. hemangioma
    a. neurilemoma
    a. odontoma
    a. sarcoma
ameloblastoma
    acanthomatous a.
    basal cell a.

calcifying a.
cystic a.
extraosseous a.
follicular a.
granular cell a.
malignant a.
melanotic a.
multicystic a.
peripheral a.
pigmented a.
plexiform a.
plexiform unicystic a.
solid a.
unicystic a.
amelogenesis imperfecta
amelogenic
amenorrhea
    a.-galactorrhea syndrome
    primary a.
    secondary a.
amentia
American Academy of Microbiology
American Association for the Advancement of Science
American Association for AIDS Research
American Association of Bioanalysts
American Association of Blood Banks
American Association for Clinical Chemistry
American Association for Clinical Immunology and Allergy
American Association of Immunologists
American Association of Neuropathologists
American Association of Pathologist Assistants
American Association of Pathologists
American Association of Pathologists and Bacteriologists
American Blood Commission
American Board of Bioanalysis
American Cancer Society
American Chemical Society
American Clinical Laboratory Association
American Hospital Association
American Joint Committee on Cancer Staging
American Medical Technologists
American Rheumatism Association

American Society of Bacteriologists
American Society for Clinical Investigation
American Society of Clinical Laboratory Technicians
American Society of Clinical Pathologists
American Society of Cytology
American Society for Experimental Pathology
American Society of Hematology
American Society for Medical Technology
American Society for Microbiology
American Society of Parasitologists
American Thoracic Society
American trypanosomiasis
American Type Culture Collection
americium
Ames
    assay
    test
Ames Lab-Tek cryostat
amethopterin
amethyst violet
AMF — automated motility factors
AmFAR — American Foundation for AIDS Research
AMG — antimacrophage globulin
    axiomesiogingival
Amh — mixed astigmatism with myopia predominating
AMI — acute myocardial infarction
    amitriptyline
    axiomesioincisal
amiantacea
amianthoid
amianthosis
amidase
    omega-a.
amide
    niacin a.
    a. synthetase
amidino
amidinotransferase
amidobenzene
amidohydrolase
amido-ligase
amidophosphoribosyltransferase
amikacin sulfate
amination

amine
    aromatic a.
    a. oxidase
    a. precursor uptake and decarboxylation
    pressor a.
aminergic nervous system
aminoacetic acid
amino acid
    acidic a.a.
    a.a. activating enzyme
    aliphatic a.a.
    amide type a.a.
    a.a. analyzer
    a.a. assay
    branched-chain a.a's
    glucogenic a.a.
    hydrogen type a.a.
    hydroxyamino type a.a.
    imino type a.a.
    ketogenic a.a.
    modified a.a.
    nonessential a.a.
    a.a. screen
aminoacidemia
α-amino-acidohydrolase
aminoacidopathy
D-aminoacid oxidase
L-aminoacid oxidase
aminoaciduria
    branched-chain a.
    renal a.
aminoacridine
9-aminoacridine
5-aminoacridine hydrochloride
aminoacyl
    a. adenylate
    a.-histidine dipeptidase
    a.-tRNA hydrolase
α-aminoadipate
α-aminoadipic acid
α-aminoadipicaciduria
aminoanthraquinone
amino apheresis machine
o-aminoazotoluene
p-aminoazobenzene
aminobenzene
aminobenzoic acid
ρ-aminobenzoic acid
p-aminobiphenyl
aminobutyrate aminotransferase
γ-aminobutyric acid
aminocaproic acid

aminodeoxyglucose
    a. acetyltransferase
    a. kinase
aminodeoxyglucosephosphate
    a. acetyltransferase
    a. isomerase
aminodimethylaniline
p-aminodimethylaniline
p-aminodiphenyl
aminoglutaric acid
aminoglutethimide
aminoglycoside
aminohippurate
p-aminohippurate clearance
amino-hippuric acid
aminohydroxybenzoic acid
aminohydroxypropylidine phosphate
aminoisobutyrate
aminoisobutyric acid
β-aminoisobutyric aciduria
2-aminoisovaleric acid
aminoketone dye
aminolevulinate dehydratase
δ-aminolevulinic acid
aminomalonate decarboxylase
aminomethane
aminomethyl
aminometradine
aminomutase
    leucine a.
2-amino-5-nitrothiazole
aminopenicillanic acid
6-aminopenicillanic acid
aminopentamide
aminopeptidase
    a. cytosol
    leucine a.
p-aminophenol
aminophylline
aminopropionitrile
aminopterin
aminopurine
aminopyridine
aminopyrine breath test
aminosalicylic acid
aminosuccinic acid
amino sugar
Aminosyn
aminotransferase
    alanine a.
    aminobutyrate a.

    aspartate a.
    glutamine-ketoacid a.
    mitochondrial aspartate a.
    ornithine a.
    ornithine-oxo-acid a.
    valine a.
3-aminotriazole
aminotripeptidase
aminuria
amiodarone-associated thyroiditis
amiphenazole
amisometradine
amitosis
amitotic
amitriptyline
amitriptyline and nortriptyline assay
amitrole
AML — acute monocytic leukemia
          acute myelocytic leukemia
          acute myelogenous leukemia
AMLS — antimouse lymphocyte
          serum
AMM — agnogenic myeloid metaplasia
          ammonia
ammeter
AMML — acute myelomonocytic leukemia
ammonemia
Ammon's horn
ammonia
    a. hemate
    a. nitrogen
ammoniacal
    a. silver nitrate test
    a. silver solutions
    a. urine
ammoniated mercury
ammonia-lyase
    L-histidine a.-l.
ammoniemia
ammonium
    a. biurate crystals
    a. carbonate
    a. chloride
    a. hydroxide
    a. magnesium phosphate crystals
    a. molybdate
    a. oxalate
    a. phosphomolybdate
    a. salt, quaternary
    a. sulfamate

AMINO ACIDS
(The 20 α-amino acids specified by the genetic code)

NAME	SYMBOLS*	STRUCTURAL FORMULA
Alanine	Ala	A	$\begin{array}{c} NH_2 \\ | \\ HOOC-CH-CH_3 \end{array}$
Arginine	Arg	R	$\begin{array}{c} NH_2 \qquad\qquad\qquad NH \\ | \qquad\qquad\qquad\qquad \| \\ HOOC-CH-CH_2-CH_2-CH_2-NH-C \\ \qquad\qquad\qquad\qquad\qquad\qquad\quad \backslash NH_2 \end{array}$
Asparagine	Asn	N	$\begin{array}{c} \qquad\qquad\qquad O \\ \qquad\qquad\qquad \| \\ NH_2 \qquad\quad C-NH_2 \\ | \qquad\quad / \\ HOOC-CH-CH_2 \\ | \\ NH_2 \end{array}$
Aspartic Acid	Asp	D	$\begin{array}{c} HOOC-CH-CH_2-COOH \\ | \\ NH_2 \end{array}$
Cysteine	Cys	C	$\begin{array}{c} HOOC-CH-CH_2-SH \\ | \\ NH_2 \end{array}$
Glutamic Acid	Glu	E	$\begin{array}{c} HOOC-CH-CH_2-CH_2-COOH \\ | \\ NH_2 \end{array}$
Glutamine	Gln	Q	$\begin{array}{c} \qquad\qquad\qquad\qquad\qquad O \\ \qquad\qquad\qquad\qquad\qquad \| \\ HOOC-CH-CH_2-CH_2-C-NH_2 \\ | \\ NH_2 \end{array}$
Glycine	Gly	G	$\begin{array}{c} HOOC-CH-H \\ | \\ NH_2 \end{array}$
Histidine	His	H	$\begin{array}{c} NH_2 \\ | \\ HOOC-CH-CH_2 \end{array}$

Isoleucine	Ile	I	$$HOOC-\underset{NH_2}{CH}-\underset{CH_3}{CH}-CH_2-CH_3$$
Leucine	Leu	L	$$HOOC-\underset{NH_2}{CH}-CH_2-\underset{CH_3}{CH}-CH_2$$
Lysine	Lys	K	$$HOOC-\underset{NH_2}{CH}-CH_2-CH_2-CH_2-CH_2-NH_2$$
Methionine	Met	M	$$HOOC-\underset{NH_2}{CH}-CH_2-CH_2-S-CH_3$$
Phenylalanine	Phe	F	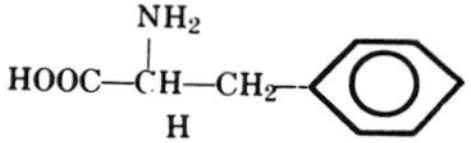 $$HOOC-\underset{NH_2}{CH}-CH_2-\phi$$
Proline	Pro	P	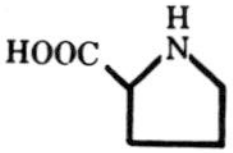 (pyrrolidine ring with N-H and HOOC)
Serine	Ser	S	$$HOOC-\underset{NH_2}{CH}-CH_2-OH$$
Threonine	Thr	T	$$HOOC-\underset{NH_2}{CH}-\underset{OH}{CH}-CH_3$$
Tryptophan	Trp	W	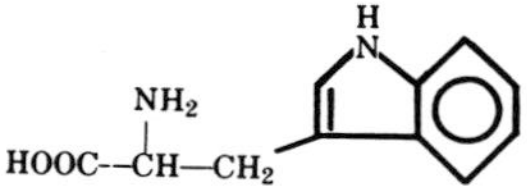 $$HOOC-\underset{NH_2}{CH}-CH_2-(indole)$$
Tyrosine	Tyr	Y	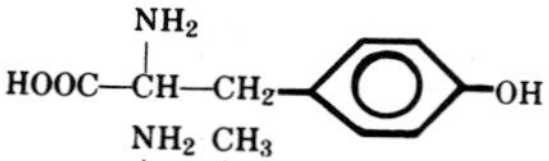 $$HOOC-\underset{NH_2}{CH}-CH_2-(C_6H_4)-OH$$
Valine	Val	V	$$HOOC-\underset{NH_2}{CH}-\underset{CH_3}{CH}-CH_3$$

* The three-letter and single-letter symbols that are used in presenting the sequence of a polypeptide or protein, e.g., Gly-Phe-Tyr. By convention, the N-terminal is shown at the left, the C-terminal at the right. For emphasis, the same formula may be written as H-Gly-Phe-Tyr-OH.

a. sulfate
a. tartrate
a. urate crystals
ammonium bromide
    a.b. alkyl aryl
    a.b. alkyl dimethyl benzyl
    a.b. alkyl dimethyl ethyl
    a.b. alkyl dimethyl ethyl-
      benzyl
    a.b. alkyl quaternary
    a.b. alkyl trimethyl
ammonium chloride
    a.c. alkyl aryl
    a.c. alkyl dimethyl benzyl
    a.c. alkyl dimethyl 3,4-
      dichlorobenzene
    a.c. alkyl dimethyl ethyl
    a.c. alkyl dimethyl ethyl-
      benzyl
    a.c. alkyl quaternary
    a.c. alkyl toluyl methyl tri-
      methyl
    a.c. alkyl trimethyl
    a.c. dialkyl dimethyl
    a.c. di-isobutyl cresolyl ethoxy
      ethyl dimethyl benzyl
    a.c. di-isobutyl phenoxy
      ethoxy ethyl dimethyl benzyl
ammoniuria
amnesia
    hysterical a.
    transient global a.
amniocentesis
amnioma
amnion nodosum
amnionitis
Amnioplastin
amniorrhea
amniotic
    a. adhesion
    a. band
    a. corpuscle
    a. fluid analysis
    a. fluid bilirubin
    a. fluid creatinine
    a. fluid embolism
    a. fluid embolus
    a. fluid lecithin/sphingomyelin
      ratio
    a. fluid pulmonary surfactant
    a. infection syndrome of Blane

a. sac
a. villi
AMO — axiomesio-occlusal
amobarbital
A-mode — amplitude modulation
    (unit)
amodiaquine hydrochloride
Amoeba
    A. buccalis
    A. cachexica
    A. coli
    A. coli mitis
    A. dentalis
    A. dysenteriae
    A. histolytica
    A. limax
    A. meleagridis
    A. urinae granulata
    A. urogenitalis
    A. verrucosa
Amoebotaenia
AMoL — acute monocytic (monoblas-
    tic) leukemia
amolanone
amorph
amorphic gene
amorphous fraction of adrenal
  cortex
amosite
amoxapine
amoxicillin
AMP — acid mucopolysaccharide
    adenosine monophosphate
    ampicillin
    average mean pressure
amp — ampere
amperage
ampere
    a.-second
    kilovolt a.
amperometry
amphetamine
    a. adipate
    a. phosphate
    a. sulfate
amphiarkyochrome
amphiarthrosis
amphibole asbestos
amphibolia
amphibolic; amphibolous
    a. fistula
    a. pathway

amphicarcinogenic
amphichroic
amphichromatic
amphicyte
amphileukemic
Amphimerus
amphinucleus
amphipath
amphipathic
amphiphile
amphiphilic
amphiprotic
amphitrichous
amphixenoses
amphochromatophil; amphochroma-
 tophile
amphochromophil; amphochro-
 mophile
amphocyte
ampholyte
amphomycin
amphophil; amphophile
 a. cell
 a. granule
amphophilic
amphoteric
 a. dye
 a. electrolyte
 a. reaction
amphotericin B
ampicillin
amplification
 a. factor
 gas a.
 gene a.
 myc oncogene a.
amplifier
 complementary symmetry a.
 Darlington a.
 logarithmic a.
amplitude
amprotropine
AMPS — abnormal mucopolysacchariduria
ampule
ampulla (pl., ampullae)
 membranous a.
 osseous a.
 rectal a.
 uterine tube a.
 a. of vas deferens
 a. of Vater

ampullar
 a. abortion
 a. pregnancy
ampullary aneurysm
ampullitis
amputating ulcer
amputation
 a. neuroma
 spontaneous a.
AMS — antimacrophage serum
 automated multiphasic
 screening
amsacrine
AMT — alpha-methyltyrosine
 American Medical Technologists
 amethopterin
 applied medical technology
amt. — amount
amu — atomic mass unit
AMV — avian myeloblastosis virus
AMV2 — avian myelocytomatosis
 virus
AMY — amylase
amyctic
amyelia
amyelinic
amyelonic
amygdalase
amygdalofugal fibers
amygdaloid nucleus
amyl
 a. acetate
 a. nitrite
amylaceous corpuscle
amylase
 alpha-a.
 beta-a.
 a. clearance
 a.-creatinine clearance ratio
 endo-a.
 pancreatic a.
 salivary a.
 serum a.
 urinary a.
amylasuria
amylemia
amyloclast
amylo-1,6-glucosidase
amyloid
 a. A
 a. angiopathy

a. bodies of prostate
a. corpuscle
a. degeneration
a. deposit
a. goiter
a. of immunoglobulin origin
a. kidney
AL (light chain) a.
a. nephrosis
a. neuropathy
β_{12}-a. protein
a. staining
transthyretin type a.
a. tumor
amyloidosis
a. cutis
adrenal a.
diffuse a.
endocrine a.
familial primary systemic a.
focal a.
hereditary a.
immunocytic a.
lichen a.
light chain–related a.
macular a.
a. of multiple myeloma
nodular a.
primary a.
reactive systemic a.
renal a.
secondary a.
senile cardiac a.
senile cerebral a.
systemic familial primary a.
systemic primary a.
amylolysis
amylolytic enzyme
amylomaltase
amylopectin
amylopectinosis
amylorrhea
amylose
alpha a.
crystalline a's
amylosuria
amyluria
amyoplasia congenita
amyosthenia
amyotonia congenita
amyotrophia
amyotrophic lateral sclerosis

amyotrophy
diabetic a.
neuralgic a.
amyous
An — anisometropia
anodal
anode
ANA — acetylneuraminic acid
antinuclear antibodies
aspartyl naphthylamide
anabasine
anabasis
anabiotic cells
anabolic steroids
anabolism promoting factor
anabolite
anacidity
anacmesis
anacrotism
anadenia ventriculi
anaerobe
facultative a's
obligate a's
anaerobia
anaerobian
anaerobiase
anaerobic
a. bacteria culture
a. bacterium
a. cellulitis
a. chamber
a. diphtheroids
a. endometrial culture
a. glycolysis
a. incubation
a. infection
a. jar
a. metabolism
a. neisseria
a. organism
a. streptococcus
a. urine specimen
anaerobiosis
anaerogenic
anagocytic
anakhré
anakmesis
anal
a. atresia
a. canal
a. fistula
a. papillitis

analbuminemia
analeptic
analgesia
analgesic
    a. nephritis
    a. nephropathy
    a. neuropathy
anallergenic serum
analog; analogue
    a. data
    folic acid a.
    a. of histidine
    homologous a.
    nucleoside a.
    pyrimidine a.
    a. signal
    somatostatin a.
analogous structures
analyser
    chemistry a.
analysis (pl., analyses)
    activation a.
    amniotic fluid a.
    automated cell image a.
    Barr body a.
    blood gas a.
    body a.
    body fluid a.
    cerebrospinal fluid a.
    chemical a.
    cluster a.
    compartmental a.
    critical path a.
    cytophotometric a.
    displacement a.
    DNA a.
    Fourier a.
    gastric a.
    genetic linkage a.
    graphic a.
    head space a.
    image display and a.
    immunochemical a.
    linear discriminant a.
    microdiffusion a.
    multimeric a.
    multivariant a.
    neutron activation a.
    Northern blot a.
    qualitative a.
    quantitative a.
    radiochemical a.

    recombinant DNA a.
    regression a.
    saturation a.
    semiquantitativvea.
    sequential a.
    sib pair a.
    Southern blot a.
    spectroscopic a.
    time series a.
    univariant a.
    a. of variance
    volumetric a.
    Western blot a.
analyte
analytic
    a. cytology
    a. ultracentrifuge
analytical
    a. balance
    a. bias
    a. chemistry
    a. electron microscope
    a. immunofiltration
    a. reagent grade
    a. toxicology
analyzer
    amino acid a.
    blood gas a.
    centrifugal a.
    chemistry a.
    desk-top a.
    ELT (euglobulin lysis time) se-
      ries hematology a.
    enzyme a.
    image a.
    infrared CO_2 a.
    kinetic a.
    light scattering a.
    multichannel a.
    oxygen a.
    oxygen gas a.
    pulse height a.
    spectrum a.
    Sysmex multichannel hematol-
      ogy a.
    Technicon a.
    wave a.
anamnesis
amamnestic response
anamorph
Ananase
anangioplasia

anangioplastic
anangioid
anaphase
anaphoresis
anaphylactic
    a. antibody
    a. shock
    a. transfusion reaction
anaphylactin
anaphylactogen
anaphylactogenesis
anaphylactoid
    a. crisis
    a. purpura
    a. reaction
    a. shock
anaphylatoxin inactivator
anaphylaxis
    aggregate a.
    complement-mediated a.
    eosinophil chemotactic factor
      of a.
    generalized a.
    local a.
    passive a.
    passive cutaneous a.
    slow-reacting substance of a.
    systemic a.
anaplasia
    monophasic a.
    polyphasic a.
Anaplasma marginale
Anaplasmataceae
anaplasmosis
anaplastic
    a. adenocarcinoma
    a. astrocytoma
    a. carcinoma
    a. cell
    a. meningioma
    a. seminoma
anaplerosis
anaplerotic
anapophysis
anarithmia
anasarca
    fetoplacental a.
anasarcous
anastalsis
anastomose
anastomosis (pl., anastomoses)
    arteriovenous a.

cholangioenteric a.
coloesophageal a.
crucial a.
enteroenteric a.
esophagogastric a.
fasciofacial a.
postcostal a.
precapillary a.
precostal a.
Roux-en-Y a.
anatherapeusis
anatomic; anatomical
    a. pathology
    a. tubercle
anatomicopathological
anatomy
    pathological a.
anatoxin
Anatrichosoma
anazoturia
ANCA — antineutrophil cytoplasmic
        antibodies
AnCC — anodal-closure contraction
anchorage
anchusin
Ancobon
anconeus muscle
anconitis
ancrod
Ancylidae
Ancylostoma
    A. braziliense
    A. caninum
    A. duodenale
Andersen's triad
Anderson-Collip test
Anderson's procedure
androblastoma
androgen
    a. excess
    a. insensitivity
    a. receptor
androgenesis
androgenic
    a. anabolic agent
    a. hormone
androgenization
andropathy
androstanediol glucuronide
androstene
androstenedione

androsterone
AnDTe — anodal-duration tetanus
anechoic
anectasis
anemia

    achlorhydric a.
    achrestic a.
    achylic a.
    acquired hemolytic a.
    acquired idiopathic sideroblastic a.
    acquired sideroachrestic a.
    acute hemolytic a.
    acute myelogenous a.
    acute posthemorrhagic a.
    Addison's a.
    addisonian a.
    angiopathic hemolytic a.
    anhematopoietic a.; anhemopoietic a.
    aplastic a.
    Arctic a.
    aregenerative a.
    asiderotic a.
    autoallergic hemolytic a.
    autoimmune hemolytic a.
    Belgian Congo a.
    Biermer's a.
    Blackfan-Diamond a.
    blood loss a.
    cameloid a.
    chlorotic a.
    chronic a.
    a. of chronic renal failure
    congenital a.
    congenital aplastic a.
    congenital aregenerative a.
    congenital atransferrinemic a.
    congenital dyserythropoietic a.
    congenital hemolytic a.
    congenital hypoplastic a.
    congenital nonspherocytic hemolytic a.
    congential pernicious a.
    congenital sideroachrestic a.
    constitutional aplastic a.
    Cooley's a.
    crescent cell a.
    deficiency a.
    Diamond-Blackfan hypoplastic a.
    dilution a.

    dimorphic a.
    diphyllobothrium a.
    drepanocytic a.
    dyserythropoietic a.
    dyshemopoietic a.
    Edelmann's a.
    Ehrlich's a.
    elliptocytic a.
    erythroblastic a.
    erythronormoblastic a.
    Estren-Damashek a.
    Faber's a.
    factor deficiency a.
    false a.
    familial erythroblastic a.
    familial hemolytic a.
    familial hypoplastic a.
    familial megaloblastic a.
    familial microcytic a.
    familial pyridoxine-responsive a.
    familial splenic a.
    Fanconi's a.
    folate deficiency a.
    folic acid a.
    genetic a.
    globe cell a.
    glucose-6-phosphate dehydrogenase deficiency a.
    a. gravis
    ground itch a.
    Hayem-Widal a.
    Heinz body hemolytic a.
    hemolytic a.
    hemolytic a. of newborn
    hemorrhagic a.
    hemotoxic a.
    hereditary hemolytic a.
    hereditary iron-loading a.
    hereditary nonspherocytic hemolytic a.
    hereditary sideroachrestic a.
    hereditary sideroblastic a.
    hereditary spherocytotic a.
    Herrick's a.
    hookworm a.
    hyperchromic a.
    hyperchromatic a.
    hypochromic a.
    hypochromic microcytic a.
    hypoferric a.
    hypoplastic a.

iatrogenic a.
icterohemolytic a.
idiopathic hypochromic a.
idiopathic myelofibrotic a.
immunohemolytic a.
a. infantum pseudoleukemic a.
infectious a.
infectious hemolytic a.
intertropical a.
iron deficiency a.
isochromic a.
isoimmune hemolytic a.
Jaksch's a.
lead a.
Lederer's a.
leukoerythroblastic a.
local a.
a. lymphatica
macrocytic a.
macrocytic achylic a.
malignant a.
Marchiafava-Micheli a.
Mediterranean a.
megaloblastic a.
megalocytic a.
metaplastic a.
microangiopathic hemolytic a.
microcytic a.
microcytic hypochromic a.
microdrepanocytic a.
milk a.
molecular a.
myelopathic a.
myelophthisic a.
neonatal a.
a. neonatorum
nonspherocytic hemolytic a.
normochromic a.
normocytic a.
nosocomial a.
nutritional macrocytic a.
osteosclerotic a.
ovalocytic a.
pernicious a.
phenylhydrazine a.
physiologic a.
polar a.
posthemorrhagic a.
primaquine-sensitive a.
primary a.
primary erythroblastic a.
primary refractory a.

protein deficiency a.
a. pseudoleukemia infantum
pure red cell a.
pyridoxine-responsive a.
radiation a.
refractory normoblastic a.
refractory sideroblastic a.
Runeberg's a.
schistocytic hemolytic a.
scorbutic a.
secondary a.
secondary refractory a.
sickle cell a.
sideroachrestic a.
sideroblastic a.
sideropenic a.
spastic a.
spherocytic a.
a. splenetica
splenic a.
spur cell a.
target cell a.
thrombopenic a.
toxic hemolytic a.
traumatic a.
trophoneurotic a.
tropical macrocytic a.
tunnel a.
vitamin deficiency a.
von Jaksch's a.
X-linked sideroblastic a.

anemic
a. anoxia
a. halo
a. hypoxia
a. infarction
a. phlebitis
anemotrophy
anencephalic
anencephaly
anenzymia catalasia
anephric
anergic
anergy
cachectic a.
clonal a.
cutaneous a.
anerythroplasia
anerythroplastic
anerythropoiesis
anerythroregenerative
anesthesia

anesthetic
anetoderma
    a. erythematosum
    Schweninger-Buzzi a.
aneucentric
aneuploid cells
aneuploidy
    chromosomal a.
aneurysm
    abdominal a.
    abdominal aortic a.
    ampullary a.
    aortic a.
    aortic arch a.
    aortic sinusal a.
    arterial a.
    arteriosclerotic a.
    arteriosclerotic aortic a.
    arteriosclerotic throm-
      bosed a.
    arteriovenous a.
    atherosclerotic a.
    axial a.
    bacterial a.
    benign bone a.
    Bérard's a.
    berry a.
    brain a.
    cardiac a.
    Charcot-Bouchard a.
    cirsoid a.
    compound a.
    congenital a.
    congenital ruptured a.
    consecutive a.
    cylindroid a.
    cystogenic a.
    diffuse a.
    dissecting a.
    ectatic a.
    embolic a.
    embolomycotic a.
    endogenous a.
    erosive a.
    exogenous a.
    false a.
    fusiform a.
    hernial a.
    intracranial a.
    luetic a.
    miliary a.
    mural a.
    mycotic a.
    a. needle
    Park's a.
    peripheral a.
    popliteal a.
    Pott's a.
    racemose a.
    Rasmussen's a.
    Richet's a.
    Rodrigues's a.
    ruptured a.
    saccular a.
    sacculated a.
    serpentine a.
    syphilitic a.
    thoracic a.
    thrombosed a.
    thrombosed arteriosclerotic a.
    traction a.
    traumatic a.
    true a.
    tubular a.
    varicose a.
    ventricular a.
aneurysmal; aneurysmatic
    a. bone cyst
    a. dilatation
    a. sac
    a. varix
aneusomatic
ANF — alpha-naphthoflavone
      antinuclear factor
ang — angiogram
"angel dust" abuse
"angel of death" mushrooms
angiasthenia
angiectasia; angiectasis
    congenital dysplastic a.
angiectatic
angiectopia
angiitis (pl., angiitides)
    allergic granulomatous a.
    consecutive a.
    cutaneous systemic a.
    hypersensitivity a.
    leukocytoclastic a.
    a. livedo reticularis
    necrotizing a.
angina
    agranulocytic a.
    Ludwig's a.
    lymphatic a.

a. lymphomatosa
monocytic a.
neutropenic a.
a. pectoris
Prinzmetal's a.
Vincent's a.
anginal
angioataxia
angioblast
angioblastic meningioma
angioblastoma
angioblastomatous meningioma
angiocardiography
angiocentric
a. immunoproliferative lesion
angiocholecystitis
angiochondroma
Angio-Conray
angiocholitis
angiocyst
angiodermatitis
angiodysplasia
papular a.
angiodystrophy; angiodystrophia
angioedema
hereditary a.
angioelephantiasis
angioendothelioma
angioendotheliomatosis
systemic proliferating a.
angiofibrolipoma
angiofibroma
juvenile a.
nasopharyngeal a.
angiofibrosis
angiofollicular mediastinal lymph node hyperplasia
angiogenesis
a. factor
tumor a.
angioglioma
angiogliomatosis
angiogram
fluorescein a.
angiogranuloma
angiography
angiohemophilia
angiohyalinosis hemorrhagica
angiohypertonia
angiohypotonia
angioimmunoblastic lymphadenopathy

angioinfarction
angioinvasive
a. adenoma
a. encapsulated carcinoma
a. tumor
angiokeratoma
a. corporis diffusum universalis
Fordyce's a.
Mibelli's a.
angiokeratosis
angioleiomyoma (pl., angioleiomyomata)
angioleucitis
angiolipofibroma
angiolipoma
angiolith
angiolithic degeneration
angiolupoid
angiolymphangioma
angiolymphoid hyperplasia
angioma
a. arteriale racemosum
arteriovenous a.
capillary a.
cavernous a.
cherry a.
a. cutis
fissural a.
hypertrophic a.
a. lymphaticum
petechial a's
a. serpiginosum
spider a.
telangiectatic a.
a. venosum racemosum
venous a.
angiomatoid tumor
angiomatosis
congenital dysplastic a.
encephalotrigeminal a.
intravascular a.
retinal a.
angiomatous meningioma
angiomegaly
angiomyofibroma
angiomyolipoma
angiomyoma
angiomyoneuroma
angiomyopathy
angiomyosarcoma
angiomyxoma
angioneuromyoma

angioneuropathy
angioneurotic edema
angionoma
angio-osteohypertrophy syndrome
angiopancreatitis
angioparalysis
angioparesis
angiopathic hemolytic anemia
angiopathy
    amyloid a.
    congenital dysplastic a.
    congophilic a.
    diabetic a.
angioplasty
    balloon a.
    laser a.
    laser thermal a.
    transluminal coronary a.
angioreninoma
angioreticuloendothelioma
angioreticuloma
angiorrhexis
angiosarcoma
    hepatic a.
angiosclerosis
angioscopy
angioscotoma
angiosis
angiospasm
angiospastic
angiostenosis
angiostrongyloidiasis
Angiostrongylus
    A. cantonensis
    A. costaricensis
angiostroph
angiotelectasis; angiotelectasia
angiotensinase
angiotensin-converting enzyme
angiotensinogen
angiotomy
angitis; angiitis
angle
    angry back a.
    a. closure glaucoma
    critical a.
    iridocorneal a.
    a. of incidence
    a. of reflection
    a. of refraction
    solid a.
angstrom

Angström's
    law
    unit
angular conjunctivitis
angulation
angulus
anhemolytic streptococcus
anhemopoietic anemia
anhidrosis
anhidrotic ectodermal dysplasia
anhydrase
    carbonic a.
anhydration
anhydride
    acetic a.
    acid a.
    cyclic lysine a.
    mixed a.
    phthalic a.
anhydrous alcohol
Anichkov's; Anitschkow's
    cell
    myocyte
anicteric hepatitis
anileridine
aniline
    a. blue
    a. dye
    a. fuchsin
    a. gentian violet
    lactophenol a.
anilingus
anilinism
anilinophil; anilinophile
anilinophilous
animal
    a. cell culture
    Houssay a.
    a. protein factor
    sentinel a.
    a. virus
animatum
    contagium a.
    virus a.
anion
    cyanide a.
    a. exchange chromatography
    a. exchange resin
    a. gap
    a. interference
anionic dye
anionotropy

aniridia
anisakiasis
Anisakis marina
anise oil
O-anisidine
anisindione
anisochromasia
anisochromia
anisocytic erythrocyte
anisocytosis
anisohypercytosis
anisohypocytosis
anisokaryosis
anisoleukocytosis
anisomorphic gliosis
anisonucleolinosis
anisonucleosis
anisopoikilocytosis
anisotropic
anisotropine
anisotropy
Anitschkow's (Anichkov's)
    cell
    myocyte
ankle
    a. joint
    a. ligament
ankyloblepharon
ankylocolpos
ankyloglossia
ankyloproctia
ankylosing
    a. hyperostosis
    a. spondylitis
ankylosis
    bony a.
    cricoarytenoid joint a.
    extracapsular a.
    fibrous a.
    intracapsular a.
    osseous a.
    stapedial a.
Ankylostoma
ankyrin
anlagen
    genital a.
    urogenital a.
ANLL — acute nonlymphocytic leu-
    kemia
Ann Arbor Staging Classification
anneal
Annelida

annellophore
annexitis
annotto
annular pancreas
annulate lamellae
annulus (pl., annuli)
    Zinn's a.
AnOC — anodal opening contraction
anococcygeal
anochromasia
anodal
anode voltage
anodic stripping voltammetry
anodontia
anodyne
anomalad
anomalous
    a. muscle band
    a. origin
    a. vascular distribution
    a. venous connection
    a. venous drainage
anomaly
    Alder-Reilly a.
    Alder's a.
    "bell-clapper" a.
    Chédiak-Higashi a.
    Chédiak-Steinbrinck-Higashi
        a.
    congenital a.
    DiGeorge's a.
    Ebstein's a.
    Freund's a.
    Hegglin's a.
    May-Hegglin a.
    Pelger-Huët a.
    Pelger-Huët nuclear a.
    pseudo-Pelger a.
    Shone's a.
    Uhl's a.
    Undritz a.
    vascular a.
anomer
anomeric
anonymous myobacterium
Anopheles maculipennis
anophthalamia
Anoplocephala
Anoplocephalidae
Anoplura
anorchia; anorchism

anorectal
    a. herpes
    a. syphilis
anorectic
anorectum
anorexia nervosa
anoscopic
anosmia
anosteoplasia
anostosis
ANOVA — analysis of variance
anovular
anovulation
anovulatory
anoxemia
anoxemic
anoxia
    altitude a.
    anemic a.
    anoxic a.
    fulminating a.
    histotoxic a.
    hypoxic a.
    myocardial a.
    a. neonatorum
    oxygen affinity a.
    a. reaction
    stagnant a.
anoxic
    a. anoxia
    a. encephalopathy
ANP — atrial natriuretic peptide
ANS — antineutrophilic serum
    arteriolonephrosclerosis
    autonomic nervous system
ansa (pl., ansae)
    a. cervicalis
    a. hypoglossi
    a. lenticularis
    a. peduncularis
    a. subclavia
Ansamycin
ansaparamedian fissure
Ansbacher unit
anserina
    cutis a.
anserine bursitis
ansiform
Antabuse
antacid
antagonism
    bacterial a.

    metabolic a.
    microbial a.
    salt a.
antagonist
    β-adrenergic a.
    competitive a.
    enzyme a.
    insulin a.
    metabolic a.
    narcotic a.
    sulfonamide a.
antazoline
antebrachial
antebrachium
antecedent
    plasma thromboplastin a.
antecubital
    a. region
    a. space
anteflexion
antegrade
antemortem
antenatal
antepartum hemorrhage
antephase
anterior
    acute a. poliomyelitis
    a. axillary line
    complete a. dislocation
    a. displacement
    a. external arcuate fibers
    a. horn cell
    a. lateral myocardial infarct
    a. pituitary extract
    a. pituitary hormone
    a. superior iliac spine
    a. synechia
    a. wall infarction
    a. wall myocardial in-
        farction
anterodorsal
anterofacial dysplasia
anterograde conduction
anterolateral
anteromedial
anteroposterior
    a. dysplasia
    a. facial dysplasia
anteroseptal myocardial infarct
anteroventral
anteversion
anteverted

anthelix
anthelmintic
anthelmycin
anthocyanidin
anthocyanin
Anthomyia
    A. canicularis
    A. incisura
    A. manicata
    A. salatrix
    A. scalaris
Anthomyiidae
anthophyllite
anthracemia
anthracene blue
6,10-anthracenedicarboxyaldehyde
anthracic
anthracin
anthracoid
anthracometer
anthraconecrosis
anthracosilicosis
anthracosis
    a. linguae
    pulmonary a.
anthracotic
    a. pigment
    a. tuberculosis
anthracycline cardiotoxicity
anthralin
anthramycin
anthranilate
anthranilic acid
anthrapurpurin
anthraquinone dye
anthrarobin
anthrax
    a. bacillus
    cutaneous a.
    a. septicemia
anthropoid
anthropometric assessment
anthroponosis (pl., anthroponoses)
anthropozoonosis
anti-3d autoantibody
antiachromotrichia factor
antiacroydnia factor
antiallotype
antiandrogen
antianemic principle
antiantibody
antiasthmatic

antibacterial
    a. agent
    a. agent susceptibility test
anti-basement
    a.-b. membrane glomerulone-
        phritis
    a.-b. membrane nephritis
antibiosis
antibiotic
    a.-associated pseudomembra-
        nous colitis
    bactericidal a.
    bacteriostatic a.
    broad-spectrum a.
    a. level
    macrolide a.
    oral a.
    polyene a.
    a. sensitivity
antibody (pl., antibodies)
    ABO a.
    acetylcholine receptor a.
    adrenal a.
    adrenocortical a.
    agglutinating a.
    allantoin-D a.
    anaphylactic a.
    antiacetylcholine receptor a.
    anti–basement membrane a.
    anticardiac a.
    anticardiolipin a.
    anticentromere a.
    anti-*Chlamydia* a.
    anticoagulant a.
    anticytoplasmic a.
    anti-DNA a.
    a.-antigen complex
    a.-dependent cell-mediated cy-
        totoxicity
    anti-HIV a.
    antihormone a.
    anti-idiotype a.
    anti-La a.
    antimicrosomal a.
    antimitochondrial a.
    antineutrophil cytoplasmic a.
    antinuclear a.
    antiphospholipid a.
    antiplatelet a.
    anti-receptor a.
    anti–red cell a.
    anti-Ro a.

anti–SS-A a.
anti–SS-B a.
anti–smooth muscle a.
anti–T-cell a.
antithyroglobulin a.
antithyroid a.
anti-*Toxoplasma* a.
antitubular basement membrane a.
autologous a.
bispecific a.
blocking a.
B-lymphocyte a.
a. catabolism
centromere a.
chimaeric a.
clonal a.
cold-reacting a.
complement-fixing a.
complement-reacting a.
cross-reacting a.
cytophilic a.
cytotoxic a.
cytotropic a.
115 D8 a.
darkfield fluorescent a.
a. deficiency syndrome
desmoplakian a.
a. detection
DF3 a.
Donath-Landsteiner a.
Duffy's a., Fy^a, Fy^b
erythrocyte-absorbing a's
a. excess zone
ferritin-conjugated a's
ferritin-coupled a's
fluorescent antinuclear a.
fluorescent treponemal a.
Forssman a.
Fy a.
α-globulin a.
gp 24 a.
gp 120/160 a.
a. half-life
hemagglutinating a.
hemagglutinating anti-penicillin a.
hemagglutination-inhibition a.
heterocytotropic a.
heterogenetic a.
heterophilic a.
homocytotropic a.

hybridoma a.
I and i a.
a. identification
idiotype a.
IgM a.
incomplete a.
inhibiting a.
islet cell a.
isophil a.
Jo1 a.
Kidd a.
kidney-fixing a.
labeled a.
leukoagglutinating a.
Lewis a., Le^a, Le^b
Lutheran a.
lymphocytotoxic a.
M$_2$ a.
measles a.
microsomal a.
microsomal thyroid a.
mitochondrial a.
monoclonal a.
mouse-human chimaeric a.
nephrotoxic a.
neutralizing a.
nuclear a.
oc-125 a.
P a.
Paul-Bunnell a.
P-K (Prausnitz-Küstner) a.
polyclonal a.
Prausnitz-Küstner a.
precipitating a.
reaginic a.
Rh a.
saline a's
Scl-70 a.
skin-sensitizing a.
thyroid colloidal a.
thyroid microsomal a.
a. titer
TSH-displacing a.
univalent a.
antibody-absorption
fluorescent treponemal a.-a.
antibody-forming cells
antibody reaction
blocking a.r.
endogenous antigen cell–bound a.r.
endogenous antigen-circulating a.r.

endogenous antigen-transferred a.r.

endogenous antigen-transferred cell–bound a.r.

heterophil a.r.

transferred antigen cell–bound a.r.

transferred antigen–transferred a.r.

antibombesin

anticholera serum

anticholinergic poisoning

anticholinesterase

anticoagulant

    circulating a.

    a.-citrate-dextrose

    a.-citrate-phosphate-dextrose

    lupus a.

    lupus-type a.

    a. therapy

anticoagulated

anticoagulation

    CD a.

    I a.

    i a.

    La a.

    leukocyte function–associated a.

    leukocyte function–related a.

    prostate-specific a.

    RNP a.

    Ro a.

    tumor a.

    very late activation a.

anticoagulative

anticoagulin

anticodon

anticolibacillary

anticollagenase

anticolloidoclastic

anticomplementary serum

anticonvulsant

anticytoplasmic

    a. antibody

    a. autoantibodies

anti-D

antideoxyribonuclease

antidepressant

    tricyclic a.

antidiphtheria serum

antidiphtheritic globulin

antidiuretic

    a. hormone

    a. hormone deficiency

    a. substance

anti-DNA antibody assay

anti-DNAse B assay

antidote

antidromic

antiemesis

antiepithelial membrane antigen

antiestrogen

anti-extractable nuclear antigens

anti-factor

    a.-f. I disorder

    a.-f. II disorder

    a.-f. III disorder

    a.-f. V disorder

    a.-f. VIII disorder

    a.-f. IX disorder

    a.-f. X

    Roger a.-f.

antifibrinogen

antifibrinolysin

antifibrinolytic

antifol

    Baker's a.

antifolate

antifolic

antifungal agent

anti-GBM (glomerular basement membrane) disease

antigen

    ABO a.

    A a.

    a_1 a.

    a_2 a.

    acetone-insoluble a.

    acquired a.

    AFP (α-fetoprotein) a.

    allogenic a.

    alum-precipitated a.

    AM (alpha chain marker) a.

    a.-antibody complex

    a.-antibody reaction

    antiepithelial membrane a.

    anti-extractable nuclear a.

    a.-antiglobulin reaction

    antithetical a.

    Australia a.

    autologous a.

    B a.

    bacterial a.

bacterial killing a.
B-cell a.
a.-binding region
a.-binding site
a. blood group system
Boivin a.
C a.
CA a.
CA 2 (colloid) a.
CA 15-3 a.
CA 19-9 a.
CA-50 a.
CA-125 a.
CALLA (common acute
    lymphoblastic leukemia) a.
capsular a.
carcinoembryonic a.
Cartwright a.
CD a.
CD-5 a.
CEA (carcinoembryonic) a.
Ch^a a.
Chido Rodgers a.
colloid a.
Colton a.
common acute lymphoblastic
    leukemia a.
common leukocyte a.
compound a.
conjugated a.
core a.
cross-reacting a.
cryptococcal a.
Cs^s a.
D a.
delta a.
Diego a.
differentiation-specific a.
Dombrock a.
Duffy's a.
E a. (red cell antigen of the
    Rh blood group)
early a.
endogenous a.
env a.
epithelial membrane a.
epithelial structural a.
Epstein-Barr nuclear a.
erythrocyte a.
exogenous a.
extractable nuclear a.
Factor VIII coagulant a.

Factor VIII-related a.
fetal a.
febrile a.
α-fetoprotein a.
flagellar a.
Forssman a.
Frei's a.
Fy a.
gag a.
Gm a.
Gross virus a.
H (with film) a.
HAV (hepatitis A virus) a.
HBcAG (hepatitis B core) a.
HBeAG (hepatitis B e) a.
HBsAG (hepatitis B surface)
    a.
HDAg (hepatitis D) a.
hepatitis a.
hepatitis-associated a.
heterogenetic a.
heterologous a.
Heymann a.
histocompatibility a.
HIV (human immunodefi-
    ciency virus) a.
HLA (human leukocyte) a.
homologous a.
human thymus lymphocyte a.
H-Y (histocompatibility) a.
Ia a.
I and i a.
isogeneic a.
isophile a.
Ja a.
Ja$_a$ a.
Jk (Kidd) a.
Jo-1 a.
K a.
Kaproski's a.
Kell a's
Kidd a.
Km a.
Knop's a.
Kveim a.
Kveim-Stilzbach a.
Landsteiner-Wiener a.
leukocyte common a.
Leu-M1 a.
Lewis a's
Luke a.
Lutheran a.

Sjögren syndrome
anti-Ro, anti-La

Lw a.
Ly a.
lymphocyte-detected membrane a.
lymphogranuloma venereum a.
Lyt a.
M a.
matrix a.
membrane a.
merozoite a.
Miltenberger a.
Mitsuda a.
mouse-specific lymphocyte a.
myeloid a.
N a.
nuclear a.
nucleoprotein a.
O (without film) a.
oncofetal a.
Oz a.
P a.
p24 a.
pancreatic oncofetal a.
panhematolymphoid a.
platelet-specific a.
Pr a.
a. presentation
a.-presenting cell
private a.
a. processing
proliferating cell nuclear a.
prostate-specific a.
protein C a.
public a.
Qa a.
recall a.
a. recognition
Rg a.
Rh a.
Rho a.
Rh_o (D) a.
Ro a.
Roger's a.
rose bengal a.
Scianna a.
Sd^a a
SD (serologically defined) a.
senescent erythrocyte a.
sequestered a.
serologically defined a.
serum hepatitis a.

S and s a.
single human leukocyte a.
Sm-Burrell a.
Smith (Sm) a.
soluble a.
Sp (Pr) a.
a.-specific helper factor
a.-specific suppressor factor
squamous cell carcinoma a.
SS (Sjögren's syndrome) a.
Swann a.
T a.
TA-4 (squamous cell carcinoma) a.
Tac a.
T-cell a.
Thomson-Friedenreich a.
thymus-dependent a.
thymus-independent a.
thymus-leukemia a.
tissue a.
tissue polypeptide a.
tissue-specific a.
TL (thymic leukemia) a.
Tn a.
transplantation a.
treponemal a.
tumor a. (T a.)
tumor-associated rejection a.
tumor-specific a.
tumor-specific transplantation a.
U a.
a. unit
V a.
Vi (*Salmonella typhii*) a.
viral capsid a.
von Willebrand's a.
Wassermann a.
Wright's a.
xenogeneic a.
Xg a.
Xga a.
Xk^a a.
YK^a a.
Yt^a a.
Yt^b a.
Z a.
antigenemia
antigenemic
antigenic
    a. assay

a. antibody lattice formation
a. binding receptor
a. competition
a. component
a. deletion
a. determinant
a. determination
a. drift
a. modulation
a. shift
a. structural grouping
a. variation
antigenicity
antigenotherapy
antiglobulin
    a. reaction
    a. reagent
    a. test
antiglomerular
    a. basement membrane glomer-
      ulonephritis
antigravity reflexes
antihemagglutinin
antihemolysin
antihemolytic
antihemophilic
    a. factor
    a. factor A
    a. factor B
    a. factor C
    a. globulin A
    a. globulin B
    a. plasma
antihemorrhagic
antiheparin factor
antihepatic serum
antiheterolysin
antihistamine
anti-histone
antihormone antibody
antihuman
    a. globulin
    a. globulin test
    a. lymphocyte serum
antihyaluronidase
    a. assay
    a. titer
antithymocyte
    a. globulins
    a. serum
antihypercholesterolemia
antihypertensive

anti-icteric
anti-idiotype
anti-immunoglobulin
anti-infective
anti-inflammatory corticoid
anti-inhibitor coagulation complex
anti-invasin
anti-isolysin
antilewisite
    British a.
antileukemic
antileukocytic
antileukoprotease
antilymphocyte
    a. globulin
    a. plasma
    a. serum
antimacrophage
    a. globulin
    a. serum
antimalarial
antimatter
antimeningococcus serum
antimetabolite
    purine a.
antimicrobial
    a. susceptibility testing
    a. synergy
antimicrosomal antibodies
antimitochondrial antibody
antimode
antimoniotungstate
antimony
    a. chloride
    a. dimercaptosuccinate
    a. hydride
    a. poisoning
    a. potassium tartrate
    a. trichloride
antimorph
antimorphic
antimüllerian hormone
antimutagen
antimycobacterial
antineoplastic
antineutrino
antineutrophilic serum
antinociceptive
antinuclear
    a. antibodies
    a. factor
anti-oncogene

antioncotic
antioxidant
antiparallel
antiparasitic
antiparietal cell antibody assay
antiparticle
antiperistaltic
antipernicious anemia factor
antipertussis serum
antiphospholipid antibody
antiphylaxis
antiplaque serum
antiplasmin
    a_2-a.
antiplatelet
    a. antibodies
    a. serum
    a. therapy
antipneumococcus serum
antiporcine
antiport
antiproaccelerin
antiproliferative
antiprotease
antiprothrombin
antiprotozoal
anti-*Pseudomonas* human plasma
antipsychotic
antipurine
antipyrogenic
antipyrimidine
antipyrine
antirabies serum
antireceptor antibodies
antireticular cytotoxic serum
antiretroviral
anti-Rh
    a.-R. agglutinin
    a.-R. titer
antiscarlatinal serum
antisense
antisepsis
antiseptic
antiserum (pl., antisera)
    human thymus a.
    monospecific a.
    monovalent a.
    multivalent a.
    polyvalent a.
    rat thymus a.
anti–smooth muscle antibody
antisnake venom

antistaphylococcal serum
antistaphylolysin
antistreptococcic
antistreptococcin
antistreptococcus serum
antistreptokinase
antistreptolysin
    a. O
    a. test
    a. titer
antisubstance
antitetanic serum
antitetanus toxin
antithetical antigens
antithrombin
    a. deficiency
    a. III
    normal a.
antithromboplastin
antithymocyte
    a. globulin
    a. serum
antithyroglobulin antibody
antithyroid antibody
antitoxic unit
antitoxin
    diphtheria a.
    tetanus a.
antitoxoplasma antibody test
anti-*Toxoplasma* antibodies
antitragus
antitrypsin deficiency
α_1-antitrypsin phenotyping
antitryptic
    a. index
    a. reaction
antituberculin
antituberculosis
antitubular basement membrane antibody
antitumor
    a. enzyme
    a. macrophage
antitumorigenesis
antivenin
    North American coral snake a.
    a. unit
antivenom
antivenomous serum
antiviral immunity
antityphoid serum
Anton's test

Antopol-Goldman lesion
ANTR — apparent net transfer
  rate
antral gastritis
antrectomy
antrum (pl., antrums, antra)
  ethmoid a.
  gastric a.
  mastoid a.
  maxillary a.
  nasal a.
  pyloric a.
  tympanic a.
Antrypol
ANTU — alpha-naphthylthiourea
anuclear
anucleated
anulus (pl., anuli)
  a. fibrosus of aorta
anuresis
anuria
anus
  imperforate a.
  melanocarcinoma of a.
  a. of Rusconi
  a. vesicalis
  vestibular a.
  a. vestibularis
  vulvovaginal a.
anxiety neurosis
anxiolytic
AO — acridine orange
  anodal opening
  anterior oblique
  aorta
  aortic opening
  axio-occlusal
  opening of the atrioventricu-
    lar valves
AOC — anodal-opening contraction
AOCl — anodal-opening clonus
AOD — arterial occlusive disease
AOP — anodal-opening picture
aorta
  abdominal a.
  ascending a.
  coarctation of a.
  cystic medial necrosis of as-
    cending a.
  descending thoracic a.
  double-barreled a.
  medial necrosis cystica of a.

  postductal coarctation of a.
  preductal coarctation of a.
  thoracic a.
aortic
  a. aneurysm
  a. arch
  a. arch arteritis
  a. arch syndrome
  a. atresia
  a. bodies
  a. body tumor
  a. cusp
  a. dissection
  a. hemorrhage
  a. impedance
  a. incompetence
  a. insufficiency
  a. internal elastic membrane
  a. isthmus
  a. lymph node
  a. plexus
  a. pulmonary window
  a. regurgitation
  a. ring
  a. septal defect
  a. stenosis
  a. tunica adventitia
  a. tunica intima
  a. tunica media
  a. valve
  a. valve replacement
  a. valve stenosis
aortica
  glomera a.
aorticorenal
  a. ganglion
  a. plexus
aorticosympathetic paraganglioma
aortitis
  bacterial a.
  Döhle-Heller a.
  giant cell a.
  luetic a.
  nummular a.
  rheumatoid a.
  syphilitic a.
aortocoronary
aortogram
aortography
  abdominal a.
  catheter a.
  selective visceral a.

thoracic a.
translumbar a.
aortoiliac occlusive disease
aortorenal bypass
aortosclerosis
AOS — anodal-opening sound
AOTe — anodal-opening tetanus
AP — acid phosphatase
acute proliferative
alkaline phosphatase
aminopeptidase
angina pectoris
antepartum
anterior pituitary
anteroposterior
appendix
arterial pressure
association period
axiopulpal
A & P — anterior and posterior
auscultation and percussion
APA — aldosterone-producing adenoma
aminopenicillanic acid
antipernicious anemia factor
APACHE — Acute Physiology and
Chronic Health Eval-
uation
apallic syndrome
apathy
Apathy's gum syrup medium
apatite
a.-associated large joint lysis
a. calculus
APB — atrial premature beat
auricular premature beat
APC — acetylsalicylic acid, phenacetin, caffeine
activated protein cell
adenoidal-pharyngeal-
conjunctival
antigen-presenting cell
aspirin, phenacetin, caffeine
atrial premature contraction
APC-C — aspirin, phenacetin, and
caffeine with codeine
APC virus
APCD — adult polycystic disease
APD — action-potential duration
atrial premature depolar-
ization

APE — aminophylline, phenobarbital, ephedrine
anterior pituitary extract
apeidosis
aperture
inferior a.
Key-Retzius lateral a.
lateral a.
median a.
numerical a.
orbital a.
piriform a.
Apeẃ virus
apex (pl., apexes, apices)
vaginal a.
APF — anabolism-promoting factor
animal protein factor
Apgar score
APGL — alkaline phosphatase activity of the granular leukocytes
APH — antepartum hemorrhage
anterior pituitary hormone
aphagia
aphakia
aphasia
motor a.
sensory a.
subcortical a.
transcortical a.
aphasmid
aphemia
apheresis
aphonia
APHP — anti-*Pseudomonas* human
plasma
aphtha (pl., aphthae)
aphthosis
genital a.
aphthous
a. fever
a. stomatitis
a. ulcer
a. ulceration
aphthovirus
apiamine
APIC — Association for Practitioners
in Infection Control
apical
a. abscess
a. canaliculi
a. dendrite

a. granuloma
a. murmur
apicitis
Apium
APL — acute promyelocytic leu-
            kemia
        anterior pituitary–like
aplanatic
a. lens
a. objective
aplasia
adrenal a.
congenital thymic a.
erythroid a.
Estren-Damashek familial a.
germ cell a.
germinal a.
gonadal a.
granulocytic a.
hematopoietic a.
megakaryocytic a.
nuclear a.
pure red cell a.
retinal a.
thymic-parathyroid a.
urothelial a.
aplasmic
aplastic
a. anemia
a. bone marrow
a. crisis
a. lymph
APN — acute pyelonephritis
apnea
deglutition a.
posthyperventilation a.
sleep a.
traumatic a.
apneusis
APO — apolipoprotein
apobiosis
apochromatic
apocodeine
apocrine
a. adenoma
a. carcinoma
a. cell
a. cystadenoma
a. hidrocystoma
a. metaplasia
a. miliaria
a. sweat gland

Apocynum
apoenzyme
apoferritin
apolipoprotein
A
A-I
A-ii
B
B-48
B-100
C
C-I
C-II
C-III
D
E
"thin line" a.
apomorphine hydrochloride
aponeurosis (pl., aponeuroses)
pharyngeal a.
aponeurositis
aponeurotic
a. fibroma
a. fibromatosis
apophyseal joint
apophysis (pl., apophyses)
apophysitis tibialis adolescentium
Apophysomyces elegans
apoplasmatic
apoplectic
a. coma
a. stroke
apoplexy
adrenal a.
pituitary a.
spät a.
apoprotein
apoptosis
aposiderin
aposome
apothecium
APP — alum-precipitated pyridine
app. — appendix
apparatus
Abbé-Zeiss a.
absorption a.
Barcroft's a.
chromidial a.
ciliary a.
Horsley-Clarke a.
juxtaglomerular a.
lacrimal a.
respiratory a.

Roughton-Scholander a.
subneural a.
Tiselius's a.
urogenital a.
Van Slyke's a.
vasomotor a.
vestibular a.
apparent power
appearance
    ground-glass a.
    Maltese cross a.
    tram-track a.
appendage
appendiceal
    a. abscess
    a. artery
    a. crypt
    a. lymphoid nodule
    a. mucous membrane
appendicitis
    actinomycotic a.
    acute a.
    acute gangrenous a.
    acute suppurative a.
    catarrhal a.
    chronic a.
    focal a.
    gangrenous a.
    helminthic a.
    lumbar a.
    obstructive a.
    stercoral a.
    subperitoneal a.
    suppurative a.
    verminous a.
appendicolithiasis
appendicular
appendix (pl., appendices, appen-
    dixes)
    a. epididymidis
    epiploic a.
    fibrous a.
    a. testis
    vermiform a.
APPG — aqueous procaine penicillin
    G
apple jelly nodules
applied science
appliqué form
apposition
appositional growth

approach
    Denker-Kahler a.
appropriate for gestational age
approximate lethal concentration
approx. — approximately, approxi-
    mation
approximately
approximation
APR — amebic prevalence rate
apraxia
aprobarbital
apron
    pudendal a.
apronalide
aprotic solvent
APRT — adenine phosphoribosyl
    transferase
APT — alum-precipitated toxoid
APTT — activated partial thrombo-
    plastin time
Apt test
aptyalism
APUD — amine precursor uptake
    and decarboxylation
apudoma
    esophageal a.
apyknomorphous
aqua (pl., aquae)
    a. regia
aquagenic urticaria
aqueduct
    cerebral a.
    a. of cochlea
    a. of Cotunnius
    a. of Fallopius
    a. of midbrain
    a. of Sylvius
    a. veil
    vestibular a.
aqueous
    a. humor
    a. mounting media
    a. solution
aquocobalamin
aquosa
    polyemia a.
AR — alarm reaction
    analytical reagent
    aortic regurgitation
    Argyll Robertson (pupil)
    artificial respiration
    ascorbic reductase

Ar — argon
ARA — American Rheumatism Association
ara-A — adenine arabinoside
L-arabinose dehydrogenase
arabinose operon
arabinoside
    adenine a.
    adenosine a.
    cytosine a.
arabinosuria
D-arabitol dehydrogense
L-arabitol dehydrogenase
ara-C — cytosine arabinoside
arachidonate
    a. 5-lipoxygenase
    a. 12-lipoxygenase
arachidonic acid
Arachis hypogaea
Arachnia propionica
arachnid
Arachnida
arachnodactyly
    contractural a.
arachnoid
    a. cap cell
    a. granulation
    intracranial a.
    a. mater
    spinal a.
    a. villi
arachnoidea
arachnoidism
arachnoiditis
arachnolysin
aramite
Arantius
    duct of A.
aratracheal
arborescence
arborescent
arborization block
arboviral
    a. encephalitis
    a. virus disease
arbovirus
ARC — AIDS-related complex
    anomalous retinal correspondence
arcade
    vascular a.
Arcanobacterium

arceau rhythm
arch
    aortic a.
    branchial a.
    faucial a.
    hyoid a.
    mandibular a.
    zygomatic a.
archencephalon
archiblast
archicerebellum
archil
arch-loop-whorl
arciform
arctation
Arctic anemia
arcuate
    a. artery
    a. fasciculus
    a. fiber
    a. nucleus
    a. nucleus, medulla oblongata
    a. periventricular nucleus
arcus senilis
ARD — acute respiratory disease
    anorectal dressing
ARDS — acute respiratory distress syndrome
    adult respiratory distress syndrome
area (pl., areae, areas)
    AI a.
    AII a.
    auditory association a.
    auditory receiving a.
    body surface a.
    brain a.
    Broca's a.
    cortical a.
    a. cribrosa
    entorhinal a.
    fusion a.
    gustatory receiving a.
    motor speech a.
    parastriate a.
    periamygdaloid a.
    a. postrema
    prepiriform a.
    primary somatomotor a.
    regulated a.
    sensory association a.
    SI a.

SII a.
somatosensory a.
a. striata
supplementary motor a.
taste receiving a.
visual association a.
visual receiving a.
areata; areatus
arecoline
areflexia
aregenerative anemia
arenaceous
arenation
Arenaviridae
arenavirus
areola (pl. areolae)
    Chaussier's a.
areolar
    a. connective tissue
    a. gland
areolitis
ARF — acute renal failure
        acute respiratory failure
Arg — arginine
arg — argentum
Argas
    A. persicus
    A. reflexus
argasid
Argasidae
argentaffin; argentaffine
    a. cell
    a. granules
    a. Masson
    a. reaction
    a. stain
argentaffinoma
argentation
Argentinian hemorrhagic fever virus
argentophil; argentophile
argentum
arginase
arginine
    a. carboxypeptidase
    a. deaminase
    a. glutamate
    a. hydrochloride
    a. insulin tolerance test
    a. monohydrochloride
    suberyl a.
    a. vasopressin
argininemia

argininosuccinase
argininosuccinate
    a. lyase
    a. lyase assay
    a. synthetase
    a. synthetase deficiency
argininosuccinic
    a. acidemia
    a. aciduria
arginyl
argon laser
Argyll Robertson pupil
argyremia
argyria
argyrophil; argyrophile
argyrophilic
    a. cells
    a. fibers
argyrosis
arhinencephalia
Arias-Stella
    cells
    effect
    phenomenon
    reaction
ariboflavinosis
Arizona
    A. arizonae
    A. hinshawii
ARM — artificial rupture of mem-
        branes
Armanni-Ebstein
    cells
    change
    kidney
Armed Forces Institute of Pathology
armed macrophage
Armigeres obturbans
Armillifer
    A. armillatus
    A. moniliformis
armored heart
Arneth's
    classification
    count
    formula
    index
    stages
Arnold-Chiari malformation
Arnold's bodies
aromatase

aromatic
    a. acid
    a. amine
    a. compound
    a. hydrocarbon
    a. ring
aromatization
arousal threshold
arrangement
    Ig gene a.
arrector (pl., arrectores)
    a. pili muscle
arrest
    cardiac a.
    deep transverse a.
    developmental a.
    epiphyseal a.
    hematopoietic maturation a.
    maturation a.
    mitotic a.
    sinus a.
    spermatogenic a.
    spermatogenic matura-
       tion a.
arrhenoblastoma
arrhinencephaly
arrhythmia
    cardiac a.
ARS — AIDS-related syndrome
    antirabies serum
arsanilic acid
arsenate
Arsenazo III dye
arsenic
    butter of a.
    a. keratosis
    a. neuropathy
    a. pigmentation
    a. poisoning
    a. polyneuropathy
    a. stain
    a. trioxide
    a. trisulfide
arsenical
    a. neuropathy
    a. polyneuropathy
arsenite
arsine gas
arsphenamine
arsthinol
ART — absolute retention time
    automated reagin test

artefact
Artemisia
    A. *absinthium*
    A. *maritima*
arteria comitans
arterial
    a. anastomosis
    a. aneurysm
    a. blood
    a. blood collection
    a. blood gases
    a. blood pressure
    a. capillaries
    a. cone
    a. embolism
    a. hemangioma
    a. hypertension
    a. hypoxemia
    a. line culture
    a. nephrosclerosis
    a. occlusive disease
    a. PCO_2 (carbon dioxide partial
       pressure)
    a. PO_2 (oxygen partial
       pressure)
    a. pressure
    a. puncture technique
    a. sclerosis
    a. spider
    a. thrombosis
    a. thrombus
    a. venous oxygen difference
arteriocapillary sclerosis
arteriogram
arteriography
arteriola (pl., arteriolae)
arteriolar
    a. nephrosclerosis
    a. sclerosis
    a. thrombonecrosis
arteriole
    afferent a.
    efferent a.
arteriolith
arteriolitis
    hyperplastic a.
    necrotizing a.
arteriolonecrosis
arteriolonephrosclerosis
arteriolosclerosis
    hyaline a.
arteriolosclerotic

arteriomalacia
arteriomyomatosis
arterionephrosclerosis
arteriopathy
    hypertensive a.
    plexogenic pulmonary a.
arterioplania
arteriosclerosis
    hyperplastic a.
    hypertensive a.
    intimal a.
    medial a.
    Mönckeberg's a.
    nodular a.
    a. obliterans
    peripheral a.
    senile a.
arteriosclerotic
    a. aneurysm
    a. aortic aneurysm
    a. cardiovascular disease
    a. gangrene
    a. heart disease
    a. retinopathy
    a. thrombosed aneurysm
arteriostenosis
arteriosus
    persistent truncus a.
arteriotomy
arteriovenous
    a. aneurysm
    a. angioma
    a. carbon dioxide difference
    a. communication
    a. fistula
    a. hemangioma
    a. malformation
    a. oxygen difference
arteritis (pl., arteritides)
    aortic arch a.
    coronary a.
    cranial a.
    giant cell a.
    a. nodosa
    a. obliterans; obliterating a.
    rheumatic a.
    rheumatoid a.
    syphilitic a.
    Takayasu's a.
    temporal a.
artery (pl., arteries)
    anterolateral striate a.

anteromedial perforating a.
carotid a.
Cohnheim's a.
elastic a.
end a.
ethmoid a.
gastric a.
gastroepiploic a.
hepatic a.
Huebner's recurrent a.
ileal a.
ileocolic a.
innominate a.
jejunal a.
lacrimal a.
lenticulostriate a.
maxillary a.
mesenteric a.
Mueller's a.
muscular a.
obturator a.
occipital a.
omphalomesenteric a.
ovarian a.
parietal a.
penile a.
perforating anterolateral a.
pipestem a.
pericardial a.
pre-rolandic a.
pulmonary a.
renal a.
sphenopalatine a.
splenic a.
striate a.
ulnar a.
umbilical a.
urethral a.
uterine a.
Zinn's a.
arthragra
arthralgia
    rheumatic a.
    a. saturnina
arthritic calculus
arthritis (pl., arthritides)
    atrophic a.
    calcium crystal deposition a.
    chronic absorptive a.
    chronic proliferative a.
    chronic villous a.
    chylous a.

a. deformans
degenerative a.
a.-dermatitis syndrome
exudative a.
filarial a.
gonococcal a.
gouty a.
hemophilic a.
hypertrophic a.
Jaccoud's a.
juvenile rheumatoid a.
migratory a.
a. mutilans
mycotic a.
navicular a.
neuropathic a.
a. nodosa
ochronotic a.
proliferative a.
psoriatic a.
rheumatoid a.
septic a.
suppurative a.
tuberculous a.
a. uratica
vertebral a.
arthrocele
arthrocentesis
arthrochalasis multiplex congenita
arthrochondritis
arthroconidia
Arthroderma
arthrodesis
    Moberg's a.
arthrogram
Arthrographis langeroni
arthrography
arthrogryposis
arthrokatadysis
arthrolith
arthrolithiasis
arthro-onychodysplasia
arthro-ophthalmopathy
    hereditary progressive a.
arthropathy
    Charcot's a.
    chondrocalcific a.
    hydroxyapatite a.
    Jaccoud's a.
    neurogenic a.
    neuropathic a.
    osteopulmonary a.

reactive a.
    tabetic a.
arthrophyma
arthroplasty
Arthropoda
arthropod-borne viral disease
arthropod-borne virus encephalitis
arthroscintigraphy
arthroscope
arthroscopy
arthrosis
arthrospore
arthrosynovitis
arthrotomy
arthrotropic
Arthus reaction
articular
    a. calculus
    a. capsule
    a. cartilage
    a. chondrocalcinosis
    a. disc
    a. gout
    a. rheumatism
articularis
    a. cubiti muscle
    a. genus muscle
articulated
articulation
artifact
    electrical a.
    fixation a.
    movement a.
    shock a.
artificial
    a. abortion
    a. dialysis
    a. kidney
    a. melanin
    a. respiration
Artyfechinostomum
ARV — AIDS-related virus
Arvin
aryepiglottic fold
arylamine acetyltransferase
arylaminopeptidase
arylesterase
aryl-ester hydrolase
arylformamidase
aryl 4-hydroxylase
arylsulfatase-A test
aryl-sulfotransferase

arytenoid
>   a. cartilage
>   a. gland
arytenoiditis
AS — acetylstrophanthidin
>   alveolar sac
>   androsterone sulfate
>   antistreptolysin
>   aortic stenosis
>   arteriosclerosis
>   astigmatism
>   atherosclerosis
As — arsenic
ASA — acetylsalicylic acid
>   Adams-Stokes attack
>   argininosuccinic acid
>   arylsulfatase-A
ASB — American Society of Bacteriologists
asbestoid
asbestos
>   amphibole a.
>   a. body
>   chrysotile a.
>   a. transformation
asbestosis
ascariasis serological test
ascaricidal
ascaricide
ascarid
ascarides
Ascaridoidea
Ascaris
>   A. *alata*
>   A. *canis*
>   A. *lumbricoides*
>   A. *mystax*
>   A. *pneumonitis*
>   A. *suis*
>   A. *suum*
Ascarops
ascending
>   a. aorta
>   a. cervical artery
>   a. cholangitis
>   a. chromatography
>   a. colon
>   a. degeneration
>   a. limb, Henle's loop
>   a. pharyngeal artery
>   a. pyelonephritis

ascertainment
>   complete a.
>   incomplete a.
>   multiple a.
>   single a.
>   truncate a.
Aschheim-Zondek
>   hormone
>   test
Aschoff's
>   body
>   cell
>   nodule
Aschoff-Rokitansky sinus
Aschoff-Tawara node
ASCI — American Society for Clinical Investigation
ascites
>   a. adiposus
>   chyliform a.
>   chylous a.; a. chylosus
>   fatty a.
>   gelatinous a.
>   hemorrhagic a.
>   hydremic a.
>   milky a.
>   pseudochylous a.
Ascit. Fl. — ascitic fluid
ascitic
>   a. agar
>   a. fluid
ascitogenous
ASCLT — American Society of Clinical Laboratory Technicians
ASCO — American Society of Clinical Oncology
Ascobolaceae
ascocarp
ascomycete
Ascomycetes
Ascomycotina
ascorbate cyanide test
ascorbemia
ascorbic
>   a. acid
>   a. acid test
>   a. reductase
ascospore-forming fungus
ascotrophosome
ASCP — American Society of Clinical Pathologists

ascus (pl., asci)
ASCVD — arteriosclerotic cardiovascular disease
　　　　atherosclerotic cardiovascular disease
ASD — aldosterone secretion defect
　　　atrial septal defect
Aselli's pancreas
asemia
ASEP — American Society for Experimental Pathology
asepsis
aseptic
　　　a. meningitis
　　　a. necrosis
asexual reproduction
ASF — aniline, sulfur, formaldehyde
ASH — American Society of Hematology
　　　asymmetrical septal hypertrophy
AsH — hypermetropic astigmatism
ASHA — American Speech and Hearing Association
Ashby's differential agglutination method
ASHD — arteriosclerotic heart disease
asialia
asialoglycoprotein
Asiatic cholera
asiderosis
asiderotic anemia
ASIS — anterior superior iliac spine
ASK — antistreptokinase
Askanazy's cell
Ask-Upmark kidney
Askin's tumor
ASL — antistreptolysin
ASLO — antistreptolysin-O
ASM — American Society for Microbiology
AsM — myopic astigmatism
ASMI – anteroseptal myocardial infarct
ASMT — American Society for Medical Technology
ASN — alkali-soluble nitrogen
Asn — asparagine
ASO — antistreptolysin-O
　　　arteriosclerosis obliterans
　　　allele-specific oligonucleotide

ASO probes
ASO titer — antistreptolysin-O titer
ASP — American Society of Parasitologists
　　　American Society of Pathologists
　　　area systolic pressure
Asp — aspartic acid
asparagic acid
asparaginase
asparagine
asparagine-ketoacid aminotransferase
asparaginic acid
asparaginyl
aspartate
　　　a. amino transaminase
　　　a. aminotransferase
　　　a. aminotransferase assay
　　　a. carbamoyltransferase
　　　a. kinase
　　　a. transaminase
D-aspartate oxidase
aspartic acid
aspartokinase
aspartyl
aspartylacetylglucosaminidase
aspartylglucosamine
aspartylglucoasminuria
aspect
　　　dorsal a.
　　　ventral a.
aspergillin
　　　otomycosis a.
aspergilloma
aspergillosis
　　　allergic bronchopulmonary a.
　　　colonizing a.
　　　invasive a.
Aspergillus
　　　A. *amsteloidami*
　　　A. *auricularis*
　　　A. *barbae*
　　　A. *bouffardi*
　　　A. *candidus*
　　　A. *carneus*
　　　A. *clavatus*
　　　A. *concentricus*
　　　A. *fisherii*
　　　A. *flaux*
　　　A. *flavus*
　　　A. *fumigatus*
　　　A. *giganteus*

A. *glaucus*
A. gliocladium
A. mucoroides
A. nidulans
A. niger
A. niveus
A. ochraceus
A. oryzae
A. parasiticus
A. pictor
A. repens
A. restrictus
A. sulphureus
A. sydowi
A. terreus
A. versicolor
Aspergillus antibody tests
Aspergillus serology
aspermatism
aspermatogenesis
    induced a.
aspermia
aspheric
asphyxia
asphyxial
asphyxiant
    chemical a.
asphyxiating
    a. thoracic chondrodystrophy
    a. thoracic dysplasia
    a. thoracic dystrophy
asphyxiation
aspidium oleoresin
aspirate
    bronchotracheal a.
aspiration
    a. biopsy
    a. biopsy cytology
    bone marrow a.
    a. cytology
    foreign body a.
    gastric a.
    meconium a.
    a. pneumonia
    a. pneumonitis
    suprapubic needle a.
    tracheal a.
    transcutaneous needle a.
    transthoracic a.
    transtracheal a.
    uterine a.
    vacuum a.

aspirator
    Cavitron ultrasonic surgical a.
    water a.
aspirin
    a. tolerance test
    a. toxicity
asplenia
asplenic
asporogenic
asporous
ASR — aldosterone secretion rate
    aldosterone secretory rate
ASS — anterior superior spine
assassin bug
assay
    acetaminophen a.
    acetylcholinesterase a.
    acid phosphatase a.
    adenosine deaminase a.
    adrenocorticotropic hormone a.
    alanine aminotransferase a.
    albumin a.
    alpha$_1$-antitrypsin a.
    alpha$_1$-fetoprotein a.
    Ames a.
    amino acid a.
    amitriptyline and nortriptyline a.
    anti-DNA antibody a.
    anti-DNase B a.
    antigenic a.
    antihyaluronidase a.
    antimitochondrial antibody a.
    antiparietal cell antibody a.
    argininosuccinate lyase a.
    aspartate aminotransferase a.
    bacterial killing a.
    Beckman a.
    benzene a.
    benzodiazepine a.
    bilirubin a.
    biologic a.
    biological a.; bioassay
    biotin a.
    blastogenesis a.
    Boyden chamber a.
    butanol extractable iodine a.
    calcium a.
    calcium ionized a.

camphor a.
carbamazepine a.
carbon dioxide concentration a.
carbon disulfide a.
carbon tetrachloride a.
catecholamine a.
cell-mediated lympholysis a.
cerebrospinal fluid a.
ceruloplasmin a.
chemiluminescence a.
chemotaxis a.
chlordiazepoxide a.
chlorohydrocarbon a.
chlorpromazine a.
cholinesterase a.
chorionic gonadotropin a.
citric acid a.
clonogenic a.
coagulation factor a.
competitive protein-binding a.
complement a.
complement-binding a.
compressed spectral a.
coproporphyrin a.
CPB (competitive protein-binding) a.
C-reactive protein a.
CSA (compressed spectral) a.
cytochrome b_5 reductase a.
DDT a.
depramine a.
diquat a.
disulfiram a.
doxepin hydrochloride a.
drug-screening a.
E (erythrocyte) rosette a.
EAC (erythrocyte, antibody, and complement rosette) a.
endorphin a.
enzyme a.
enzyme-linked immunosorbent a.
epinephrine and norepinephrine a.
Epstein-Barr virus antibody a.
ethchlorvynol a.
ethosuximide a.
Falcon a.
fatty a.
fluoroacetate a.
fluorocarbon a.

follicle-stimulating hormone a.
glucosephosphate isomerase a.
glucosylceramidase a.
glutathione reductase a.
glutethimide a.
Guthrie bacterial inhibition a.
halogenated hydrocarbon a.
haloperidol a.
halothane a.
haptoglobin a.
hemagglutination inhibition a.
hemoglobin a.
hemolytic plaque a.
hexachlorophene a.
Histoplasma antibody a.
17-hydroxycorticosteroid a.
5-hydroxyindoleacetic acid a.
human tumor clonogenic a.
hydroxyproline a.
iditol dehydrogenase a.
imipramine a.
immune a.
immune adherence hemagglutination a.
immunochemical a.
immunoconcentration a.
immunoenzymometric a.
immunofluorescence a.
immunofluorescent a.
immunometric a.
immunoradiometric a.
isocitrate dehydrogenase a.
isoniazid a.
isopropanol a.
Jaffe's a.
Jerne plaque a.
17-ketogenic steroid a.
17-ketosteroid a.
lactate dehydrogenase a.
leukotactic a.
lidocaine a.
lipoprotein a.
Lowry a.
luteinizing hormone a.
lymphocyte microcytotoxicity a.
lymphocytotoxic a.
lysergic acid diethylamide a.
lysozyme a.
macroglobulin a.
metanephrine a.
methanol a.

methaqualone a.
methemalbumin a.
p-methoxyamphetamine a.
3,4-methylenedioxyam-
    phetamine a.
methylphenidate a.
metronidazole a.
microbiological a.
microcytotoxicity a.
microhemagglutination a.
microlymphocytotoxicity a.
mucoprotein a.
nephelometric inhibi-
    tion a.
opiate a.
organothiophosphate a.
ornithine carbamoyltrans-
    ferase a.
oxalic a.
pantothenic acid a.
paraquat a.
pepsinogen a.
phencyclidine a.
phenobarbital a.
phenothiazine a.
phenylalanine a.
phenylbutazone a.
phenytoin a.
6-phosphogluconate dehydroge-
    nase a.
phospholipid a.
phosphorus a.
plaque-forming cell a.
polychlorinated biphenyl a.
polyethylene glycol precipita-
    tion a.
porphobilinogen a.
pregnanediol a.
primidone a.
procainamide a.
properdin (factor P) a.
propoxyphene a.
propranolol a.
protein-bound iodine a.
protoporphyrin a.
protriptyline a.
pyrimethamine a.
pyruvate kinase a.
quinidine a.
quinine a.
radial partition immunofluoro-
    metric a.

radioenzymatic a.
radioimmunoprecipitation a.
radioligand a.
radioreceptor a.
Raji cell a.
Raji cell radioimmune a.
renal venous renin a.
selenium a.
serotonin a.
staphylococcal protein A–
    binding a.
sulfonamide a.
sulfonylurea a.
superoxide a.
TBG (thyroxine-binding globu-
    lin) a.
tellurium a.
thallium a.
theophylline a.
thiamine a.
thiamphenicol a.
thioridazine a.
thyroxine a.
TPI (*Treponema pallidum* immo-
    bilization) a.
transferrin a.
transketolase a.
Treponema pallidum hemaggluti-
    nation a.
triiodothyronine a.
triosephosphate isomerase a.
tyrosine a.
urobilinogen a.
uromucoid a.
uropesinogen a.
uroporphyrin a.
vitamin A and carotene a.
volatile organic substances a.
warfarin a.
zinc a.
assembly
    Ig gene a.
assessment
    anthropometric a.
    immunocompetence a.
assimilation limit
Assmann's tuberculous infiltrate
association
    a. constant
    a. fibers
Association for the Advancement of
    Medical Instrumentation

Association of Clinical Scientists
Association for Practitioners in Infection Control
association constant
associative reaction
assortative mating
     negative a.m.
     positive a.m.
assortment
     independent a.
AST — aspartate aminotransferase
Ast — astigmatism
astasia-abasia
astatine
asteatosis
aster
asterixis
Asterococcus
asteroid body
Asth. — asthenopia
asthenia
     neurocirculatory a.
asthenopia
     neurasthenic a.
     retinal a.
     tarsal a.
asthma
     allergic a.
     alveolar a.
     atopic a.
     bronchial a
     cotton dust a.
     a. crystals
     emphysematous a.
     essential a.
     grinders' a.
     intrinsic a.
     Millar's a.
     millers' a.
     miners' a.
     nonreaginic a.
     potters' a.
     steam-fitters' a.
     stone-strippers' a.
asthmatic bronchitis
astigmatism
asthmaticus
     status a.
Astler-Coller rectal system
ASTO — antistreptolysin-O
astomatous

Astracyanine
Astrafer
astragaloid joint
astringent
astroblast
astroblastoma
astrocoele
astrocyte
     fibrillar a.
     fibrillary a.
     fibrous a.
     gemistocytic a.
     pilocytic a.
     plasmatofibrous a.
     protoplasmic a.
     a. staining
astrocytic glioma
astrocytoma
     anaplastic a.
     cerebellar a.
     fibrillary a.
     fibrous a.
     gemistocytic a.
     hypothalamic a.
     malignant a.
     pigmented pilocytic a.
     pilocytic a.
     piloid a.
     a. protoplasmaticum
     protoplasmic a.
astrocytosis
astroglia
astrokinetic
astrosphere
astrovirus
Astwood's test
ASV — anodic stripping voltammetry
     antisnake venom
asymbolia
asymmetric
     a. carbon atom
     a. septal hypertrophy
asymmetrical
     a. chondrodystrophy
     a. karyokinesis
     a. septal hypertrophy
asymmetry
asymptomatic
     a. bacteriuria
     a. coccidioidomycosis
     a. proteinuria
asymptote

asynapsis
asynchronism
asynchrony
     nuclear-cytoplasmic a.
asynechia
asynergia
asystematic
asystole
AT — antitrypsin
AT-III — antithrombin III
AT_{10} — dihydrotachysterol
At — astatine
ATA — anti-*Toxoplasma* antibodies
     atmosphere absolute
     aurintricarboxylic acid
Atabrine
ataxia
     acute bronchial cerebellar a.
     acute cerebellar a.
     familial cerebellar a.
     Friedreich's a.
     hereditary cerebellar a.
     hereditary spinal a.
     a.-pancytopenia syndrome
     a.-telangiectasia
ataxic
ATCC — American Type Culture
          Collection
ATD — asphyxiating thoracic dys-
          trophy
ATE — adipose tissue extract
ATEE — acetyltyrosine ethyl ester
atelectasis
     absorption a.
     compression a.
     contraction a.
     a. neonatorum
     obstructive a.
     primary a.
     round a.
     secondary a.
atelia
ateliosis
ateliotic
Atelosaccharomyces
ATG — antithymocyte globulin
          antithyroglobulin
A_2 thalassemia
atheroembolism
atherogenesis
atherogenic
atherogenicity

atheroma
atheromatosis
atheromatous
     a. degeneration
     a. embolism
     a. embolus
     a. plaque
atherosclerosis
     aortic a.
atherosclerotic
     a. aneurysm
     a. cardiovascular disease
     a. heart disease
     a. vascular disease
atherosis
atherothrombosis
atherothrombotic
athetoid movement
athetosis
athetotic gait
athlete's foot
athletic heart
atherectomy
athrepsia
athreptic immunity
athrombia
AT III — antithrombin III
ATL — adult T-cell leukemia
          adult T-cell lymphoma
          antitension line
atlas
ATLL — adult T-cell leukemia-
          lymphoma
atmosphere absolute
atmospheric
     a. monitoring
     a. pressure changes
ATN — acute tubular necrosis
at. no. — atomic number
atocia
atom
     asymmetric carbon a.
atomic
     a. absorption
     a. absorption spectropho-
          tometry
     a. mass
     a. mass unit
     a. number
     a. spectrum
     a. weight
     a. weight unit

atomization
atonic ureter
atony
atopen
atopic
>a. allergen
>a. allergy
>a. asthma
>a. dermatitis
>a. keratoconjunctivitis

atopy
ATP — adenosine triphosphate
ATPase — adenosinetriphosphatase
ATPase
>calcium-activated A.
>magnesium-activated A.
>A. stain

ATP-creatine-*N*-phosphotransferase
ATP pyrophosphohydrolase
ATPS — ambient temperature and
>>pressure, saturated
atransferrinemia
Atrax robustus
atresia
>anal a.
>aortic a.
>biliary a.
>choanal a.
>congenital a.
>duodenal a.
>epididymal a.
>esophageal a.
>extrahepatic biliary a.
>follicular a.
>intestinal a.
>mitral a.
>prepyloric a.
>pulmonary a.
>tricuspid a.
>ureteral a.
>vaginal a.
>valvular a.

atresic
atretic follicle
atretocystia
atretogastria
atr. fib. — atrial fibrillation
atrial
>a. anomalous bands
>a. appendage
>a. arrhythmia
>a. fibrillation

>a. flutter
>a. gallop
>a. infarction
>a. myxoma
>a. natriuretic peptide
>a. premature beat
>a. premature contraction
>a. premature depolarization
>a. septal defect
>a. septum

atrichous
atriodigital dysplasia
atriomegaly
atrioventricular
>a. block
>a. bundle
>a. canal cushion
>a. node
>a. synchrony
>a. valve

atrium (pl., atria)
>accessory a.

Atropa
atrophedema
atrophia
>acne a.

atrophia maculosa varioliformis cutis
atrophic
>a. arthritis
>a. candidiasis
>a. chronic gastritis
>a. endometrium
>a. fenestration
>a. gastritis
>a. glossitis
>a. inflammation
>a. lichen planus
>a. pharyngitis
>a. rhinitis
>a. thrombosis
>a. vulvitis

atrophicans
>acrodermatitis chronica a.

atrophied
atrophoderma
>a. albidum
>a. maculatum
>a. neuriticum
>a. pigmentosum
>a. reticulatum

atrophy
>acquired a.

acute yellow a.
adrenal a.
brown a.
cellular a.
Charcot-Marie-Tooth muscular a.
circumscribed a.
compensatory a.
cyanotic a.
cystic a.
denervation a.
disuse a.
essential a.
exhaustion a.
fatty a.
focal a.
gelatinous a.
granular a.
group a.
hypertropic polyneuritic-type muscular a.
infantile muscular a.
ischemic muscular a.
Kienböck's a.
knife blade a.
Leber's optic a.
lobar cerebral a.
macular a.
marantic a.
mucinous a.
muscular a.
myelopathic muscular a.
neuritic a.
neurogenic muscular a.
neurotropic a.
olivocerebellar a.
olivopontocerebellar a.
optic a.
peroneal muscular a.
polyneuritic-type hypertrophic muscular a.
postmenopausal a.
pressure a.
progressive muscular a.
progressive spinal muscular a.
red a.
senile cystic endometrial a.
serous a.
simple a.
subtotal villose a.
Sudeck's a.

testicular a.
traction a.
traumatic a.
yellow a.
atropine suppression test
ATS — antitetanic serum
antithymocyte serum
arteriosclerosis
attachment
a. plaque
spindle a.
attack
Adam-Stokes a.
micturition a.
a. rate
transient ischemic a.
attapulgite
attenuated
a. culture
a. tuberculosis
a. virus
attenuation
attenuator
attraction sphere
attribute
at. vol. — atomic volume
at. wt. — atomic weight
atypia
cellular a.
glandular a.
koilocytotic a.
urothelial a.
atypical
a. adenoma
a. fibrous histiocytoma
a. fibroxanthoma
a. hyperplasia
a. insulin
a. lipoma
a. lymphocytes
a. melanocytic hyperplasia
a. mycobacterium
a. pneumonia
a. primary pneumonia
a. regeneration
a. repetitive spike-and-slow waves
a. tuberculosis
a. verrucous endocarditis
atypism
AU — Angström unit
antitoxin unit

arbitrary units
azauridine
Au — Australia antigen
    gold
Au Ag — Australia antigen
Auberger blood group system
Auchencloss-Madden mastectomy
Auchmeromyia luteola
audioanalysis
auditory
    a. artery
    a. canal
    a. evoked potential
    a. meatus
    a. nerve
    a. ossicle
    a. pathway
    a. projection
    a. radiation
    a. stimulation
    a. tube
    a. vein
    a. vesicle
Auer's
    bodies
    rods
Auerbach's plexus
Auger
    effect
    electron
augmentation
augmented
    a. histamine test
    a. secretin test
AUL — acute undifferentiated leukemia
AUO — amyloid of unknown origin
aural polyp
auramine
    a. O fluorescent stain
    a.-rhodamine stain
aurantiasis
Aureobasidium pullulans
aur. fib. — auricular fibrillation
auricle
    cervical a.
    left a. of heart
    right a. of heart
auricular
    a. appendage
    a. artery, posterior
    a. branch, tenth cranial nerve

    a. branch, vagus nerve
    a. cartilage
    a. chondritis
    a. docimasia
    a. fibrillation
    a. line
    a. lymph node, anterior
    a. lymph node, posterior
    a. nerve, greater
    a. point
    a. region
    a. tachycardia, paroxysmal
auricularis
auriculotemporal
aurintricarboxylic acid
aurochromoderma
Aurococcus
aurotherapy
aurothioglucose
auscultatory
    a. gap
    a. precussion
Auspitz sign
Austin Flint murmur
Austin and Van Slyke's method
Australia antigen
Australian
    X disease
    X encephalitis virus
Australorbis glabratus
autacoid
autoadsorption
autoagglutination
    enzyme a. factor
autoagglutinin
    cold a.
autoallergic hemolytic anemia
autoallergy
autoanalyzer
    sequential multichannel a.
autoantibody
    anti-3d a.
    anti-H a's
    anti-I a's
    anti-i a's
    anti-P a's
    anti-Pr a-s
    anti-Sp a's
    antineutrophil cytoplasmic a.
    antiplatelet a's
    cold a's

hemagglutinating cold a.
platelet a's
thymocytotoxic a.
warm a.
autoanticomplement
autoantigen
autoantitoxin
autoassay
Autobac system
autobiotic
autoblast
autobody
autocatalysis
autochthonous
autoclasis; autoclasia
autoclave
autocoid
autocorrelation function
autocrine
    a. hypothesis
    a. growth factor
    a. motility factor
autocytometer
    Fisher a.
autocytotoxin
autoerythrophagocytosis
autofluorescence
autofluoroscope
autogeneic
autogenic graft
autogenous vaccine
autograft
autohemagglutination
autohemagglutinin
autohemolysin
autohemolysis test
autohemotherapy
autoimmune
    a. adrenalitis
    a. chronic hepatitis
    a. disease
    a. encephalomyelitis
    a. gastritis
    a. glomerulonephritis
    a. hemolytic anemia
    a. hepatitis
    a. hyperthyroidism
    a. hypophysitis
    a. leukopenia
    a. myositis
    a. orchitis
    a. pancytopenia

    a. panhypopituitarism
    a. panleukopenia
    a. reaction
    a. response
    a. sialadenitis
    a. thrombocytopenia
    a. thrombocytopenic purpura
    a. thyroiditis
    a. thyrotoxicosis
autoimmunity
autoimmunocytopenia
autoinfection
autoinoculable
autoinoculation
autoisolysin
autokinesis
autoleukoagglutinin
autologous
    a. antigen
    a. blood
    a. bone marrow transplant
    a. graft
    a. hemagglutinin
    a. lymphoma
autologous transfusion
    predeposit a.t.
autolysis
autolysosome
autolytic enzyme
automated
    a. activated partial thrombo-
      plastin
    a. bacteriology
    a. cell image leukocyte counter
    a. differential leukocyte
      counter
    a. immunoassay
    a. immunoprecipitation
    a. motility factors
    a. multiphasic screening
    a. reagin test
    a. slide staining
automatic
    a. cell
    a. tissue processing
automaticity
    junctional a.
automation
    blood cell count a.
    clinical chemistry a.
    differential leukocyte count a.

microbiology a.
radioimmunoassay a.
Automeris io
AutoMicrobic system
automutagen
autonomic
    a nervous system
    a. neuropathy
    a. plexus
auto-oxidation
auto-oxidizable
autoparenchymatous metaplasia
autophagic vacuole
autophagocytosis
autophagosome
autophagy
autoplast
autoplex
autoploidy
autoprothrombin
    a. I
    a. II
    a. IIA
    a. III
    a. C
autopsy
autoradiograph
autoradiography
    contact a.
    dip-coating a.
    film stripping a.
    thick-layer a.
    two-emulsion a.
autoradiolysis
autoreactive lymphocyte
autoregulation
Auto SCAN system
autosensitization
autosomal
    a. dominant disorders
    a. dominant inheritance
    a. dominant polycystic kidney
    a. gene
    a. heredity
    a. recessive disorders
    a. recessive inheritance
    a. recessive polycystic kidney
autosome translocation
autosplenectomy
autothromboagglutinin
autotomography
autotoxemia

autotoxicosis
autotransformer
    variable a.
autotransfusion
autotrepanation
autotroph
    facultative a.
    obligate a.
autotrophic
    a. bacterium
    a. fixation
autovaccination
auxanography
auxesis
auxochrome
auxocyte
auxospore
auxotroph
auxotrophic mutation
AV — alveolar duct
AV or A-V — arteriovenous
    atrioventricular
A-V
    A-V aneurysm
    A-V block
Av. — average
    avoirdupois
AV/AF — anteverted/anteflexed
avalanche ionization
Avantage system
avascular necrosis
AVCS — atrioventricular conduction
    system
average
    a. deviation
    a. gradient
    a. life
    Walsh's a.
    weighted a.
AVF — arteriovenous fistula
AVH — acute viral hepatitis
aviadenovirus
avian
    a. erythroblastosis virus
    a. myeloblastosis virus
    a. myelocytomatosis virus
    a. sarcoma
    a. tubercle bacillus
Avicenna's gland
avidin
    a.-antigen conjugate
    a.-biotin system

avidity testing
Avipoxvirus
avirulence
avirulent
avitaminosis
AVM — arteriovenous malformation
AVN — atrioventricular node
Avogadro's number
avoirdupois
AVP — arginine vasopressin
AVR — aortic valve replacement
AVRP — atrioventricular refractory
               period
A-V shunt — arteriovenous shunt
avulsed wound
avulsion
AW — anterior wall
AWI — anterior wall infarction
AWMI — anterior wall myocardial in-
               farction
awu — atomic weight unit
axenic
axial aneurysm
axidothymidine
axilla (pl., axillae)
axillary
       a. artery
       a. fascia
       a. glands
       a. line
       a. lymph node
       a. nerve
       a. projection
       a. region
       a. vein
axiolateral
axis (pl., axes)
       cell a.
       celiac a.
       a. cylinder
       esophageal a.
       a. oculi
       pituitary hypothalamic a.
       renal-adrenal a.
       renin-aldosterone a.
       renin-angiotensin a.
       a. of rotation
axoaxonic
axodendritic
axolemma
axon
       fusimotor a.

a. hillock
myelinated a.
a. staining method
unmyelinated a.
axonal
       a. degeneration
       a. demyelination
       a. reaction
       a. spheroid
axoneme
axonopathy
axonotmesis
axoplasm
axoplasmic flow
axtreonam
Ayoub-Shklar method
Az — azote (French for nitrogen)
azacyclonol hydrochloride
azacytidine
azaguanine
azamethonium bromide
azan stain
azanator maleate
azanidazole
azapetine phosphate
azarabine
azaserine
azatadine maleate
azathioprine
6-azauracil
6-azauridine
azeotrope
azeotropic solution
azeotropy
azg. — azaguanine
azide
3'-azido-3'deoxythymidine
azidothymidine
azine dye
azinphosmethyl
aziridine
aziridinyl
azlocillin
azlocillinylbenzoquinone
azo — a prefix indicating presence of
        the group —N:N—
       a. coupling reaction
       a. dye
azobenzene reductase
azobilirubin
azocarmine B; azocarmine G
       a. dyes

azoic dye
azolitmin paper
azoospermia
azophloxin
azoprotein
azote
azotemia
    chloropenic a.
    extrarenal a.
    hypochloremic a.
    nonrenal a.
    postrenal a.
    prerenal a.
    renal a.
azotemic
Azotobacter
azotomycin
azotorrhea

azoturia
azovan blue
AZT — Aschheim-Zondek
    test
    azidothymidine
azul
AZUR — azauridine
azure A/B/C stains
azure-eosin stain
azuresin
azurophil; azurophile
azurophilic granule
azygoesophageal
azygos
    a. lobe
    a. vein
azygous
azymia

B

B — bacillus
    Baume's scale
    Benoist's scale
    bicuspid
    boron
    buccal
    whole blood
B. — *Brucella*
BA — bacterial agglutination
    betamethasone acetate
    blocking antibody
    bovine albumin
    brachial artery
    bronchial asthma
    buccoaxial
Ba — barium
Babcock tube
Babes-Ernst granules
Babesia microti
babesiasis
babesiosis serological test
Babes's
    node
    nodule
Babinski's
    reflex
    sign

baby
    blue b.
    collodion b.
BAC — blood alcohol concentration
    buccoaxiocervical
bacampicillin hydrochloride
Bachman-Pettit test
Bachman test
Bacillaceae
bacillary
    b. dysentery
    b. embolism
    b. emulsion (tuberculin)
    b. hemoglobinuria
bacille Calmette-Guerin
bacille Calmette-Guerin vaccine
bacillemia
bacilliform
bacilluria
Bacillus
    B. *acidi lactici*
    B. *aerogenes capsulatus*
    B. *aertrycke*
    B. *alvei*
    B. *ambiguus*
    B. *anthracis*
    B. *botulinus*

B. brevis
B. bronchisepticus
B. cereus
B. circulans
B. coli
B. diphtheriae
B. dysenteriae
B. enteritidis
B. faecalis alcaligenes
B. influenzae
B. larvae
B. leprae
B. licheniformis
B. mallei
B. megaterium
B. necrophorus
B. oedematiens
B. oedematis maligni
B. pertussis
B. pestis
B. pneumoniae
B. polymyxa
B. proteus
B. pseudomallei
B. pumilus
B. pyocyaneus
B. sphaericus
B. stearothermophilus
B. subtilis
B. suipestifer
B. tetani
B. tuberculosis
B. tularense
B. typhi
B. typhosus
B. welchii
B. whitmori

bacillus (pl., bacilli)
　b. abortivus equinus
　acid-fast bacilli
　aerobic spore-forming bacilli
　anthrax b.
　avian tubercle b.
　Bang's b.
　Battey b.
　Boas-Oppler b.
　Bordet-Gengou b.
　bovine tubercle b.
　Calmette-Guérin b.
　coliform b.
　colon b.
　diphtheria b.

diphtheroid bacilli
Döderlein's b.
Ducrey's b.
dysentery bacilli
enteric b.
Escherich's b.
Fick's b.
Flexner's b.
Flexner-Strong b.
Friedländer's b.
Frisch b.
fusiform b.
Gärtner's b.
Ghon-Sachs b.
glanders b.
gram-negative bacilli
gram-positive bacilli
Hansen's b.
Hofmann's b.
human tubercle b.
Johne's b.
Klebs-Löffler b.
Klein's b.
Koch's b.
Koch-Weeks b.
leprosy b.
Morax-Axenfeld b.
Morgan's b.
Newcastle-Manchester b.
Nocard's b.
paracolon bacilli
Pfeiffer's b.
plague b.
Preisz-Nocard b.
pseudotuberculosis b.
rhinoscleroma b.
Schmitz's b.
Schmorl's b.
Shiga's b.
smegma b.
Sonne-Duval b.
spore-forming bacilli
Strong's b.
swine rotlauf b.
tap water b.
tetanus b.
timothy b.
tubercle b.
typhoid b.
vole b.
Weeks' bacillus
Welch's b.
Whitemore's b.

bacillus Calmette-Guérin therapy
bacitracin
    b. differential disk test
    b. disk
    zinc b.
back
    b. fascia
    functional b.
    b. pressure
    saddle b.
    b. subcutaneous tissue
backalgia
backbone
backcross
backflow
background
    b. count
    flame b.
    b. interference
    b. radiation
    smear b.
backlash
backscatter peak
backward chaining
backwash ileitis
baclofen
bact. — bacterium
Bactec system
bacteremia
    bacteroides b.
    gonococcal b.
    gram-negative b.
    meningococcal b.
    myobacterial b.
    nosocomial b.
    pneumococcal b.
bacteria (see also bacterium)
    anaerobic b.
    gram-negative b.
    gram-positive b.
    higher b.
    indigenous b.
    intermediate coliform b.
    lactic acid b.
bacteria-free stage of bacterial endocar-
    ditis
bacterial
    b. adherence
    b. agar method
    b. agglutination
    b. aneurysm
    b. antagonism

    b. antigen
    b. antigen detection method
    b. aortitis
    b. capsule
    b. culture
    b. culturing
    b. cystitis
    b. dissociation
    b. encephalitis
    b. endaortitis
    b. endarteritis
    b. endocarditis
    b. enterocolitis
    b. enzymes
    b. epiglottiditis
    b. exotoxins
    b. filter
    b. genetics
    b. hemolysin
    b. infection
    b. killing assay
    b. lawn
    b. meningitis
    b. nephritis
    b. opsonin
    b. overgrowth syndrome
    b. pathogenicity
    b. pericarditis
    b. peritonitis
    b. pneumonia
    b. prostatitis
    b. serology
    b. shock
    b. sialedinitis
    b. spore
    b. staining
    b. susceptibility testing
    b. tracheobronchitis
    b. transformation
    b. transfusion reaction
    b. urinary cast
    vegetation
    b. virus
    Week's b.
bactericholia
bactericidal
    b. antibiotic
    b. concentration
bactericide
bactericidin
bacterid
    pustular b.

bacteriemia
bacterin
bacterioagglutinin
bacteriocin
bacteriocinogen
bacterioclasis
bacteriogenic agglutination
bacterioid
bacteriologic
bacteriological index
bacteriologist
bacteriology
    automated b.
    clinical diagnostic b.
    sanitary b.
    systematic b.
bacteriolysin
bacteriolysis
bacteriolytic amboceptor
Bacterionema matruchotii
bacterio-opsonin
bacteriopexy
bacteriophage
    b. genetics
    Lambda b.
    b. typing
bacteriophytoma
bacterioplasmin
bacterioprecipitin
bacteriopsonic
bacteriopsonin
bacteriorhodopsin
bacteriostasis
bacteriostat
bacteriostatic
    b. agent
    b. antibiotic
bacteriotherapy
bacteriotoxemia
bacteriotoxic
bacteriotropic
bacteriotropin
Bacterium
    B. aerogenes
    B. aeruginosum
    B. anitratum
    B. cholerae suis
    B. cloacae
    B. coli
    B. dysenteriae
    B. mirabilis
    B. pestis bubonicae

    B. sonnei
    B. subgroup B
    B. tularense
    B. typhosum
bacterium (pl., bacteria)
    acid-fast b.
    aerobic b.
    anaerobic b.
    autotrophic b.
    beaded b.
    bifid b.
    chemoautotrophic b.
    chemoheterotrophic b.
    chromogenic b.
    denitrifying b.
    endogenous b.
    exogenous b.
    facultative b.
    gram-negative b.
    gram-positive b.
    hemophilic b.
    heterotrophic b.
    hydrogen b.
    lysogenic b.
    mesophilic b.
    nitrifying b.
    organotropic b.
    psychrophilic b.
    pyogenic b.
    rough b.
    smooth b.
    sulfur b.
    thermophilic b.
    toxigenic b.
    water b.
bacteriuria
    significant asymptomatic b.
bacteroid
Bacteroidaceae
Bacteroides
    B. corrodens
    B. fragilis
    B. funduliformis
    B. fusiformis
    B. gingivalis
    B. melaninogenicus
    B. ochraceus
    B. oralis
    B. pneumosintes
    B. praeacutus
    B. ruminicola
    B. serpens

B. *splanchnicus*
B. *thetaiotaomicron*
B. *ureolyticus*
B. *vulgatus*
Bacteroides septicemia
bacteruria
Bactocil
Bactometer
Bactrim
BAEE — benzoyl arginine ethyl ester
        benzylarginine ethyl ester
Baehr-Lohlein lesion
BAEP — brain stem auditory evoked
        potential
BAG — buccoaxiogingival
bagassosis
bag-box circuit
bag fiber
Baggenstoss change
BAIB — beta-aminoisobutyric acid
Bainbridge reflex
Bakamjian deltopectoral flap
Baker counter
Baker's
    acid hematein
    acid hematein test
    antifol
    cyst
    formol calcium
    pyridine extraction
    pyridine extraction test
    Sudan black method
BAL (British antilewisite) dimercaprol
Balamuth's
    buffer solution
    culture medium
balance
    acid-base b.
    analytical b.
    calcium b.
    enzyme b.
    fluid b.
    genic b.
    keratotic b.
    microchemical b.
    nitrogen b.
    semimicro b.
    b. translocation
balanced
    b. polymorphism
    b. salt solution

balanitis
    b. circinata
    b. circumscripta plasmacellu-
        laris
    b. gangrenosa
    keratotic b.
    micaceous b.
    pseudoepitheliomatous b.
    b. xerotica obliterans
    Zoon's b.
balanoposthitis
balantidial
    b. colitis
    b. dysentery
balantidiasis
Balantidium coli
Balbiani's
    body
    chromosome
    nucleus
    ring
baldness
Balfour's gastroenterostomy
Balkan
    grippe
    nephropathy
ball
    chondrin b.
    fungus b.
    hair b.
    pleural fibrin b's
    b. thrombus
ballismus
ballistic movements
ballistocardiogram
ballistocardiography
balloon
    b. angioplasty
    b. catheter
    b. cell
    b. cell melanoma
    b. cell nevus
    b. dilator
    Shea-Anthony antral b.
    sinus b.
ballooning
    b. colliquation
    b. degeneration
ballottement
ball value
    b.v. obstruction
    b.v. thrombus

balsam
    Canada b.
    friars' b.
    Peruvian b.
    silver b.
    tolu b.
Balser's fatty necrosis
Bamberger's
    albuminuria
    sign
BAME — benzoylarginine methyl
        ester
Bancroft's
    filarial worm
    filariasis
Bancroftian filariasis
band
    A b.
    alpha$_1$ b.
    anomalous muscle b.
    Büngner's b's
    b. cell
    centromeric b's
    chromosome b's
    contraction b.
    b. form
    b.-form granulocyte
    H b.
    I b.
    b. keratopathy
    Ladd's b.
    M b.
    moderator b.
    monoclonal b.
    b. neutrophil
    Soret b.
    b. spectrum
    theta b.
banding
    BrDu (bromodeoxyuridine) b.
    C (centromeric) b.
    chromosome b.
    G (Giemsa) b.
    high-resolution b.
    N (nuclear stain) b.
    oligoclonal b.
    prometaphase b.
    Q (quinacrine) b.
    R (reverse) b.
    T (telomere) b.
Bandl's ring
bandpass filter

Bang's bacillus
B antigen
Banti's spleen
Bantu siderosis
BAO — basal acid output
BAP — blood agar plate
bar
    chromatoidal b.
    hyoid b.
    labial b.
    lingual b.
    median b.
    median b. of Mercier
    Passavant's b.
    sternal b.
    terminal b's
baragnosis
Barbados leg
barber's itch
barbital
barbiturate
    b. level
    b. spindle
Barcroft's apparatus
bare lymphocyte syndrome
Bargen's streptococcus
baritosis
barium
    b. enema
    b. esophagram
    b. fluosilicate
    b. sulfate
    b. test
barn
Barnett-Bourne acetic alcohol silver
    nitrate method
barometer
barometric pressure
barophilic
baroreceptor
baroreflex failure
barosinusitis
barotrauma
Barr
    bodies
    body analysis
    body test
barrel chest
barreling distortion
Barrett's
    epithelium
    esophagus

metaplasia
ulcer
barrier
blood-air b.
blood-brain b.
blood-cerebral fluid b.
blood-gas b.
blood-testis b.
blood-thymus b.
connective tissue b.
b. filter
filtration b.
gastric mucosal b.
hematoencephalic b.
histohematic connective tissue b.
b.- layer cell
testis b.
Barrnett-Seligman
dihydroxydinaphthyl disulfide method
indoxyl esterase method
Barroso-Moguel and Costero silver method
bartholinitis
Bartholin's
abscess
cyst
gland
Bartlett procedure
Bartonella bacilliformis
Bartonellaceae
bartonellosis
Bart's
hemoglobin; hemoglobin B.
vibrator
baruria
basal
b. acid output
b. body
Bruch's b. membrane
b. ganglia
b. granule
b. lamina
b. metabolic rate
b. metabolism
b. nuclei
b. plate
b. projection
b. region
b. squamous cell carcinoma
b. striations

b. tuberculosis
b. vein
basal cell
b.c. acanthoma
b.c. adenoma
b.c. ameloblastoma
b.c. carcinoma
b.c. dysplasia
b.c. epithelioma
b.c. hyperplasia
b.c. nevus
b.c. nevus syndrome
b.c. papilloma
basaloid carcinoma
basaloma
base
blood buffer b.
Brönsted-Lowry b.
buffer b.
complementary b's
conjugate
b. deficit
b. excess
b. ionization constant
KCN (potassium cyanide) broth b.
Lewis b.
b. pair
b. pairing
pressor b.
purine b's
pyrimidine b's
b. ratio
Schiff b.
baseline steady state
basement membrane capillaries
bas-fond
BASH — body acceleration given synchronously with the heartbeat
basic
b. dye
b. fuchsin
b. fuchsin–methylene blue stain
b. magenta
basicaryoplastin
basichromatin
basichromiole
basicytoplasm
Basidiobolaceae

Basidiobolus
　　B. haptosporus
　　B. ranarum
Basidiomycetes
Basidiomycotina
basidium (pl., basidia)
basilar
　　b. artery
　　b. membrane
　　b. region, pons
　　b. white matter
basilic vein
basiocciput
basiparaplastin
basipetal
basis (pl., bases)
　　b. cerebri
　　b. pedunculi
　　b. pulmonis
basisphenoid
basket
　　b. cell
　　fiber b's
Baso — basophil
basocyte
basocytopenia
basocytosis
basoerythrocyte
basoerythrocytosis
basometachromophil; basometachro-
　　mophile
basopenia
basophil; basophile
　　b. adenoma
　　beta b.
　　b. cell
　　b. chemotactic factor
　　b. Crooke-Russell b's
　　b. degranulation test
　　delta b.
　　b. granule
　　polymorphonuclear b.
basophilia
　　Grawitz' b.
　　pituitary b.
　　punctate b.
basophilic
　　b. adenoma
　　b. degeneration
　　b. erythroblast
　　b. erythrocyte
　　b. granular degeneration

　　b. granule
　　b. granulocyte
　　b. hyperplasia
　　b. leukemia
　　b. leukocyte
　　b. leukocytosis
　　b. leukopenia
　　b. marrow
　　b. megakaryocyte
　　b. metamyelocyte
　　b. myelocyte
　　b. normoblast
　　b. promyelocyte
　　b. stippling
basophilism
　　Cushing's b.
　　pituitary b.
basophilocyte
basophilocytic leukemia
basophilopenia
basoplasm
basosquamous carcinoma
bassorin
BAT — brain-adjacent tumor
batch processing
bath
　　antipyretic b.
　　carbon dioxide b.
　　Finsen's bath
　　flotation b.
　　foam b.
　　immersion b.
　　sedative b.
bathing trunk nevus
bathochrome
bathochromic shift
bathophenanthroline
bathorhodopsin
bathrocephaly
bathycardia
bathygastry
Battey
　　bacillus
　　-type mycobacterium
battledore placenta
baud
Bauer reaction
Baurer's chromic acid leucofuchsin
　　stain
Baumé's scale
Baumgartner method

Bayes's
    rule
    theorem
Bayle's granulations
Bayliss effect
BB — blood bank
    blood buffer base
    "blue bloaters" (emphysema)
    breakthrough bleeding
    breast biopsy
    buffer base
BBB — blood–brain barrier
    bundle branch block
BBT — basal body temperature
BC — bactericidal concentration
    bone conduction
    buccocervical
BCB — brilliant cresyl blue
BCD — binary-coded decimal
BCDF — B-cell differentiation factor
BCE — basal cell epithelioma
B-cell
    B.-c. acute
    B.-c. acute lymphoblastic leukemia
    B.-c. antigen
    B.-c. antigen receptor
    B.-c. bursal-derived cell
    B.-c. chronic lymphocytic leukemia
    B.-c. differentiation factor
    B.-c. function
    B.-c. growth factor I, II
    B.-c. immunoglobulin
    B.-c. leukemia
    B.-c. lymphoma
    B.-c. malignancy
    B.-c. markers
    B.-c. mitogens
    B.-c. neoplasm
    B.-c. stimulating factor 1, 2
    B.-c. tolerance
BCF — basophil chemotactic factor
BCG — bacille Calmette-Guerin
    (vaccine)
    ballistocardiogram
    bicolor guaiac (test)
    bromocresol green
BCGF — B-cell growth factor
BCME — bis(chloromethyl) ether
BCNU — bischloroethylnitrosourea
    bischloronitrosourea

BCP – basic calcium phosphate
BCP-D — bromocresol purple desoxycholate
BD — base deficit
    bile duct
    buccodistal
Bdellonyssus bacoti
Bdellovibrio
BDG — buffered desoxycholate glucose
BE — bacillary emulsion (tuberculin)
    bacterial endocarditis
    base excess
    bovine enteritis
Be — beryllium
bead
    magnetic b's
beaded
    b. bacterium
    b. hair
beading
beaker
beam
    electron b.
    b. splitting
Beard test
beat
    apex b.
    capture b's
    dropped b.
    ectopic b.
    fusion b.
    premature b.
    reciprocal b's
Beau's lines
Beauvaria
beauvariosis
Beaver direct smear method
Becker's
    muscular dystrophy
    nevus
    stain for spirochetes
Beckman assay
Beckmann thermometer
Beck's triad
beclomethasone dipropionate
becquerel
Bednar tumor
Bedsonia
beef tapeworm
Beer's law
beeturia

bee venom (toxin)
behavioral genetics
behenate
behenic acid
Behla's bodies
Behnken's unit
BEI — butanol-extractable iodine
BEI test
bejel
bel
Belascaris
Belganyl
Belgian Congo anemia
belladonna tincture
bell-clapper anomaly
Bellini's papillary duct
Bell-Magendie law
Bell's palsy
belly
      prune b.
bemegride
benactyzine hydrochloride
Bence Jones
      albumin
      albumosuria
      cylinders
      myeloma
      protein
      protein test
      proteinuria
      reaction
Benditt hypothesis
bendroflumethiazide
bends
Benedict-Hopkins-Cole reagent
Benedict's
      reagent
      solution
      test
Bengston's method
benign
      b. albuminuria
      b. bone aneurysm
      b. chronic bullous dermatosis
      b. dyskeratosis
      b. epithelial odontogenic
        tumor
      b. epithelial tumor
      b. epithelioma
      b. familial icterus
      b. fibrous mesothelioma
      b. glycosuria

b. hypertension
b. intracranial hypertension
b. juvenile melanoma
b. lymphadenosis
b. lymphocytoma cutis
b. lymphoepithelial lesion
b. lymphogranulomatosis
b. lymphoma
b. mediastinal lymph node hyperplasia
b. mesenchymoma
b. mesothelioma of genital
  tract
b. monoclonal gammopathy
b. mucosal pemphigoid
b. mucous membrane pem-
  phigus
b. neoplasm
b. nephrosclerosis
b. prostatic hyperplasia
b. prostatic hypertrophy
b. teratoma
b. tertian malaria
b. tumor
Bennett's sulfhydryl method
Bennhold's Congo red method, stain
Benois' scale
benoxaprofen
benoxinate hydrochloride
Benoy scale
Bensley's
      aniline-acid fuchsin–methyl
        green method
      osmic dichromate fluid
      safranin acid violet
bent head defect
bentiromide test
bentonite flocculation test
benzaldehyde dehydrogenase
benzalkonium chloride
benzanthracene
Benzathin
benzene
      b. assay
      b. hexachloride
      isopropyl b.
benzeneamine
1,2-benzenedicarboxylic acid
benzestrol
benzethonium
benzidine
      b. method for myoglobin perox-
        idase

    b. oxidase
    b. test
benzimidazole
benzo [a]pyrene
benzoate
    caffeine sodium b.
    estradiol b.
benzocaine
benzodepa
benzodiazepine
    b. assay
benzoflavine
benzoic acid
benzoin
benzol
benzomethamine
benzomorphin
benzonatate
benzopurpurine
benzopyrene
benzoquinone
benzo sky blue method
benzoyl
    b. chloride
    b. oil red
    b. peroxide
benzoylaminoacetic acid
benzoylation
benzoylcholine
benzoylcholinesterase
benzoylecgonine
benzoylglycine
N-benzoyl-L-tyrosyl-p aminobenzoic a.
benzphetamine hydrochloride
benzpyrene
benzpyrinium bromide
benzquinamide
benzthiazide
benztropine mesylate
benzydroflumethiazide
benzyl
    b. alcohol
    b. benzoate
    b. bromide
    b. carbinol
    b. fumarate
    b. mandelate
    b. succinate
benzylamine
o-benzyl-parachlorophenol
benzylpenicillin
benzylpenicilloyl polylysine

bephenium hydroxynaphthoate
Bérard's aneurysm
berberine
Bereitschafts potential
bergamot oil
Bergeron's chorea
Berger's
    focal glomerulonephritis
    rhythm
Bergey's classification
Bergh's staging system
Bergmann's glia
Berg's
    chelate removal method
    stain
beriberi
    wet b.
Berkefeld filter
berkelium
Berlin blue
Bernstein test
Bernthsen's methylene violet
berry
    b. aneurysm
    b. cell
Berson test
Berthelot's
    procedure
    reaction
    reagent
Bertiella
    B. mucronata
    B. studeri
Bertini's renal columns
berylliosis
beryllium
    b. granuloma
    b. granulomatosis
Bessey-Lowry unit
Bessey-Lowry-Brock unit
Bessman anemia classification
Best's carmine stain
beta
    b. agglutinin
    b.-aminoisobutyric acid
    b.-aminoisobutyricaciduria
    b. band
    b. basophil
    b. blocker
    b.-butoxy-beta-
        thiocyanodiethyl ether
    b.-carotene

b. chain
b.-cholestanol
b. decay
b. emitter
b.-endorphin
b.-globulin
b.-glucuronidase
b. granule
b. hemolysis
b.-hemolytic streptococcus
11-b.-hydroxylase inhibition
b.-hypophamine
b.-interferon
b.-lactamase
b.-lactose
b.-lipoprotein
b.-lysin
b. metachromasia
b.$_2$-microglobulin
b. motoneurons
b.-naphthylamine
b. particles
b.-phenylisopropylamine
b.-pleated sheet
b.-pyridyl-carbinol
b. radiation
b. ray
b. receptor
b. staphylolysin
b. streptococcus
b. substance
b. thalassemia
b.-thalassemia trait
b.-thiocyanoethyl
b.-thromboglobulin
beta-adrenergic
b.-a. antagonist
b.-a. blocking agent
b.-a. receptor
beta cells of the odenohypophysis
betacyaninuria
betaglobin gene
betaglobulin
steroid-binding b.
betaine
b. aldehyde dehydrogenase
b. homocysteine methyl-
transferase
betamethasone
betamicin sulfate
betanaphthol
beta-oxybutyria

betatron
betazole hydrochloride
betel cancer
bethanechol chloride
Bethesda
method
unit
Bethesda-Ballerup group of *Citrobacter*
Betke-Kleihauer test
Betke stain
Bettendorff's test
Betula
Betz cells
Beutler test
BeV — billion electron volts
Bevan-Lewis cell
bezoar
Bezold-Jarisch reflex
Bezold's
abscess
reflex
BF — blastogenic factor
blood flow
B/F — bound-free ratio
bf — bouillon filtrate (tuberculin)
BFC — benign febrile convulsion
BFP — biologic false-positive
BFR — biologic false-positive reactor
blood flow rate
bone formation rate
BFT — bentonite flocculation test
BFU-E — burst-forming unit-
erythroid
BG — blood glucose
blood group
bone graft
buccogingival
BGG — bovine gamma globulin
BGH — bovine growth hormone
BGP — beta-glycerophosphatase
BGSA — blood granulocyte-specific
activity
BGTT — borderline glucose toler-
ance test
BH — benzalkonium and heparin
BHA — butylated hydroxyanisole
BHC — benzene hexachloride
bhCG — beta-human chorionic go-
nadotropin
BHI — brain-heart infusion
BHS — beta-hemolytic streptococcus
BHT — butylated hydroxytoluene

BH/VH — body hematocrit–venous
              hematocrit ratio
BI — bacteriological index
       burn index
Bi — bismuth
biallylamicol
Bial's
       reagent
       test
bias
       analytical b.
       forward b.
       reverse b.
biased estimate
biatriatum
       cor pseudotriloculare b.
       cor triloculare b.
bibulous
bicameral abscess
bicarbonate
       blood b.
       b. buffer
       b. buffer system
       plasma b.
       b. of soda
       standard b.
       b. titration test
bicellular
biceps
       b. brachii muscle
       b. femoris muscle
       b. femoris superior muscle
       b. tendon
bichloride
       mercury b.
Bicillin
bicipital
bicipitoradialis
biclonal gammopathy
bicolor guaiac test
biconcave
biconvex
bicornuate
bicoronal flap
bicuspid aortic valve
bidermoma
bidiazotized benzidine method
BIDLB — block in the posteroinferior
              division of the left
              branch
Biebrich
       scarlet
       scarlet-picroaniline blue

Bielschowsky's
       method
       stain
Biermer's anemia
bifascicular block
bifid
       b. bacterium
       b. scrotum
       b. thumb
       b. tongue
       b. ureter
       b. uterus
Bifidobacterium
       B. bifidum
       B. eriksonii
       B. infantis
bifurcation
bigeminal
bigeminy
       ventricular b.
BIH — benign intracranial hyper-
              tension
BIL — bilirubin
bil. — bilateral
bilat. — bilateral
bilateral
       b. breast cancer
       b. otitis media
       b., symmetrical and
              equal
       b. symmetry
bilayer
       lipid b.
bile
       b. acids
       b. acid test
       b. acid tolerance test
       b. canaliculi
       b. capillaries
       b. cast
       b. duct
       b. esculin agar
       b. esculin hydrolysis test
       b. extravasation
       b. fluid examination
       b. infarct
       b. lake
       b. nephrosis
       b. peritonitis
       b. pigment demonstration in
              tissue
       b. pigment hemoglobin

b. pigments
b. pigment test
b. salt agar
b. salt breath test
b. salt deficiency syndrome
b. salts
b. salts sucrose
b. solubility test
b. stasis
b. thrombus
white b.

bile duct
b.d. adenoma
b.d. canaliculus
b.d. carcinoma
common b.d.
b.d. cystadenoma
cystic b.d.
extrahepatic b.d.
hepatic b.d.
interlobular b.d.
intrahepatic b.d.
b.d. plate malformation

bile ductule
intralobular b.d.
periportal b.d.

Bilharzia
bilharzial
b. carcinoma
b. deposition pigment
b. dysentery
b. granuloma
b. pigment deposition

bilharziasis
bilharzioma
biliary
b. achalasia
b. atresia
b. calculus
b. cirrhosis
b. colic
b. ectasia
b. fistula
b. obstruction
b. system
b. tract disease
b. xanthomatosis

bilineage leukemia
biliousness
bilious remittent malaria
bilirubin
amniotic fluid b.

b. assay
conjugated b.
delta b.
direct reacting b.
b. encephalopathy
b. glucuronide
indirect reacting b.
minimum concentration of b.
neonatal b.
b. pigment
serum b.
b. test, direct, indirect
b. tolerance test
unconjugated b.
b.-uridine diphosphate-
glucuronyl transferase
urine b.
volume of distribution of b.

bilirubinate crystals
bilirubinemia
hereditary nonhemolytic b.

bilirubinuria
biliuria
biliverdin globin
biliverdin reductase
Billroth's
cords
gastroenterostomy
operation

bilobate placenta
bilobed
b. flap
b. lung

biloculare
cor b.

bilocular stomach
Bilopaque
bimetal thermometer
bimodal
bimolecular
binary
b. acid
b. addition
b. code
b. coded decimal
b. digit
b. fission
b. variate

binasal hemianopsia
binding
b. energy
protein b.

Binet staging system
binocular microscope
binomial
    b. coefficient
    b. distribution
    b. nomenclature
binuclear
binucleate
binucleation
binucleolate
Binz's test
bioaccumulation
bioactive leukotrienes
bioassay
bioavailability
bioblast
biochemical
    b. biopsy
    b. energetics
    b. genetics
    b. profile
    b. screening
biochemistry
biochemorphology
biocytin
biodegradability
biodegradable
bioenergetics
bioequivalence
biofeedback
biogenesis
biogenetic
biogenic amine hypothesis
biohazard
    b. sign
    b. symbol
biologic
    b. assay
    b. false-positive
    b. false-positive reaction
    b. half-life
    b. response modifier
biological
    b. alkylating agent
    b. assay
    b. clock
    b. marker
    b. standard unit
Biological Stain Commission
biology
    cellular b.

    molecular b.
    population b.
bioluminescence
biomarker
biomass
biomechanical preparation
biomechanics
biomedical
    b. engineering
    b. science
biomembrane
biometrician
biometry
biomodulator
biomolecule
Biomphalaria glabrata
Biondi-Heidenhain stain
bionics
bionucleonics
biophysics
bioplasm
bioplast
biopsy
    aspiration b.
    biochemical b.
    bite b.
    bone b.
    bone marrow b.
    brush b.
    chorionic villus b.
    closed pleural b.
    cone b.
    contralateral b.
    core needle b.
    cytological b.
    endoscopic b.
    excisional b.
    exploratory b.
    fine-needle b.
    incisional b.
    intranasal b.
    large-bore needle b.
    lymph node b.
    mediastinoscopic b.
    Menghini needle b.
    muscle b.
    needle b.
    needle core b.
    open b.
    open lung b.
    percutaneous needle b.
    pleural b.

pre-excisional b.
punch b.
renal b.
scalene node b.
sponge b.
sternal b.
surface b.
synovial b.
testicular b.
thin-needle b.
transbronchial b.
transbronchial lung b.
trephine b.
Tru-Cut b.
wedge b.
biopterin
bioptome
biopyoculture
biospectrometry
biospectroscopy
biosynthesis
pyrimidine b.
biosynthetic pathway
biotaxis
biotin
b. assay
b. deficiency
biotinidase
biotinyl
biotinylation
biotoxin
biotransformation
biotype
BIP — bismuth iodoform paraffin
biparental inheritance
biparietal
bipedal lymphangiography
bipedicle flap
biperiden
biphasic
biphenamine
biphenotypic leukemia
biphenotypy
biphenyl
polychlorinated b.
p-biphenylamine
biphosphate
fructose b.
biplane fluoroscopy
bipolar
b. cell
b. needle electrode

b. neuron
b. spindle
b. staining
Bipolaris
bipyridyl
Birbeck's granules
Birch-Hirschfeld stain
birdseed agar
bird's nest lesion
birefringence
crystalline b.
flow b.
form b.
strain b.
birefringent crystals
birthmark
strawberry b.
vascular b.
birth rate
bisacodyl tannex
bisalbuminemia
bisantrene
bischloroethylnitrosourea
bis(2-chloroethyl) sulfide
bis(chloromethyl) ether
bischloronitrosourea
bis-(p-chlorophenoxy) methane
bis-(p-chlorophenyl) ethanol
1-1-bis-(p-chlorophenyl)-2-
nitrobutane
1-1-bis(p-chlorophenyl)-2-
nitropropane
bis-(p-chlorophenyl) trichloroethanol
bis-(diethylthiocarbamyl) disulfide
bis-(dimethylamino)- phosphorus anhydride
bis-(dimethylthiocarbamyl) disulfide
bisection
bisexual
bishydroxycoumarin
Bismarck
brown R
brown Y
bismuth
b. aluminate
b. iodide
b. iodoform paraffin
b. pigmentation
b. subcarbonate
b. subgallate
b. subnitrate
b. subsalicylate

b. sulfite agar
b. triiodide
b. violet
bisphosphatidylglycerol
bisphosphoglycerate
    b. mutase
    b. phosphatase
    b. synthase
1,3-bisphosphoglycerate
2,3-bisphosphoglycerate
bisphosphoglyceric acid
bisphosphoglyceromutase
bis-trimethylsiltrifluoroacetamide
bis-trimethylsilylacetamide
bisulfate
bisulfide
    carbon b.
bisulfite
    menadione sodium b.
bitartrate
    levarterenol b.
bitemporal hemianopsia
bithionol
Bithynia
Bitot's spots
biundulant milk fever
    virus
biuret
    b. method
    b. reaction
    b. reactive material
    b. test
bivalency
    monogamous b.
bivalent
    heteromorphic b.
    homomorphic b.
biventriculare
    cor triloculare b.
bixin
bizarre leiomyoma
Bizzozero's
    corpuscles
    platelets
    red cells
BJP — Bence Jones protein
Bk — berkelium
BL — baseline
    Bessey-Lowry (units)
    bleeding
    blood loss

buccolingual
Burkitt's lymphoma
black
    b. adenoma
    b. box
    b. cancer
    b. currant rash
    b. fever
    b. fly
    b. hairy tongue
    b. jaundice
    b. lead
    b. lung
    b. lung disease
    b. measles
    b. periodic acid method
    b. piedra
    b. plaque
    Sudan b. B
    b. tongue
    b. urine
    b. widow spider
blackbody radiation
Blackfan-Diamond anemia
blackwater fever
bladder
    b. agenesis
    atonic b.
    atonic neurogenic b.
    b. autonomous b.
    cloacogenic b.
    denervated b.
    b. endometriosis
    b. exstrophy
    fasciculated b.
    b. lavage
    low-compliance b.
    b. neck contracture
    b. neck obstruction
    neurogenic b.
    paralytic b.
    septal b.
    spastic b.
    "superficial" b.
    tabetic b.
    tear drop b.
    b. tumor
    urinary b.
blanch
bland
    b. embolism

b. embolus
b. infarct
b. infarction

blast
b. cell leukemia
b. chest
b. crisis
b. injury
b. leukemia
b. transformation

blastema
nephrogenic b.
nodular renal b.
renal b.

blastic transformation
blastin
blastoconidia
blastocyst
Blastocystis hominis
blastocyte
blastocytoma
blastoderm
blastogenesis assay
blastogenic factor

blastoma
pluricentric b.
pulmonary b.
unicentric b.

blastomatosis
blastomere
blastomogenic

Blastomyces
B. *brasiliensis*
B. *coccidioides*
B. *dermatitidis*

Blastomycetes
blastomycin

blastomycosis
cutaneous b.
European b.
North American b.
pulmonary b.
b. serology
South American b.

blastosphere
blastospore
blastostroma
blastula (pl., blastulae)
blastulation
Blatta
Blattella
Blattidae

BLB (Bessey-Lowry-Brock) unit
bleach

bleb
emphysematous b.
b. formation

bleeder

bleeding
breakthrough b.
b. diathesis
estrogen withdrawal b.
functional b.
gastrointestinal b.
implantation b.
occult b.
placentation b.
b. polyp

bleeding time
Duke's method of calculating b.t.
Ivy's method of calculating b.t.

blennadenitis
blennorrhagia
blennorrhagic inflammation

blennorrhea
inclusion b.
b. neonatorum

blennuria
Blenoxane
bleomycin sulfate
blepharitis ulcerosa
blepharoconjunctivitis
blepharoncus
blepharoplast
blepharoptosis
BLG — beta-lactoglobulin

blind
b. fistula
single b.
b. test

blindness
color b.
night b.
word b.

blink responses

blister
blood b.
fever b.
herpetic b.
Marochetti's b's
pharyngeal b.

BLN — bronchial lymph nodes

Bloch's reaction
block
    adrenergic b.
    alveolar-capillary b.
    arborization b.
    A-V (atrioventricular) b.
    bundle branch b.
    caudal b.
    celiac plexus b.
    cell b.
    complete heart b.
    complete left bundle branch b.
    complete right bundle
      branch b.
    b. diagram
    diffusion b.
    epidural b.
    incomplete bundle branch b.
    intercostal b.
    intraspinal b.
    methadone b.
    nerve b.
    paracervical b.
    parasacral b.
    paravertebral b.
    perineural b.
    sacral b.
    second-degree heart b.
    sinoatrial b.
    stellate b.
    subarachnoid b.
    sympathetic b.
    third-degree heart b.
    tubal b.
    uterosacral b.
    vagal b.
    ventricular b.
    Wenckebach b.
blockade
    adrenergic b.
    adrenergic neuron b.
    alpha b.
    alpha-adrenergic b.
    beta-adrenergic b.
    cholinergic b.
    narcotic b.
    renal b.
    reticuloendothelial b.
    virus b.
blocker
    beta b.

blocking
    adrenergic b.
    b. antibody
    b. antibody reaction
    b. filter
Blondheim test
blood
    b. agar
    b. agar plate
    b.-air barrier
    b. albumin
    b. alcohol
    b. alcohol concentration
    anticoagulated b.
    arterial b.
    arterialized b.
    autologous b.
    b. bank
    b. banking
    b. bicarbonate
    b. blister
    b.-brain barrier
    b. buffer base
    b. buffering capacity
    b. calculus
    capillary b.
    b. cast
    b. cell
    b. cell count
    b. cell count automation
    b.-cerebral fluid barrier
    b. chemistry
    citrated b.
    b. clot
    b. clot lysis time
    b. coagulation disorder
    b. component
    cord b.
    b. corpuscle
    b. count
    b. crisis
    b. crystals
    b. culture
    b. cyst
    b. cytolysate
    defibrinated b.
    b. derivative
    b. disk
    b. dust
    b. dyscrasia
    b. extravasation
    b. factor

b. filters
fixed b. film
b. flow
b. fluke
b. gas analysis
b.-gas barrier
b. gases
b. ghost
b. glucose
b. granulocyte-specific activity
b. group
b. group agglutinins
b. group chimera
b. group incompatibility
b. grouping
b. group–specific substance A
   and B
b. group substances
b. group systems
b. indices
b. islands
b. lancet
b. loss
b. loss anemia
b. lymph
mixed venous b.
b. mole
b. motes
occult b.
oxygen capacity of b.
oxygen content of b.
peripheral b.
b. plasma
b. plasma fractions
b. plastid
b. plate
platelet-poor b.
b. platelet thrombus
b. poisoning
b. pool scan
b. pressure
b. quotient
red venous b.
b. retinol
b. serum
sludged b.
b. smear
b. smear morphology
b. specimen
splanchnic b.
b. spots
strawberry-cream b.

b. substitute
b. sugar
b.-testis barrier
b.-thymus barrier
b. transfusion
b. tumor
b. type
b. typing
b. urea clearance
b. urea nitrogen/creatinine
   ratio
b. urea nitrogen test
venous b.
b. vessel
b. volume
b. volume measurements
b. volume nomogram
b. warming
whole b.
blood cell
   erythrocytic b.c.
   granulocytic b.c.
   lymphocytic b.c.
   megakaryocytic b.c.
   monocytic b.c.
   plasma b.c.
   plasmacytic b.c.
blood count
   complete b.c.
   differential white b.c.
   Schilling's b.c.
bloodless
blood serum
   glycerin b.s.
   Löffler's b.s.
blood vessel
   embryonic b.v.
   vitelline b.v.
Bloor's test
blot
   enzyme-linked immunoelectro-
     transfer b.
   b. test
blotting
   Northern b.
   Southern b.
   Western b.
Blount's test
blowback
blowout pipet
Bloxam's test

BNP = brain natriuretic peptide
* 3 types of BNP — ANP (atrial type), NTproANP; BNP
(brain type) BNP & NTProBNP; N-terminal pro B type, & C type   body   105

BLP — Boothby, Lovelace, Bulbulian
    (mask)
bl. pr. — blood pressure
BLU — Bessey-Lowry units
blue
    alkaline methylene b.
    anthracene b.
    b. baby
    Biebrich scarlet-picroaniline b.
    "b. bloaters" (emphysema)
    b. bodies
    bromothymol b.
    bromphenol b.
    carbolic methylene b.
    cotton b.
    dextran b.
    dianil b.
    b. diaper syndrome
    b. dome cyst
    b. edema
    lactophenol cotton b.
    methylene b.
    molybdenum b.
    b. nevus
    b. pus
    b. rubber-bleb disease
    b. rubber-bleb nevi
    b. spot
    tetrabromophenol b.
    thymol b.
    toluidine b.
    tungsten b.
    Turnbull b.
    Unna's alkaline methylene b.
bluebottle fly
Blumberg's sign
blunt duct adenosis
blush
    papillary b.
BLV — bovine leukemia virus
B (bursa derived) lymphocyte
BM — basement membrane
    body mass
    bone marrow
    bowel movement
    buccomesial
BMC test strip
BMG — benign monoclonal gammo-
    pathy
bmk — birthmark
B-mode unit
BMR — basal metabolic rate

BMT — bone marrow transplantation
BN — branchial neuritis
BNO — bladder neck obstruction
BNPA — binasal pharyngeal airway
BNS – benign nephrosclerosis
BO — bucco-occlusal
B & O — belladonna and
    opium
Boas-Oppler
    bacillus
    lactobacillus
Boas' test
BOBA — beta-oxybutyric acids
Bochdalek's foramen
Bodansky unit
Bodian's
    copper-protargol stain
    method
Bodin-Gibb staging system
Bodo
    B. caudatus
    B. saltans
    B. urinaria
Bodonidae
body
    acetone b.
    acidophilic b.
    alcoholic hyaline b's
    Alder b's
    Alder-Reilly b's
    alkapton b's
    amyloid b's of prostate
    b. analysis
    aortic b's
    Arnold's b's
    asbestos b.
    Aschoff's b.
    asteroid b's
    Auer's b's
    Balbiani's b.
    Barr b's
    basal b.
    Behla's b's
    brassy b.
    Cabot's ring b's
    Call-Exner b's
    cancer b's
    carotid b.
    b. cavity
    chromaffin b.
    chromatin b's
    chromatinic b.

Civatte's b.
colloid b.
conchoidal b.
contact b.
Councilman hyaline b.
Councilman's b's
Cowdry b's
Cowdry type A intranuclear inclusion b's
Cowdry type I inclusion b's
creola b's
Deetjen's b's
demilune b.
dense b.
Döhle's inclusion b's
Donné's b's
Donovan's b's
Dutcher b.
Ehrlich's inner b.
elementary b.
embryoid b's
erectile b's
ferruginous b's
fibrin b.
fibrous b.
b. fluid analysis
foreign b.
fuchsin b's
Gamna-Favre b's
Gandy-Gamna B's
Gordon's b.
Guarnieri's b's
Heinz b's
Heinz-Ehrlich b's
b. hematocrit—venous hematocrit ratio
hematoxylin b.
hematoxyphil b's
Herring b's
Hirano b's
Howell-Jolly b's
Howell's b's
HX b's
hyaline b.
immune b's
inclusion b's
intraocular foreign b.
intrauterine foreign b.
b. joint
Jolly's b's
jugular b's
juxtarestiform b.

ketone b's
Lafora's b's
Lallemand's b's
Leishman-Donovan b's
Lewy b.
Luse b's
Mallory's b's
malpighian b's
mammillary b.
Maragiliano b.
b. mass
May-Hegglin b.
melon seed b.
membranous cytoplasmic b.
metachromatic b's
metallic foreign b.
Meyers-Kouvenaar b's
Michaelis-Gutmann b's
mineral foreign b.
mineral oil foreign b.
molluscum b.
Mott b's
multilamellar b.
multivesicular b.
Negri b's
Nissl b's
nuclear inclusion b.
onion b's
oval fat b.
oxyphil inclusion b's
Pappenheimer b.
phi b.
Pick's b's
Plimmer's b's
polar b.
polyglucosan b's
psammoma b's
residual b.
retained foreign b.
rice b.
Russell's b's
Schaumann's b's
Schiller-Duval b's
sclerotic b's
b.-section radiography
selenoid b.
spiculated b's
b. substance isolation system
b. surface area
b. temperature
b. temperature, ambient pressure, saturated

thermostable b.
Todd b's
threshold b.
Trousseau-Lallemand b's
tuffstone b.
ultimobranchial b.
Verocay b.
b. wall
Weibel-Palade b's
Wesenberg-Hamazaki b.
wolffian b.
Wolf-Orton b's
x (xanthine) b's
X chromatin b's
yellow b.
zebra b.
BOEA — ethyl biscoumacetate
Boeck-Drbohlav-Locke egg-serum
   medium
Boeck's sarcoid
Boehmer's hematoxylin
Boettcher cells
Bohn's nodule
Bohr
   effect
   equation
   magneton
Bol. — pill (bolus)
Boletus
Boling burner
Bollinger granules
bolus
   b. alba
   alimentary b.
BOM — bilateral otitis media
bombardment
Bombay
   blood group
   phenotype
bombesin
Bombidae
Bombus californicus
Bonanno's test
bond
   chemical b.
   coordinate covalent b.
   covalent b.
   disulfide b.
   electron pair b.
   b. energy
   high-energy b.
   hydrogen b.

ionic b.
metallic b.
peptide b.
pi b.
sigma b.
bonding
bone
   b. abscess
   cancellous b.
   capitate b.
   carpal b.
   cartilage b.
   b. cell
   b. chip
   compact b.
   b. conduction
   cortex b.
   cranial b.
   b. crystal alteration
   b. cyst
   dermal b.
   b. dysplasia
   epihyal b.
   ethmoid b.
   b. exostosis
   facial b.
   b. formation rate
   frontal b.
   giant cell tumor of b.
   b. Gla protein
   b. graft
   hamate b.
   heterotopic b.
   hyoid b.
   b. infarct
   innominate b.
   lamellar b.
   lunate b.
   marble b's
   b. marrow
   b. matrix alteration
   b. metastasis
   b. morphogenetic protein
   occipital b.
   palatine b.
   parietal b.
   pelvic b's
   petrous b.
   pisiform b.
   remodeling b.
   b. resorption
   b. scan

scaphoid b.
b. sclerosis
sesamoid b.
sphenoid b.
b. spur
tarsal b.
temporal b.
trabecular b.
trapezial b.
trapezoidal b.
triangular b.
b. tumor
zygomatic b.
bone marrow
    b.m. aspiration
    b.m. biopsy
    b.m. depression
    b.m. differential count
    b.m. embolism
    b.m. embolus
    b.m. imprint
    megaloblastic b.m.
    b.m. scan
    b.m. suppression
    b.m. transplantation
bongkrekic acid
Bonnet's plexus
Bonsignore test
bony
    b. ankylosis
    b. callus
    b. heart
Boolean
    algebra
    factor analysis
    function
Boophilus annulatus
booster dose
Boothby, Lovelace, Bulbulian (mask)
borate
borax
Borchgrevink method
border
    brush b.
borderline
    b. glucose tolerance test
    b. leprosy
Bordetella
    B. bronchiseptica
    B. parapertussis
    B. pertussis

Bordetella pertussis nasopharyngeal
    culture
Bordet-Gengou
    agar
    bacillus
    medium
    phenomenon
    potato blood agar
Bordet's amboceptor
boric acid
borism
borneol
bornyl chloride
boroglycerin
boron
    b. carbide
    b. trifluoride-methanol
    b. trioxide
borosilicate glass
Borrelia
    B. aegyptica
    B. anserina
    B. berbera
    B. buccalis
    B. burgdorferi
    b. carteri
    B. caucasica
    B. duttonii
    B. hermsii
    B. hispanica
    B. kochii
    B. neotropicalis
    B. novyi
    B. parkeri
    B. persica
    B. recurrentis
    B. refringens
    B. theileri
    B. turicatae
    B. venezuelensis
    B. vincentii
borreliosis
    Lyme b.
Borrel's blue stain
Borrmann's classification
Borst-Jadassohn intraepidermal
    basal cell epithelioma
boss
    parietal b's
bosselated
bosselation
Boston exanthem

bothridium
bothriocephaliasis
Bothriocephalus
bothrium
Bothrops atrox serine proteinase
botryoid
    b. rhabdomyosarcoma
    b. sarcoma
botryoides
    sarcoma b.
botryomycosis
botryomycotic
Bottcher's crystal
bottle
    Roux's b.
botulin
botulinum toxin
botulism
Botzmann's
    constant
    equation
Bouchard's nodes
bougie
bougienage
Bouguer's law
bouillon filtrate (tuberculin)
Bouin's
    fixative
    fluid
    picroformal-acetic
      fixative
bound-free ration
bound serum iron
bouton
    b. de passage
    b. en passant
    synaptic b.
    terminal b.
    b's termineaux
boutonneuse fever
Bovicola
bovine
    b. albumin
    b. enteritis
    b. gamma globulin
    b. growth hormone
    b. leukemia virus
    b. malaria
    b. papilloma virus
    b. red blood cells
    b. serum albumin
    b. tubercle bacillus

bovinum
    cor b.
Bowditch staircase phenomenology
bowel
    b. bypass syndrome
    b. obstruction
bowel sounds
    hyperactive b.s.
    hypoactive b.s.
bowenoid papulosis
Bowen's precancerous dermatosis
Bowers-McComb unit
Bowie stain
Bowman's
    capsule
    glands
    lamina
    membrane
Boyden chamber assay
Boyle's law
BP — back pressure
    benzpyrene
    blood pressure
    bronchopleural
    buccopulpal
    bypass
bp — base pair
    boiling point
BPD — bronchopulmonary dysplasia
BPH — benign prostatic hypertrophy
BPL — beta-propiolactone
BPO — benzylpenicilloyl
Bq — becquerel
BR — bilirubin
Br — bromine
Br. — *Brucella*
brachial
    b. artery
    b. fascia
    b. lymph node
    b. neuritis
    b. plexus
    b. vein
brachialis muscle
brachiocephalic
    b. artery
    b. vein
brachioradialis
    b. muscle
    b. reflex
brachium
    b. conjunctivum

inferior b.
b. points
Bracht-Wachter lesion
brachycephalic
brachydactyly
brachymesomelia-renal syndrome
brachytherapy
Bradshaw's
    albumosuria
    test
bradyarrhythmia
bradycardia
    junctional b.
    nodal b.
    sinus b.
    b.-tachycardia syndrome
bradykinin
bradylalia
Bragg
    curve
    reflection
brain
    b. abscess
    b. aneurysm
    b. artery
    b. death
    b. death syndrome
    b. edema
    fungal b.
    b. necrosis
    olfactory b.
    respirator b.
    b. sand
    b. scan
    b. stem
    b. stem auditory evoked potential
    b. stem glioma
    b. stem reflexes
    b. tumor
    b. waves
brain-heart
    b.-h. infusion
    b.-h. infusion agar
    b.-h. infusion broth medium
Brain Tumor Study Group
braking radiation
branch
    left bundle b.
    lingual b.
    right bundle b.
branched calculus

branched-chain
    b.-c. aminoaciduria
    b.-c. keto acid
    b.-c. α-ketoacid decarboxylase
    b.-c. α-ketoacid dehydrogenase
    b.-c. ketoaciduria
    b.-c. ketonuria
brancher
    b. enzyme deficiency
    b. glycogenosis
branchial
    b. arch
    b. cleft
    b. cleft cyst
    b. cleft sinus
    b. cyst
    b. fistula
    b. neuritis
    b. pouch
    b. region
branching
    b. decay
    b. enzyme
    b. fraction
    b. ratio
branchiogenous cancer
branchioma
branchiomeric paraganglioma
branchio-oto-renal syndrome
Brand-Legal nitroprusside reaction
Branhamella catarrhalis
Brasil's fixative
Braun and Jaboulay's gastroenterostomy
brazilein
Brazilian trypanosomiasis
brazilin
BRBC — bovine red blood cells
BrdU — 5-bromodeoxyuridine
"bread-and-butter" pericarditis
break
    isochromatid b.
breakbone fever
breakdown
    protein b.
    Zener's b.
breaker
    circuit b.
    vacuum b.
breakthrough bleeding
breast
    b. abscess

b. biopsy
b. carcinoma
Cooper's irritable b.
b. cyst
cystic disease of b.
cystic hyperplasia of b.
fascial b.
fibrocystic disease of b.
funnel b.
ipsilateral b.
neural b.
papillomatosis of b.
pigeon b.
proemial b.
b. reconstruction
shotty b.
b. specimen radiography
tension cyst of b.
topographic b.
vascular b.
breast cancer
adenoid cystic b.c.
advanced b.c.
bilateral b.c.
carcinoid b.c.
ductal b.c.
glycogen-rich clear b.c.
inflammatory b.c.
in situ b.c.
intracystic b.c.
lobular b.c.
male b.c.
mamographically occult b.c.
medullary b.c.
microinvasive b.c.
mucinous b.c.
multicentric b.c.
multifocal b.c.
oat cell b.c.
occult b.c.
papillary b.c.
preclinical b.c.
signet ring cell b.c.
squamous cell b.c.
sudoriferous b.c.
tubular b.c.
breast tumors
benign epithelial b.t's
malignant b.t's
breath analysis test
breathing
b. frequency

Kussmaul b.
b. zone
Brecher-Cronkite method
Brecher's new methylene blue technique
breech presentation
breeder reactor
breeding
random b.
Breed smear
bregma
bremsstrahlung
Brenner
nodules
tumor
Breslow's thickness
Breus mole
brevicollis
Brewer's infarcts
bridge
conjugation b.
cytoplasmic b.
intercellular b.
myocardial b.
protoplasmic b.
b. rectifier
salt b.
Wheatstone b.
bridging
b. hepatic necrosis
b. necrosis
b. vein
bridle
brightfield microscopy
brilliant
b. cresyl blue
b. crocein
b. green
b. green agar
b. green bile salt agar
b. purpurin
b. vital red
b. yellow
Bristol's hemoglobin
British
antilewisite
thermal unit
brittle bone disease
BRM — biologic response modifier
biuret-reactive material

broad
> b.-beta disease
> b. fish tapeworm
> b. ligament
> b.-spectrum antibiotic
> b. urinary cast

broadening
> peak b.

Broca's area

Broders'
> classification
> grading system
> index

Brodie's
> abscess
> knee

broken
> b. cell preparation
> b. compensation
> b. leukocyte

bromate

brombenzyl cyanide

bromcresol
> b. green indicator
> b. method
> b. purple indicator
> b. purple desoxycholate

bromelain; bromelin

bromide
> cetyltrimethylammonium b.
> glycopyrronium b.
> hexamethonium b.
> methyl b.
> valethamate b.

bromine isotope

brominism

bromism

bromisovalum

bromocriptine
> b. mesylate
> b. suppression test

bromodeoxyuracil

5-bromodeoxyuridine

bromoderma

bromodiphenhydramine hydrochloride

bromoiodism

bromomethane

bromphenol
> b. blue indicator
> b. test

2-bromo-4-phenyl phenol

brompheniramine maleate

Brompton's mixture

Bromsulphalein test

bromthymol blue indicator

bronchi

bronchial
> b. adenoma
> b. artery
> b. aspirate anaerobic culture
> b. asthma
> b. breathing
> b. calculus
> b. candidiasis
> b. carcinoid
> b. carcinoid tumor
> b. carcinoma
> b. cartilage
> b. casts
> b. cells
> b. cyst
> b. epithelium
> b. lavage
> b. lumen
> b. lymph node
> b. mucous gland
> b. mucus
> b. pneumonia
> b. polyp
> b. submucosa
> b. tree
> b. vein
> b. washing cytology

bronchiectasia sicca

bronchiectasic

bronchiectasis
> cylindrical b.
> cylindroid b.
> dry b.
> follicular b.
> fusiform b.
> saccular b.

bronchiectatic

bronchioalveolar
> b. adenocarcinoma
> b. carcinoma
> b. intravascular tumor
> b. lavage

bronchiolar
> b. adenocarcinoma
> b. carcinoma
> b. cell

bronchiole
> alveolar b.

respiratory b.
terminal b.
bronchiolectasia
bronchiolectasis
bronchiolitis
exudative b.
b. fibrosa obliterans
obliterative b.
proliferative b.
viral b.
bronchiolization
bronchiolo-alveolar carcinoma
bronchiostenosis
bronchitic
bronchitis
acute b.
asthmatic b.
chronic b.
croupous b.
fibrinous b.
obliterative b.; b. obliterans
plastic b.
pseudomembranous b.
bronchium
bronchoalveolar
b. carcinoma
b. lavage
bronchoalveolitis
bronchoaspergillosis
bronchoblastomycosis
bronchocandidiasis
bronchocavernous
bronchoconstriction
bronchoconstrictor
bronchodilatation
bronchodilator
bronchoedema
bronchoesophageal fistula
bronchoesophagoscopy
bronchofibroscopy
bronchogenic
b. adenocarcinoma
b. cancer
b. carcinoma
b. cyst
bronchogram
bronchography
Cope method of b.
broncholith
broncholithiasis
bronchomalacia
bronchomycosis

bronchopancreatic
bronchopathy
bronchopleural fistula
bronchopneumonia
acute b.
acute hemorrhagic b.
confluent b.
diffuse b.
focal b.
hemorrhagic b.
necrotizing b.
Pseudomonas b.
sequestration b.
staphylococcal b.
subacute b.
tuberculous b.
viral b.
bronchopneumopathy
bronchopulmonary
b. aspergillosis
b. dysplasia
b. lavage
b. segment
b. sequestration
bronchoradiography
bronchoscopic smear
bronchoscopy
fiberoptic b.
bronchospasm
bronchospirography
bronchospirometry
differential b.
bronchostenosis
bronchotracheal aspirate
bronchovascular
bronchus
cardiac b.
lingular b.
segmental b.
Brönsted-Lowry
acid
base
bronze diabetes
Brooke's tumor
bropirimine
broth
brain-heart infusion b.
chopped meat b.
decarboxylase b.
enrichment b.
gram-negative b.
hippurate b.

indole-nitrate b.
malonate b.
methyl b.
Middlebrook's b.
Mueller-Hinton b.
nitrate b.
nutrient b.
selenite b.
sodium chloride b.
sorbitol phenol-red b.
thioglycollate b.
Todd-Hewitt b.
trypticase soy b.
trypticase soy with agar b.
Voges-Proskauer b.
Brown
    dermatome
    method
brown
    b. adipose tissue
    b. atrophy
    Bismarck b. R
    Bismarck b. Y
    b. edema
    b. fat
    b. induration of lung
    b. recluse spider
    b. tumor
Brown-Brenn
    stain
    technique
brownian movement
Brown-Pearce tumor
BRP — bilirubin production
Brucella
    B. abortus
    B. bronchiseptica
    B. canis
    B. melitensis
    B. suis
brucella agglutination test
Brucellaceae
brucellin
brucellosis agglutinins
Bruch's
    basal membrane
    glands
brucine
Brudzinski's sign
Brugia
    B. malayi
    B. microfilariae
Brug's filariasis

bruise
bruising
bruit
brunescent cataract
Brunhilde virus
brunneroma
brunnerosis
Brunner's glands
Brunn's epithelial nests
brush
    b. border
    endometrial b.
Bruton's agammaglobulinemia
Bryce's sign
BS — blood sugar
        breath sounds
BSA — bismuth-sulfite agar
        body surface area
        bovine serum albumin
BSAP — brief short-action potential
BSB — body surface burned
BSDLB — block in the anterosuperior division of the left branch
BSE — bilateral, symmetrical, and equal
BSF — back scatter factor
        B-lymphocyte stimulating factors
BSI — bound serum iron
BSO — bilateral salpingo-oophorectomy
B-5 sodium acetate-sublimate formalin
BSP — Bromsulphalein
BSP excretion test
BSR — basal skin resistance
BSS — balanced salt solution
        buffered saline solution
BT — bladder tumor
        bleeding time
        brain tumor
BTB — breakthrough bleeding
BTPS — body temperature, ambient pressure, saturated
BTR — Bezold-type reflex
BTU — British thermal unit
BU — Bodansky unit
bubo
        climatic b.
        tropical b.
bubonic plague
bubonulus

buccal
>   b. branch
>   b. cavity
>   b. cheek flap
>   b. gland
>   b. mucosa
>   b. nerve
>   b. region
>   b. smear
>   b. smear for sex chromatin
>   evaluation
>   b. tablet

buckthorn poisoning

Bucky
>   diaphragm
>   grid

Bucky-Potter diaphragm

buclizine hydrochloride

budding

Budd's cirrhosis

BUDR — bs-bromodeoxy-uridine

buffer
>   b. action
>   b. amplifier
>   b. base
>   bicarbonate b.
>   bonate b.
>   cacodylate b.
>   b. capacity
>   Holmes's alkaline b.
>   Krebs-Ringer bicarbonate b.
>   phosphate b.
>   protein b.
>   secondary b.
>   Sorensen's phosphate b.
>   b. system
>   tricine b.
>   *tris*(hydroxymethyl)amino-
>   methane b.
>   b. value
>   veronal b.

buffered
>   b. charcoal yeast extract agar
>   b. desoxycholate glucose
>   b. neutral formalin
>   b. saline solution

buffering
>   secondary b.

buffy
>   b. coat
>   b. coat micromethod
>   b. coat smear study

Bulan

bulb
>   duodenal b.
>   end b.
>   Held's b.
>   Krause's end b.
>   olfactory b.
>   Rouget's b.
>   sinovaginal b.
>   tungsten b.
>   vaginal b.

bulbar
>   b. conjunctiva
>   b. palsy

bulbitis

bulbocapnine

bulbocavernous gland

bulbopontine

bulbospiral

bulbospongiosus reflex

bulbourethral glands

bulbus (pl., bulbi)
>   b. cordis
>   b. oculi
>   b. penis

bulimia

Bulimus fuchsianus

Bulinus

bulla (pl., bullae)
>   intraepidermic b.
>   pulmonary b.
>   subepidermic b.

Bullis fever

bull neck

bullosis diabeticorum

bullous
>   b. cystitis
>   b. dermatosis
>   b. disease
>   b. edema
>   b. edema vesicae
>   b. emphysema
>   b. eruption
>   b. granulomatous
>   inflammation
>   b. impetigo
>   b. inflammation
>   b. lichen planus
>   b. myringitis
>   b. pemphigoid

"bull's eye" granule

BUN — blood urea nitrogen

BUN/creatinine ratio
bunamiodyl
bundle
- b. bone
- b. branch block
- hair b.
- b. of His

bungarotoxin
- I-125–labeled b.

Büngner's bands
bunion
Bunostomum
Bunsen
- burner
- coefficient

Bunyamwera virus
Bunyaviridae
bunyavirus
buoyant density
buphthalmos
bupivacaine hydrochloride
buprenorphine
Burchard-Liebermann reaction
Burdach's tract
buret; burette
Burkitt-like lymphoma
Burkitt's
- acute lymphoblastic leukemia
- lymphoma
- tumor

burn
- b. culture
- first-degree b.
- fourth-degree b.
- full-thickness b.
- b. index
- inhalation b.
- partial-thickness b.
- screen b.
- second-degree b.
- b. shock
- superficial b.
- third-degree b.
- ultraviolet b.

burner
- Boling b.
- Bunsen b.
- laminar flow b.

Burow's solution
burr cell

bursa
- Achilles b.
- anserine b.
- b. of biceps femoris superior muscle
- b. bicipitoradialis; bicipitoradial b.
- b. of calcaneal tendon
- b. of extensor carpi radialis brevis muscle
- b. of Fabricius
- iliac b.
- infrahyoid b.
- infrapatellar b.
- intermuscular b.
- ischial b.
- omental b.
- b. of piriformis muscle
- retrohyoid b
- retromammary b.
- sacral b.
- b. of semimembranosus muscle
- subacromial b.
- subcutaneous b.
- subdeltoid b.
- subfascial b.
- submuscular b.
- subtendinous b.
- suprapatellar b.
- b. of tensor veli palatini muscle
- trochanteric b.

"bursa-equivalent" tissue
bursal
- b. abscess
- b. cyst

bursitis
- anserine b.
- iliopectineal b.
- ischiogluteal b.
- prepatellar b.
- septic b.
- traumatic b.
- trochanteric b.

burst
- b.-forming unit-erythroid
- metabolic b.
- respiratory b.
- b. suppression

Buruli ulcer
BUS — Bartholin's, urethral, Skene's (glands)

Buschké-Löwenstein
  giant condyloma
  tumor
Busse's saccharomyces
busulfan; busulphan
butabarbital sodium
butadiene
butane
butanoic acid
butanol
  b.-extractable iodine assay
  b.-extractable iodine test
2-butanone
butaperazine
Butchart staging system
butene
butethamine hydrochloride
butopyronoxyl
butorphanol tartrate
butoxypolypropylene glycol
butter
  b. of antimony
  b. of arsenic
butterfat
"butterfly" rash
Butter's cancer
buttonhole stenosis
butyl
  b. acetate
  b. alcohol
  b. aminobenzoate
  b. carbitol
  b. chloride
  b. methacrylate
  b. nitrite
N-butyl acetanilide
butyleneglycol dehydrogenase
butylidene chloride
butylmethyl ketone

butylphenamide
butyraceous
butyrate coenzyme A transferase
Butyribacterium
butyric acid
butyroid tumor
butyrophenone
butyrous colony
butyryl
butyrylcholine
butyryl-coenzyme A dehydrogenase
buyo cheek cancer
BV — biologic value
  blood vessel
  blood volume
  bronchovesicular
BVH — biventricular hypertrophy
BVI — blood vessel invasion
B virus hepatitis
BVV — bovine vaginitis virus
BW — birth weight
  body water
  body weight
Bwamba
  fever
  fever virus
BX — biopsy
BYE — Barile-Yaguchi-Eveland (culture medium)
bypass
  aortorenal b.
  b. capacitor
  cardiopulmonary b.
  coronary artery b.
  fundoesophageal b.
  intestinal b.
  jejuno-esophageal b.
  jejunoileal b.
byssinosis
byte

C — calculus
    calorie (large)
    carbohydrate
    carbon
    cervical
    complement
    compound
    contracture
    coulomb
    curie
    cytidine
    cytosine
C. — cathodal
    cathode
    Celsius
    centigrade
    clearance
    clonus
    closure
    color sense
    congius (gallon)
    contraction
    cylinder
C. — *Clostridium*
    Cryptococcus
c. — calorie (small)
    contact
    curie
C_{alb} — albumin clearance
C_{am} — amylase clearance
C_{cr} — creatinine clearance
C_{in} — insulin clearance
C_{pah} — para-aminohippurate
    clearance
C_u — urea clearance
C antigen
CA — cancer
    carcinoma
    cardiac arrest
    cathode
    cervicoaxial
    chronological age
    cold agglutinin
    common antigen
    coronary artery
    corpora amylacea
    croup-associated (virus)
    cytosine arabinoside
CA-2 (colloid antigen)
CA 15-3 antigen

CA 19-9 antigen
CA-50 antigen
CA-125 antigen — *nl is < 30*
Ca — calcium
    cancer
    cathodal
    cathode
CAA — regular constitutional aplastic anemia
CAB — coronary artery bypass
CABG — coronary artery bypass graft
Cabot's ring bodies
cacao oil
CACC — cathodal closure contraction
cachectic
    c. anergy
    c. endocarditis
cachectin
Cache Valley virus
cachexia
    cancerous c.
    c. exophthalmica
    c. hypophysiopriva
    malarial c.
    c. reaction
    Simmonds's c.
    c. strumipriva
    c. suprarenalis
    thyroid c.
    uremic c.
cachexin
cacocholia
cacodylate buffer
cacodylic acid
cacoethic
cactinomycin
cacumen
CAD — coronary artery disease
cadaver donor
cadaveric spasm
cadaverine
cadence
    counting c.
cadmium
    c. sulfide
    c. telluride detector
CADTe — cathodal-duration tetanus
café au lait spots
caffeic acid
caffeine sodium benzoate

CAG — chronic atrophic gastritis
CAH — chronic active hepatitis
      congenital adrenal hyperplasia
CAHD — coronary atherosclerotic heart disease
CAHEA — Committee on Allied Health Education and Accreditation
Cahn-Ingold-Prelog sequence rules
caisson disease
Cajal's
      astrocyte stain
      cell
      formol ammonium bromide solution
      gold-sublimate method
      uranium silver method
cake kidney
Cal. — large calorie
cal. — small calorie
calabar swelling
calamine
calamus scriptorius
C/alb — albumin clearance
calcaneal osteochondritis
calcaneus (pl., calcanei)
calcar
      c. avis
      c. femorale
      c. pedis
calcareous
      c. degeneration
      c. infiltration
      c. metastasis
calcarine
      c. artery
      c. fissure
calcariuria
calcein
calcemia
calcicosis
calciferol
calcific
      c. aortic stenosis
      c. concretions
      c. dystrophy
      c. nodular aortic stenosis
      c. nodular stenosis
      c. stenosis
calcification
      dystrophic c.

      focal c.
      medial c.
      metastatic c.
      mitral annulus c.
      mitral valve c.
      Mönckeberg's c.
      Mönckeberg's medial c.
      pathologic c.
      soft tissue c.
calcified
      c. cartilage
      c. granuloma
      c. granulomatous inflammation
calcifying
      c. ameloblastoma
      c. epithelial odontogenic tumor
      Malherbe's c. epithelioma
      c. pancreatitis
calcinosis
      c. circumscripta
      c. cutis
      dystrophic c.
      c. intervertebralis
      reversible c.
      tumoral c.
      c. universalis
calcinuric diabetes
calciorrhachia
calciotropism
calcipenia
calcipexic
calcipexis; calcipexy
calciphilia
calciphylaxis
      systemic c.
      topical c.
calcite
calcitonin
      c. gene-related peptide
      c. mRNA (messenger RNA)
      c. peptide
      c.-producing cell
      c. testing
calcitriol
calcitropic
calcium
      c. 45
      c. acetate formalin
      c.-activated ATPase
      c. aminosalicylate
      c. arsenate

c. arsenite
c. assay
Baker's formol c.
c. balance
c. benzoate
c. bilirubinate crystals
c. calculus
c. carbimide, citrated
c. carbonate
c. carcinate
c. caseinate
c. caustic alkali
c. chloride
c. compound
c. crystal deposition arthritis
c. cyanamide
c. cyanide
c. deposit demonstration
c. deposition
c. disodium edathamil
c. disodium edetate
endogenous fecal c.
c. gluconate
c. gout
c. hydrogen phosphate crystals
c. hydroxyapatite
c. ion
c. ionized assay
ipodate c.
c. isotope
c. lactate
c. leucovorin
c. orotate
c. oxalate
c. oxalate calculus
c. oxalate test
c. pantothenate
c. phosphate
phosphate calculus
c. polysulfide
c. pyrophosphate
c. pyrophosphate dihydrate
   crystals
c. red
c. salts
c.-sodium channel
c. test
c. time
c. undecylenate
c. urate crystals
calciuria
calcivirus
calcofluor white

calcoglobulin
calcospherite
calculated
   c. osmolality
   c. serum osmolality
calculosis
calculous
   c. cystitis
   c. pigment
calculus (pl., calculi)
   apatite c.
   arthritic c.
   articular c.
   biliary c.
   blood c.
   branched c.
   bronchial c.
   calcium c.
   calcium oxalate c.
   calcium phosphate c.
   cardiac c.
   cholesterol c.
   combination c.
   coral c.
   cystine c.
   decubitus c.
   dendritic c.
   dental c.
   encysted c.
   fibrin c.
   fusible c.
   gastric c.
   hemic c.
   indigo c.
   intestinal c.
   joint c.
   lacrimal c.
   mammary c.
   matrix c.
   mixed c.
   mulberry c.
   nephritic c.
   oxalate c.
   pancreatic c.
   pharyngeal c.
   pigment c.
   pleural c.
   pocketed c.
   preputial c.
   primary renal c.
   prostatic c.
   renal c.

salivary c.
secondary renal c.
staghorn c.
struvite c.
urate c.
uric acid c.
urinary c.
uterine c.
vesical c.
xanthic c.
Caldwell-Moloy
classification
method
Caldwell projection
calefacient
calentura; calenture
caliber
calibrate
calibration
c. curve
film density c.
calibrator
dose c.
calicectasis
calicivirus
caliculus
lacrimal c.
caliectasis
California encephalitis
C.e. virus
C.e. virus titer
californium
calix (pl., calices)
CALLA — common acute lymphoblastic leukemia an-
tigen
Call-Exner bodies
calling sequence
Calliphora vomitoria
Calliphoridae
Callison's fluid
Callitroga
callosal
callosity
callosomarginal
callosum
callus
bony c.
central c.
definitive c.
ensheathing c.

myelogenous c.
provisional c.
Calmette-Guérin bacillus
calmodulin
calomel
calomel electrode
calor
c. febrilis
c. fervens
c. innatus
c. mordicans
caloradiance
calorescence
caloric
c. deficiency
c. quotient
calorie
gram-c.
large c.
small c.
calorigenesis
calorigenic action
calorimeter
calorimetry
calotte
calsequestrin
calusterone
calutron
calvacin
calvaria
Calvatia gigantea
calycectasis
calyectasis
Calymmatobacterium
C. *donovania*
C. *granulomatis*
calyx (pl., calyces)
c. chlorata
major c.
minor c.
renal c.
c. sulfurata
CAM — chorioallantoic membrane
contralateral axillary metastasis
C/am — amylase clearance
cambium layer
cameloid anemia
camera
gamma c.
c. lucida
c. oculi

c. pulpi
scintillation c.
CAMP — cyclophosphamide, Adriamycin, methotrexate, and procarbazine
CAMP factor
CAMP test
cAMP — adenosine 3′,5′-cyclic phosphate
cyclic adenosine monophosphate
cAMP-dependent protein kinase
Campbell's cruciate sulcus
campesterol
Camp-Gianturco method
camphene
camphor assay
camphorism
camptocormia
Campylobacter
    C. cinaedi
    C. coli
    C. fennelliae
    C. fetus
    C. fetus enteritis
    C. fetus intestinalis
    C. fetus jejuni
    C. gastritis
    C. jejuni
    C. pylori
    C. sputorum
Campylobacter septicemia
campylobacteriosis
Canada balsam
canal
    adductor c.
    anal c.
    auditory c.
    cervical c.
    Cloquet's c.
    endocervical c.
    femoral c.
    Hering's c.
    Hunter's c.
    hyaloid c.
    Hyrtl's c.
    inguinal c.
    interfacial c.
    internal auditory c.
    Lambert's c.
    Nuck's c.
    Schlemm's c.

semicircular c.
spiral c.
Sucquet-Hoyer c.
Volkmann's c.
canalicular adenoma
canaliculus (pl., canaliculi)
    apical c.
    bile canaliculi
    bile duct c.
    innominate c.
    intercellular c.
    lacrimal c.
    mastoid c.
    secretory c.
    Thiersch's canaliculi
    tympanic c.
canalization
canalized thrombus
Canavalia
canavalin
canavaninosuccinic acid
cancellous
    c. bone
    c. tissue
cancer
    acinar c.
    acinous c.
    adenoid c.
    c. à deux
    alveolar c.
    aniline c.
    apinoid c.
    c. atrophicans
    betel c.
    black c.
    branchiogenous c.
    breast c.
    bronchogenic c.
    Butter's c.
    buyo cheek c.
    cecal c.
    cerebriform c.
    cervical lymph node c.
    chimney sweep's c.
    chondroid c.
    cloacogenic c.
    colloid c.
    colorectal c.
    conjugal c.
    cystic c.
    dendritic c.
    dermoid c.

encephaloid c.
c. en cuirasse
endometrial c.
endothelial c.
epidermoid c.
epithelial c.
esophageal c.
extragonadal germ cell c.
familial c.
glandular c.
green c.
hematoid c.
c. in situ
c. juice
kang c.; kangri c.
lymph node c.
medullary thyroid c.
melanotic c.
mesenchymal c.
metastatic c.
mouse c.
mule-spinner's c.
non–small-cell lung c.
occult c.
ovarian c.
pancreatic c.
paraffin c.
parietal c.
periampullary c.
peritoneal c.
pipe-smoker's c.
pitch-worker's c.
prostatic c.
renal c.
retrograde c.
scar c.
schistosomal bladder c.
scirrhous c.
small-cell lung c.
solanoid c.
spider c.
c. staging
stump c.
telangiectatic c.
testicular c.
tubular c.
uroepithelial c.
uterine c.
villous duct c.
Cancer and Acute Leukemia Group
canceration
canceremia

cancericidal
cancerigenic
Cancer Information Service
cancerocidal
cancerous cachexia
cancra
cancriform
cancroid
cancrum (pl., cancra)
    c. nasi
    c. oris
candela
candicidin
Candida
    C. *albicans*
    C. *albidus*
    C. *esophagitis*
    C. *glabrata*
    C. *guilliermondii*
    C. *krusei*
    C. *laurentii*
    C. *lusitaniae*
    C. *luteolus*
    C. *meningitis*
    C. *mesenterica*
    C. *parakrusei*
    C. *parapsilosis*
    C. *proctitis*
    C. *pseudotropicalis*
    C. *stellatoidea*
    C. *stomatitis*
    C. *tropicalis*
    C. *vini*
    C. *viswanathii*
candidal
    c. cystitis
    c. endocarditis
    c. esophagitis
    c. granuloma
    c. meningitis
    c. vaginitis
candida precipitin test
candidemia
candidiasis
    acute pseudomembranous c.
    atrophic c.
    bronchial c.
    cutaneous c.
    disseminated c.
    hepatosplenic c.
    mucocutaneous c.

pulmonary c.
c. serologic test
candidid
candidin
candidosis
candiduria
canescent
Canis
canities
canker sore
cannabinoid
cannabis
cannabism
Cannon-Bard theory
Cannon's ring
cannula
cannulation
venous c.
canrenoate potassium
canrenone
cantharidin
canthomeatal line
canthus (pl., canthi)
inner c.
outer c.
CAO — chronic airway obstruction
caoutchouc pelvis
CAP — capsule
cellulose acetate phthalate
chloramphenicol
College of American
Pathologists
cystine aminopeptidase
cap
c. cell
head c.
phrygian c.
pyloric c.
skull c.
TBG (thyroxine-binding globulin) c.
capacitance
membrane c.
capacitation
capacitive reactance
capacitor
bypass c.
ceramic c.
coupling c.
disk c.
electrolytic c.
filter c.
junction c.

Mylar c.
output c.
paper c.
variable c.
capacity
blood buffering c.
buffer c.
dye-binding c.
forced vital c.
inspiratory reserve c.
iron-binding c.
latent iron-binding c.
storage c.
total iron-binding c.
trypsin-inhibitory c.
unsaturated iron-binding c.
unsaturated vitamin B_{12}–binding c.
capillarectasia
Capillaria
C. *hepatica*
C. *philippinensis*
capillariasis
capillaritis
capillarity
capillaropathy
capillary
c. action
c. angioma
arterial c's
basement membrane c's
bile c's
c. blood
continuous c's
c. electrophoresis
c. embolism
endothelial c's
erythrocytic c's
fenestrated c's
c. flames
c. fragility
c. fragility test
glomerular c's
c. hemangioma
c. loops
c. lymphangioma
lymphatic c's
c. nevus
secretory c's
sinusoidal c's
c. telangiectasia
venous c's

capillus
capistration
capita
capitate
capitis
    pityriasis c.
Caplan's nodules
capneic
Capnocytophaga
capnohepatography
capobenate sodium
capon-comb-growth test
capotement
capping
caprate
    cellulose c.
capreomycin
capric acid
caproic acid
caprylate
    zinc c.
caprylic acid
capsicum
capsid
capsomer
capsula adiposa
capsular
    c. antigen
    c. cell
    c. cirrhosis of liver
    c. ligament
    c. space
capsule
    adrenal c.
    articular c.
    bacterial c.
    Bowman's c.
    c. cell
    external c.
    extreme c.
    Glisson's c.
    hepatic c.
    internal c.
    kidney c.
    lens c.
    lymph node c.
    Müller's c.
    ovarian c.
    pituitary c.
    prostatic c.
    salivary gland c.
    splenic c.

    thymic c.
    thyroid c.
    tonsillar c.
capsulitis
    adhesive c.
    hepatic c.
capsuloma
    renal c.
captamine hydrochloride
captodiamine hydrochloride
capture
    c. cross section
    electron c.
    radiative c.
caput (pl., capita)
    c. medusae
    c. quadratum
    c. succedaneum
Carazzi's hematoxylin
carbachol
carbamate
    calcium c.
    ethyl c.
    c. kinase
carbamazepine assay
carbamide
carbamino-carbon dioxide
carbamino compound
carbaminohemoglobin
carbamoyl
    c. phosphate
    c.-phosphate synthetase
    c.-phosphate synthetase I deficiency
carbamoylaspartate
carbamoylation
carbamoyltransferase
    ornithine c.
carbamylation
    extracorporeal c.
carbamyl phosphate
carbamylurea
carbanion
carbarsone oxide
carbaryl carbaspirin calcium
carbazochrome salicylate
carbazole
carbenicillin
    c. disodium
    c. indanyl sodium
    c. phenyl sodium

c. potassium
c. sodium
carbenoxolone sodium
carbetapentate citrate
carbhemoglobin
carbide
carbimazole
carbinol
carbinoxamine maleate
Carbitol
carbohemoglobin
carbohydrate
    accumulation of c's
    c. disks
    c. fermentation test
    c. identification test
    c. inversion
    c. metabolism index
    c. utilization test
carbohydrate-induced hyperlipidemia
carbohydraturia
carbolfuchsin
    c. stain
    c. methylene blue staining
        method
carbolic
    c. acid
    c. methylene blue
carbolineum
carbolism
carbol-thionin stain
carboluria
carbolxylene
carbomycin
carbon
    c. bisulfide
    c. dioxide
    c. dioxide absorbent
    c. dioxide acidosis
    c. dioxide combining power
    c. dioxide combining power
        test
    c. dioxide concentration
    c. dioxide concentration assay
    c. dioxide content
    c. dioxide dissociation curve
    c. dioxide electrode
    c. dioxide fixation
    c. dioxide narcosis
    c. dioxide output
    c. dioxide poisoning
    c. dioxide pressure

c. dioxide production
c. dioxide response curve
c. dioxide tension
c. disulfide
c. disulfide assay
c. disulfide poisoning
c. gelatin mass
c. inorganic compound
c. isotope
c. monoxide
c. monoxide fractional uptake
c. monoxide hemoglobin
c. monoxide poisoning
c. oxysulfide
c. particles
radioactive c.
c. resistor
c. tetrachloride
c. tetrachloride assay
c. tetrachloride poisoning
c. trichloride
carbon 11
carbon 12
carbon 13
carbon 14
carbonate
    calcium c.
    c. dehydratase
    ferrous c.
carbon dioxide
    solid c.d.
carbon-film resistor
carbonic
    c. acid
    c. anhydrase
    c. anhydrase inhibitor
    c. dichloride
carbonium ion
carbon monoxide
    fractional uptake of c.m.
carbonuria
    dysoxidative c.
carbonyl
    c. chloride
    c. hemoglobin
    nickel c.
carbophenothion
carboprost
Carborundum
Carbowax
carboxydismutase
Carboxydomonas

γ-carboxyglutamate
γ-carboxyglutamic acid
carboxyhemoglobin
carboxyhemoglobinemia
carboxyhemoglobinuria
carboxylase
    acetyl-CoA c.
    propionate c.
    propionyl-CoA c.
    pyruvate c.
carboxylate
    c. ion
    pyrrolidone c.
carboxylation
carboxylesterase
carboxylic
    c. acid
    c. ester hydrolase
carboxyl terminal
carboxyltransferase
carboxymethylcellulose sodium
carboxypeptidase
α-carboxypeptide aminoacidohydrolase
carboxyphthalatoplatinum
carboxypolypeptidase
    arginine c.
carboxysulfhemoglobin
carboxyterminal
carbromal
carbuncle
    kidney c.
    malignant c.
    renal c.
carbuncular
carbunculosis
carcinelcosis
carcinemia
carcinoembryonic antigen
carcinogen
    chemical c.
    complete c.
    epigenetic c.
    genotoxic c.
    industrial c.
    radiation c.
    viral c.
carcinogenesis
    chemical c.
    multistage c.
carcinogenic
    c. chemicals
    c. hydrocarbon

carcinoid
    c. breast cancer
    bronchial c.
    c. of bronchus
    c. flush
    c. heart disease
    c. syndrome
    c. tumor
carcinolytic
carcinoma (pl., carcinomas or carcinomata)
    acinar c.
    acinar cell c.
    acinic cell c.
    acinose c.; acinous c.
    adenocystic c.
    adenoid cystic c.
    adenoid squamous cell c.
    c. adenomatosum
    adenosquamous c.
    adnexal c.
    adrenal cortical c.
    aldosterone-producing c.
    aldosterone-secreting c.
    alveolar c.
    alveolar cell c.
    ameloblastic c.
    anaplastic c.
    angioinvasive encapsulated c.
    apocrine c.
    basal cell c., alveolar
    basal cell c., comedo
    basal cell c., cystic
    basal cell c., morphea-like
    basal cell c., multicentric
    basal cell c., nodulo-ulcerative
    basal cell c., pigmented
    basal cell c., sclerosing
    basal cell c., superficial
    basaloid c.
    basal squamous cell c.
    c. basocellulare
    basosquamous c.; basisquamous c.
    bile duct c.
    bilharzial c.
    breast c.
    bronchial c.
    bronchioalveolar c.
    bronchiolar c.
    bronchioloalveolar c.

bronchogenic c.
cerebriform c.
ceruminous c.
cholangiocellular c.
chorionic c.
choroid plexus c.
clear cell c.
cloacogenic c.
collision c.
colloid c.
colorectal c.
congenital c.
cortisol-producing c.
cribriform c.
c. cutaneum
cylindromatous c.
cystic c.
duct c.; ductal c.
ductal c. in situ
c. durum
eccrine c.
Ehrlich's ascites c.
embryonal c.
embryonal cell c.
encephaloid c.
c. en cuirasse
endometrial c.
endometrioid c.
c. of endometrium
epibulbar c.
epidermoid c.
epimyoepithelial c.
c. epitheliale adenoides
Epstein-Barr nasopharyngeal c.
c. erysipelatoides
c. ex mixed tumor
exophytic c.
c. expleomorphic adenoma
c. ex ulcere
familial c.
fibrinolamellar c.
fibrolamellar hepatocellular c.
fibrolamellar liver cell c.
follicular c.
gastric c.
gelatinous c.
giant cell c.
c. gigantocellulare
glandular c.
glassy cell c.
glycogen-rich clear cell c.
granulosa cell c.

hematoid c.
hepatobiliary c.
hepatocellular c.
hepatocellular bile duct c.
Hürthle cell c.
hyaline c.
infiltrating duct c.
infiltrating lobular c.
inflammatory c.
c. in situ
insular c.
intercalated duct c.
intermediate c.
intraductal c.
intraepidermal c.
intraepithelial c.
intralaryngeal c.
intratracheal c.
intraurothelial c.
invasive lobular c.
islet cell c.
juvenile embryonal c.
kangri burn c.
Krompecher's c.
Kulchitzky-cell c.
large cell c.
latent c.
lateral aberrant thyroid c.
lenticular c.
c. lenticulare
leptomeningeal c.
lipomatous c.
liver cell c.
lobular c.
lobular c. in situ
lymphoepithelial c.
c. mastoides
c. medullare
medullary c.
c. melanodes
melanotic c.
meningeal c.
Merkel's cell c.
mesometanephric c.
mesonephric c.
metaplastic c.
metastatic c.
metatypical c.
microinvasive c.
micropapillary c.
mixed c.
mixed hepatocellular c.

mixed medullary-follicular c.
mixed papillary-follicular c.
c. molle
mucinous c.
mucoepidermoid c.
c. mucosum
c. myxomatodes
neuroendocrine c.
noninfiltrating lobular c.
nonkeratinizing c.
non–small-cell c.
non–small-cell lung c.
oat cell c.
occult c.
odontogenic c.
oncoplastic c.
c. ossificans
Paget's c.
pancreatic c.
papilla of Vater c.
papillary c.
papillary serous c.
papillary transitional cell c.
periampullary c.
pharyngeal c.
pleomorphic c.
polypoid c.
poorly differentiated c.
porta hepatis c.
prickle cell c.
primary c.
primary intraosseous c.
prostatic c.
recurrent c.
renal cell c.
reserve cell c.
residual c.
rete testis c.
reticular cell c.
salivary duct c.
c. sarcomatodes
sarcomatoid c.
scar c.
schneiderian c.
scirrhous c.
sclerosing c.
c. scroti
sebaceous c.
secondary c.
secretory c.
signet cell c.
signet-ring cell c.

c. simplex
c. in situ
small-cell c.
solanoid c.
solid c.
spheroidal cell c.
spindle cell c.
c. spongiosum
squamous cell c.
sudoriferous c.
superficial multicentric basal
     cell c.
sweat gland c.
c. telangiectaticum
c. telangiectodes
terminal duct c.
thymic c.
thyroid c.
trabecular c.
transitional cell c.
tuberous c.
tubular c.
tubulolobular c.
undifferentiated c.
undifferentiated epidermoid c.
undifferentiated squamous
     cell c.
urachal c.
urothelial transitional cell c.
uterine corpus c.
vaginal squamous c.
varicoid c.
verrucous c.
villous c.
c. villosum
virilizing c.
Walker c.
warty c.
wolffian duct c.
yolk sac c.
carcinomatoid
carcinomatosus
     leptomeningeal c.
     meningeal c.
carcinomatous
     c. cirrhosis
     c. encephalomyelopathy
     c. implants
     c. meningoencephalopathy
     c. myelopathy
     c. myopathy
     c. neuromyopathy

c. pericarditis
c. polyneuropathy
carcinophobia
carcinosarcoma
  embryonal c.
  renal c.
  Walker c.
carcinosis
  miliary c.
  c. pleurae
  pulmonary c.
carcinostatic
carcinous
cardia
  gastric c.
cardiac
  c. albuminuria
  c. aneurysm
  c. arrest
  c. arrhythmia
  c. bronchus
  c. calculus
  c. catheterization
  c. cirrhosis
  c. conduction alteration
  c. conduction system
  c. cycle
  c. decompensation
  c. dilation
  c. disease
  c. diuretic
  c. edema
  c. enlargement
  c. enzymes
  c. epithelium
  c. failure
  c. fibrillation
  c. glycoside
  c. hemoptysis
  c. heterotaxia
  c. histiocyte
  c. index
  c. injury
  c. isoenzyme
  c. lymphoma
  c. massage
  c. murmur
  c. muscle
  c. myxoma
  c. nerve
  c. neuralgia
  c. output curve

c. plexus
c. polyp
c. prosthesis
c. rate alteration
c. rhythm alteration
c. sclerosis
c. shunt detection
c. shunting
c. silhouette
c. sound alteration
c. standstill
c. tamponade
c. thrombosis
c. valve
c. valve myxomatosis
c. valvular malformation
c. valvular regurgitation
cardialgia
cardiasthenia
cardiectasis
cardinal
cardioangiography
Cardiobacterium hominis
cardiocentesis
cardiochalasia
cardiocyte
cardioesophageal
  c. junction
  c. sphincter
cardiogenesis
cardiogenic shock
Cardiografin
cardiogram
cardiography
Cardio-Green
cardiolipin
  c. natural lecithin
  c. synthetic lecithin
cardiolith
cardiology
cardiomalacia
cardiomegaly
cardiomyoliposis
cardiomyopathy
  Adriamycin c.
  alcoholic c.
  cardiotoxic c.
  catecholamine c.
  congestive c.
  dilated c.
  hypertrophic c.
  hypothyroid c.

idiopathic c.
ischemic c.
obstructive hypertrophic c.
peripartum c.
periportal c.
primary c.
restrictive/infiltrative c.
secondary c.
thyrotoxic c.
cardionecrosis
cardionector hypothesis
cardiopathy
cardioplegia
cardioptosia
cardiopulmonary
c. bypass
c. resuscitation
cardiospasm
cardiosphygmograph
cardiotachometer
cardiothoracic (ratio)
cardiotocography
cardiotoxic myolysis
cardiotoxicity
anthracycline c.
cardiotropic drugs
cardiovascular
c. accident
c. control centers
c. disease
c. malformation
c. murmur
c.-renal cerebrovascular resistance
c. renal disease
c. syphilis
c. system
cardiovascular disease
arteriosclerotic c.d.
hypertensive c.d.
cardioversion
cardioverter
cardiovirus
carditis
rheumatic c.
streptococcal c.
verrucous c.
Carey's Ranvier technique
Carica papaya
caries
dental c.

carina (pl., carinae)
c. of trachea
c. of vagina
carinate
carinatum
pectus c.
cariogenesis
carious
carisoprodol
carmalum
carmine
alizarin c.
alum c.
chrome alum c.
c. dye
c. gelatin mass
indigo c.
lithium c.
Schneider's c.
carminic acid
carminomycin
carminophil; carminophile
carminophilous
carmustine
carnaceous
carneous
c. degeneration
c. mole
Carney's
procedure
triad
carnification
carnitine
c. acetyltransferase
c. palmitoyl transferase
Carnivora
carnosinase
carnosine
carnosinemia
carnosinuria
carnosity
Carnoy's fixative
carotenase
carotene
carotenemia
carotenoid
provitamin A c's
carotic
caroticotympanic
carotid
c. artery
c. body
c. body tumor

c.-cavernous fistula
c. nerve
c. paraganglioma
c. plexus
c. sheath
c. sinus
c. sinus nerve
c. sinus stimulation
c. sinus syncope
c. sinus syndrome
c. tracing
carotinemia
carpal
    c. bone
    c. tunnel
    c. tunnel decompression
    c. tunnel syndrome
carphenazine maleate
carphology
Carpoglyphus passularum
carpometacarpal joint
carpophalangeal
carpocarpal dysplasia
carprofen
carpus curvus
carrier
    c. cell
    female c.
    c.-free
    c. gas
    c.-mediated transport
    c. protein
Carr-Price reaction
cartesian
    c. coordinates
    c. nomogram
cartilage
    articular c.
    arytenoid c.
    auricular c.
    c. bone
    bronchial c.
    calcified c.
    corniculate c.
    costal c.
    cricoid c.
    cuneiform c.
    epiglottic c.
    fibroelastic c.
    greater alar c.
    c.-hair hypoplasia
    hyaline c.

c. lacunae
laryngeal c.
lateral nasal c.
c. matrix alteration
Meckel's c.
metaplastic c.
nasal c.
nasal septal c.
Santorini's c.
thyroid c.
tracheal c.
vomeronasal c.
cartilaginous
    c. exostosis
    c. joint
    c. metaplasia
    c. rest
Cartwright's
    antigen
    blood group system
    test
caruncle
    amniotic c's
    hymenal c's
    lacrimal c.
    papillomatous c.
    sublingual c.
    urethral c.
caruncula (pl., carunculae)
    c. sublingualis
carvacrol
caryochrome
casanthranol
cascade
    electron c.
    metastatic c.
cascara sagrada
case
    c.-control study
    c. fatality rate
    c. history
    index c.
caseating
    c. granuloma
    c. granulomatous inflammation
    c. inflammation
caseation necrosis
casein
    c. agar
    c.-calcium
    c. hydrolysate
    serum c.

caseinate
    calcium c.
caseous
    c. abscess
    c. degeneration
    c. inflammation
    c. necrosis
    c. osteitis
    c. pericarditis
    c. pneumonia
    c. tubercle
    c. tuberculosis
Casoni's intradermal test
cassette
cast
    bile c.
    blood c.
    bronchial c's
    coma c.
    corrosion c.
    decidual c.
    endometrial c.
    epithelial c.
    false c.
    fatty c.
    fibrinous c.
    granular c.
    hemoglobin c.
    hyaline c.
    inclusion c's
    mucous c.
    pigmented c's
    red cell c's
    renal c.
    spurious c.
    tube c.
    urinary c.
    waxy c.
    white cell c's
Castellanella castellani
Castellania
Castellani's test
Castenada technique
casting
Castleman's giant lymph node hyperplasia
Castle's intrinsic factor
castor
    c. bean
    c. oil
castrate

castration
    c. cells
    female c.
    male c.
    parasitic c.
CAT — chlormerodrin accumulation test
    computed axial tomography
    computerized axial tomography
cat
    c. liver fluke
    c. unit
catabasis
catabiosis
catabolic
catabolism
    antibody c.
    heme c.
catabolite
    c. activator protein
    c. repression
cataclysm
catacrotic limb
catacrotism
catagenesis
catalase test
catalepsy
catalysis
    contact c.
catalyst
    negative c.
catalytic
catalyze
catalyzer
catamenia
catamnesis
cataphasia
cataphoresis
cataphoretic
cataphylaxis
cataplectic
cataplexy
catapophysis
cataract
    brunescent c.
    cortical c.
    glaucomatous c.
    intumescent c.
    morgagnian c.
    posterior subcapsular c.
    senile c.

Soemmering's c.
subcapsular c.
catarrh
catarrhal
   c. appendicitis
   c. conjunctivitis
   c. dysentery
   c. gastritis
   c. inflammation
   c. ophthalmia
catatonia
catatonic schizophrenia
catatorulin test
catatrichy
cat-bite fever
cat-cry syndrome
catechin
catechinic acid
catechol
   c. O-methyl transferase
   c. oxidase
catecholamine
   c. assay
   c. cardiomyopathy
   c. excess
   c. metabolite
   c.-secreting tumor
   c. test
catechuic acid
categorical data
Catenabacterium
caterpillar cell
cath. — cathartic
   catheter
   catheterize
catharsis
cathemoglobin
cathepsin
catheptic enzyme
catheretic
catheter
   balloon c.
   Foley c.
   Groshong c.
   Gruentzig balloon c.
   Hickman c.
   indwelling c.
   prostatic c.
   Swan-Ganz c.
   toposcopic c.
catheterization
   cardiac c.

indwelling vascular c.
retrourethral c.
ureteral c.
urethral c.
cathexis
cathodal opening tetanus
cathode
   c. ray
   c.-ray tube
cathodoluminescence
cation
   c.-anion difference
   c. channel
   c.-exchange chromatography
   c.-exchange resin
   c. interference
cationic dye
cationogen
cat liver fluke
cat-scratch disease
cat's-eye syndrome
cauda (pl., caudae)
   c. equina
   c. nuclei caudati
caudad
caudal
   c. area
   d. displacement
   c. duplication
   c. myotome
caudalis
caudalizing agent
caudate
   c. lobe
   c. nucleus
   c. vein
cauliflower ear
Caulobacter
caumesthesia
causalgia
causative
cause
   constitutional c.
   c. of death
   predisposing c.
   proximate c.
   c.-specific death rate
caustic
cauter
cauterant
cauterization
cautery

CAV — congenital absence of vagina
  congenital adrenal virilism
caveola (pl., caveolae)
cavernitis
  fibrous c.
cavernoscopy
cavernositis
cavernous
  c. angioma
  c. hemangioma
  c. lymphangiectasis
  c. lymphangioma
  c. plexus
  c. sinus
CA virus
cavitary pulmonary lesion
cavitating inflammation
cavitation
Cavitron ultrasonic surgical aspirator
cavity
  absorption c's
  accessory sinus c.
  amniotic c.
  body c.
  chorionic c.
  cranial c.
  endometrial c.
  exocoelomic c.
  glenoid c.
  inflammatory c.
  laryngeal c.
  nasal c.
  nasopharyngeal c.
  oral c.
  pelvic peritoneal c.
  pericardial c.
  peritoneal c.
  pharyngeal c.
  pleural c.
  renal pelvic c.
  c. resonator
  serous c.
  thoracic c.
  tympanic c.
  upper respiratory tract c.
  urinary bladder c.
cavography
  inferior vena c.
cavum (pl., cava)
  c. septic pellucidi
  c. vergae
cavus

CB — chronic bronchitis
Cb — columbium
CBA — chronic bronchitis with
  asthma
CB (chocolate blood) agar
C-banding
  C-b. stain
CBC — complete blood count
CBD — common bile duct
CBF — cerebral blood flow
  coronary blood flow
CBG — corticosteroid-binding globulin
  cortisol-binding globulin
CBS — chronic brain syndrome
CBV — central blood volume
  circulating blood volume
  corrected blood volume
CC — cardiac cycle
  chief complaint
  compound cathartic
  cord compression
  costochondral
  creatinine clearance
cc — cubic centimeter
CCA — chick-cell agglutination
  chimpanzee coryza agent
  choriocarcinoma
  common carotid artery
CCAT — conglutinating complement
  absorption test
CCC — cathodal-closing contraction
  chronic calculous cholecystitis
CCCl — cathodal-closure clonus
C cell hyperplasia
C cells
CCF — cephalin-cholesterol flocculation
  compound comminuted fracture
  congestive cardiac failure
  crystal-induced chemotactic
  factor
CCK — cholecystokinin
CCK-PZ — cholecystokinin-
  pancreozymin
c. cm. — cubic centimeter
C_3 complement
C_4 complement
C3 convertase
CCP — ciliocytophthoria

C/cr — creatinine clearance
CCTe — cathodal-closure tetanus
CCU — Cherry-Crandall units
    Coronary Care Unit
CCV — conductivity cell volume
CCW — counterclockwise
CD — cadaver donor
    cardiac disease
    cardiac dullness
    cardiovascular disease
    circular dichroism
    cluster of differentiation
    common duct
    conjugata diagonalis
    consanguineous donor
    curative dose
    cystic duct
CD_{50} — median curative dose
Cd — cadmium
    caudal
    coccygeal
cd — candela
CDA — congenital dyserythropoietic
    anemia
CD 5 antigen
CDC — Centers for Disease Control
    and Prevention
    chenodeoxycholate
CDE — canine distemper encephalitis
    chlordiazepoxide
    common duct exploration
CDH — ceramide dihexoside
    congenital dislocation of the
    hip
CDL — chlorodeoxylincomycin
cDNA — complementary DNA
cDNA clone
cDNA library
CDP — cytidine diphosphate
CDP-choline
CDP diacylglycerol
CDP-diglyceride
CDR — complementarity-
    determining region
CE — California encephalitis
    cardiac enlargement
    chick embryo
    cholesterol esters
    contractile element
Ce — cerium
CEA — carcinoembryonic antigen
    crystalline egg albumin

ceanothus extract
cebocephalus
cebocephaly
cecal cancer
cecectomy
cecitis
cecosigmoidostomy
cecostomy
cecum (pl., ceca)
    minor c.
cedar oil
Cedecea davisae
CEDIA — cloned enzyme donor im-
    munoassay
CEEV — Central European encephali-
    tis virus
CEF — chick embryo fibroblast
cefaclor
cefadroxil
cefamandole
cefaparole
cefatrizine
cefazaflur sodium
cefazolin
cefoperazone
ceforanide
cefotaxime
cefoxitin
ceftazidime
ceftriaxone
Cel — Celsius
Celebes vibrio
celestin blue B
Celestin's tube
celiac
    c. artery
    c. axis
    c. crisis
    c. disease
    c. ganglion
    c. lymph node
    c. plexus
    c. rickets
    c. sprue
celiectomy
celiocentesis
celioma
celiomyositis
celioparacentesis
celiopathy
celioscopy
celitis

cell

A c.
absorption c.
absorptive c.
acanthoid c's
accessory c's
acidophil c.
acidophilic c's
acinar c.
c. adhesion molecular deficiency
adipose c.
adrenal cortical c.
adrenocorticotropic c.
adventitious c.
algoid c.
alpha c's
alveolar c.
amacrine c's
amphophil c.
anabiotic c's
anaplastic c.
aneuploid c's
Anichkov's (Anitschkow's) c.
anterior horn c.
antibody-forming c's
antigen-presenting c.
anti-parietal c.
apocrine c.
argentaffin c's
argyrophilic c's
Arias-Stella c's
Armanni-Ebstein c's
Aschoff's c.
Askanazy's c.
automatic c.
c. axis
B c's
balloon c.
band c's
barrier-layer c.
basal c.
basket c.
basophilic c.
berry c.
beta c's
Betz c's
Bevan-Lewis c.
bipolar c.
Bizzozero's red c's
blast c.
c. block preparation

blood c's
c. body
Boettcher c's
bone c.
bovine red blood c's
bronchial c's
bronchiolar c.
buffy-coated c's
burr c.
C c's
Cajal c.
calciform c.
calcitonin-producing c.
cameloid c.
cap c.
capsular c.
capsule c.
carrier c.
Casperson type B c's
castration c's
caterpillar c.
caudate c's
centroacinar c's
chalice c.
chief c.
chromaffin c's
chromophobe c.
chronic c. leukemia
chronic lymphosarcoma c.
circulating c's
circulating reticuloendothelial c's
Clara c's
clear c.
cleavage c.
cleaved c.
c. coat
colloid c's
columnar c.
comet c.
committed progenitor c's
concentrated red c's
Conway c.
corticotroph c.
c. count
c. counter
crenated c's
crescent c.
Crooke's c's
crystal c.
cuboidal c's
c. culture

Custer's c's
c. cycle
c.-cycle determination
c.-cycle inhibitor
c. cycle time
cytotoxic c.
cytotoxic T c's
daughter c.
decidual c's
decoy c.
delta c's
dendritic epidermal c's
c. differentiation
c. division
Dorothy Reed c's
Downey's c's
dust c.
Edelmann's c.
effector c's
electrochemical c.
electrolytic c.
endocrine c's
endothelial c's
enterochromaffin c's
c. envelope
ependymal c's
epithelial c's
epithelioid c.
erythrocytic blood c.
erythroid c's
erythropoietin-responsive c.
eukaryotic c's
excitable c.
exudation c.
Fañana's c.
Ferrata's c's
flame c.
foam c.
follicular c's
foreign body giant c.
Foulis' c.
c.-free system
frozen red c's
fuchsinophil c.
fusiform c's
c. fusion
galvanic c.
gametoid c's
gamma c's
ganglion c's
Gaucher's c.
Gegenbaur's c.

germ c.
germinal c.
ghost c.
giant c.
gitter c.
Gley's c's
glia c.
glitter c's
globoid c.
glomerular c.
glomus c.
goblet c.
gonadotropic c.
Graham's c's
granulocytic blood c.
granulosa c's
granulosa-lutein c's
H c.
H-2^b mouse c's
hair c.
hairy c's
Hargraves' c.
heart failure c's
Heidenhain's c's
HeLa c's
helmet c.
helper c.
helper T c's
hematopoietic stem c.
heteromeral c's
high-peroxidase c's
hilar c's
hilus c's
hobnail c.
Hodgkin's c.
Hofbauer c's
homozygous typing c.
horizontal c. of retina
horse red blood c's
Hürthle c's
hybrid c.
hyperchromatic c.
hyperplastic c's
I c.
immunocompetent c's
immunologically activated c.
immunologically competent c.
immunoreactive c's
inclusion c's
c. inclusions
inducer T c.
interfollicular c.

interstitial c's
intimal c.
intracytoplasmic inclusion c's
irreversibly sickled c.
irritation c.
islet c's
c. junction
juvenile c.
juxtaglomerular c's
K c's
karyochrome c's
K-B c.
killer c.
c. kinetics
Kulchitsky's c's
Kupffer's c's
L c's
labile c's
lacunar c's
LAK c's
Langerhans's c.
Langerhans's giant c.
Langhans's giant c's
Langhans-type giant c's
LE (lupus erythematosus) c.
Leber's c's
Leishman's chrome c's
lepra c.
leukemic c's
leukocyte-poor red blood c's
Leydig's c.
Leydig's interstitial c's
light c.
c. line
Lipschütz c.
littoral c.
Loevit's c.
lupus erythematosus c.
lutein c's
Lyl B c.
lymph c.
lymphadenoma c's
lymphocytic blood c's
lymphoid c's
lymphoid stem c.
lymphokine-activated killer c's
lymphoreticular c's
Marchand's c.
c. marker
Martinotti's c's
mast c's
c.-mediated immune response

c.-mediated immunity
c.-mediated lympholysis assay
megakaryocytic blood c.
c. membrane
Merkel-Ranvier c's
Merkel's c.
mesenchymal c's
mesothelial c's
metallophil c's
Mexican hat c.
Meynert's c's
microglial c.
migratory c's
Mikulicz's c's
mirror-image c.
mitochondrion rich c.
monkey kidney c's
monocytic blood c's
monocytoid c.
mononuclear c's
monosomic c's
Mott c.
c's of Müller
multipotential stem c's
myeloid c.
myeloma c.
myoepithelial c.
Nageotte's c's
natural killer c's
navicular c's
c. nests
neuroendocrine c's
neuroglial c's
neurosecretory c.
nevus c.
Niemann-Pick c.
NIH 3T3 c's
NK (natural killer) c's
nodal c's
noncleaved c.
non-erythroid c's
nucleated red blood c.
null c's
oat c.
OKT c's
olfactory c's
osseous c.
osteoprogenitor c.
oxyntic c.
oxyphil c.
P c's
pacemaker c.

packed c's
packed red blood c's
Paget's c.
pagetoid c's
palatine c's
pancreatic polypep-
    tide c's
Paneth's c's
parafollicular c's
paraluteal c's
parathyroid chief c.
parathyroid oxyphil c.
parathyroid transitional c.
parathyroid wasserhelle c.
parenchymal hepatic c's
parenchymatous c.
parietal c.
pathologic c.
pediculated c's
peptic c.
periglomerular c's
perineuronal satellite c.
peritubular contractile c.
pessary c.
phagocytic c.
pheochrome c.
photoconductive c.
photovoltaic c.
physaliferous c's
picket c.
Pick's c's
placental c's
plaque-forming c.
plasma c's
plasma blood c.
plasmacytic blood c.
pluripotent myeloid stem c.
pluripotential c's
pluripotential stem c's
PNH (paroxysmal nocturnal he-
    moglobinuria) c's
polychromatic c.
polychromatophil c.
pre-B c.
precursor c.
primitive neuroblastic c.
primordial germ c.
primordial sex c.
principal c.
progenitor c's
c. proliferation
pseudo-Gaucher c.

pseudoxanthoma c.
pulmonary epithelial c's
pulpar c.
Purkinje's c's
pus c.
pyrrol c.
RA (ragocyte) c.
Raji c's
red c.
red blood c.
Reed-Sternberg giant c.
Renshaw c.
reserve c.
resting c.
reticular c.
reticuloendothelial c.
reticulum c's
rhagiocrine c.
Rh-negative c's
Rieder c's
Rindfleisch's c's
rod c's
rosette-forming c's
Rouget's c.
Russell-Crooke c.
c. salvage
c. sap
sarcogenic c's
scavenger c.
Schultze's c's
Schwann's c.
secretory c.
sedimented red c's
segmented c.
seminal vesicle c's
seminoma c's
c. separation methods
septal c.
serous c.
Sertoli's c.
sex c.
Sézary c's
Sézary-Lutzner c's
shadow c's
sheep red c's
sickle c.
sickle c. β-thalassemia
sickled c.
signet-ring c.
silver c.
sinusoidal endothelial c.
skein c.

small cleaved c.
small noncleaved c.
small uncleaved c.
smudge c's
solitary c.
somatic c.
somatostatin c.
spiculated c.
spider c.
spindle c.
spindly squamoid c.
spur c.
squamous c.
squamous epithelial c's
stab c.
stable c's
stave c's
stem c's
Sternberg-Reed c.
Sternberg's giant c's
stichochrome c.
stipple c.
c. strain
strap c.
suppressor c's
suppressor T c's
c. surface receptor
sustentacular c's
sympathicotrophic c's
syncytial giant c's
synovial stromal c's
T c's
T4 c's
T8 c's
tadpole c.
tanned red c.
target c's
tart c.
tautomeral c.
T-cytotoxic c.
teardrop c.
technetium Tc-99m blood c's
tegmental c's
tetracarcinoma c's
theca c's
T-helper c's
thymic epithelial c's
thymic reticulum c.
thymus c.
totipotential c.
Touton giant c.
c. transformation

transitional c's
transitional epithelial c's
trisomic c's
T-suppressor c.
tufted c.
tumor c's
Türk's c.
tympanic c's
Type I c.
Type II c.
Tzanck c's
ultimobranchial c's
c. ultrastructure
umbrella c's
unipotential stem c's
unit c.
urothelial c's
vacuolated c.
vasoformative c's
viral inclusion c's
c. volume
c. volume profile
von Hansemann c's
von Kupffer c's
c. wall
c. wall–deficient
Warthin-Finkeldey c's
washed red c's
wasserhelle c.
water-clear c.
c. web
white c.
white blood c.
whole blood c's
xanthoma c.
zenoplated tumor c's
zymogenic c's
cell count
    viable c.c.
Cellfalcicula
cell line
    BeWo choriocarcinoma c.l.
    established c.l.
    glioblastoma c.l.
cellobiase
cellobiose/mannitol sugar permeability
    test
celloidin
cellophane tape method
celloscope
cellula

cellular
- c. adaptation
- c. atrophy
- c. atypia
- c. biology
- c. blue nevus
- c. cloning
- c. degeneration
- c. differentiation
- c. dysplasia
- c. edema
- c. embolism
- c. hybridization
- c. hypertrophy
- c. hypoxia
- c. immune deficiency
- c. immunity
- c. immunity deficiency syndrome
- c. immunodeficiency
- c. inclusions
- c. infiltration
- c. injury
- c. kinetics
- c. membranes
- c. necrosis
- c. neurofilaments
- c. oncogenes
- c. pathology
- c. polyp
- c. spill
- c. swelling
- c. tumor

cellularity
- granulocytic c.

cellulase
cellulicidal
cellulite
cellulitic phlegmasia
cellulitis
- anaerobic c.
- clostridial c.
- eosinophilic c.
- gangrenous c.
- necrotizing c.
- pelvic c.
- phlegmonous c.
- streptococcal c.

cellulocutaneous plaque
cellulofibrous
cellulose
- c. acetate electrophoresis
- c. acetate phthalate
- c. caprate
- c. membranes
- microcrystalline c.
- oxidized c.
- c. phosphate
- c. tape
- tetranitrate c.

cellulosity
Cellvibrio
- *C. flavescens*
- *C. fulvus*
- *C. mixtus*
- *C. ochraceus*
- *C. vulgaris*

celoschisis
celosomia
Celsius
- C. temperature scale
- C. thermometer

cement
- intracellular c.
- c. line
- c. substance

cemental dysplasia
cementification
cementifying fibroma
cementoblast
cementoblastoma
cementocyte
cementoma
- true c.

cemento-ossifying fibroma
cementum
cenobium
censored observation
Cent. — centigrade
cent. — centimeter
center
- cardiovascular control c's
- chiral c.
- follicular c.
- germinal c.
- satiety c.
- sweat c.

Centers for Disease Control and Prevention
centigrade
- c. temperature scale
- c. thermometer

centigram
centiliter
centimeter
- cubic c.

gram-c.
    c.-gram-second system
centimorgan
centipede
centipoise
centistoke
central
    c. blood volume
    c. callus
    c. canal
    c. chemoreceptor
    c. core disease
    c. excitatory state
    c. hemorrhagic necrosis
    c. inhibitory state
    c. lesion
    c. limit theorem
    c. necrosis
    c. nervous system
    c. nervous system tuberculosis
    c. nervous system tumors
    c. neuron
    c. osteitis
    c. pneumonia
    c. pontine myelinolysis
    c. processing unit
    c. retinal artery
    c. tendency
    c. venous pressure
Central European encephalitis virus
centralis
centric fusion
Centriflo filter
centrifugal
    c. analyzer
    c. flotation
    c. force
centrifugalization
centrifugalize
centrifugation
    density gradient c.
centrifuge
centrilobular
    c. emphysema
    c. necrosis
centriole
centripetal force
centroacinar
    c. cells
    c. emphysema
centroblast
centroblastic/centrocytic lymphoma

centrocyte
centrocytic lymphoma
centromere
    c. banding stain
    c. interference
centromere/kinetochore antibody
centromeric
    c. bands
    c. DNA
    c. index
centronuclear myopathy
centroplasm
centrosome
centrosphere
centrum (pl., centra)
Centruroides
cenurosis
cenurus
CEP — congenital erythropoietic por-
      phyria
cephacetrile sodium
Cephaelis
cephalad
cephalexin
cephalgia
cephalic
    c. index
    c. vein
cephalin-cholesterol flocculation test
cephalin flocculation test
cephaloglycin
cephalogram
cephalohematocele
cephalohematoma
cephalomegaly
cephalometer
cephalometry
    fetal c.
    roentgen c.
    ultrasonic c.
cephalonia
cephalo-oculocutaneous telangiectasia
cephalopathy
cephalopelvic disproportion
cephalopelvimetry
Cephalopoda
cephaloridine
cephalosporin
Cephalosporium
    C. falciforme
    C. granulomatis
cephalostat

cephalothin
cephalothoracopagus
cephamycin
cephapirin
Ceph. floc. — cephalin flocculation
cephradine
cera
ceramic capacitor
ceramidase
ceramide
    galactosyl c.
    D-glucose c.
    c. glucoside
    glycosyl c.
    c. hexoside
    c. lactoside
    c. lactoside lipidosis
    c. lactosidosis
    lactosyl c.
    c. trihexosidase
Cerankov radiation
Ceratophyllus
Ceratopogonidae
cercaria (pl., cercariae)
cercarial dermatitis
Cercomonas
Cercopithecus
Cercospora apii
cercosporamycosis
cerebellar
    c. agenesis
    c. artery
    c. ataxia, familial
    c. ataxia, hereditary
    c. biventral lobule
    c. ciliary body
    c. cortex
    c. declive
    c. dentate nucleus
    c. dyssynergia
    c. emboliform nucleus
    c. fasciculus uncinatus
    c. fastigial nucleus
    c. fimbriate nucleus
    c. fissure
    c. folium
    c. globose nucleus
    c. gracile lobule
    c. hemangioblastoma
    c. lenticular nucleus
    c. lobe
    c. motor tectal nucleus

c. peduncle
c. posterior inferior ansiform
    lobule
c. posterior lobe
c. pressure cone
c. pyramis
c. region
c. roof nucleus
c. sarcoma
c. tonsil
c. tuber
c. vein
c. vermis
c. white matter
cerebellomedullary cistern
cerebello-olivary
cerebellopontine angle meningioma
cerebellorubrospinal
cerebellovestibular fibers
cerebellum agenesis
cerebral
    c. abscess
    c. amyloidosis
    c. aneurysm
    c. arcuate fibers
    c. artery thrombosis
    c. atrophy
    c. blood flow
    c. cortex
    c. cortex perfusion rate
    c. death
    c. dorsum
    c. dysplasia
    c. edema
    c. embolism
    c. epidural abscess
    c. fissure
    c. gliomatosis
    c. glucose oxygen quotient
    c. gray matter
    c. hemangioma
    c. hemisphere
    c. hemorrhage
    c. herniation
    c. infarct
    c. infarction
    c. ischemia
    c. lacunae
    c. laminar necrosis
    c. medial surface
    c. metabolic rate
    c. metabolic rate of glucose

c. metabolic rate of oxygen
c. mucormycosis
c. neuroblastoma
c. pachymeningitis
c. palsy
c. peduncle
c. stroke
c. superolateral surface
c. thrombosis
c. toxoplasmosis
c. vascular accident
c. vein
c. ventricle
c. white matter
cerebralis
    adiposis c.
cerebriform
    cancer
    c. nucleus
cerebris
    mycetismus c.
cerebritis
cerebrocuprein
cerebrohepatorenal syndrome
cerebronic acid
cerebrosclerosis
cerebroside
    c.-galactosidase
    c.-glucosidase
    c. lipidosis
    c. sulfate
    c. sulfatide
cerebrosidosis
cerebrospinal
    c. meningitis
cerebrospinal fluid
    c.f. analysis
    c.f. assay
    c.f. culture
    c.f. electrophoresis
    c.f. IgG synthesis rate
    c.f. myelin basic protein
    c.f. oligoclonal bands
    c.f. pressure
    c.f. protein
    c.f. protein electrophoresis
cerebrotendinous
    c. cholesterinosis
    c. xanthoma
    c. xanthomatosis
cerebrovascular
    c. accident
    c. obstructive disease

cerebrum
Cerenkov's radiation
Cerithidea
cerium oxalate
ceroid
    c. lipofuscinosis
    c. pigment
    c. storage disease
ceroma
ceroplasty
cerous oxalate
certainty factor
certified
    c. stains
    c. standards
Certified Laboratory Assistant
Cerubedine
cerulea
    macula c.
cerulein
ceruloplasmin assay
cerumen
ceruminal
ceruminoma
ceruminous
    c. adenoma
    c. carcinoma
    c. gland
cerveau isolé
cervical
    c. adenitis
    c. artery
    c. branch
    c. canal
    c. culture
    c. cutaneous nerve
    c. diverticulum
    c. dysplasia
    c. epidermidization
    c. esophagus
    c. fascia
    c. fistula
    c. flap
    c. ganglion
    c. gland
    c. hygroma
    c. intraepithelial neoplasia
    c. lamina propria
    c. lymphatics
    c. lymph node
    c. lymphoepithelial cyst
    c. mucous membrane

c. mucus
c. myotome
c. nerve
c. plexus
c. polyp
c. rib syndrome
c. scraper
c. secretion
c. smear
c. somatosensory evoked potential
c. spinal cord
c. spondylosis
c. thymoma
c. vaginal cytology
c. vein
c. vertebrae
c. vertebral joint
cervicitis
    cystic chronic c.
    follicular c.
    gonococcal c.
cervicoaxial
cervicobrachial neuralgia
cervicofacial actinomycosis
cervico-occipital neuralgia
cervix (pl., cervices)
    incompetent c.
    c. uteri
    uterine c.
CES — central excitatory state
cesarean section
cesium
Cestoda
cestode
cestodiasis
cetaben sodium
cetalkonium chloride
cetiedil citrate
cetocycline hydrochloride
Cetraria
cetrimide-citrate-saline solution
cetrimonium bromide
cetyl
cetylpyridinium chloride
cetylpyridinium chloride test
cetyltrimethylammonium bromide
cevadine
CF — carbolfuchsin
    cardiac failure
    carrier-free
    certainty factor

    chemotactic factor
    chest and left leg
    Chiari-Frommel syndrome
    Christmas factor
    citrovorum factor
    complement fixation
    complement-fixing
    contractile force
    cystic fibrosis
C-F
CF antibody titer
Cf — californium
cf. — compare
CFA — complement-fixing antibody
    complete Freund adjuvant
CFF — critical flicker fusion test
c.f.f. — critical fusion frequency
C-fiber nociceptor
CFP — chronic false-positive
    cystic fibrosis of the pancreas
CFT — complement-fixation test
CFU-C — colony-forming unit (culture)
CFU-E — colony-forming unit (erythroid)
CFU-G — colony-forming unit (granulocyte)
CFU-L — colony-forming unit (lymphoid)
CFU-M — colony-forming unit (megakaryocyte)
CFU/mL — colony-forming units/mL
CFU-S — colony-forming unit (spleen)
CFWM — cancer-free white mouse
CG — Cardio-Green
    chorionic gonadotropin
    chronic glomerulonephritis
    colloidal gold
    phosgene (choking gas)
Cg or cg — centigram
CGD — chronic granulomatous disease
CGL — chronic granulocytic leukemia
cgm — centigram
cGMP — cyclic guanosine monophosphate
CGN — chronic glomerulonephritis
CG/OQ — cerebral glucose oxygen quotient

CGP — choline glycerophosphatide
chorionic growth hormone prolactin
circulating granulocyte pool
CGRP — calcitonin gene-related peptide
CGS or cgs — centimeter-gram-second
cgs system
cgs unit
CGT — chorionic gonadotropin
CGTT — cortisone glucose tolerance test
CH — cholesterol
crown-heel
Ch-antigen
CHA — congenital hypoplastic anemia
cyclohexylamine
Chabertia
Chaddock's sign
Chaetoconidium
Chaetomium
chafe
Chagas' disease serological test
chagoma
chain
    alpha c.
    beta c.
    branched c.
    electron transport c.
    c. fiber
    H c.; heavy c.
    invariant c.
    c. isomerism
    J (joining) c.
    kappa c.
    L c.; light c.
    lambda c.
    nuclear c.
    polypeptide c.
    c. reaction
    respiratory c.
    sympathetic c.
μ-chain disease
chaining
    backward c.
chalasia
chalaza
chalazion (pl., chalazia)
chalcogen
chalcogenide

chalcone
chalcosis
chalicosis
challenge
chalone
chamaecephaly
chamber
    Abbé-Zeis counting c.
    anaerobic c.
    Boyden c.
    Finn c.
    Fuchs-Rosenthal c.
    hyperbaric c.
    ionization c.
    multiwire proportional c.
    stiffness c.
    Thoma's counting c.
    vitreous c.
    Zappert counting c.
Chamberland filter
Champy's fixative
chancre
    hard c.
    mixed c.
    monorecidive c.
    c. redux
    soft c.
    sporotrichositic c.
    tularemic c.
chancriform
    c. pyoderma
    c. syndrome
chancroid
chancroidal ulcer
chancrous
change
    Armanni-Ebstein c.
    Baggenstoss c.
    Crooke's hyalin (hyaline) c.
    decidual c.
    degenerative c.
    harlequin color c.
    hydropic c.
    orange peel c.
    polycystic c.
    Tenney c's
Chang's aniline-acid fuchsin method
channel
    acetylcholine c.
    blood c's
    calcium-sodium c.
    cation c.

fast c.
gated c.
ligand-gated c.
lymph c's
perineural c.
potassium c.
protein c.
slow c.
thoroughfare c.
voltage-gated c.
channeling immunoassay
character
    acquired c.
    c. density
    dominant c.
    mendelian c.
    monogenic c.
    primary sex c.
    recessive c.
    secondary sex c.
    sex-conditioned c.
    sex-limited c.
    sex-linked c.
    X-linked c.
    Y-linked c.
characteristic
    c. curve
    c. fluorescent ray
    c. rays
    receiver operating c.
charcoal
    activated c.
Charcot-Böttcher crystals
Charcot-Bouchard aneurysm
Charcot-Leyden crystals
Charcot-Marie-Tooth muscular dystrophy
Charcot-Neumann crystals
Charcot-Robin crystals
Charcot's
    arthropathy
    joint
    triad
charge
    electric c.
    elementary c.
    ionic c.
    space c.
    c.-transfer complex
charged particle
Charles's law
charring

chart
    alignment c.
    flow c.
    Levey-Jennings control c.
    pedigree c.
    quality c.
    c. recorder
    Snellen c.
chassis
chaulmoogra oil
Chaussier's areola
CHB — complete heart block
CHD — congenital heart disease
            congestive heart disease
            coronary heart disease
ChE — cholinesterase
check
    alert c.
    delta c.
    c. digit
    limit c.
    linearity c.
    parity c.
    previous valve c.
checkerboard method
Chédiak-Higashi anomaly
Chédiak-Steinbrinck-Higashi anomaly
Chédiak's test
cheesy pus
cheilitis
cheilosis
cheiragra
cheirarthritis
chelate
chelating agent
chelation
    c. test
    c. therapy
cheloid
Chem. — chemotherapy
chemical
    c. adsorption
    c. affinity
    c. analysis
    c. asphyxiant
    c. bond
    c. carcinogen
    c. carcinogenic
    c. cystitis
    c. equation
    c. equilibrium
    c. incompatibility

c. inhibition isoamylase test
c. interference
c. irritant
c. mediators
c. meningitis
c. peritonitis
c. pneumonia
c. pneumonitis
c. reaction
c. styptic
c. synapse
c. waste
chemiluminescence
c. assay
c. test
cheminosis
chemiosmotic hypothesis
chemisorption
chemistry
analytical c.
c. analyzer
blood c.
clinical c.
inorganic c.
organic c.
physical c.
physiologic c.
c. profile
c. tests
chemoattractant
chemoautotroph
chemoautotrophic bacteria
chemocoagulation
chemodectoma
chemodifferentiation
chemoheterotroph
chemoheterotrophic bacteria
chemoimmunology
chemokinesis
chemolithotroph
chemoluminescence
chemoorganotroph
chemoreceptor
central c.
peripheral c.
c. tumor
chemoresistance
chemosensitive
chemostasis
pure c.
chemostat
chemosterilant

chemosynthesis
chemotactic
c. activity
c. factor
c. peptide
chemotactin
chemotaxin
chemotaxis assay
chemotherapeutic index
chemotherapy
induction c.
neoadjuvant c.
topical c.
chemotransmitter
chemotroph
chemotropism
chemstrip test
chenodeoxycholate
chenodeoxycholic acid
chenodeoxycholylglycine
Chenopodium
chenopodium oil
Chen's test
cherry
c. angioma
c. method
c. red spot
Cherry-Crandall procedure
cherubic facies
cherubism
chest
alar c.
barrel c.
blast c.
cobbler's c.
foveated c.
pterygoid c.
tetrahedron c.
Cheyletiella parasitovorax
Cheyne-Stokes respiration
CHF — congestive heart failure
CHH — cartilage-hair hypoplasia
Chiari's
malformation
net
network
chiasm
chiasma (pl., chiasmata)
chick-cell agglutination
chick embryo fibroblast
chicken
c. fat clot
c. louse

chickenpox virus
Chick-Martin test
chiclero ulcer
Chido Rodgers antigen
Chido test
chief
    c. agglutinin
    c. cell
    c. cell adenoma
Chievitz's organ
Chiffelle and Putt method
chiggers
chikungunya
    c. fever
    c. fever virus
chilblain lupus
childbed fever
childhood hemolytic-uremic syndrome
childhood-type tuberculosis
Chilomastix mesnili
chilopod
Chilopoda
chimaeric antibodies
chimera
    blood group c.
    dispermic c.
    heterologous c.
    homologous c.
    isologous c.
    radiation c.
chimerism
chimney sweep's cancer
chimpanzee coryza agent
Chinese liver fluke
Chinese restaurant syndrome
chiniofon
chip
    bone c.
    c. fracture
    prostatic c's
chiral
    c. center
    c. crystal
chirality
Chiroptera
chi-squared
    c. distribution
    c. test
chitin
CHL — chloramphenicol
Chlamydia
    C. oculogenitalis
    C. pneumoniae
    C. psittaci
    C. trachomatis
chlamydia
    c. culture
    c. group titer
Chlamydiaceae
chlamydial
    c. disease
    c. infection
    c. urethritis
chlamydiosis
Chlamydobacteriaceae
Chlamydobacteriales
Chlamydophrys
chlamydospore
Chlamydozoaceae
Chlamydozoon
chloasma bronzinum
chlophedianol hydrochloride
chloracne
chloral
    c. betaine
    c. hydrate
chlorambucil
chloramine-T
chloramphenicol
chloranil
chloranilate method
chlorasol
chlorate
    potassium c.
chlorazanil hydrochloride
chlorazol
    c. black E
    c. black E stain
chlorbenside
chlorcyclizine hydrochloride
chlordane
chlordantoin
chlordecone
chlordiazepoxide
    c. assay
    c. hydrochloride
chloremia
chlorhexidine
chloric acid
chloride
    ammonium c.
    benzalkonium c.
    calcium c.
    carbonyl c.

cobaltous c.
dansyl c.
edrophonium c.
gold c.
hydrogen c.
magnesium c.
c. methods
palladium c.
c. plate test
platinum c.
polyvinyl c.
pralidoxime c.
c. shield
c. shift
sodium c.
vinyl c.
zinc c.
chloridimetry
chloridometer
chloriduria
chlorinated
  c. hydrocarbon
  c. hydrocarbon pesticide
chlorine isotope
chlorisondamine chloride
chlormerodrin
  c. accumulation test
  c. Hg 197
  c. Hg 203
chlormezanone
chloroacetaldehyde
chloroacetate esterase reaction
chloroacetic acid
chloroacetone
chloroacetophenone
chloroallyl diethyldithiocarbamate
chloroanemia
chloroaniline
Chlorobacteriaceae
Chlorobacterium
chlorobenzene
chlorobenzilate
Chlorobium
1-chloro-3-bromopropene-1
chlorobutanol
Chlorochromatium
chlorocresol
2-chlorodeoxyadenosine
chlorodiallylacetamide
chlorodiethylacetamide
chlorodimethyl phenoxy ethanol
chlorodinitrobenzene

chloroethanol
chloroethylene oxide
chlorofluorocarbon
chloroform
  c.-methanol
  methyl c.
  c. poisoning
chloroguanide hydrochloride
chlorohydrin
  ethylene c.
chlorohydrocarbon assay
chloroleukemia
chlorolymphosarcoma
chloroma
p-chloromercuribenzoate
p-chlorometacresol
chloromethane
Chloromycetin
chloromyeloma
1-chloro-1-nitroethane
1-chloro-1-nitropropane
chloropenia
chloropenic azotemia
p-chlorophenol
chlorophenol red
chlorophenothane
chlorophenoxyacetic acid
chlorophenoxy herbicides
p-chlorophenyl-*p*-chlorobenzyl sulfide
3-(*p*-chlorophenyl)-1,1-dimethyl urea
chlorophenyl dimethylurea trichloroacetate
chloro-*o*-phenyl phenol
p-chlorophenyl phenyl sulfone
chlorophyllase
chlorophyllin
chlorophyll unit
chloropicrin
Chloropidae
chloroplast
chloroprocaine hydrochloride
chloropropylene oxide
chloropsia
chloroquine
chlorosis
chlorothen citrate
chlorothiazide
Chlorothion
chlorothymol
chlorotic anemia
chlorotoloxyacetic acid
chlorotrianisene

chlorous acid reagent
chlorovinyldichloroarsine
chloroxine
chloroxylenol
chlorphenesin carbamate
chlorpheniramine maleate
chlorphenoxamine hydrochloride
chlorphentermine hydrochloride
chlorpromazine assay
chlorpropamide
chlorprothixene
chlorquinaldol
chlortetracycline hydrochloride
chlorthalidone
chlorthion
chloruresis
chloruria
chlorzoxazone
CHN — central hemorrhagic necrosis
CHO — carbohydrate
choana (pl., choanae)
choanal
    c. atresia
    c. polyp
chocolate
    c. agar
    c. blood agar
    c. cyst
choke
    ophthalmovascular c.
chol. — cholesterol
cholagogue
cholaneresis
cholangiectasis
cholangioadenoma
cholangiocarcinoma
cholangioenteric anastomosis
cholangiofibrosis
cholangiogram
cholangiography
    delayed operative c.
    direct c.
    infantile obstructive c.
    intravenous c.
    operative c.
    percutaneous transhepatic c.
    postoperative c.
cholangiole
cholangiolitic
    c. cirrhosis
    c. hepatitis
cholangiolitis

cholangioma
cholangiopancreatography
    endoscopic retrograde c.
    hilar c.
    peripheral c.
cholangiopathy
cholangiostomy
cholangiotomogram
cholangitis; cholangeitis
    ascending c.
    destructive sclerosing c.
    primary sclerosing c.
    sclerosing c.
    suppurative c.
cholanthrene
cholate
cholecalciferol
cholechromopoiesis
cholecyst
cholecystagogue
cholecystangiography
cholecystectasia
cholecystenterostomy
cholecystitis
    acalculous c.
    acute c.
    acute hemorrhagic c.
    chronic c.
    chronic calculous c.
    emphysematous c.
    follicular c.
    gangrenous c.
    glandularis proliferans c.
    xanthogranulomatous c.
cholecystocholangiography
cholecystocolostomy
cholecystoduodenal fistula
cholecystoduodenostomy
cholecystogastrostomy
cholecystogram
    oral c.
cholecystography
    intravenous c.
    oral c.
cholecystoileostomy
cholecystojejunostomy
cholecystokinase
cholecystokinin pancreozymin
cholecystolithiasis
cholecystosis
    hyperplastic c.
choledochal cyst

choledochitis
choledochoduodenostomy
choledochoenterostomy
choledochogram
choledochography
choledocholith
choledocholithiasis
choledochostomy
choledochus
choleglobin
cholegraphy
cholehemia
cholelith
cholelithiasis
cholemia
cholemic nephrosis
choleophosphatase
cholepathia
choleperitoneum
choleperitonitis
cholepoiesis
cholera
    Asiatic c.
    pancreatic c.
    c. sicca
Choleraesuis salmonella
choleragen
choleraphage
cholera-red reaction
choleresis
choleretic
cholescintigram
chol. est. — cholesterol esters
cholestanetriol
cholestasia
cholestasis
    extrahepatic c.
    familial recurrent c.
    hepatocellular c.
    intrahepatic c.
    neonatal c.
    obstructive c.
    pure c.
cholestatic
    c. hepatitis
    c. jaundice
cholesteatoma
    intracranial c.
cholesteremia
cholesterinemia
cholesterinosis
    cerebrotendinous c.

cholesterinuria
cholesterohistechia
cholesterol
    c. calculus
    c. clefts
    c. deposition
    c. desmolase
    c. embolism
    c. esterase
    c. ester storage disease
    c. gallstone
    c.-lecithin flocculation test
    low-density lipoprotein c.
    c. oxidase
    c.-phospholipid ratio
    c. polyp
    c. staining methods
    c. test
    total c.
cholesterolemia
cholesterolestersturz
cholesterolopoiesis
cholesterolosis
    extracellular c.
cholesteroluria
cholesteryl ester hydrolase
cholesterosis
    extracellular c.
cholestyramine resin
choleuria
cholic acid
cholicele
choline
    c. acetyltransferase
    c. dehydrogenase
    c. kinase
    lysophosphatidyl c.
cholinephosphate cytidylyltransferase
cholinephosphotransferase
cholinergic
    c. blockade
    c. blocking agent
    c. fibers
    c. receptors
    c. urticaria
cholinesterase
    c. assay
    c. inhibitors
    c. test
    true c.
cholinolytic
Cholografin

chololith
chololithiasis
chololithic
choloplania
cholothorax
choloyl-coenzyme A synthetase
choluria
Chondodendron
chondralgia
chondralloplasia
chondrification
chondrify
chondrin ball
chondritis
    auricular c.
chondroblast
chondroblastic osteosarcoma
chondroblastoma
chondrocalcinosis
    articular c.
chondrocyte
    isogenous c's
chondrodermatitis nodularis chronica
    helicis
chondrodysplasia
    hereditary deforming c.
    c. punctata
chondrodystrophia
    c. calcificans congenita
    c. congenita punctata
chondrodystrophic dwarfism
chondrodystrophy
    asphyxiating thoracic c.
    asymmetrical c.
    hereditary deforming c.
chondroectodermal dysplasia
chondrofibroma
chondrohypoplasia
chondroid
    c. cancer
    c. metaplasia
    c. syringoma
chondroitin
    c. sulfate
    c. sulfate A
    c. sulfate staining
chondroma
    extraskeletal c.
    juxtacortical c.
    periosteal c.
chondromalacia
    c. fetalis

    laryngeal c.
    systemic c.
chondromatosis
    synovial c.
chondromatous
    c. exostosis
    c. giant cell tumor
    c. hamartoma
chondrometaplasia
chondromucoprotein
chondromyxoid fibroma
chondromyxoma
chondro-osteodystrophy
chondropathy
chondrophyte
chondroporosis
chondrosarcoma
    clear cell c.
    dedifferentiated c.
    juxtacortical c.
    myxoid c.
    periosteal c.
    peripheral c.
    synovial c.
chondrosis
chondrosulfatase
chondrotropic hormone
chondrus
CHOP — cyclophosphamide,
        hydroxydaunomycin,
        Oncovin (vincristine),
        and prednisone
chopped meat medium
chorda (pl., chordae)
    chordae tendineae cordis
    c. tympani
chordal fibrosarcoma
chorda-mesoderm
chordee
chorditis
chordoblastoma
chordoid tumor
chordoma
chorea
    Huntington's c.
    Sydenham's c.
choreic
choreiform
choreoacanthocytosis
choreoathetosis
chorioadenoma destruens
chorioallantoic membrane
chorioamnionitis

chorioangioma
choriocarcinoma
    gestational c.
chorioepithelioma
chorioma
choriomeningitis
    lymphatic c.
    lymphocytic c.
chorion
    abnormal c.
    c. frondosum
    c. laeve
    mature abnormal c.
    primitive c.
    shaggy c.
chorionic
    c. carcinoma
    c. cavity
    c. epithelioma
    c. melanoma
    c. plate
    c. somatomammotropin
    c. villi
    c. villus biopsy
chorionic gonadotropin
    c.g.-alpha subunit
    c.g. assay
    c.g.-beta subunit
    c.g. growth hormone prolactin
    c.g. hit
Chorioptes
chorioretinitis
chorista
choristoblastoma
choristoma
choroid
    c. lamina basalis
    c. plexus
    c. plexus carcinoma
    c. plexus papilloma
choroidal
choroideremia
choroiditis
Chr. — *Chromobacterium*
chr. — chronic
Christeller reaction
Christensen's urea agar
Christison's formula
Christmas factor
chromaffin
    c. body
    c. cells

    c. hormone
    c. paraganglioma
    c. reaction test
    c. tumor
chromaffinoma
    medullary c.
chromaffinopathy
chromaphil
chromargentaffin
chromate
    c. method
    c. stain for lead
chromated serum albumin
chromatic
    c. aberration
    c. radiation
chromatica
    trichomycosis c.
chromatid
    c. gap
    c. interference
    nonsister c's
    sister c's
chromatin
    c. bodies
    c. dust
    c. granules
    heteropyknotic c.
    c.-negative
    c. network
    nucleolar-associated c.
    nucleolus-associated c.
    oxyphil c.
    c. particles
    c.-positive
    c. reservoir
    sex c.
    X c.
    Y c.
chromatinic body
chromation
chromatism
chromatofocusing
chromatogram
chromatograph
    gas c.
chromatography
    adsorption c.
    affinity c.
    anion exchange c.
    ascending c.
    cation exchange c.

gas c.
gas-liquid c.
gas-solid c.
gel-filtration c.
gel-permeation c.
high-performance liquid c.
high-pressure liquid c.
hydrophobic c.
instant thin-layer c.
ion exchange c.
liquid-liquid c.
molecular exclusion c.
molecular sieve c.
paper c.
SDS-gel filtration c.
size-exclusion c.
thin-layer c.
two-dimensional c.
vapor-phase c.
chromatokinesis
chromatolysis
chromatometer
chromatopectic
chromatopexis
chromatophil; chromatophile
chromatophilia
chromatophilic; chromatophilous
    c. granules
chromatophobia
chromatophore
chromatophorotropic hormone
chromatotaxis
chromaturia
chrome
    c. alum
    c. alum carmine
    c. alum hematoxylin-phloxine
      method
    c. alum hematoxylin-phloxine
      stain
    c. red
    c. violet
    c. violet CG
    c. yellow
chromic
    c. acid
    c. phosphate colloid
chromidial net
chromium
    c. acid
    c. phosphate colloid
    c. poisoning

    c. sulfate
    c. trioxide
chromium 51
chromium 51 ethylenediaminetetra-
    acetic acid
chromium 51–labeled albumin
chromium sesquioxide
Chromobacterium
    C. *amethystinum*
    C. *janthinum*
    C. *marismortui*
    C. *typhiflavum*
    C. *violaceum*
chromoblastomycosis
chromocenter
chromocholoscopy
chromocystoscopy
chromocyte
chromogen
    Porter-Silber c's
chromogenesis
chromogenic
    c. bacterium
    c. cephalosporin test
chromogranin protein
Chromohalobacter marismortui
chromolytic method
chromomere
chromometer
chromomycosis
chromonar hydrochloride
chromonema (pl., chromonemata)
chromonucleic acid
chromopectic
chromopexis
chromophage
chromophil; chromophile
    c. adenoma
    c. granule
chromophilia
chromophilic; chromophilous
chromophobe
    c. adenoma
    c. cell
    c. granules
chromophobia
chromophobic
chromophore
chromophoric; chromophorous
chromoprotein
chromosomal
    c. aberration

c. abnormality
c. aneuploidy
c. bands
c. breakage syndrome
c. deletion
c. derangement
c. inversion
c. linkage
c. malformation syndrome
c. mutagen
c. nondisjunction
c. RNA

chromosome
c. aberration
c. abnormality
accessory c's
acrocentric c.
c. alteration
c. analysis
Balbiani's c.
c. band
c. banding
c. complement
derivative c.
dicentric c.
gametic c.
heteromorphic c's
homologous c.
c. map
marker c.
meiotic c.
metacentric c.
metaphase c's
c. nomenclature
Philadelphia c.
polytene c.
ring c.
sex c.
somatic c.
submetacentric c.
c. translocation
c. trisomy
X c.
Y c.

chromotoxic
chromotrichial factor
chromotrope
chromotropic acid
chromoxane
c. cyanin R
c. pure blue B
c. pure blue BLD

chronaxie; chronaxy
chronic
c. abscess
c. absorptive arthritis
c. acholuric jaundice
c. active hepatitis
c. adhesive pachymeningitis
c. airway obstruction
c. allograft rejection
c. anemia
c. appendicitis
c. atrophic gastritis
c. atrophic polychondritis
c. atrophic thyroiditis
c. atrophic vulvitis
c. basophilic leukemia
c. brain syndrome
c. bronchitis
c. calculous cholecystitis
c. cell leukemia
c. cholecystitis
c. cicatrizing enteritis
c. cold agglutinin disease
c. constrictive pericarditis
c. cystic mastitis
c. discoid lupus erythematosus
c. eczema
c. eosinophilic leukemia
c. familial icterus
c. familial jaundice
c. filariasis
c. glomerulonephritis
c. granulocytic leukemia
c. granulomatous disease
c. hepatitis
c. hypertrophic gastritis
c. hypertrophic vulvitis
c. idiopathic jaundice
c. idiopathic megacolon
c. inflammation
c. inflammatory dermatosis
c. interstitial hepatitis
c. interstitial nephritis
c. interstitial salpingitis
c. ischemic heart disease
c. leukemia
c. lingual papillitis
c. liver disease
c. lung disease
c. lymphatic leukemia
c. lymphocytic leukemia
c. lymphosarcoma

c. lymphosarcomatous leukemia
c. membranous glomerulonephritis
c. meningitis
c. monoblastic leukemia
c. monocytic leukemia
c. myelocytic leukemia
c. myelogenous leukemia
c. myeloid leukemia
c. myelomonocytic leukemia
c. nephritis
c. nonleukemic myelosis
c. nonspecific lymphadenitis
c. obstructive lung disease
c. obstructive pulmonary disease
c. pancreatitis
c. passive congestion
c. persistent hepatitis
c. proliferative arthritis
c. proliferative periorchitis
c. prostatitis
c. pulmonary emphysema
c. pyelonephritis
c. renal disease
c. renal failure
c. respiratory failure
c. rheumatism
c. subdural hematoma
c. superficial gastritis
c. thyroiditis
c. ulcer
c. ulcerative colitis
c. ulcerative proctitis
c. villous arthritis
chronological age
chrono-oncology
chronotropic
chronotropism
chrotoplast
chrysene
chrysiasis
chrysocyanosis
chrysoidin
Chrysomyia
chrysophoresis
Chrysops
Chrysosporium
chrysotherapy
chrysotile asbestos

CHS — Chédiak-Higashi syndrome
        cholinesterase
Chvostek's sign
chylangioma
chylaqueous
chyle
        c. corpuscle
        c. cyst
        c. peritonitis
chylemia
chyliform ascites
chylocele
        parasitic c.
chyloderma
chylomediastinum
chylomicron (pl., chylomicra, chylomicrons)
        lipoprotein c.
        c. remnants
chylomicronemia
chylopericarditis
chylopericardium
chyloperitoneum
chylopleura
chylopneumothorax
chylorrhea
chylothorax
chylous
        c. arthritis
        c. ascites
        c. effusion
        c. fistula
        c. hydrothorax
        c. urine
chyluria
        tropical c.
chymase
chyme
chymodenin
chymosin
chymotrypsin
chymotrypsinogen
CI — cardiac index
        cardiac insufficiency
        cerebral infarction
        chemotherapeutic index
        colloidal iron
        color index
        coronary insufficiency
        crystalline insulin
Ci — curie
Ciaccio-positive lipids

Ciaccio's
    fluid
    glands
    method
    stain
Cib. (cibus) — food
cicatricial
    c. horn
    c. kidney
    c. pemphigoid
cicatrix (pl., cicatrices)
cicatrizant
cicatrization
cicatrizing enterocolitis
Cicuta
cicutoxin
CID — cytomegalic inclusion disease
CIDS — cellular immunity deficiency
        syndrome
CIE — countercurrent immunoelectro-
        phoresis
CIEP — counterimmunoelectro-
        phoresis
CIF — clone-inhibiting factor
ciguatera
ciguatoxin
Ci-hr — curie-hour
cilia dysmotility
ciliary
    c. apparatus
    c. artery
    c. body
    c. crown
    c. dysentery
    c. dyskinesis syndrome
    c. ganglion
    c. gland
    c. muscle
    c. nerve
    c. plicae
    c. process
    c. ring
Ciliata
ciliate
    c. dysentery
    intestinal c's
ciliocytophthoria
Ciliophora
ciliorum
cilium (pl., cilia)
Cillobacterium
cimetidine

Cimex lectularius
CIN — cervical intra-epithelial neo-
        plasia
        chronic interstitial nephritis
C/in — insulin clearance
cinchonidine sulfate
cinchophen
cinclisis
cineangiocardiography
cineangiography
        radionuclide c.
cinebronchography
cinedensigraphy
cinefluorography
cinemicrography
cinepazet maleate
cinephlebography
cineradiography
cinerea
cinerins
cineurography
cingulate
        c. fasciculus
        c. gyrus
        c. sulcus
cingulum (pl., cingula)
cinoxacin
C. I. (color index) number
ciprofloxacin
circ. — circulation
circadian
        c. quotient
        c. rhythm
circinata
circinate retinopathy
circle
        c. of confusion
        c. of Willis
circuit
        c. breaker
        delay c.
        c. gate
        open c.
        paper c.
        Papez c.
        parallel c.
        reflex c.
        reverberating c.
        series c.
        short c.
circuitry
circular dichroism

circulating
  c. anticoagulant
  c. antithromboplastin disorder
  c. atypical lymphocytes
  c. blood volume
  c. cells
  c. DNA
  c. granulocyte pool
  c. immune complex nephritis
  c. reticuloendothelial cells
circulation
  pulmonary c.
  c. rate
  c. time
circulatory
  c. collapse
  c. failure
  c. insufficiency
  c. overload
  c. system
circulus (pl., circuli)
circumanal
circumarticular
circumaxillary
circumcallosal
circumcision
circumferential implantation
circumflex
  c. artery
  c. iliac vein
  c. radial artery
  c. ulnar artery
  c. vein
circummarginata
  placenta c.
circumnevic vitiligo
circumscribed
  c. atrophy
  c. edema
  c. inflammation
  c. peritonitis
circumscripta
  osteoporosis c.
circumvallate
  c. placenta
cirrhogenous; cirrhogenic
cirrhosis
  alcoholic c.
  biliary c.
  Budd's c.
  capsular liver c.
  carcinomatous c.

cardiac c.
cholangiolitic c.
congestive c.
cryptogenic c.
diffuse septal c.
fatty c.
Glisson's c.
Hanot's c.
Indian childhood c.
juvenile c.
Laennec's c.
macronodular c.
micronodular c.
necrotic c.
nutritional c.
obstructive c.
pigment c.
pigmentary c.
pipestem c.
portal c.
posthepatic c.
posthepatitic c.
postnecrotic c.
primary biliary c.
stasis c.
toxic c.
cirrhotic
  c. glomerulosclerosis
  c. liver
cirrus (pl., cirri)
cirsocele
cirsoid
  c. aneurysm
  c. varix
cirsomphalos
CIS — carcinoma in situ
      central inhibitory state
cis configuration
cisplatin
cistern
  basal c.
  great c.
  subarachnoidal c's
  terminal c's
cisterna (pl., cisternae)
  c. ambiens
  c. cerebellomedullaris
  c. chiasmatica
  c. chyli
  c. corpus callosum
  c. fossae lateralis
  c. interpeduncularis

c. lamina terminalis
c. magna
perinuclear c.
c. pontis
subsarcolemmal c.
c. superioris
terminal c.
cisternal puncture
cisternography
    radionuclide c.
cis-trans test
cistron
Citellus
citrate
    c. agar gel electrophoresis
    c. agar slant
    c. carbetapentate
    c. condensing enzyme
    cupric c.
    ferric c.
    c. intoxication
    iron ammonium c.
    c. lithium
    c.-phosphate dextrose
    c.-phosphate dextrose adenine
    c. synthase
    c. test
    thiosulfate c.
    trisodium c.
citrated blood
citreoviridin
citric acid
    c.a. assay
    c.a. cycle
Citrobacter
    Bethesda-Ballerup group of C.
    C. diversus
    C. freundii
citron
citrophosphate
citrovorum factor
citrulline
citrullinemia
citrullinuria
Civatte's
    body
    poikiloderma
CIXU — constant infusion excretory
    urogram
CJD — Creutzfeldt-Jakob disease
CK — creatine kinase
CL — chest and left arm

Cl — chlorine
Cl esterase inhibitor
Cl. — Clostridium
cl — centiliter
CLA — Certified Laboratory
    Assistant
    cyclic lysine anhydride
cladosporiosis
Cladosporium
    C. bantianum
    C. carrionii
    C. cladosporoides
    C. mansonii
    C. trichoides
    C. werneckii
Cladothrix
clamoxyquin hydrochloride
clamp
    Doyen's c.
    Payr c.
    Rankin c.
    c. technique
Clara
    cells
    hematoxylin
clarificant
clarification
clarify
Clark-Collip procedure
Clarke's
    cell
    column
    fluid
    nucleus
Clark's
    electrode
    level
    oxygen electrode
    rule
    test
CLAS — congenital localized absence
    of skin
clasmatocyte
clasmatocytosis
clasmatodendrosis
clasmatosis
classical
    c. complement pathway
    c. hemophilia
    c. osteosarcoma
    c. seminoma
classic vasculitis

CK-MB-isoenzyme of creatine kinase w/ muscle & brain subunits (cardiac)

classification
  American Urological System cancer staging c.
  Ann Arbor staging c.
  Arneth's c.
  Bergey's c.
  Bessman anemia c.
  Borrmann's c.
  Broder's c.
  Caldwell-Moloy c.
  Denver c.
  Duke's c.
  FIGO (International Federation of Gynecology and Obstetrics) c.
  Fredrickson dyslipoproteinemia c.
  French-American-British leukemia c.
  Gell and Coombs c.
  Jansky's c.
  Jensen's c.
  Kauffman-White c.
  Kiel c.
  Lancefield c.
  Lauren c.
  Lennert c.
  Lukes and Butler c.
  Lukes-Collins c.
  McNeer c.
  Ming's c.
  Moss's c.
  Paris c.
  Portmann c.
  Rappaport c.
  Runyon's c.
  Rye c.
  Seattle c.
  Sebileau's c.
clastogenic
clathrate
clathrin
Clathrochloris
Clathrocystis
Clauberg
  test
  unit
claudication
  intermittent c.
  venous c.
clause
  Delaney c.

Clauss method
claustrum (pl., claustra)
clausura
clava
clavate
clavi
Claviceps
clavicle
clavicular
claviculus
clavipectoral
clavulanate
clavus (pl., clavi)
claw
    griffin c.
clawfoot
clawhand
Clay Adams Ultra-Flow 100 counter
CLBBB — complete left bundle branch block
CLD — chronic liver disease
        chronic lung disease
clean-catch collection method
clearance
    albumin c.
    p-aminohippurate c.
    amylase c.
    blood urea c.
    creatinine c.
    Diodrast c.
    endogenous creatinine c.
    exogenous creatinine c.
    free water c.
    hepatic c.
    hippurate c.
    immune c.
    insulin c.
    interocclusal c.
    inulin c.
    iron c.
    iron plasma c.
    maximum urea c.
    osmodal c.
    osmolal c.
    plasma c.
    renal c.
    standard urea c.
    thyroidal c.
    total body c.
    urea c.
clear cell
    c.c. acanthoma

c.c. adenocarcinoma
c.c. adenoma
c.c. carcinoma
c.c. chondrosarcoma
c.c. cystadenoma
c.c. hidradenocarcinoma
c.c. hidradenoma
c.c. intraductal hyperplasia
c.c. sarcoma
c.c. tumor
clearing
    c. factor lipase
    c. factors
    c. medium
clear plaque mutation
cleavage
    c. cell
    heterolytic c.
    homolytic c.
    c. of ovum
    c. product
cleaved cell
cleft
    branchial c.
    cholesterol c's
    c. glans penis
    Larrey's c.
    c. leaflet, mitral valve
    c. leaflet, tricuspid valve
    Maurer's c's
    c. palate
    primary synaptic c.
    secondary synaptic c.
    subneural c's
cleidocranial, clidocranial
    c. dysostosis
    c. dysplasia
cleidocranialis dysostosis
cleistothecium
Cleland's reagent
clemastine
clemizole
    c. hydrochloride
    c. penicillin
Cleveland procedure
click
    ejection c.
    midsystolic c.
clidinium bromide
climacteric
    delayed c.
climatic bubo

clindamycin
cline
clinical
    c. bacteriology
    c. chemistry
    c. chemistry automation
    c. chemistry quality control
    c. cytogenetics
    c. diagnosis
    c. diagnostic bacteriology
    c. genetics
    c. laboratory
    c. medicine
    c. microbiology quality control
    c. pathology
    c. spectrometry
    c. spectroscopy
    c. spectrum
    c. toxicology
    c. trials
Clinical Laboratory Improvement Act
Clinical Laboratory Management
    Association
Clinical Laboratory Scientist
clinician
clinicopathologic conference
Clinilab
Clinistix
Clinitest
clinography
Clinoril
clinoscope
clip
    alligator c.
Clitocybe
clitoral
    c. cavernous body
    c. dorsal nerve
    c. ligament
    c. prepuce
clitoridal
    c. artery
    c. fascia
clitoris
clitoritis
    smegma c.
clitoromegaly
clival meningioma
clivus metastases
CLL — chronic lymphatic leukemia
           chronic lymphocytic leu-
           kemia

CLMA — Clinical Laboratory Management Association
cloaca (pl., cloacae)
    persistent c.
cloacal membrane
cloacogenic
    c. bladder
    c. cancer
    c. carcinoma
clock
    biological c.
    real-time c.
clofazimine
clofibrate
clomiphene
    c. citrate
    c. test
clomipramine hydrochloride
clonal
    c. anergy
    c. antibodies
    c. marker
clonality
clonazepam
clone
    cDNA c.
    genomic c.
    genomic DNA c's
    c.-inhibiting factor
cloned enzyme donor immunoassay
clonic
clonidine
    c. hydrochloride
    c. suppression test
cloning
    cellular c.
    gene c.
    c. inhibitory factor
    molecular c.
    c. vector
clonogenic assay
clonorchiasis
Clonorchis sinensis
clonotype
clonotypic
clonus
Cloquet's
    canal
    lymph node
clorazepate
clorexolone
cloroperone hydrochloride

clorophene
closed
    c. dislocation
    c. fracture
    c. loop obstruction
    c.-loop reflex
clostridia
clostridial
    c. cellulitis
    c. colitis
    c. exotoxin
    c. infection
    c. myonecrosis
    c. myositis
    c. toxins
clostridiopeptidase
clostridium (pl., clostridia)
Clostridium
    C. bifermentans
    C. botulinum
    C. butyricum
    C. clostridiiforme
    C. clostridioforme
    C. difficile
    C. histolyticum
    C. histolyticum collagenase
    C. innocuum
    C. novyi
    C. perfringens
    C. ramosum
    C. ramosus
    C. septicum
    C. sordelli
    C. sphenoides
    C. tetani
    C. welchii
closure
    delayed primary c.
clot
    antemortem c.
    blood c.
    chicken fat c.
    fibrin c's
    c. lysis
    c. lysis time
    postmortem c.
    c. reaction
    c. retraction
    c. retraction time
clotrimazole
clottage

clotting
    c. factor
    c. time
Cloudman melanoma
cloudy
    c. swelling
    c. swelling degeneration
    c. urine
clove oil
cloxacillin sodium
cloxyquin
CLSL — chronic lymphosarcomatous leukemia
CLT — clot lysis time
clubbed
    c. digits
    c. fingers
    c. toes
clubbing
clubfoot
clubhand
clumping
cluster analysis
Clutton's joints
clysis
clyster
cM — centimorgan
CM — capreomycin
    chloroquine-mepacrine
    cochlear microphonic
    costal margin
Cm — curium
cm — centimeter
cm^3 — cubic centimeter
CMB — carbolic methylene blue
CMC — carboxymethylcellulose
    critical micelle concentration
CM-cellulose
CMF — chondromyxoid fibroma
    Cytoxan, methotrexate, 5-fluorouracil
CMGN — chronic membranous glomerulonephritis
CMI — carbohydrate metabolism index
    cell-mediated immunity
CMID — cytomegalic inclusion disease
c/min — cycles per minute

CML — chronic myelocytic leukemia
    chronic myelogenous leukemia
CMM — cutaneous malignant melanoma
cmm — cubic millimeter
CMN — cystic medial necrosis
CMN-AA — cystic medial necrosis of the ascending aorta
CMO — cardiac minute output
cMO — centimorgan
CMoL — chronic monocytic (monoblastic) leukemia
C-MOPP — cyclophosphamide, nitrogen mustard, Oncovin (vincristine), procarbazine, and prednisone
CMOS — complementary metal oxide semiconductor
CMP — cardiomyopathy
    cytidine monophosphate
CMR — carpometacarpal ratio
    cerebral metabolic rate
    crude mortality ratio
CMRG — cerebral metabolic rate of glucose
CMRO — cerebral metabolic rate of oxygen
CMRR — common mode rejection ratio
CMU — chlorophenyldimethylurea
CMV — cytomegalovirus
CN — cyanide anion
    cyanogen
C3 Nef (C3 nephritic factor)
Cnephia
CNHD — congenital nonspherocytic hemolytic disease
CNL — cardiolipin natural lecithin
CNP — continuous negative pressure
CNS — central nervous system
CNSHA — congenital nonspherocytic hemolytic anemia
CNV — conative negative variation
    contingent negative variation
CO — carbon monoxide
    cardiac output
    cervicoaxial
    coenzyme
    compound
    corneal opacity

CO$_2$ — carbon dioxide
CoA — coenzyme A
coacervate
coacervation
coag. — coagulation
coagglutination
coagula
coagulable
coagulant
coagulase
    c. plasma
    c. test
coagulate
coagulated albumin
coagulating enzyme
coagulation
    acute disseminated intra-
      vascular c.
    c. deficiency
    diffuse intravascular c.
    disseminated intravascular c.
    exogenous anticoagulant c.
    c. factor (I to XIII)
    c. factor assay
    c. factor inhibitors
    c. factor transfusion
    fibrinolysin c.
    c. inhibitor
    c. necrosis
    c. pathways
    plasmin c.
    c. system
    c. test
    c. time
    c. time test
coagulative
    c. myocytolysis
    c. necrosis
    c. thrombosis
coagulin
coagulogram
coagulopathy
    consumption c.
    consumptive c.
    intravascular consumption c.
coagulum (pl., coagula)
coalesce
coalescence
coal-miner's lung
coal tar
coal worker's pneumoconiosis
coarctate retina

coarctation
    c. of aorta
    postductal c. of the aorta
    preductal c. of the aorta
coarsening
coat
    buffy c.
    cell c.
coating fixative
cobalamin
    c. adenosyltransferase
    c. concentrate
cobalophilin
cobalt
    c. isotope
    c. salipyrine
    c. 60
cobaltinitrite method
cobaltous chloride
cobamide
cobbler's chest
Cobe/IBM-2997 machine
Cobe Spectra machine
cobra
    c. venom
    c. venom factor
    c. venom solution
COBS — cesarean-obtained barrier-
      sustained
COC — cathodal opening clonus
      cathodal opening con-
        traction
      coccygeal
cocaine
    c. hydrochloride
    c. metabolite
co-capping
cocarboxylase
cocarcinogen
cocarcinogenesis
coccal
cocci
    gram-negative c.
    gram-positive c.
Coccidia
coccidial enteritis
coccidian protozoan
coccidioidal granuloma
Coccidioides immitis
coccidioidin
coccidioidin test
coccidioidoma

coccidioidomyces
coccidioidomycosis
  c. antibodies
  asymptomatic c.
  extrapulmonary c.
  latent c.
  primary extrapulmonary c.
  progressive c.
  pulmonary c.
  secondary c.
coccidiosis
Coccidium hominis
coccidium (pl., coccidia)
coccinella
coccinellin
coccobacillus
coccobacteria
coccoid
coccus (pl., cocci)
coccygeal
  c. fistula
  c. glomus
  c. ligament
  c. plexus
coccygeus
coccygodynia
coccyx (pl., coccyges)
Cochin China diarrhea
cochineal
cochlea
cochlear
  c. duct
  c. hydrops
  c. nerve
  c. nucleus
  c. root
  c. spiral canal
  c. window
Cochliomyia hominivorax
cocillana
cockscomb
  c. polyp
  c. ulcer
COCL — cathodal opening clonus
cocoa butter
Coct. (*coctio*) — boiling
coctoprecipitin
cocultivation
cocurrent
COD — cause of death
code
  degenerate c.

  gene c.
  genetic c.
  Hollerith c.
  mnemonic c.
  object c.
  OP (osmostic pressure) c.
  operation c.
  resistor color c.
  triplet c.
coded aperture imaging
codeine
  c. phosphate
  c. sulfate
coding
  c. factor
  c. triplet
cod liver oil
Codman's
  triangle
  tumor
codocyte
codominance
codominant
  c. genes
  c. inheritance
codon
  initiation c.
  start c.
  stop c.
  termination c.
coefficient
  absorption c.
  binomial c.
  Bunsen c.
  conversion c.
  correlation c.
  creatinine c.
  decay c.
  diffusion c.
  dilution c.
  distribution c.
  extinction c.
  extraction c.
  hygienic laboratory c.
  inbreeding c.
  isotonic c.
  lethal c.
  Long's c.
  mass attenuation c.
  molar absorption c.
  molar extinction c.
  osmotic c.

THE GENETIC CODE

UUU	UCU	UAU	UGU
AAA	AGA	ATA	ACA
phe	ser	tyr	cys
UUC	UCC	UAC	UGC
GAA	GGA	GTA	GCA
phe	ser	tyr	cys
UUA	UCA	UAA	UGA
TAA	TGA	TTA	TCA
leu	ser	*term*	*term*
UUG	UCG	UAG	UGG
CAA	CGA	CTA	CCA
leu	ser	*term*	trp
CUU	CCU	CAU	CGU
AAG	AGG	ATG	ACG
leu	pro	his	arg
CUC	CCC	CAC	CGC
GAG	GGG	GTG	GCG
leu	pro	his	arg
CUA	CCA	CAA	CGA
TAG	TGG	TTG	TCG
leu	pro	gln	arg
CUG	CCG	CAG	CGG
CAG	CGG	CTG	CCG
leu	pro	gln	arg
AUU	ACU	AAU	AGU
AAT	AGT	ATT	ACT
ile	thr	asn	ser
AUC	ACC	AAC	AGC
GAT	GGT	GTT	GCT
ile	thr	asn	ser
AUA	ACA	AAA	AGA
TAT	TGT	TTT	TCT
ile	thr	lys	arg
AUG	ACG	AAG	AGG
CAT	CGT	CTT	CCT
met *(init)*	thr	lys	arg
GUU	GCU	GAU	GGU
AAC	AGC	ATC	ACC
val	ala	asp	gly
GUC	GCC	GAC	GGC
GAC	GGC	GTC	GCC
val	ala	asp	gly
GUA	GCA	GAA	GGA
TAC	TGC	TTC	TCC
val	ala	glu	gly
GUG	GCG	GAG	GGG
CAC	CGC	CTC	CCC
val *(init)*	ala	glu	gly

oxygen utilization c.
partition c.
Pearson's c.
phenol c.
product-moment c.
rank correlation c.
regression c.
Rideal-Walker c.
sample correlation c.
sedimentation c.
c. of selection

solubility c.
Spearman's rank correlation c.
Svedberg's sedimentation c.
temperature c.
urohemolytic c.
urotoxic c.
c. of variation
velocity c.
volume c.
coelenterate
coeloblastula

coelom; celom
      extraembryonic c.
      intraembryonic c.
coelomic
      c. cavity
      c. epithelium
coenurus
coenzyme
      c. A
      c. factor
      c. I
      c. II
      c. Q
      c. R
coenzymometer
coeur en sabot
cofactor
      heparin c.
      platelet c.
      platelet c. I
      platelet c. II
      ristocetin c.
      c. of thromboplastin
      c. V
Coffey-Humber treatment
cognate
      c. interaction
      c. recognition
cognition
COGTT — cortisone-primed oral glu-
            cose tolerance test
cogwheel respiration
COHB — carboxyhemoglobin
coherent smallpox
cohesion
cohesive
      c. end
      c. termini
Cohnheim's
      artery
      theory
cohort
      c. labeling
      c. study
coil
      paranemic c.
      plectonemic c.
      primary c.
      random c.
      relational c.

      secondary c.
      standard c.
coincidence
      c. correction
      c. error
      c. sum peak
coin lesion
coinlike
coinosite
coitus
Colcemid
Colcher-Sussman method
colchicine
      quinine c.
COLD — chronic obstructive lung
            disease
cold
      c. abscess
      c. agglutination
      c. agglutinin
      c. agglutinin screen
      c. agglutinin syndrome
      c. agglutinin test
      c. agglutinin titer
      c. autoabsorption
      c. autoagglutinin
      c. autoantibodies
      c. gangrene
      c. hemagglutinin
      c. hemoglobinuria
      c. hemolysin test
      c. injury
      c. intolerance
      c.-knife conization
      c. lesion
      c. microtome
      c. nodule
      c. pack
      c.-reacting antibody
      c. receptor
      c.-sensitive mutation
      c. ulcer
coldsore
colectasia
coleitis
Coleman-Schiff reagent
Coleoptera
coleoptosis
Cole's hematoxylin
colestipol hydrochloride
Coley's toxin

coli
>Holophyra c.
>melanosis c.
>pseudomelanosis c.
coli-aerogenes group
colibacillary
colibacillemia
colibacilluria
colibacillus
colic
>biliary c.
>endemic c.
>intestinal c.
>c. intussusception
>menstrual c.
>pancreatic c.
>renal c.
>uterine c.
>verminous c.
colicin
colicinogen
coliform bacillus
colinearity
colipase
>pancreatic c.
coliphage
colistimethate sodium
colistin
>c.–nalidixic acid agar
>c. sulfate
colitis
>acute ulcerative c.
>amebic c.
>antibiotic-associated pseudo-
>membranous c.
>balantidial c.
>chronic ulcerative c.
>clostridial c.
>collagenous c.
>c. cystica profunda
>c. cystica superficialis
>granulomatous c.
>c. gravis
>hemorrhagic c.
>ischemic c.
>mucous c.
>c. polyposa
>pseudomembranous c.
>radiation c.
>regional c.
>spastic c.
>transmural c.

>ulcerative c.
>uremic c.
colitose
colitoxemia
colitoxicosis
colitoxin
coliuria
collagen
>c. degeneration
>c. disease
>c. fibril alteration
>fibrillar c.
>fibrous long-spacing c.
>interstitial c.
>intimal c.
>c. matrix
>segmental long-spacing c.
>c.-staining method
>c. vascular disease
collagenase
>*Clostridium histolyticum* c.
collagenoblast
collagenocyte
collagenolysis
collagenosis
>systemic c.
collagenous
>c. colitis
>c. fibers
collapse
>circulatory c.
>massive c.
>structure c.
>c. therapy
collar button
>c.b. abscess
>c.b. lesion
collateral
>c. eminence
>c. sulcus
>c. ulnar artery
>c. ventilation
collecting
>c. duct
>c. tubule
College of American Pathologists
colliculitis
colliculus (pl., colliculi)
>inferior c.
>c. seminalis
>superior c.
collidine

collier's lung
colligative
collimate
collimation
collimator
colliquation
    ballooning c.
    reticulating c.
colliquative
    c. albuminuria
    c. degeneration
    c. necrosis
collision
    c. carcinoma
    c. tumor
collodion
    c. baby
    c. filter
colloid
    c. adenocarcinoma
    c. adenoma
    c. antigen
    c. body
    c. cancer
    c. carcinoma
    c. cells
    c. corpuscle
    c. cyst
    c. degeneration
    c. goiter
    c. milium
    c. osmotic hemolysis
    c. osmotic lysis
    c. shock
    c. silica
    thyroid c.
    c. tumor
colloidal
    c. dispersion
    c. electrolyte
    c. gold
    c. gold test
    c. iron stain
    c. osmotic pressure
    c. silicon dioxide
colloidoclasia
"colloidophagy"
colloid osmotic lysis
collum (pl., colla)
coloboma (pl., colobomas, colobomata)
colocholecystostomy

colocolostomy
colocutaneous fistula
colocynth
coloesophageal anastomosis
coloileal fistula
colon
    ascending c.
    c. bacillus
    descending c.
    giant c.
    irritable c.
    lead-pipe c.
    mesenteric c.
    rectosigmoid c.
    sigmoid c.
    transverse c.
    c. tumor
colonic
    c. conduit
    c. crypts of Lieberkühn
    c. epithelium
    c. fistula
    c. glands
    c. lumen
    c. mucous membrane
    c. mucus
    c. muscularis propria
    c. polyp
    c. serosa
    c. smear
    c. solitary lymphoid nodule
    c. submucosa
    c. subserosa
    c. vomitus
colonization
    c. infection
    jejunal c.
colonizing aspergillosis
colonorrhagia
colonoscope
colonoscopy
colony
    bacterial c's
    butyrous c.
    D (dwarf) c.
    daughter c.
    disgonic c.
    dwarf c.
    effuse c.
    H (thin film) c.
    M (mucoid) c.
    matte c.
    motile c.

mucoid c.
O (without film) c.
R (rough) c.
raised c.
rough c.
S (smooth) c.
satellite c.
smooth c.
c.-stimulating activity
c.-stimulating factor
colony-forming
    c.-f. unit
    c.-f. unit-culture
    c.-f. unit-erythroid
    c.-f. unit-granulocyte
    c.-f. unit-granulocyte-
      macrophage
    c.-f. unit-lymphoid
    c.-f. megakaryocyte
    c.-f. units/mL
    c.-f. unit-spleen
colopexy
coloplication
coloproctitis
coloptosis; coloptosia
coloproctostomy
color
    c. blindness
    complementary c.
    c. index
    c. index number
    primary c.
    spectral c.
    c. vision
Colorado
    tick fever
    tick fever virus
color-contrast microscope
colorectal
    c. adenocarcinoma
    c. cancer
    c. carcinoma
    c. polyp
colorectitis
colorimeter
colorimetric
colorimetry
color index number
colosigmoidostomy
colostomy
colostrum
    c. corpuscle
    c. gravidarum

Colour Index
colovaginal fistula
colovesical fistula
colpatresia
colpectasia
colpitis
colpocystitis
colpocytogram
colpocytology
colpohyperplasia
    c. cystica
    c. emphysematosa
colpomicroscope
colposcope
colposcopy
Colton antigen
Colton blood group system
Columbia blood agar
Columbia-SK virus
columbium
columella (pl., columellae)
columellate
column
    Bertini's renal c's
    Clarke's c.
    fornix c.
    Morgagni's c.
    vertebral c.
columna (pl., columnae)
columnar
    c. cell
    c. epithelium
coma
    alcoholic c.
    apoplectic c.
    c. cast
    c. de passé
    diabetic c.
    hepatic c.
    hyperglycemic c.
    hypoglycemic c.
    irreversible c.
    metabolic c.
    myxedematous c.
    nonketotic hyperosmolar c.
    uremic c.
    c. vigil
Comamonas terrigena
comatose
comb-growth test
combination calculus

combined
- c. hyperlipidemia
- c. immunodeficiency
- c. modality therapy
- c. pituitary function test
- c. systems disease
- c. ventricular hypertrophy

comb rhythm

combustible
- c. gas
- c. gas detector
- c. liquid
- c. vapor

combustion

comedo (pl., comedones)
- c. nevus

comedocarcinoma

comedomastitis

comedones

comet cell

commensal

commensalism

comminuted fracture

Commission on Office Laboratory
Assessment

commissura (pl., commissurae)

commissural myelotomy

commissure
- anterior c.
- aortic c.
- Forel's c.
- habenular c.
- hippocampal c.
- inferior colliculus c.
- laryngeal c.
- mitral valve c.
- oral c.
- posterior c.
- pulmonic valve c.
- superior colliculus c.
- tricuspid valve c.

committed progenitor cells

Committee on Allied Health Education and Accreditation

common
- c. antigen
- c. bile duct
- c. carotid artery
- c. cold virus
- c. excretory duct
- c. facial vein
- c. iliac artery
- c. iliac vein
- c. leukocyte antigen
- c. logarithm
- c. mode rejection ratio
- c. mode signal
- c. pathway of coagulation
- c. peroneal nerve
- c. reference
- c. storage
- c. tendon sheath
- c. variable agammaglobuli-nemia
- c. variable hypogammaglobuli-nemia
- c. variable immunodeficiency
- c. wart

communicable

communicating hydrocephalus

commutator

compact bone

comparative pathology

comparison
- c. eyepiece
- c. film
- c. microscopes
- c. operation

compartment
- muscular c.
- vascular c.

compartmental
- c. analysis
- c. syndrome

compatibility
- ABO c.
- c. test
- c. tests in vivo

compatible

Compazine

compensated
- c. acidosis
- c. alkalosis
- c. eyepiece
- c. hemolysis
- c. shock

compensation
- broken c.
- dosage c.
- c. neurosis
- temperature c.

compensatory
- c. atrophy
- c. cardiac hypertrophy

c. emphysema
c. hyperplasia
c. hypertrophy
c. polycythemia
c. regeneration
competence
embryonic c.
immunologic c.
competition
antigenic c.
c. hybridization
competitive
c. antagonist
c. inhibition
c. protein-binding assay
compile time
compiler
optimizing c.
complement
c. activation
c. assay
c. binding assay
c. chemotactic factor
chromosome c.
c. components
c. deficiency state
dominant c.
endocellular c.
c. fixation
c.-fixation test
c.-fixing antibody
c. inactivation
c. level
c. lysis sensitivity test
c.-mediated anaphylaxis
c.-mediated cytotoxicity
c. profile
c. receptor 1, 2, 3, 4
c. sequence
c. system
c. total
c. unit
whole c.
complemental inheritance
complementarity
dominant c.
complementary
c. bases
c. colors
c. deoxyribonucleic acid
c. DNA
c. genes

c. hypertrophy
c. metal oxide semiconductor
logic
c. symmetry amplifier
complementation
complement-fixation
Reiter protein c.-f.
Treponema pallidum c.-f.
complementophil
complete
c. abortion
c. anomalous venous drainage
c. anterior dislocation
c. antibody
c. blood count
c. carcinogen
c. dislocation
c. fistula
c. heart block
c. inferior dislocation
c. left bundle branch block
c. obstruction
c. penetrance
c. posterior dislocation
c. reaction of degeneration
c. right bundle branch block
c. superior dislocation
complex
activated c.
acyl-plasminogen streptokinase
activator c.
c. adrenal endocrine disorder
AGR (aniridia, genitourinary
malformations, and mental
retardation) c.
AIDS-related c.
antigen-antibody c.
anti-inhibitor coagulation c.
B-chain gene c.
charge-transfer c.
dementia c.
Eisenmenger's c.
c. endocrine disorder
factor X c.
familial juvenile nephronophthisis–medullary cystic disease c.
Ghon c.
c. globulin
Golgi's c.
c. gonadal endocrine disorder
hapten-carrier c.

HLA (human leukocyte antigen) c.
immune c.
iron carbohydrate c.
junctional c.
major histocompatibility c.
membrane attack c.
Meyenburg's c.
minor histocompatibility c.
nephronophthisis–uremic medullary cystic disease c.
c. number
c. odontoma
PAP (peroxidase-antiperoxidase) c.
c. pituitary endocrine disorder
primary c.
prothrombin c.
ribonucleoprotein c.
ribosome-lamella c.
RNP (ribonucleoprotein) c.
sicca c.
steroid-receptor c.
synaptonemal c.
c. thyroid endocrine disorder
triple symptom c.
tubular immune c.
VATER (vertebral defects, imperforate anus, tracheoesophageal fistula, and radial and
renal dysplasia) c.
vitamin B c.
von Meyenburg's c.
complexity
compliance
dynamic c.
specific c.
static c.
complication
complotype
component
antihemophilic c.
blood c.
complement c's
late positive c.
M (myeloma or macroglobulinemia) c.
P c.
plasma thromboplastin c.
secretory c.
serum amyloid A c.
serum amyloid P c.

splanchnic motor c.
splanchnic sensory c.
thromboplastic plasma c.
composite
c. lymphoma
c. tumor
composition
c. resistor
c. tumor
compound
acetone c.
acyclic c.
aliphatic c.
c. aneurysm
c. antigen
aromatic c.
c. B (corticosterone)
binary c.
carbamino c.
carbon inorganic c.
c. comminuted fracture
condensation c.
c. cyst
diazo c.
c. dislocation
c. E (cortisone)
endothermic c.
exothermic c.
c. F (cortisol)
c. fracture
c. gland
c. granular corpuscle
heterocyclic c.
Hurler-Scheie c.
isocyclic c.
c. leukemia
meso c.
c. microscope
c. multiple fractures
c. nevus
nonpolar c's
c. odontoma
organomercury c.
organometallic c.
organophosphate c's
organophosphorous c's
polar c.
c. presentation
c. Q
c. S
saturated c.
secretory c.
substitution c.

tertiary c.
c. tumor
c. X
compressed
c.-air illness
c. fracture
c. gas storage
c. spectral assay
compression
c. atelectasis
cord c.
c. injury
pericardial c.
compromised
Compton
edge
effect
photon
compulsion
computed tomography
computer
general-purpose c.
c. graphics
computerization
computerized
c. axial tomography
c. transaxial tomography
COMT — catechol-O-methyl transferase
ConA — concanavalin A
conc. — concentrated
concentration
concanavalin A
concatenate
concatenation
concave
concentrate
granulocyte c.
intrinsic factor c.
lyophilized c.
marine protein c.
platelet c.
porcine c.
concentrated
concentration
approximate lethal c.
bactericidal c.
blood alcohol c.
carbon dioxide c.
critical micelle c.
hazardous c.
hydrogen ion c.

hydroxyl c.
ionic c.
lethal c.
limiting isorrheic c.
M (maximum) c.
mass c.
maximum permissible c.
maximum urinary c.
MC (maximum cell) c.
mean cell hemoglobin c.
mean corpuscular hemoglobin c.
minimal bactericidal c.
minimal inhibitory c.
minimal isorrheic c.
minimal lethal c.
minimum bactericidal c.
minimum complete-killing c.
minimum detectable c.
minimum inhibitory c.
minimum lethal c.
minimum mycoplasmacidal c.
molar c.
c. procedures
radioactive c.
renal vein renin c.
c.-response curve
substance c.
c. test
total L-chain c.
concentric
c. fibroma
c. hypertrophy
concept
second messenger c.
conception
retained products of c.
conceptional age
concha (pl., conchae)
conchoidal bodies
concomitant
concordance
concrement
concrescence
concretio
c. cordis
c. pericardii
concretion
calcific c.
concurrent
concussion

condensans
  osteitis c.
condensation
  c. compound
  c. fibrosis
  c. polymer
condenser
  Abbé's c.
  cardioid c.
  darkfield c.
  paraboloid c.
condensing
  c. osteitis
  c. vacuole
condition
  steady-state c.
  sufficient c.
conditional
  c. jump
  c. lethal mutation
  c. probability
conditioned stimulus
conductance
  airway c.
conduction
  anterograde c.
  cardiac c.
  c. deafness
  c. defect
  c. electron
  c. ratio
  saltatory c.
  c. system
  c. time
  c. velocity
  volume c.
conductivity
  c. cell volume
  thermal c.
  water c.
conductometry
conductor
conduit
  colonic c.
  ileal loop c.
  interstitial c.
  intestinal c.
  isoperistaltic c.
  urinary c.
condylar displacement
condyle
  mandibular c.

condylectomy
condyloma (pl., condylomata)
  c. acuminatum
  Buschke-Löwenstein giant c.
  flat c.
  c. latum
  pointed c.
condylomatous
cone
  c. biopsy
  c. pressure
  c. shell
confabulation
conference
  clinicopathologic c.
confidence
  c. interval
  c. level
configuration
  cis c.
  trans c.
confluent
  c. bronchopneumonia
  c. inflammation
  c. pneumonia
  c. reticulate papillomatosis
  c. smallpox
conformation
conformational determinant
conformer
confusion
  circle of c.
congener
congenic
congenital
  c. absence
  c. absence of vagina
  c. achromia
  c. adrenal hyperplasia
  c. adrenal virilism
  c. afibrinogenemia
  c. agammaglobulinemia
  c. anemia
  c. aneurysm
  c. anomaly
  c. aplastic anemia
  c. aregenerative anemia
  c. atransferrinemia
  c. atresia
  c. carcinoma
  c. contracture
  c. cyst

c. defect
c. deformity
c. dislocation
c. duplication
c. dyserythropoietic anemia
c. dysphagocytosis
c. dysplastic angiectasia
c. dysplastic angiomatosis
c. dysplastic angiopathy
c. ectodermal defect
c. ectodermal dysplasia
c. elephantiasis
c. epulis
c. erythropoietic porphyria
c. familial icterus
c. familial jaundice
c. generalized fibromatosis
c. glaucoma
c. goiter
c. heart disease
c. Heinz body hemolytic anemia
c. hemidysplasia
c. hemolytic anemia
c. hemolytic icterus
c. hemolytic jaundice
c. hepatic fibrosis
c. hydronephrosis
c. hyperaldosteronism
c. hyperbilirubinemia
c. hypophosphatasia
c. hypoplastic anemia
c. leukemia
c. leukopenia
c. lipodystrophy
c. lipoid hyperplasia
c. lymphedema
c. malformation
c. megacolon
c. mesoblastic nephroma
c. methemoglobinemia
c. myopathy
c. nephromegaly
c. nevus
c. nonspherocytic hemolytic disease
c. pancytopenia
c. pernicious anemia
c. porphyria
c. pterygium
c. pyloric stenosis
c. renal hyperplasia
c. renal hypoplasia
c. rubella syndrome
c. ruptured aneurysm
c. sebaceous hyperplasia
c. sideroachrestic anemia
c. stenosis
c. sutural alopecia
c. syphilis
c. syphilitic orchitis
c. thymic aplasia
c. thymic dysplasia
c. torticollis
c. total lipodystrophy
c. toxoplasmosis
c. virilizing adrenal hyperplasia

congestion
    chronic passive c.
    hepatic c.
    hypostatic c.
    passive c.
    pulmonary c.
    pulmonary venous c.
    venous c.

congestive
    c. cardiac failure
    c. cardiomyopathy
    c. cirrhosis
    c. edema
    c. heart disease
    c. heart failure
    c. splenomegaly

conglobate gland
conglutin
    immune c.
conglutinating complement absorption test
conglutination reaction
conglutinin
conglutinogen-activating factor
Congo
    C. Corinth
    C. floor maggot
    C. red
    C. red paper
    C. red stain
    C. red test
    C. rubrum C.
congophilic angiopathy
conical
conidia
conidial

Conidiobolus
    C. coronatus
    C. incongruus
conidioma
conidiophore
conidiospore
conidium (pl., conidia)
coniine
coniofibrosis
coniolymphastasis
coniophage
coniosis
Coniosporium
coniosporosis
coniotoxicosis
Conium
conization
    cold-knife c.
conjoined twins
conjugal cancer
conjugase enzyme
conjugate
    c. acid
    c. acid-base pairs
    c. base
    c. focus
    c. gaze
    c. redox pair
conjugated
    c. bilirubin
    c. estriol
    c. hyperbilirubinemia
    c. protein
conjugation map
conjugative plasmid
conjunctiva (pl., conjunctivae)
    c. and sclera
    bulbar c.
    lymphatics of c.
    ocular c.
    palpebral c.
    tunica c.
conjunctival
    c. culture
    c. fungus culture
    c. hyperemia
conjunctivitis
    adenoviral c.
    adult gonococcal c.
    allergic c.
    angular c.
    catarrhal c.

    follicular c.
    granular c.
    herpetic c.
    inclusion c.
    meningococcal c.
    c. neonatorum
    phlyctenular c.
    swimming pool c.
    trachoma-inclusion c.
    tularemic c.
    vernal c.
    viral c.
    welder's c.
conjunctivoma
connection
    anomalous venous c.
    intertendinous c.
connective
    c. tissue nevus
    c. tumor
connective tissue
    c.t. barrier
    dense elastic c.t.
    dense fibrous c.t.
    c.t. disease
    endocervical c.t.
    exocervical c.t.
    histohematic c.t. barrier
    loose areolar c.t.
    mammary interlobular c.t.
    mammary intralobular c.t.
    mucous c.t.
connector
    Luer c.
conoid ligament
Conray
consanguineous
    c. donor
    c. mating
consanguinity
consciousness disturbance
consecutive
    c. aneurysm
    c. angiitis
consensual light reflex
consensus sequence
console
consolidation therapy
conspecific
constant
    absorption c.
    acid ionization c.

affinity c.
Ambard's c.
association c.
base ionization c.
Botzmann's c.
decay c.
dielectric c.
disintegration c.
dissociation c.
equilibrium c.
Faraday's c.
gas c.
intrinsic association c.
ionization c.
Planck's c.
radioactive c.
rate c.
c. region
solubility product c.
velocity c.
constipation
constitution
constitutional
    c. aplastic anemia
    c. cause
    c. dwarf
    c. hepatic dysfunction
    c. hyperbilirubinemia
    c. psychopathic inferiority
    c. thrombopathy
    c. ulcer
constitutive
    c. enzyme
    c. heterochromatin
    c. heterochromatin method
    c. mutation
constriction
    primary c.
    secondary c.
constrictive
    c. endocarditis
    c. pericarditis
constrictor pharyngeus muscle
constructable
construction
constructive
    c. interference
    c. proof
consultation system
consumption
consumptive
    c. coagulopathy
    oxygen c.

contact
    c. activation product
    c. autoradiography
    c. catalysis
    c. dermatitis
    c. inhibition
    c. sensitivity
contagion
contagious infection
contagium
    c. animatum
    c. vivum
containment
contaminant
contaminated
contamination
contents
    carbon dioxide c.
    gastrointestinal c.
contiguity
contiguous
continence
continent
contingency table
contingent negative variation
continua
    acrodermatitis c.
    epilepsia partialis c.
continuous
    c. capillaries
    c. distending pressure
    c. endothelium
    c. flow culture
    c. function
    c. murmur
    c. negative pressure
    c. phase
    c. positive airway pressure
    c. spectrum
    c. variable
    c. x-ray spectrum
contour
contoured
Contracaecum
contraception
contraceptive
    oral c.
contracted
    c. erythrocyte
    c. kidney
    c. leukocyte
    c. muscle

contractile
- c. force
- c. protein
- c. reserve
- c. ring
- c. vacuole

contractility

contraction
- c. atelectasis
- c. band necrosis
- isovolumetric c.
- isovolumic c.
- c. time
- uterine c.

contracture
- bladder neck c.
- congenital c.
- c. deformity
- Dupuytren's c.
- ischemic c.
- organic c.
- Volkmann's c.

contrafissura

contraindication

contralateral
- c. axillary metastasis
- c. biopsy

contrast
- c. echocardiography
- c. media
- c. media reaction
- c. medium
- c. stain

contrasuppression

contrecoup

control
- c. animal
- c. experiment
- c. group
- ignition source c.
- c. materials
- motor c.
- negative c.
- c. panel
- positive c.
- process c.
- quality c.
- spill c.
- c. system
- c. unit

controlled
- c. access laboratory
- c. substance

Controlled Substances Act

contuse

contused wound

contusion
- cerebral c.
- contrecoup c.
- wind c.

conus (pl., coni)
- c. arteriosus
- c. elasticus
- c. medullaris
- c. papillary muscle
- c. terminalis

convalescence

convalescent serum

convallamarin

convallarin

convection

convergence
- multimodal c.

conversational mode

conversion
- c. coefficient
- c. electron
- internal c.
- c. hysteria
- Mantoux c.
- c. ratio
- tumor c.

convertase
- C3 c.

converter
- analog-to-digital c.
- D/A c.
- voltage-to-frequency c.

convertin

converting enzyme

convex

convexity meningiomas

convoluted
- c. tubule
- c. T-cell lymphoma

convolution

convulsant

convulsion

convulsive shock therapy

Conway cell

coolant

cooled-knife method

Cooley's
- anemia
- trait

Coomassie brillant blue
Coombs's
    serum
    test
Cooper's
    irritable breast
    irritable testis
    ligament
    suspensory ligament
coordinate
    cartesian c.
    c. covalent bond
    polar c.
    spherical polar c.
coordination
    c. compound
    c. number
co-oximeter
COP — colloid osmotic pressure
    Cytoxan, Oncovin, prednisone
coparaffinate
COPD — chronic obstructive pulmonary disease
Cope method bronchography
Copepoda
Coplin jar
copolymer
copper
    c. acetoarsenite
    c. arsenate
    c. deposit demonstration
    c. intoxication
    c. naphthenate
    c. oxidase
    c. oxychloride sulfate
    c. 3-phenyl salicylate
    radioactive c.
    c. reduction test
    c. storage protein
    c. sulfate
    c. sulfate method
    c. undecylenate
copperhead
coprecipitin
copremesis
Coprinus
coproantibody
coprohematology
coprolith
coprology
coproma

Copromastix prowazeki
Copromonas subtilis
coprophagia
coprophil
coproporphyria
    free erythrocyte c.
    hereditary c.
coproporphyrin
    c. assay
    free erythrocyte c.
    c. test
    urinary c.
coproporphyrinogen
    c. decarboxylase
    c. oxidase
coproporphyrinuria
coprostanol
coprostasis
coprosterol
coprozoic ameba
Co Q — coenzyme Q
cor
    c. adiposum
    c. biloculare
    c. bovinum
    c. mobile
    c. pendulum
    c. pseudotriloculare
    c. pseudotriloculare biatriatum
    c. pulmonale
    c. triatriatum
    c. triloculare biatriatum
    c. triloculare biventriculare
CORA — conditioned orientation reflex audiometry
coracobrachialis muscle
coracoid
coral calculus
corallin
    yellow c.
Corbin technique
cord
    Billroth's c's
    c. bladder
    c. blood
    c. blood screen
    c. compression
    c. factor
    hepatic c's
    lumbar spinal c.
    lumbosacral spinal c.
    prolapsed umbilical c.

ruptured umbilical c.
seminiferous c.
sex c's
spermatic c.
spinal c.
umbilical c.
vocal c.
cordal
    c. fibroma
    c. histiocytoma
    c. leiomyosarcoma
    c. lipoma
    c. liposarcoma
    c. mesothelioma
    c. rhabdomyosarcoma
cordectomy
cording
    c. factor
cordis
cordotomy
    spinothalamic c.
Cordylobia anthropophaga
core
    air c.
    c. antigen
    magnetic c.
    c. memory
    mesenchymal villous c.
    c. needle biopsy
    c. pneumonia
corectasis
coremium
corepressor
coriamyrtin
Corinth
    Congo C.
coriphosphine O
Cori's cycle
corium
cornea
corneal
    c. opacity
    c. reflex
    c. ulcer
    c. vascularization
corneoscleral
corneous
Corner-Allen
    test
    unit
corniculate cartilage
cornification

cornified
corn meal agar
cornoid lamella
cornu (pl., cornua)
    c. cutaneum
corona (pl., coronas, coronae)
    c. ciliaris
    c. of glans penis
    c. radiata
    c. veneris
coronal
    c. flap
    c. plane
    c. suture
coronary
    c. arteritis
    c. artery
    c. artery bypass graft
    c. artery disease
    c. atherosclerotic heart disease
    c. blood flow
    c. embolism
    c. heart disease
    c. insufficiency
    c. ligament
    c. ostial stenosis
    c. prognostic index
    c. sinus
    c. thrombosis
    c. vein
coronavirus
coroner
coronoid
coroscopy
corpora
    c. amylacea
    c. arenacea
    c. lutea
    c. lutea cysts
    c. quadrigemina
corporis
corps ronds
corpulence; corpulency
cor pulmonale
corpus (pl., corpora)
    c. albicans
    c. amylaceum
    c. atreticum
    c. callosum
    c. cavernosum clitoridis
    c. cavernosum penis
    c. coccygeum

c. fimbriatum
c. fornicis
c. hemorrhagicum
c. hemorrhagicum cyst
c. luteum
c. luteum hematoma
c. luteum hormone unit
c. pancreatis
c. spongiosum
c. striatum
c. uteri

corpuscle
amniotic c.
amylaceous c.; amyloid c.
Bizzozero's c.
blood c.
chyle c.
colloid c.
colostrum c.
compound granular c.
Donné's c's
dust c's
Eichhorst's c's
exudation c.
ghost c.
Gierke's c's
Gluge's c's
Golgi-Mazzoni c.
Golgi's c.
Hassall's c.
Hayem's c.
inflammatory c.
lymph c.; lymphatic c.;
    lymphoid c.
Meissner's c.
Merkel's c.
Mexican hat c.
molluscum c.
Norris' c's
paciniform c's
pessary c.
phantom c.
plastic c.
pus c.
red c.
renal c.
reticulated c.
Ruffini's c.
salivary c.
shadow c.
third c.
Traube's c.

Vater-Pacini c.
white c.
Zimmermann's c.

corpuscular
c. lymph
c. radiation

corpusculum (pl., corpuscula)

corrected
c. blood volume
c. dextrocardia
c. retention time
c. reticulocyte count
c. sedimentation rate
c. transposition

correction
Allen's c.
coincidence c.

correlation coefficient

corresponding ray

Corrigan's pulse

corrin ring

corrinoid

corrosion
c. cast
c. preparation

corrosive gastritis

corrosivity

cort. — cortex

cortex (pl., cortices)
adrenal c.
multinodular adrenal c.
nodular adrenal c.
renal c.

cortical
c. achromia
c. bone
c. cataract
c. DC potential
c. defect
c. hormone
c. labyrinth
c. necrosis
c. nephron
c. osteitis
c. retention
c. stromal fibrosis
c. stromal hyperplasia

corticifugal

corticipetal

corticobulbar tract

corticocancellous

corticocollicular

corticoid
      anti-inflammatory c.
corticomedullary ratio
corticopontine
corticorubral
corticospinal tract
corticosteroid
      c.-binding globulin
      c.-binding protein
corticosterone
corticostriate fibers
corticothalamic
corticotrope, corticotroph
corticotrophic, corticotropic
      c. adenoma
      c. cell
corticotrophin, corticotropin
      c.-like intermediate lobe
         peptide
      c.-releasing factor
      c.-releasing hormone
cortin
Cortinarius orellanus
Corti's
      ganglion
      organ
cortisol
      c.-binding globulin
      c.-producing carcinoma
      c. production rate
      c. secretion rate
      urinary free c.
cortisone
      c. acetate
      c.-glucose tolerance test
      c.-primed oral glucose toler-
        ance test
      c. reductase
cortol
cortolone
Cortrosyn
corymbiform
corynebacteria
Corynebacteriaceae
corynebacterial exotoxin
Corynebacterium
      C. *acnes*
      C. *belfantii*
      C. *diphtheriae*
      C. *enzymicum*
      C. *equi*
      C. *genitalium*

      C. *haemolyticum*
      C. *hoagii*
      C. *hofmannii*
      C. *infantisepticum*
      C. *minutissimum*
      C. *mycetoides*
      C. *necrophorum*
      C. *parvulum*
      C. *pseudodiphtheriticum*
      C. *pseudotuberculosis*
      C. *pseudotuberculosis-ovis*
      C. *pyogenes*
      C. *renale*
      C. *tenuis*
      C. *ulcerans*
      C. *vaginale*
      C. *xerosis*
coryneform group
coryza
coryzavirus
cos
cosine
Cosmegen
cosmic
      c. radiation
      c. rays
cosmid
costa (pl., costae)
costal
      c. cartilage
      c. element
      c. pleura
      c. pleurisy
costochondral
costochondritis
costoclavicular
costotransverse joint
costovertebral
      c. angle
      c. joint
Cost Sterling blood group system
cosynthase
      uroporphyrinogen III c.
cosyntropin test
COTe — cathodal opening tetanus
cothromboplastin
cotinine
Cotlove titrator
cotransport
cotrimoxazole
cotton
      c. blue

collodion c.
c.-dust asthma
c.-fiber embolism
salicylated c.
c.-wool spot
cotyledon
cough
dry c.
c. plate
productive c.
c. reflex
smoker's c.
c. swab technique
whooping c.
coulomb
Coulomb's law
coulometer
coulometric titration
coulometry
Coulter's
counter
thrombocounter
whole blood lysing kit
coumachlor
Coumadin
coumaric anhydride
coumarin
Councilmania
C. dissimilis
C. lafleuri
Councilman's
bodies
hyaline body
lesion
counseling
genetic c.
count
absolute eosinophil c.
Addis c.
agar plate c.
Arneth's c.
background c.
blood c.
blood cell c.
bone marrow differential c.
cell c.
complete blood c.
corrected reticulocyte c.
c. density
differential c.
differential leukocyte c.
eosinophil c.

filament-nonfilament c.
c. information density
platelet c.
proportional c.
c. rate
c. rate meter
red blood c.
red blood cell c.
reticulocyte c.
Schilling blood c.
scintillation c.
spinal fluid leukocyte c.
total ridge c.
white blood cell c.
white cell c.
counter
automated differential leukocyte c.
Baker c.
binary c.
cell c.
Clay Adams Ultra-flow 100 c.
Coulter's c.
Duke's cell c.
electronic cell c.
c. electrophoresis
frequency c.
Geiger c.
Geiger-Müller c.
Hemalog c.
Hematrak c.
c. immunoelectrophoresis
ion c.
liquid scintillation c.
proportional c.
radiation c.
ring c.
ripple c.
scintillation c.
shift c.
synchronous c.
counterclockwise
countercurrent
c. extraction
c. immunoelectrophoresis
c. mechanism
counterimmunoelectrophoresis
counterpulsation
counterstain
countertransport
sodium-lithium c.

counting
      c. cadence
      c. chamber
      photon c.
      c. plate
counting chamber
      Abbé-Zeiss c.c.
counts per minute
coup
      c. de fouet
      en c. de sabre
      c. de sang
      c. de soleil
      c. sur coup
couple
      redox c.
coupler
      acoustic c.
coupling
      c. capacitor
      c. defect
      excitation-contraction c.
      fixed c.
Courvoisier's
      law
      sign
covalence
covalent bond
covariance
coverglass method
coverslip
Cowdria
Cowdry
      bodies
      type A intranuclear inclusion
         body
cowperitis
Cowper's
      cyst
      gland
cowpox virus
coxa (pl., coxae)
      c. magna
      c. plana
      c. valga
      c. vara
coxal region
coxalgia
Coxiella burnetii
coxitis
coxodynia
Cox proportional hazards model

Coxsackie virus A, Type 1; B, Type 1
coxsackievirus
      c. A
      c. B.
Cox vaccine
coyotillo
cozymase
CP — cerebral palsy
      chemically pure
      chloropurine
      chloroquine and primaquine
      chronic pyelonephritis
      closing pressure
      cochlear potential
      coproporphyrin
      creatine phosphate
C/P — cholesterol-phospholipid ratio
C3PA — C3 proactivator
C3PAase — C3 proactivator con-
         vertase
cP — centipoise
CPA — cerebellar pontine angle
      chlorophenylalanine
C/pah — *p*-aminohippurate clearance
CPAP — continuous positive airway
         pressure
CPB — cardiopulmonary bypass
      competitive protein-binding
      (assay)
CPC — cetylpyridinium chloride
      chronic passive congestion
      clinicopathologic conference
CPD — cephalopelvic disproportion
      citrate-phosphate-dextrose
CPDA — citrate-phosphate-dextrose-
         adenine
CPE — chronic pulmonary em-
         physema
      cytopathic effect
C-peptide
CPG — coproporphyrinogen
CPI — coronary prognostic index
CPIB — chlorophenoxyiso-butyrate
CPK — creatine phosphokinase
cpm — counts per minute
CPN — chronic pyelonephritis
CPP — cyclopentenophenanthrene
CPPB — continuous positive-pressure
         breathing
CPPD — calcium pyrophosphate dihy-
         drate

CPR — cardiopulmonary resuscitation
       cerebral cortex perfusion rate
       cortisol production rate
cps — cycles per second
CPZ — chlorpromazine
CQ — chloroquine-quinine
       circadian quotient
C1q immune complex detection
C1q radioassay
CR — chest and right arm
       chloride
       conditioned reflex
       creatinine
       crown-rump
Cr — chromium
CRA — central retinal artery
       colorectal adenocarcinoma
crab
       c. eye
       c. hand
       c. louse
       c. yaws
Crabtree's effect
cracked heels
Craigie's tube method
cramp discharge
cran. — cranial
craniad
cranial
       c. arteritis
       c. bone
       c. cavity
       c. duplication
       c. dura mater
       c. epidural space
       c. insufflation
       c. meningocele
       c. monocephalus duplication
       c. nerve
       c. neuralgia
       c. pia mater
       c. subarachnoid space
       c. subdural space
craniectomy
craniobuccal
craniocarpotarsal
       c. dysplasia
       c. dystrophy
craniocaudal projection
craniocleidodysostosis
craniodiaphyseal dysplasia
craniofacial dysostosis

craniofenestria
craniolacunia
craniometaphyseal dysplasia
craniometry
craniopagus
craniopathy
       metabolic c.
craniopharyngeal
craniopharyngioma
craniorachischisis
cranioschisis
craniosclerosis
cranioscopy
craniostenosis
craniosynostosis
craniotabes
craniotomy
cranium (pl., craniums, crania)
crassamentum
crater
crateriform
craw-craw
CRBBB — complete right bundle
       branch block
CRD — chronic renal disease
       complete reaction of de-
       generation
C-reactive
       C-r. protein assay
       C-r. protein test
cream
       leukocyte c.
crease
       palmar c.
       simian c.
creat. — creatinine
creatinase
creatine
       c. kinase
       c. kinase isoenzyme electropho-
       resis
       c. kinase isoenzymes
       c. phosphate
       c. phosphokinase
       c. phosphokinase Bi
       c. phosphokinase MB
       c. phosphotransferase
       c. test
creatinemia
creatininase
creatinine
       amniotic fluid c.

c. clearance
c. clearance test
c. coefficient
creatinuria
Credé's
method
ointment
creeping
c. eruption
c. ulcer
CREG — cross-reactive group
cremasteric
c. fascia
c. muscle
c. reflex
cremaster muscle
crena (pl., crenae)
crenate
crenated cell
crenation
crenocyte
crenocytosis
crenulate
creola bodies
crepitans
tenosynovitis c.
crepitation
crepitus
crescent
c. cell
c. cell anemia
epithelial c.
glomerular c.
pressure c.
c. sign
sublingual c.
crescentic
c. glomerulonephritis
c. glomerulopathy
cresol
isopropyl c.
c. red
crest
iliac c.
maxillary c.
pubic c.
c. time
CREST (calcinosis cutis, Raynaud's
phenomenon, esophageal dysfunction, sclerodactyly, and telangiectasia) syndrome

cresyl
c. blue
c. blue brilliant
c. fast violet
c. violet
c. violet acetate
c. violet stain
cresylic acid
cretinism
neurologic c.
CRF — chronic renal failure
corticotropin-releasing factor
CRH — corticosteroid-releasing
hormone
cribriform
c. carcinoma
c. pattern
c. plate
cribrosa
area c.
cricoid cartilage
cricopharyngeal
cri du chat syndrome
Crimean hemorrhagic fever virus
criminal abortion
crinin
crinophagy
Crippa's lead tetra-acetate method
crisis (pl., crises)
addisonian c.
adrenal c.
anaphylactoid c.
aplastic c.
blast c.
blood c.
celiac c.
deglobulinization c.
hemolytic c.
hypertensive c.
megaloblastic c.
myelocytic c.
salt-losing c.
sickle-cell c.
splenic sequestration c.
thyroid c.
vaso-occlusive c.
crisis/storm
thyrotoxic c.
crista (pl., cristae)
c. ampullaris
c. galli

c. supraventricularis
c. urethra
criterion (pl., criteria)
    Fajans-Conn c.
    Haagensen and Stout c.
    Jones' c.
    Siperstein c.
Crithidia luciliae
critical
    c. angle
    c. flicker frequency
    c. fusion frequency
    c. illumination
    c. mass
    c. micelle concentration
    c. path analysis
    c. region
    c. temperature
CRM — cross-reacting material
cRNA — chromosomal RNA
crocein
    brilliant c.
crocidolite
cromolyn sodium
Crooke-Russell basophils
Crooke's
    cell
    hyaline change
    hyaline degeneration
cross
    c. activation
    c.-assembler
    c.-compiler
    c.-fire treatment
    c. hybridization
    c.-linking
    c. product
    c.-reacting agglutinin
    c.-reacting antigen
    c.-reacting material
    c. reaction
    c.-reactivity
    c.-resistance
    c.-sectional echocardiography
    c.-sectional survey
    c. sensitization
    three-point c.
    c. wall
crossed
    c. adductor reflex
    c. extension reflex

c. grid
c. immunoelectrophoresis
crossmatch
crossmatching
crossover frequency
crotalin
Crotalus
crotamiton
crotin
crotonase
croton oil
crot value
croup-associated virus
croupous
    c. bronchitis
    c. inflammation
    c. lymph
    c. membrane
    c. pharyngitis
Crouzon's craniofacial dysostosis
crowded cell index
crowding effect
crown-heel length
crown-rump length
CRP — C-reactive protein
CRS — Chinese restaurant syndrome
CRST — calcinosis cutis, Raynaud's
        phenomenon, sclero-
        dactyly, and telangiec-
        tasia
CRT — cathode ray tube
cruciate
    c. ligament
    c. lobe
    c. sulcus
crucible
crude
    c. mortality ratio
    c. rate
    c. urine
cruor (pl., cruores)
crural
cruris
crus (pl., crura)
    c. cerebri
    c. fornix
    c. penis
crush
    c. injury
    c. kidney
    c. preparation
    c. syndrome

crusta (pl., crustae)
    c. inflammatoria
    c. phlogistica
Crustacea
CRV — central retinal vein
cryalgesia
cryoablation
cryobank
cryobiology
cryocautery
cryocrit
cryofibrinogen
cryofibrinogenemia
cryogammaglobulin
cryogenic
cryoglobulin
cryoglobulinemia
    crystal c.
cryohydrocytosis
Cryokwik
cryopathic hemolytic syndrome
cryophile
cryoprecipitate
cryoprecipitated antihemophilic factor
cryoprecipitation
cryopreservation
cryopreserved leukocyte
cryoprobe
cryoprotectant
cryoprotein
cryoscope
cryoscopy
cryostat
    Ames Lab-Tek c.
cryosurgery
cryothalamotomy
cryotherapy
crypt
    c. abscesses
    anal c.
    appendiceal c.
    colonic c.
    Lieberkühn's c's
    Luschka's c's
    Morgagni's c.
    rectal c.
    small intestinal c.
    tonsillar c's
cryptenamine
cryptic enzyme
cryptitis
Cryptococcaceae

cryptococcal
    c. antigen
    c. antigen titer
    c. meningitis
    c. meningoencephalitis
cryptococci
cryptococcoma
cryptococcosis
Cryptococcus
    C. albidus/albidus
    C. albidus/diffluens
    C. capsulatus
    C. epidermidis
    C. gilchristi
    C. histolyticus
    C. hominis
    C. laurentii
    C. luteolus
    C. meningitidis
    C. neoformans
    C. terreus
Cryptococcus antibody titer
cryptogenic
    c. cirrhosis
    c. infection
    c. pyemia
    c. septicemia
cryptoglioma
cryptoleukemia
cryptolith
cryptomenorrhea
cryptophthalmos
    c. syndrome
cryptorchidism
    prepubertal c.
cryptorchid testis
cryptorchism
cryptosporidial
    c. enteritis
    c. infection
cryptosporidiosis
    biliary c.
Cryptosporidium listeria
Cryptostroma corticale
cryptostromosis
cryptoxanthin
cryptozoite
crys. — crystal
crystal
    acetylsulfadiazine c's
    acetylsulfamethoxazole c's
    ammonium biurate c's

ammonium magnesium phosphate c's
ammonium urate c's
asthma c's
birefringent c's
blood c's
Böttcher's c's
calcium bilirubinate c's
calcium hydrogen phosphate c's
calcium urate c's
c. cell
Charcot-Böttcher c's
Charcot-Leyden c's
Charcot-Neumann c's
Charcot-Robin c's
chiral c.
CPPD (calcium pyrophosphate dihydrate) c's
c. cryoglobulinemia
cystine c's
c. deposition disease
dicalcium hydrogen phosphate c's
Florence's c's
hematin c's
hematoidin c's
hydroxyapatite c.
indigotin c's
knife-rest c's
leukocytic c's
Leyden's c's
liquid c's
c. of Lubarsch
Lubarsch's c's
magnesium phosphate c's
meglumine diatrizoate c's
monosodium urate c's
oxalate c's
potassium urate c's
radiograph media c's
Reinke c's
rhomboid c's
rock c.
scintillation c.
sodium urate c's
sperm c's; spermin c's
thorn apple c's
triple phosphate c's
twin c.
urate c's
uric acid c's

c. urinary cast
urine sediment c's
c. violet
Virchow's c's
whetstone c's
crystalline
c. aggregate, nuclear
c. amyloses
c. birefringence
c. egg albumin
c. insulin
c. lens
c. macromolecule alteration
crystallization
crystalloglobulinemia
crystallography
x-ray c.
crystalloid
Charcot-Böttcher c's
crystalluria
CS — cesarean section
chondroitin sulfate
chorionic somatomammotropin
conditioned stimulus
coronary sinus
corticosteroid
cycloserine
C & S — conjuctiva and sclera
culture and sensitivity
Cs — cesium
CSA — canavaninosuccinic acid
chondroitin sulfate A
colony-stimulating activity
compressed spectral assay
Cs antigen
CSC — coup sur coup
CSF — cerebrospinal fluid
colony-stimulating factor
CSH — chronic subdural hematoma
cortical stromal hyperplasia
CSL — cardiolipin synthetic lecithin
CSM — cerebrospinal meningitis
CSN — carotid sinus nerve
CSR — Cheyne-Stokes respiration
corrected sedimentation rate
cortisol secretion rate
CSS — carotid sinus stimulation
CST — convulsive shock therapy
cST — centistoke
C-Stix test
CT — cardiothoracic (ratio)
carotid tracing

carpal tunnel
cerebral thrombosis
chlorothiazide
circulation time
clotting time
coagulation time
collecting tubule
computed tomography
computerized tomography
connective tissue
contraction time
Coombs's test
coronary thrombosis
corrected transposition
crest time
cytotechnologist
CTA — chromotropic acid
CTAB — cetyltrimethylammonium
     bromide
CTAT — computerized transaxial to-
     mography
CTBA — cetrimonium bromide
CTC — chlortetracycline
CTCL — cutaneous T-cell lymphoma
CTD — carpal tunnel decompression
     congenital thymic dysplasia
Ctenocephalides canis
C-terminal
ctetosome
CTFE — chlorotrifluoroethylene
CTH — ceramide trihexoside
C-thyroglobulin
CTL — cytologic T lymphocyte
CT number
CTP — cytidine triphosphate
CTR — cardiothoracic ratio
CTX — Cytoxan
C-type retrovirus
CTZ — chemoreceptor trigger zone
     chlorothiazide
Cu — copper
C/u — urea clearance
cubic
    c. centimeter
    c. millimeter
cubital
    c. fossa
    c. lymph node
    c. vein
cubitus
    c. valgus
    c. varus

cuboid
cuboidal
CUC — chronic ulcerative colitis
cu cm — cubic centimeter
cuff
    perivascular c.
cuffing
CUG — cystourethrogram
     cytidine-uridine-guanosine
cul-de-sac
    conjunctival c.
    Douglas's c.
    dural c.
    c. smear
culdocentesis
culdoscope
culdoscopy
Culex
Culicidae
Culicoides
Cullen's sign
culling
culmen
cultivation
culture
    adenovirus c.
    aerobic c.
    anaerobic c.
    anaerobic bacteria c.
    animal cell c.
    attenuated c.
    bacterial c.
    blood c.
    bone marrow c.
    cell c.
    cerebrospinal fluid c.
    cervical c.
    chorioallantoic c.
    continuous flow c.
    direct c.
    flask c.
    gonorrhea c.
    gravity-settling c.
    hanging-block c.
    hanging-drop c.
    c. medium (pl., c. media)
    microbiologic c.
    mixed c.
    mixed lymphocyte c.
    nasopharyngeal c.
    needle c.
    organ c.

plate c.
primary c.
pure c.
radioisotropic c.
secondary c.
c. and sensitivity
sensitized c.
shake c.
slant c.
slope c.
spinal fluid c.
smear c.
stab c.
stock c.
stool c.
streak c.
stroke c.
synchronized c.
throat c.
thrust c.
tissue c.
tube c.
type c.
urine c.
culture media *(see also* Appendix 3)
culture medium (pl., culture media)
nonpermissive c.m.
permissive c.m.
culturing
bacterial c.
cu mm — cubic millimeter
cumulated activity ratio
cumulative
c. action
c. distribution
c. effect
c. genes
cumulus (pl., cumuli)
c. oophorus
ovarian c.
cuneate nucleus
cuneiform
c. cartilage
c. lobe
cuneus
cunnilingus
Cunninghamella
C. bertholetiae
C. elegans
Cunninghamellaceae
CuO — cupric oxide
cupping

cuprein enzymes
cupremia
cupric ion–inhibited acid phosphatase
cupriuresis
cuprous
curare
curariform
curarization
curative dose
curdy pus
curet
curettage
endometrial c.
curette
curie-hour
curietherapy
curium
Curling's ulcer
current
alternating c.
dark c.
diffusion c.
direct c.
c. gain
pacemaker c.
c. regulator
saturation c.
three-phase c.
Curschmann's spiral
cursor
curvature
greater c. of stomach
lesser c. of stomach
spinal c.
curve
Bragg's c.
calibration c.
carbon dioxide dissociation c.
carbon dioxide response c.
cardiac output c.
cell survival c.
characteristic c.
compensation-response c.
dose-response c.
dye-dilution c.
epidemic c.
c. fitting
Frank-Starling c.
H and D c.
indicator-dilution c.
Kaplan-Meier survival c.
logarithmic c.

multiple event c.
oxygen-dissociation c.
oxygen-hemoglobin dissocia-
    tion c.
precipitin c.
pressure-volume c.
Price-Jones c.
regression c.
standard c.
Starling's c.
venous return c.
ventricular function c.
whole-body titration c.
Curvoisier's gastroenterostomy
Curvularia
    C. geniculata
    C. lunata
cushingoid facies
Cushing's
    basophilism
    reflex
    ulcer
cushion
    intimal c.
cuspid
    deciduous c.
    mandibular c.
    maxillary c.
Custer's cell
customary temperature scale
cutaneomandibular polyoncosis
cutaneomucouveal syndrome
cutaneous
    c. anergy
    c. anthrax
    c. branch
    c. candidiasis
    c. emphysema
    c. fistula
    c. fluids
    c. fungus
    c. gland
    c. hamartoma
    c. hemorrhoids
    c. horn
    c. infection
    c. leishmaniasis
    c. leprosy
    c. lupus erythematosus
    c. lymphoid hyperplasia
    c. lymphoplasia
    c. malformation

c. malignant melanoma
c. meningioma
c. metastasis
c. mucous gland
c. myiasis
c. nerve
c. nociceptors
c. reaction
c. receptor
c. systemic angiitis
c. T-cell lymphoma
c. tuberculosis
c. vasculitis
cutdown
Cuterebra
cuticle
cuticulum
cutireaction
cutis
    c. anserina
    atrophia maculosa varioli-
        formis c.
    c. elastica
    c. hyperelastica
    c. laxa
    c. verticis gyrata
cutoff
    c. frequency
    Roche c.
cutter
    agar c.
cutting
    section c.
cuvet; cuvette
    c. oximeter
Cuvier's duct
CV — cardiovascular
    cell volume
    central venous
    cerebrovascular
    coefficient of variation
    color vision
    conjugata vera (conjugate
        diameter of pelvic inlet)
    corpuscular volume
    cresyl violet
CVA — cardiovascular accident
    cerebrovascular accident
    costovertebral angle
CVD — cardiovascular disease
    color vision deviant

CVH — combined ventricular hypertrophy
    common variable hypogammaglobulinemia
CVI — common variable immunodeficiency
C virus — Coxsackie virus
CVO — conjugata vera obstetrica (obstetric conjugate diameter of pelvic inlet)
CVOD — cerebrovascular obstructive disease
CVP — cell volume profile
    central venous pressure
    cyclophosphamide, vincristine, prednisone
    Cytoxan, vincristine, prednisone
CVR — cardiovascular-renal
    cerebrovascular resistance
CVRD — cardiovascular renal disease
CVS — cardiovascular surgery
    cardiovascular system
C wave
CWDF — cell wall–deficient bacterial forms
CWI — cardiac work index
CWP — coal workers' pneumoconiosis
cwt — hundredweight
CX or cx — convex
CXR — chest x-ray film
Cy — cyanogen
cyanamide
    calcium c.
cyanate
cyanemia
cyanhemoglobin
cyanide
    c. anion
    c.-ascorbate test
    calcium c.
    ethyl c.
    hydrogen c.
    mercuric c.
    c.-nitroprusside test
    c. poisoning
    potassium c.
    vinyl c.
    zinc c.
cyanidol
cyanin

cyanmethemoglobin
cyanmetmyoglobin
cyanoacrylate
Cyanobacteria
cyanochroic; cyanochrous
cyanocobalamin
    radioactive c.
cyanogen
    c. bromide
    c. chloride
cyanoguanidine
    mercuric c.
cyanohemoglobin
cyanoketone
cyanol FF
cyanophil; cyanophile
cyanophilous
cyanophoric glycoside
cyanopia
cyanosed
cyanose tardive
cyanosis
    enterogenous c.
    false c.
    hereditary methemoglobinemic c.
    toxic c.
cyanotic
    c. atrophy
    c. atrophy of liver
    c. induration
cyanuria
cybernetics
cybrid
CYC — cyclophosphamide
cycad
Cycas
cyclacillin
cyclamate
cyclandelate
cyclase
    adenyl c.
    adenylate c.
    nucleotide c.
cyclazocine
cycle
    anovulatory c.
    biliary c.
    carbon c.
    cardiac c.
    cell c.
    citric acid c.

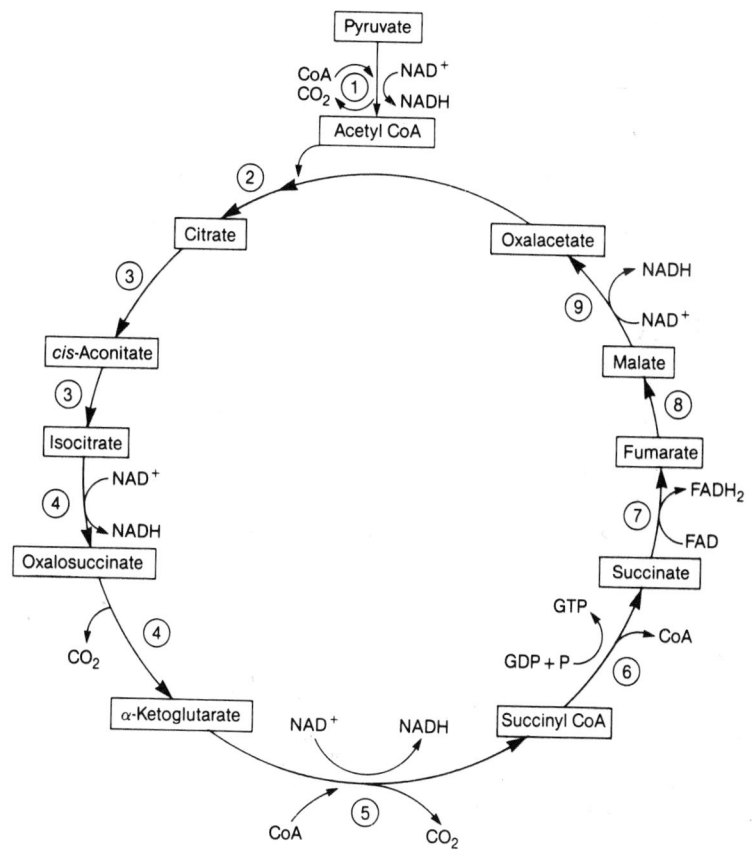

Tricarboxylic acid (Krebs') cycle

c. alteration
cAMP (adenosine monophosphate)
cAMP (adenosine monophosphate)–dependent kinase
cGMP (guanosine monophosphate)
c. hydrocarbon
c. lysine anhydride
c. neutropenia
c. nucleotides
c. tissue alteration
cyclitis
cyclitol
cyclization
cyclizine hydrochloride
Cyclo. — cyclophosphamide
cyclopropane
cycloalkane
cycloalkene
cyclobarbital
cyclobenzaprine hydrochloride
cyclobutane
cyclocryotherapy
cyclocumarol
cyclodiene hydrocarbon pesticides
cyclodimerization
cyclogeny
cyclogram
cyclohexane
methyl c.
cyclohexanol
cyclohexene oxide
cycloheximide
cyclohexylamine
2-cyclohexyl-4,6-dinitrophenol
cycloisomerase
cyclo-ligase
cyclomastopathy
cyclomethycaine sulfate
cyclonite
cyclooxygenase pathway
cyclopentamine hydrochloride
cyclopentane
cyclopentanoperhydrophenanthrene
cyclopentolate hydrochloride
cyclopentylpropionate testosterone
cyclophosphamide
Cyclophyllidea
cyclopia
cyclopropane
Cyclops

cyclops hypognathus
cyclorotary
cyclorotation
cycloscope
cycloserine
cyclosis
cyclosporin A
cyclosporine
c. poisoning
cyclothiazide
cyclothymic
cyclotron
cycrimine hydrochloride
cyesis
cylinder
axis c.
Bence Jones c's
graduated c.
Külz's c.
cylindric; cylindrical
c. bronchiectasis
c. embryo
c. epithelioma
cylindroadenoma
cylindrocellular
cylindroid
c. aneurysm
c. bronchiectasis
cylindroma
dermal eccrine c.
cylindromatous carcinoma
cylindrosarcoma
cylindruria
cymarin
cynanche
c. maligna
c. tonsillaris
cypionate testosterone
cyproheptadine hydrochloride
cyproterone acetate
cyrtometer
cys. — cystine
cyst
adrenal cortex c.
adventitious c.
allantoic c.
alveolar c.
alveolar hydatid c.
amebic c.
aneurysmal bone c.
Baker's c.
Bartholin's c.

blood c.
blue dome c.
bone c.
branchial c.
branchial cleft c.
breast c.
bronchial c.
bronchogenic c.
bursal c.
calcifying odontogenic c.
cervical lymphoepithelial c.
chocolate c.
choledochal c.
chyle c.
colloid c.
compound c.
congenital c.
corpora lutea c's
corpus hemorrhagicum c.
corpus luteum c.
cortical retention c.
Cowper's c.
daughter c.
dental follicular c.
dentigerous c.
dermoid c.
developmental c.
distention c.
duplication c.
echinococcus c.
embryonal duct c.
endometrial c.
endothelial c.
enteric duplication c.
enterogenous c's
epidermal c.
epidermal inclusion c.
epidermoid c.
epidermoid inclusion c.
epididymal c.
epithelial c.
epithelial inclusion c.
extravasation c.
exudation c.
false c.
fatty c.
fissural c.
c. fluid cytology
follicle c.
follicular c.
ganglion c.
Gartner's c.

Gartner's duct c.
gas c.
germinal epithelial inclusion c.
germinal inclusion c.
giardial c.
globulomaxillary c.
glomerular c.
Gorlin's c.
granddaughter c.
hemorrhagic c.
hepatic c's
heterotopic oral gastrointestinal c.
horn c's
hydatid c.
implantation c.
inclusion c.
inflammatory c.
involution c.
iodine c's
junctional c.
keratinous c.
Kobelt's c.
lacteal c.
luteal c.
luteinized follicular c.
lymphoepithelial c.
median raphe c.
mediastinal c.
medullary renal c.
meibomian c.
mesenteric c.
mesonephric c.
mesothelial c.
milium c.
milk c.
Morgagni's c.
mother c.
mucinous c.
mucoid c.
mucous c.
multilocular c.
multilocular hydatid c.
multiloculate hydatid c.
myxoid c.
nabothian c.
nasopalatine duct c.
necrotic c.
odontogenic c.
oil c.
oophoritic c.
osseous hydatid c.

ovarian c.
pancreatic c.
paraphyseal c.
parasitic c.
parathyroid c.
parent c.
paroophoritic c.
parovarian c.
parvilocular c.
pericardial c.
periodontal c.
phaeomycotic c.
pilar c.
piliferous c.
pilonidal c.
pneumocystic c.
proliferating trichilemmal c.
proliferation c.; proliferative c.
prostatic c.
pseudomucinous c.
pulmonary c.
radicular c.
ranular c.
Rathke's cleft c.
renal c.
renal parenchymal c.
retention c.
rete ovarii c.
saccular c.
sanguineous c.
sebaceous c.
secretory c.
sequestration c.
serous c.
simple c.
solitary c.
solitary bone c.
sperm-containing c.
sterile c.
sublingual c.
suprasellar c.
synovial c.
tapeworm c.
tarry c.
tarsal c.
tension c.
teratomatous c.
theca lutein c.
thyroglossal duct c.
thyroid c.
thyrolingual c.
Tornwaldt's c.

trichilemmal c.
tubular c.
umbilical c.
unicameral c.
unicameral bone c.
unilocular c.
unilocular hydatid c.
urachal c.
urinary c.
vitellointestinal c.
vulvar c.
wolffian c.
cystadenocarcinoma
mucinous c.
papillary c.
papillary serous c.
pseudomucinous c.
serous c.
cystadenofibroma
cystadenoma
c. adamantinum
apocrine c.
bile duct c.
clear cell c.
c. lymphomatosum
mucinous c.
oncocytic papillary c.
papillary c.
papillary c. lymphomatosum
papillary serous c.
pseudomucinous c.
serous c.
cystalgia
cystathionase
cystathionine
c. γ-lyase
c. β-synthase
cystathioninuria
cystauchenitis
cysteamine dehydrogenase
cystectasia; cystectasy
cystectomy
cysteic acid method
cysteine
c. aminotransferase
c. desulfhydrase
c. synthase
c. synthetase
cysteinesulfinate decarboxylase
cysteinyl
cysteinyl-glycine dipeptidase

cystic
- c. acute inflammation
- c. ameloblastoma
- c. artery
- c. atrophy
- c. cancer
- c. carcinoma
- c. chondromalacia
- c. chronic cervicitis
- c. chronic inflammation
- c. corpus hemorrhagicum
- c. corpus luteum
- c. cystitis
- c. degeneration
- c. dermoid teratoma
- c. diathesis
- c. disease
- c. disease of renal medulla
- c. duct
- c. dysplasia
- c. endometrial hyperplasia
- c. epithelioma
- c. fibroma
- c. fibrosis
- c. fibrosis of pancreas
- c. fibrosis tests
- c. goiter
- c. granulomatous inflammation
- c. hygroma
- c. hyperplasia
- c. hyperplasia of breast
- c. hyperplasia of endometrium
- c. inflammation
- c. kidney
- c. leiomyoma
- c. lymphangiectasis
- c. lymphangioma
- c. mastitis
- c. mastopathy
- c. medial necrosis
- c. medial necrosis of ascending aorta
- c. medionecrosis
- c. meningioma
- c. mole
- c. myxoma
- c. nephroma
- c. ovarian follicle
- c. polyp
- c. renal dysplasia
- c. teratoma
- c. vein

cysticerci
cysticercoid
cysticercosis titer
Cysticercus
- C. *acanthrotrias*
- C. *bovis*
- C. *cellulosae*
- C. *fasciolaris*
- C. *ovis*
- C. *tenuicollis*

cysticercus (pl., cysticerci)
cystides
cystidolaparotomy
cystiform
cystigerous
cystine
- c. calculus
- c. crystals
- c. reductase
- c. storage disease
- c.-tellurite blood agar
- c. trypticase agar

cystinemia
cystinosis
cystinotic leukocyte
cystinuria
- familial c.
- c. tests

cystiphorous
cystis (pl., cystides)
cystitis
- acute hemorrhagic c.
- amebic c.
- bacterial c.
- bullous c.
- calculous c.
- candidal c.
- chemical c.
- c. colli
- cystic c.
- c. cystica
- denuding c.
- emphysematous c.
- encrusted c.
- eosinophilic c.
- follicular c.
- c. follicularis
- formalin c.
- fungal c.
- giant cell c.
- glandular c.
- c. glandularis

hemorrhagic c.
honeymoon c.
Hunner's c.
inflammatory c.
interstitial c.
lupus c.
c. lymphopathia
c. pneumatoides
polypoid c.
proliferative c.
radiation c.
recurrent c.
suppurative c.
trigonal c.
tuberculous c.
ulcerative c.
viral c.
cysto. — cystoscopic examination
cystoadenoma
cystoblast
cystocarcinoma
cystocele
cystocolostomy
cystodiaphanoscopy
cystodiverticulum
cystoenterostomy
cystoepithelioma
cystofibroma
cystogastrostomy
cystogenic aneurysm
cystogram
voiding c.
cystography
radionuclide c.
retrograde c.
cystoid
c. degeneration
c. macular degeneration
cystojejunostomy
Cystokon
cystolith
cystolithiasis
cystolithic
cystoma
serous c.
cystometer
cystometrography
cystomorphous
cystomyoma
cystomyxoadenoma
cystomyxoma
cystopherous

cystoproctostomy
cystoprostatectomy
cystoptosis; cystoptosia
cystopyelitis
cystopyelonephritis
cystosarcoma
c. phyllodes
c. phylloides
cystoscope
cystoscopy
cystostomy
cystoureteritis
cystoureterogram
cystoureterography
cystourethritis
cystourethrocele
cystourethroscope
cystous
cystyl
cytapheresis
cytarabine hydrochloride
cytase
cytaster
cythemolytic icterus
cytidine
c. deaminase
c. diphosphate
c. monophosphate
c. phosphate
c. triphosphate
cytidine-5′-phosphate
cytidine-uridine-guanosine
cytidotrachelotomy
cytidylic acid
cytidylyl
cytisine
cytisism
cytoanalyzer
cytobiology
cytoblast
cytoblastema
cytocentrifugation
cytocentrifuge
cytochalasin B
cytochemical
cytochemistry
cytochrome
c. b_5 reductase
c. b_5 reductase assay
c. c oxidase
c. oxidase
c. oxidase strips

c. oxidase test
c. P450
c. peroxidase
c. reductase
ubiquinol c. reductase
cytocidal
cytocide
cytoclasis
cytoclastic
cytoclesis
cytocyst
cytode
cytodegenerative necrosis
cytodiagnosis
    exfoliative c.
cytodiagnostic urinalysis
cytodieresis
cytodifferentiation
cytodistal
cytofluorography
cytogene
cytogenetic
    c. map
    c. marker
    c. remission
cytogenetics
    clinical c.
    population c.
cytogenic gland
cytoglomerator
cytoglucopenia
cytohistogenesis
cytoid
cytokalipenia
cytokeratin
    c. polypeptide
    c. reaction
cytokine
    fibrogenic c.
cytokinesis
cytokinetic
cytokinin
cytolipin H
cytologic
    c. abnormality
    c. alteration
    c. degeneration
    c. diagnosis
    c. engulfment
    c. examination
    c. filter preparation
    c. screening

c. smear
c. specimen
c. T lymphocyte
cytology
    analytic c.
    aspiration c.
    aspiration biopsy c.
    effusion c.
    exfoliative c.
    urinary c.
cytolysate
    blood c.
cytolysin
cytolysis
    immune c.
cytolysosome
cytolytic
cytoma
cytomegalic
    c. adrenal hypoplasia
    c. inclusion disease
    c. inclusion disease cytology
    c. inclusion disease virus
cytomegalovirus
    c. antibody
    c. culture
    c. disease
    disseminated c.
    c. isolation
    c. mononucleosis
    c. retinitis
cytomegaly
    adrenal c.
cytometaplasia
cytometer
    flow c.
cytometry
    flow c.
cytomorphology
cytomorphosis
cytopathic
    c. effect
    c. inflammation
    c. virus
cytopathogenesis
cytopathogenic
cytopathologic; cytopathological
cytopathologist
cytopathology
cytopathy
cytopenia
    refractory c.

cytophagic panniculitis
cytophagous
cytophagy
cytophilic antibody
cytophotometer
cytophotometric analysis
cytophotometry
    flow c.
cytophylaxis
cytopipette
cytoplasm
    clear cell c.
    ground-glass c.
cytoplasmic
    c. aggregate
    c. alteration
    c. bridge
    c. crystalline aggregate
    c. fiber alteration
    c. fibril alteration
    c. fibrin
    c. filament alteration
    c. glia
    c. glycogen
    c. glycolytic enzyme
    c. granules
    c. inclusion
    c. inheritance
    c. lipid aggregate
    c. lipid droplet alteration
    c. macromolecular aggregate
    c. marker
    c. matrix alteration
    c. membrane
    c. organoid
    c. streaming
    c. vacuolization
cytoplast
cytopreparation
cytoreductive therapy
cytorrhyctes
cytoscopy
cytosiderin
cytosine
    arabinoside c.

guanine c.
hydroxymethyl c.
cytosis
cytoskeleton
cytosmear
cytosol
cytosome
    lipid c's
cytostasis
cytostatic
cytostome
cytostromatic
cytotactic
cytotaxia
cytotaxin
cytotaxis
    negative c.
    positive c.
cytotechnologist
cytothesis
cytotoxic
    c. antibody
    c. cell
    c. cell protein
    c. edema
    c. necrosis
    c. suppressor
    c. T cells
    c. T lymphocytes
cytotoxicity
    antibody-dependent cell-
      mediated c.
    complement-mediated c.
    lymphocyte-mediated c.
    c. test
    T-lymphocyte c.
cytotoxin
cytotrophic serum
cytotrophoblast
cytotropic antibody
    test
cytotropism
Cytoxan
cytozyme
cyturia
Czapek-Dox agar

D — deciduous
density
deuterium
deuteron
dextro
diopter
distal
dorsal
duration
vitamin D unit
D- — a prefix specifying relationship
to D-glyceraldehyde
D_{CO} — diffusing capacity for carbon
monoxide
D_L — diffusing capacity of lung
d. —day(s)
decigram
diurnal
d — dextrorotatory
DA — degenerative arthritis
developmental age
direct agglutination
disaggregated
dopamine
ductus arteriosus
DAB — dimethylaminoazobenzene
DAC — digital-to-analog converter
dacarbazine
D/A converter
dacryote
dacryoadenalgia
dacryoadenectomy
dacryoadenitis
dacryoblennorrhea
dacryocyst
dacryocystitis
dacryocystography
dacryocyte
dacryolith
Desmarres's d's
dacryoma
dacryosolenitis
DACT. — dactinomycin
dactyl
dactylitis
sickle cell d.
dactylolysis spontanea
DADDS — diacetyl diaminodiphenylsulfone
dADP — deoxyadenosine diphosphate

DAF — decay antibody-accelerating
factor
Da Fano's stain
DAG — diacylglycerol
DAGT — direct antiglobulin test
DAH — disordered action of the
heart
Dakin's solution
DALA — delta-aminolevulinic acid
dalapon
Dale-Laidlaw's clotting time method
Dalen-Fuchs nodules
dalton
Dalton's law
DAM — degraded amyloid
diacetyl monoxime
damage
diffuse alveolar d.
irradiation d.
minimal brain d.
myocardial d.
radiation d.
dammar
dAMP — deoxyadenosine monophosphate
damping
Dam unit
danazol
D and C — dilatation and curettage
dilation and curettage
dandy fever
Dandy-Walker malformation
Dane's
method
particle
stain
DANS — 1-dimethylamino-naphtha-
lene-5-sulfonyl chloride
dansyl chloride
danthron
115 D8 antibody
D antigen
dantrolene sodium
Danubian endemic familial nephropathy
Danysz phenomenon
DAO — diamine oxidase
DAP — dihydroxyacetone phosphate
direct agglutination pregnancy (test)

dapsone
DAPT — direct agglutination pregnancy test
Dapt. — Daptazole
D-arabitol dehydrogenase
Daraprim
Darier-Roussy sarcoid
Darier's sign
dark
    d. current
    d. reactions
    d. reactivation
darkfield
    d. condenser
    d. fluorescent antibody
    d. microscope
Darkshevich's nucleus
Darlington amplifier
d'Arsonval meter
dartos
Darvon
darwinian
    d. point
    d. tubercle
DAT — differential agglutination titer
    diphtheria antitoxin
    direct agglutination test
    direct antiglobulin test
data
    d. acquisition system
    analog d.
    categorical d.
    d. display
    metric d.
    d. processing
    ranked d.
    d. reduction
database
dATP — deoxyadenosine triphosphate
Datril
daughter
    d. colony
    d. cyst
daunomycin
daunorubicin
Davainea
Davaineidae
Davenport graph
Davidsohn's differential test
Dawson's encephalitis

Day's test
DB — dextran blue
    distobuccal
dB; db — decibel
DBA — dibenzanthracene
DBC — dye-binding capacity
DBCL — dilute blood clot lysis (method)
DBI — development-at-birth index
DBM — dibromomannitol
DBO — distobucco-occlusal
DBP — diastolic blood pressure
    distobuccopulpal
DC — deoxycholate
    diphenylarsine cyanide
    distocervical
    direct current; also, dc
D&C — dilatation and curettage
    dilation and curettage
DCA — deoxycholate-citrate agar
    desoxycorticosterone acetate
DCc — double concave
dCDP — deoxycytidine diphosphate
DCF — deoxycoformycin
    direct centrifugal flotation
DCG — disodium cromoglycate
DCHFB — dichlorohexafluorobutane
DCI — dichloroisoproterenol
DCIP — dichlorophenolindophenol
DCIS — ductal carcinoma in situ
DCLS — deoxycholate citrate lactose saccharose
dCMP — deoxycytidine monophosphate
D colony
DCT — direct Coombs' test
DCTMA — desoxycorticosterone trimethylacetate
dCTP — deoxycytidine triphosphate
DCTPA — desoxycorticosterone triphenylacetate
DCx — double convex
DDAVP — 1-deamino-(8-D-arginine)-vasopressin
DDC — diethyldithiocarbamic acid
DDCT — dideoxycytidine
DDD — dihydroxydinaphthyl disulfide
    dense deposit disease
    dichlorodiphenyldichloroethane

dihydroxydinaphthyl
disulfide

D-dimer

DDP — cis-diaminodichloroplatinum

DDS — diaminodiphenylsulfone
dystrophy-dystocia syndrome

DDT — dichlorodiphenyltrichloroethane

DDVP — dichlorvos
dimethyldichlorovinyl
phosphate

D&E — dilation and evacuation

DEA — dehydroepiandrosterone
diethanolamine

deactivation

deacylase
acylsphingosine d.

deacylate

dead on arrival

dead retained fetus

DEAE — diethylaminoethanol
diethylaminoethyl

DEAE-D — diethylaminoethyl
dextran

deafferentation

deafness
apoplectiform d.
conduction d.
high-frequency d.
mixed-type d.
nerve d.
tone d.

dealbation

dealcoholization

deallergization

deamidase

deaminase
adenosine d.
adenylic acid d.
arginine d.
cytidine d.
guanine d.
guanosine d.
guanylic acid d.
porphobilinogen d.

α-deaminase
histidine α-d.

deamination

deanol acetamidobenzoate

deaquation

dearterialization

death
crib d.

intrauterine d.
local d.
neonatal d.
perinatal d.
d. rate
somatic d.

DEBA — diethylbarbituric acid

Debaryomyces
D. hansenii
D. hominis
D. neoformans

debilitating

debrancher
d. deficiency
d. enzyme

debranching enzyme

débride

débridement

debris
necrotic d.

debug

debye

DEC — dendritic epidermal cell

decacurie

Decaderm

Decadron

decagram

decahydronaphthalene

decalcification

decalcify

decalcifying

decaliter

decameter

decamethonium
d. bromide
d. iodide

decannulation

decanoic acid

decantation

decapeptide

decapitation

decapsulation

decarbonization

decarboxylase
acetoacetate d.
acetolactate d.
branched-chain α-ketoacid d.
d. broth
dopa d.
glutamate d.
glutamic acid d.
histidine d.
methylmalonyl-CoA d.

ornithine d.
orotidine-5′-phosphate d.
orotidylate d.
oxaloacetate d.
uroporphyrinogen d.
decarboxylation
amine precursor uptake and d.
De Castro's fluid
decavitamin
decay
d.-activating factor
alpha d.
d. antibody-accelerating factor
beta d.
branching d.
d. coefficient
d. constant
exponential d.
d. mode
positron beta d.
d. product
radioactive d.
d. rate
d. scheme
decedent
deceration
decerebrate rigidity
decibel
decidua
basal d.
capsular d.
ectopic d.
menstrual d.
parietal d.
reflex d.
d. vera
decidual
d. alteration
d. cast
d. cells
d. change
d. endometritis
d. membrane
d. metaplasia
deciduitis
deciduoma
Loeb's d.
deciduous
d. incisor
d. molar
d. skin
decigram

decile
deciliter
milligrams per d.
decimal reduction time
decimeter
decinem
decoagulant
decode
decoder
decolorize
decompensated shock
decompensation
cardiac d.
d. injury
d. sickness
decomposition potential
decompression
carpal tunnel d.
d. injury
d. sickness
decontamination
decortication
decoy cell
decrement
decrementing response
decubation
decubitus
d. calculus
dorsal d.
d. ulcer
ventral d.
decussate
decussation
dorsal tegmental d.
d. of inferior cerebellar pe-
duncles
d. of pyramids
d. of superior cerebellar pe-
duncles
pons d.
pyramidal d.
supramammillary d.
ventral tegmental d.
dedifferentiated
d. chondrosarcoma
d. liposarcoma
dedifferentiation
DEEG — depth electroencephalogram
depth electroencephalography
depth electrography
Deelman effect

deep
>   d. agar
>   d. brachial artery
>   d. cervical lymphatics
>   d. circumflex iliac vein
>   d. infrapatellar bursa
>   d. lymphatics
>   d. middle cerebral vein
>   d. palmar arch
>   d. peroneal nerve
>   d. plantar branch
>   d. sylvian vein
>   d. temporal nerve
>   d. transverse fibers
>   d. volar arch

Deetjen's bodies
def. — deficiency
defecation
defecography
defect
>   acquired d.
>   aldosterone secretion d.
>   aortic septal d.
>   atrial septal d.
>   bent head d.
>   congenital d.
>   congenital ectodermal d.
>   cortical d.
>   coupling d.
>   ectodermal d.
>   endocardial cushion d's
>   fibrous cortical d.
>   filling d.
>   Gerbode d.
>   hydrogen-detected ventricular
>   septal d.
>   interatrial septal d.
>   interventricular septal d.
>   intraventricular conduction d.
>   iodide transport d.
>   iodotyrosine deiodinase d.
>   labyrinthine d.
>   metaphyseal fibrous d.
>   neural tube d.
>   organofaction d.
>   Passavoy d.
>   plasma d.
>   platelet d.
>   septal d.
>   serum d.
>   surgical d.

>   ventricular septal d.
>   zero d's

defective
>   d. recent memory
>   d. remote memory
>   d. virus

defense
>   host d.

defenestration
deferentitis
deferoxamine
>   d. hydrochloride
>   d. mesylate

defervescence
defibrillation
defibrillator
defibrinated blood
defibrination syndrome
defibrinogenation
deficiency
>   acquired C1 inhibitor d.
>   adenine phosphoribosyl trans-
>   ferase d.
>   adenosine deaminase d.
>   adenosylcobalamin d.
>   adenylate kinase d.
>   ADH (antidiuretic hor-
>   mone) d.
>   aldolase d.
>   alpha$_1$-antitrypsin d.
>   d. anemia
>   antithrombin d.
>   antitrypsin d.
>   argininosuccinate synthetase d.
>   biotin d.
>   brancher d.
>   C1, 2, 3, 4, 5, 6, 6-7, 7, 8, 9 d.
>   caloric d.
>   carbamoyl-phosphate synthe-
>   tase I d.
>   cell adhesion molecular d.
>   cellular immune d.
>   coagulation d.
>   debrancher d.
>   delta granule d.
>   20,22-desmolase d.
>   dihydrofolate reductase d.
>   dihydropteridine reductase d.
>   2,3-diphosphoglycerate mu-
>   tase d.
>   disaccharidase d.
>   duplication d.

enzyme d.
erythrocyte hexokinase d.
factor I, II, V, VII, VIII, IX,
    X, XI d.
Factor D, H, I d.
folate d.
folic d.
folic acid d.
formiminotransferase d.
galactokinase d.
α-galactosidase d.
β-galactosidase d.
glucocerebrosidase d.
glucose-6-phosphate dehydroge-
    nase d.
glucose-6-phosphate isomerase
    d.
glucuronyl transferase d.
glutamate formiminotrans-
    ferase d.
glutamylcysteine synthetase d.
glutathione reductase d.
glyceraldehyde-3-phosphate de-
    hydrogenase d.
gonadotropin d.
growth hormone d.
hereditary plasma thromboplas-
    tin component d.
hexosaminidase A d.
11-hydroxylase d.
17-hydroxylase d.
21-hydroxylase d.
immune d.
immunoglobulin A d.
immunoglobulin G d.
inosine phosphorylase d.
iodine d.
iron d.
lactase d.
lecithin-cholesterol acyltrans-
    ferase d.
leukocyte adhesion d.
lipoprotein lipase d.
mental d.
mineral d.
myeloperoxidase d.
Nezelof's T-cell d.
ornithine carbamoyltrans-
    ferase d.
ornithine transcarbamylase d.
phenylalanine hydroxylase d.
phosphofructokinase d.

phosphohexose isomerase d.
phosphorylase d.
plasma thromboplastin antece-
    dent d.
protein d.
prothrombin d.
pseudocholinesterase d.
pyrimidine-5'-nucleotidase d.
pyruvate kinase d.
pyruvate kinase d., erythrocyte
recessive enzymatic d.
5α-reductase d.
secondary antibody d.
selenium d.
serum prothrombin conversion
    accelerator d.
specific coagulation factor d.
sphingomyelinase d.
stable factor d.
sucrase-isomaltase d.
sulfite oxidase d.
thiamine d.
thromboplastin antecedent d.
triosephosphate isomerase d.
tuftsin d.
tyrosinase d.
tyrosine aminotransferase d.
vitamin d.
vitamin K d.
X-linked hypogammaglobuli-
    nemia with growth hor-
    mone d.
zinc d.
deficit
defined substrate
definition
    recursive d.
definitive
    d. callus
    d. erythroblast
    d. host
    d. method
    d. organism identification
deflection signal
deflorescence
defoliant
deformability
deformation
deforming
deformity
    acquired d.
    congenital d.
    hourglass d.

Klippel-Feil d.
lobster claw d.
pigeon breast d.
saddle nose d.
swan-neck d.
valgus d.
varus d.
deg. — degeneration
degree
De Galantha's method for urates
degeneracy
degenerate code
degenerated
    d. intervertebral disc
    d. intervertebral fibrocartilage
    d. meniscus
degenerating myelin demonstration
degeneration
    adipose d.
    albuminoid d.
    albuminous d.
    Alzheimer's fibrillary d.
    amyloid d.
    angiolithic d.
    ascending d.
    atheromatous d.
    axonal d.
    ballooning d.
    basophilic d.
    basophilic granular d.
    calcareous d.
    carneous d.
    caseous d.
    cellular d.
    cloudy swelling d.
    collagen d.
    colliquative d.
    colloid d.
    Crooke's hyaline d.
    cystic d.
    cystoid d.
    cystoid macular d.
    cytologic d.
    descending d.
    elastoid d.
    elastotic d.
    fatty d.
    feathery d.
    fibrinoid d.
    fibrinous d.
    fibrous d.
    floccular d.

granular d.
granulovacuolar d.
hepatolenticular d.
hyaline d.
hydatid d.
hydropic d.
lenticular progressive d.
lipid d.
lipoid d.
liquefaction d.
liquefactive d.
macular d.
medial d.
Mönckeberg's d.
mucinoid d.
mucinous d.
mucoid d.
mucoid medial d.
myelin d.
myelinic d.
myxoid d.
myxomatous d.
paraneoplastic cerebellar d.
parenchymatous d.
partial reaction of d.
pericyte d.
pigmentary d.
pseudomucinous d.
pseudotubular d.
reaction of d.
reaction to d.
red d.
reticular d.
secondary d.
senile d.
spinocerebellar d.
striatonigral d.
subacute cerebellar d.
subacute combined d.
trans-synaptic d.
vacuolar d.
vitreous d.
wallerian d.
waxy d.
Zenker's d.
degenerative
    d. arthritis
    d. change
    d. index
    d. inflammation
    d. joint disease
deglobulination crisis

deglutition
deglycerolization
Degos's acanthoma
degradation
degranulation
degree
    d's of freedom
    prism d.
    second d.
dehiscence
dehydrase
    aminolevulinic acid d.
dehydratase
    ALA (aminolevulinic acid) d.
    carbonate d.
dehydrate
dehydrated alcohol
dehydration
dehydroacetic acid
dehydroascorbic acid
dehydrobilirubin
dehydrocholesterol
    activated 7-d.
dehydrocholic acid
11-dehydrocorticosterone
dehydroepiandrosterone sulfate
dehydrogenase
    acyl-CoA d.
    adenylate kinase d.
    alcohol d.
    aldehyde d.
    d-beta-ol d.
    branched-chain α-ketoacid d.
    D-arabitol d.
    d. formaldehyde
    glucose-6-phosphate d.
    glutamate d.
    glyceraldehyde-phosphate d.
    heat-stable lactic acid d.
    hexosephosphate d.
    3-hydroxybutyrate d.
    iditol d.
    isocitrate d.
    isocitric acid d.
    isovaleryl-CoA d.
    lactate d.
    lactic acid d.
    L-arabinose d.
    L-arabitol d.
    lysine d.
    malate d.
    malic acid d.

    oxoglutarate d.
    2-oxoisovalerate d.
    phosphogluconate d.
    6-phosphoglycerate d.
    polyol d.
    proline d.
    1-pyrroline-5-carboxylate d.
    saccharopine d.
    sarcosine d.
    serum hydroxybutyrate d.
    serum isocitric acid d.
    serum lactic acid d.
    sorbitol d.
    tetrahydrofolate d.
    triosephosphate d.
    ubiquinol d.
    uracil d.
    xylitol d.
    L-xylose d.
dehydrogenate
dehydrogenation
dehydroisoandrosterone
dehydropeptidase
deiodinase
deionization
Deiters's nucleus
Dejerine-Sottas disease
dekanem
Delafield's hematoxylin
Delalutin
Delaney clause
Delatestryl
delay
    d. circuit
    d. line
delayed
    d. adrenarche
    d. climacteric
    d. hemolytic transfusion re-
      action
    d. hypersensitivity
    d. menopause
    d. primary closure
    d. puberty
    d.-type hypersensitivity
de-lead
deletion
    antigenic d.
    chromosomal d.
    intercalary d.
    interstitial d.
    d. mutation

terminal d.
d. theory
deliquescence
deliquescent
delirium (pl., deliria)
d. tremens
delivery
precipitous d.
spontaneous d.
delle
delomorphous
Delphian node
delta
d. aminolevulinic acid
d. antigen
d. band
d. base
d. beta-thalassemia
d. bilirubin
d. cell islet
d. cells
d. chain
d. check
d. granule deficiency
d. hepatitis
hepatitis d. agent
d. osmolality
d. ray
d. spathylolysin
d.-9-tetrahydrocannabinol
delta activity
intermittent rhythmic d.a.
polymorphic d.a.
Delta-Cortef
Deltasone
deltoideus muscle
deltoid ligament
deltopectoral flap
Deltra
Delves cup technique
Dem. — Demerol (meperidine)
demarcation
line of d.
Dematiaceae
dematiaceous fungi
Dematium
demecarium bromide
demeclocycline hydrochloride
demecolcine
dementia
d. complex
presenile d.

senile d.
transmissible agent d.
Demerol (meperidine)
demethylchlortetracycline
demeton
methyl d.
demilune
d. body
demineralization
Demodex folliculorum
demonstration
calcium deposit d.
copper deposit d.
degenerating myelin d.
iron-positive pigment d.
De Morgan's spots
demyelinate
demyelinating
d. disease
d. neuropathy
demyelination
axonal d.
segmental d.
demyelinization
denaturation
protein d.
denatured hemoglobin
denaturing gels
dendrite
apical d.
dendritic
d. calculus
d. cancer
d. epidermal cells
d. keratitis
d. melanocyte
d. tree
dendrodendritic
dendrophagocytosis
denervated bladder
denervation atrophy
dengue
d. fever
hemorrhagic d.
d. virus, types 1, 2, 3, 4
denitrifying bacterium
Denker-Kahler approach
Dennis's technique
de novo
d.n. fibrosis
d.n. pathway

dens (pl., dentes)
    d. in dente
dense
    d. body
    d. connective tissue
    d. deposit disease
    d. granule
densimeter
densitometer
densitometry
density
    base d.
    buoyant d.
    calcific d.
    character d.
    count d.
    count information d.
    decreased d.
    d.-dependent repair
    fiber d.
    d. function
    d. gradient centrifugation
    increased d.
    intermediate d.
    luminous flux d.
    optical d.
    radiographic d.
    scan information d.
    total body d.
    water d.
dental
    d. calculus
    d. caries
    d. fluorosis
    d. follicular cyst
    d. granuloma
    d. lamina
    d. lymph
    d. pathology
    d. plaque
    d. radiography
dentate
    d. gyrus
    d. ligament
    d. nucleus
denticle
denticulated
denticulate ligament
dentigerous
    d. cyst
    d. mixed tumor

dentin
    d. crystal alteration
    d. dysplasia
    d. formation
dentinal fluid
dentinoblast
dentinoblastoma
dentinogenesis imperfecta
dentinoma
    fibroameloblastic d.
dentinosteroid
dentistry
dentition
denucleated
denuding cystitis
Denver classification
deossification
deoxyadenosine
    d. monophosphate
    d. phosphate
    d.-5'-phosphate
deoxyadenosyl
deoxyadenylic acid
deoxycholate
    d. citrate agar
    d. citrate lactose saccharose
deoxycholic acid
deoxycholylglycine
2'-deoxycoformycin
deoxycorticoids
deoxycorticosterone acetate
11-deoxycorticosterone
11-deoxycortisol
deoxycytidine
    d. monophosphate
    d. phosphate
    d.-5'-phosphate
deoxycytidylic acid
6-deoxygalactose
2-deoxy-D-galactose
6-deoxy-L-galactose
deoxygenated hemoglobin
deoxy-D-glucose
deoxyguanosine
    d. monophosphate
    d. phosphate
    d.-5'-phosphate
2-deoxyguanosine-5'-triphosphate
deoxyguanylic acid
deoxyhemoglobin
deoxyhexose
2'-deoxy-5-iodouridine

6-deoxy-mannose
6-deoxy-β-L-mannose
deoxynucleoside triphosphate
deoxynucleotidyl transferase
deoxypentose
deoxyribonuclease (DNase)
    d. agar
    d. digestion
    d. test
    d. I
    d. II
deoxyribonucleic acid
deoxyribonucleoprotein
deoxyribonucleoside
deoxyribonucleotide
deoxyribose
deoxysugar
deoxythymidine
    d. diphosphate
    d. kinase
    d. monophosphate
    d. triphosphate
deoxythymidylate
deoxyuridine
    d. monophosphate
    d. phosphate
    d.-5'-phosphate
    d. suppression test
    d. triphosphate
deoxyuridylate
deoxyuridylic acid
Depakene
deparaffinization
dependence
    anchorage d.
    drug d.
dependent
    d. edema
    d. variable
dependovirus
dephospho-coenzyme A
    d.-CoA kinase
    d.-CoA pyrophosphorylase
dephosphorylation
depigmentation
deplasmolysis
depletion
    d. layer
    lipid d.
    ovarian ascorbic acid d.
    plasma d.
    zymogen granule d.

depolarization
depolarizer
depolymerization
deposit
    amyloid d.
    posterior corneal d's
    tooth d.
deposition
    bilharzial pigment d.
    calcium d.
    cholesterol d.
    fatty d.
    ferrocalcinotic d.
    foreign material d.
    hemosiderin d.
    iron d.
    malarial pigment d.
    particulate crystalline d.
    xanthomatous d.
depot
    fat d.
Depo-Testosterone
depressant
depressed
    d. fracture
    d. gene
    d.-type manic-depressive psy-
      chosis
depression
    bone marrow d.
    endogenous d.
    myeloid d.
    psychoneurotic d.
    reactive d.
deprivation
    d. dwarfism
    oxygen d.
deproteinization
depth
    d. dose
    d. electroencephalogram
    d. electroencephalography
    d. electrography
    d. of field
    d. of focus
deQuervain's
    tenosynovitis
    thyroiditis
DeR — reaction of degeneration
der — derivative chromosome
deradelphus

derangement
    chromosomal d.
derepression
    gene d.
    transient d.
De Ritis ratio
derivation
derivative
    blood d.
    d. chromosome
    hematoporphyrin d.
    d.-standard purified protein
derived
    d. albumin
    d. protein
Dermacentor
    D. andersoni
    D. occidentalis
    D. reticulatus
    D. variabilis
Dermacentroxenus
    D. rickettsi
    D. sibericus
    D. typhi
dermad
dermal
    d. bone
    d. duct tumor
    d. eccrine cylindroma
    d. epidermal nevus
    d. nevus
    d. papilla
    d. sinus
    d. tuberculosis
Dermanyssus gallinae
dermatan sulfate
dermatitis (pl., dermatitides)
    actinic d.
    allergic d.
    atopic d.
    d. atrophicans
    d. atrophicans diffusa
    d. atrophicans maculosa
    cercarial d.
    d. chronica atrophicans idio-
        pathica
    contact d.
    drug-related d.
    eczematoid d.
    eczematous d.
    epidural reactive d.
    erythematous d.

d. escharotica
d. exfoliativa
d. exfoliativa infantum
d. exfoliativa neonatorum
exfoliative d.
factitious d.
d. gangrenosa infantum
d. herpetiformis
lichenoid d.
d. medicamentosa
photo contact d.
phototoxic contact d.
pigmented purpuric lichenoid d.
primary irritant d.
psoriasiform d.
radiation d.
reactive d.
d. repens
Schamberg's d.
schistosome cercarial d.
seborrheic d.
spongiotic d.
stasis d.
subcorneal pustular d.
toxic d.
d. venenata
d. verrucosa
dermatoarthritis
    lipoid d.
Dermatobia hominis
dermatocele
dermatocellulitis
dermatochalasis
dermatocyst
dermatofibroma
dermatofibrosarcoma
    d. protuberans
    storiform pattern d.
dermatofibrosis lenticularis disseminata
dermatogen
dermatoglyphics
dermatographism
dermatologic
dermatology
dermatolysis
dermatoma
dermatomal herpes zoster
dermatome
    Brown d.
    Padgett d.
    Reese d.
dermatomegaly

dermatomycin
dermatomycosis
dermatomyoma
dermatomyositis
dermatopathia pigmentosa reticularis
dermatopathic
    d. lymphadenitis
    d. lymphadenopathy
dermatopathology
Dermatophagoides pteronyssinus
Dermatophilaceae
dermatophilosis
Dermatophilus
    D. congolensis
    D. penetrans
dermatophyte test medium
dermatophytid
Dermatophytin "O"
dermatophytosis
    opportunistic d.
dermatorrhexis
dermatosclerosis
dermatosis (pl., dermatoses)
    acute inflammatory d.
    benign chronic bullous d.
    Bowen's precancerous d.
    bullous d.
    chronic inflammatory d.
    dermolytic bullous d.
    genital d.
    d. papulosa nigra
    pigmentary d.
    progressive pigmentary d.
    radiation d.
    subcorneal pustular d.
dermatosome
dermatrophia; dermatrophy
dermis
dermoblast
dermographia
dermoid
    d. cancer
    d. cyst
    d. cyst of ovary
    implantation d.
    inclusion d.
    sequestration d.
    d. teratoma
    d. tumor
dermolysin
dermolysis
dermolytic bullous dermatosis

dermonecrotic
dermopathy
    diabetic d.
dermophlebitis
dermostenosis
dermostosis
dermosyphilopathy
dermovascular
derodidymus
DES — diethylstilbestrol
desacetyl vinblastine amide
desalt
desamido-NAD$^+$
desaturation
Descemet's
    membrane
    posterior lamina
descending
    d. colon
    d. degeneration
    d. hypoglossal nerve
    d. limb
    d. thoracic aorta
descensus ventriculi
desensitization
    drug d.
desensitize
deserpidine
desetope
Desferal
desferrioxamine
deshydremia
desiccant
desiccate
desiccation
desiccative
desiccator
desipramine
    d. assay
    d. hydrochloride
deslanoside
Desmarres's dacryolith
desmectasis; desmectasia
desmepithelium
desmin filaments
desmitis
desmocyte
desmocytoma
desmogenous
desmoid
    extra-abdominal d.
    d. fibromatosis

periosteal d.
d. tumor
desmolase
17,20-d.
20,22-d.
20,22-d. deficiency
desmoma
desmoneoplasm
desmoplakian antibody
desmoplasia
desmoplastic
d. fibroma
d. melanoma
d. trichoepithelioma
desmopressin
desmosine
desmosome
intercapillary d.
desmosterol
desolvation
desoxycholate
bromocresol purple d.
sodium d.
11-desoxycorticosterone
11-desoxy,17-OH-corticosterone
despeciate
despumation
desquamate
desquamation
desquamative
d. inflammatory vaginitis
d. interstitial pneumonia
d. interstitial pneumonitis
d. interstitial poisoning
destructive
d. distillation
d. interference
d. sclerosing cholangitis
desynapsis
desynchronization
desynchronized sleep
DET — diethyltryptamine
detachment
retinal d.
rhegmatogenous retinal d.
detection
antibody d.
cardiac shunt d.
detector
alpha-particle d.
cadmium telluride d.
combustible gas d.

electron capture d.
flame ionization d.
lithium-drifted d.
surface-barrier d.
thermal conductivity d.
thermoluminescent d.
d. transfer function
detergent
determinant
antigenic d.
conformational d.
immunogenic d.
isoallotypic d.
Kern's isotopic d.
KM allotypic d.
Meg isotypic d.
sequential d.
R (electrical resistance) d.
resistance d.
determination
activity d.
antigenic d.
immunogenic d.
lactate dehydrogenase isoenzyme d.
lecithin-sphingomyelin ratio d.
sex d.
detoxification
metabolic d.
detrition
detritus
detrusor
d. muscle
d. urinae
detubation
detumescence
deutan
deuteranomaly
deuteranopia
deuterium light source
deuterohemophilia
Deuteromycetes
Deuteromycota
Deuteromycotina
deuteron
deuterosome
deuterotoxin
DEV — duck embryo vaccine
devascularization
development
developmental
d. arrest

d. genetics
d. jaw cyst
d. mixoploid
d. synchronism
development-at-birth index
deviant
deviate
deviation
average d.
mean d.
mean square d.
no significant d.
relative standard d.
right axis d.
standard d.
sum of square d's
d. to the left
d. to the right
device
intrauterine d.
semiconductor d.
Surgicutt d.
devolution
dew point osmometer
Dewar flask
dexamethasone suppression test
dexbrompheniramine maleate
dexchlorpheniramine maleate
Dexedrine
dexiocardia
dexpanthenol
dextran
d. blue
iron d.
low-molecular-weight d.
dextranase
dextrin
limit d.
dextrin-1,6-glucosidase
dextrinase
dextrinosis
limit d.
dextrinuria
dextroamphetamine
dextrocardia
corrected d.
false d.
isolated d.
secondary d.
type 1 d.
type 2 d.

type 3 d.
type 4 d.
d. with situs inversus
dextrogastria
dextromethorphan hydrobromide
dextroposition of heart
dextrorotatory
dextrose
d. agar
d.-nitrogen ratio
d.-saline
d. solution mixture
d. test   d. stick
dextrosuria
dextrothyroxine sodium
dextroversion of heart
DF — decapacitation factor
deficiency factor
desferrioxamine
discriminant function
disseminated foci
df — degrees of freedom
DF3 antibody
DFDT — difluorodiphenyltrichloro-ethane
DFMO — difluoromethylornithine
DFO — deferoxamine
DFP — diisopropylfluorophos-phate
DFS — disease-free survival
DFT32 — diisofluorophosphate
DFU — dead fetus in utero
dideoxyfluorouridine
DG — deoxyglucose
diastolic gallop
diglyceride
distogingival
DGI — disseminated gonococcal in-fection
dg; dgm — decigram
dGDP — deoxyguanosine disphos-phate
dGMP — deoxyguanosine monophos-phate
dGTP — 2-deoxyguanosine-5'-triphosphate
DH — delayed hypersensitivity
DHA — dehydroepiandrosterone
dihydroxyacetone
DHAP — dihydroxyacetone phos-phate

DHAS — dehydroepiandrosterone
     sulfate
DHE — dihydroergotamine
DHEA — dehydroepiandrosterone
DHEAS — dehydroepiandrosterone
     sulfate
DHFR — dihydrofolate reductase
DHIA — dehydroisoandrosterone
DHL — diffuse histiocytic lymphoma
DHMA — dihydroxymandelic acid
dhobie itch
DHPG — 9-(1,3-dihydroxy 2-propoxy-
     methyl) guanine
DHPR — dihydropteridine reductase
DHT — dihydrotachysterol
     dihydrotestosterone
DI — diabetes insipidus
DI(2-hydroxypropyl)-nitrosamine
diabetes
     adult-onset d.
     alimentary d.
     bronzed d.
     calcinuric d.
     gestational d.
     d. innocens
     d. insipidus
     insulin-dependent d. mellitus
     juvenile d. mellitus
     juvenile-onset d.
     lipoatrophic d.
     maturity-onset d.
     d. mellitus
     Mosler's d.
     non−insulin-dependent d.
       mellitus
     phloridzin d.
     phosphate d.
     renal d.
     thiazide d.
diabetic
     d. acidosis
     d. amyotrophy
     d. angiopathy
     d. coma
     d. dermopathy
     d. gangrene
     d. glomerulopathy
     d. glomerulosclerosis
     hyperosmolar d. coma
     d. ketoacidosis
     d. lipemia
     d. microangiopathy

     d. myelopathy
     d. nephropathy
     d. neuropathy
     d. retinopathy
     d. ulcer
     d. urine
diabeticorum
     bullosis d.
     xanthoma d.
diabetogenic hormone
diacetemia
diacetate
diacetic acid
diacetonuria
diaceturia
diacetylaminoazotoluene
diacetyl reaction
diaclasis; diaclasia
diacrinous
diacylglycerol
diag. — diagnosis
Diagnex blue test
diagnosis
     clinical d.
     cytologic d.
     differential d.
     laboratory d.
     pathologic d.
     physical d.
     prenatal d.
     provocative d.
     roentgen d.
     serum d.
diagnostic
     d. sensitivity
     d. specificity
diagram
     acid-base d.
     block d.
     scatter d.
     vector d.
     Venn d.
diakinesis
dial
     vernier d.
Dialister
dialkyl
     d. dimethyl ammonium
       chloride
     d. sodium sulfosuccinate
dialysance
dialysate

dialysis
        equilibrium d.
        extracorporeal d.
        peritoneal d.
dialyzer
diamagnetic
diameter
        Mantoux d.
        mean cell d.
        mean corpuscular d.
        outside d.
diamide
diamine
        diethylene d.
        d. oxidase
diaminoacid aminotransferase
cis-diaminodichloroplatinum
p-diaminodiphenyl
diaminodiphenylsulfone
2,4-diaminophenol hydrochloride
Diamond-Blackfan anemia
diamond fuchsin
diamorphine
diamthazole dihydrochloride
Diamyl
diapedesis; diapiresis
        red cell d.
diaphane
diaphanography
diaphanometer
diaphanoscope
diaphorase
diaphoresis
diaphragm
        Akerlund d.
        Bucky d.
        Bucky-Potter d.
        eventration of the d.
        field d.
        iris d.
        Potter-Bucky d.
diaphragma
        d. pelvis
        d. sellae
        d. urogenitale
diaphragmatic
        d. hernia
        d. hiatus
        d. lymph node
        d. peritonitis
        d. pleura
diaphragmitis; diaphragmatitis

diaphyseal; diaphysial
        d. aclasis
        d. dysplasia
        d. juxtaepiphyseal exostosis
diapiresis; diapedisis
diaphysis (pl., diaphyses)
diaphysitis
diapophysis
diapositive
Diaptomus
diarrhea
        amebic d.
        Cochin China d.
        tropical d.
        viral d.
diarrheagenic E. coli
diarrheogenic tumor
diarthrosis (pl., diarthroses)
diaschisis
diascope
diaspironecrobiosis
diaspironecrosis
diastase
diastasis
diastasuria
diastatic
diastematomyelia
diastereoisomer
diastereoisomerism
diastereomer
diastole
diastolic
        d. hypertension
        d. murmur
        d. pressure
diathermy
diathesis
        cystic d.
        hemorrhagic d.
diathetic
diatom
diatomaceous
diatrizoate
        d. meglumine
        d. sodium
diauxic
diauxie
diaxon
diazepam breath test
diazine
diazinon

diazo
> d. reaction
> d. reagent
> d. stain for argentaffin granules
> d. staining method
> d. tablet

diazomethane generator
diazonium salt
diazotization
diazotize
diazoxide
dibasic
> d. acid
> d. potassium phosphate

dibenzanthracene
dibenzepin hydrochloride
dibenzothiazine
dibenzylchlorethamine
diblastula
diborane
dibothriocephaliasis
Dibothriocephalus
dibrachius
> monocephalus tetrapus d.
> monocephalus tripus d.

dibromethane
1,2-dibromethane
dibromide
> ethylene d.

dibromochloropropane
1,2-dibromoethane
dibromosalicylaldehyde
dibucaine
> d. hydrochloride
> d. number

dibutoline sulfate
dibutyl
> d. adipate
> d. phthalate
> d. succinate

DIC — diffuse intravascular coagulation
> disseminated intravascular coagulation

dic. — dicentric
dicalcium hydrogen phosphate crystals
dicarbamylamine
dicarboxylic acid
dicarboxylicaciduria
dicentric chromosome
dicephalus
> d. dipus dibrachius

> d. dipus tetrabrachius
> d. dipus tribrachius
> d. dipygus
> d. parasiticus
> d. tripus tribrachius

dicheirus
dichlobenil
dichloride
> carbonic d.
> ethylene d.
> ethylidene d.

dichlorisone
dichlorobenzene
p-dichlorobenzene
dichloro-chloroaniline-triazine
dichlorodiethyl sulfide
dichlorodiphenyldichloroethane
dichlorodiphenyltrichloroethane
dichloroethane
1,1-dichloroethane
1,2-dichloroethane
1,1-dichloroethylene
sym-dichloroethylene
dichloroethyl ether
2,6-dichloroindophenol
dichloromethane
sym-dichloromethyl ether
dichloronaphthoquinone
1,1-dichloro-1-nitroethane
dichlorophene
2,6-dichlorophenol-indophenol
2,4-dichloro-phenoxyacetic acid
dichlorophenyl dimethyl urea
dichlorophenyl methyl butylurea
dichloropropane
1,3-dichloro-2-propanol
dichloropropene
dichloropropionic acid
dichlorphenamide
dichlorvos
dichogeny
dichorionic
> d. diamniotic placenta
> d. placenta twins

dichotomize
dichotomous variable
dichotomy
dichroism
> circular d.

dichromate
> potassium d.

dichromophil; dichromophile

Dick test
dicloxacillin sodium
dicofol
Dicrocoelium dendriticum
dicrotic notch
Dictyocaulus
dictyokinesis
dictyosome
dictyotene
dicumarol
dicyanodiamine
    mercuric d.
dicyclomine hydrochloride
dicycloxylamine
Didelphis
dideoxycytidine
dideoxyfluorouridine
didymitis
Diego
    antigen
    blood group system
dieldrin
dielectric
    d. constant
    d. strength
dielectrolysis
diencephalic
    d. periventricular fibers
    d. syndrome
diencephalon
diene
diener
dienestrol
Dientamoeba fragilis
dieresis
diester
dietary protein
Dieterle's
    method
    stain
dietetic albuminuria
dietetics
diethanolamine
diethyl
    d. ether
    d. 2-chlorovinyl phosphate
    d. dithiocarbamate
    d. *p*-nitrophenyl phosphate
    d. sulfate
    d. toluamide
    d. xanthogen disulfide

diethylamide
    lysergic acid d.
diethylamine
diethylaminoethyl cellulose
diethylcarbamazine citrate
diethyldithiocarbamate
1,4-diethylene dioxide
diethylene glycol
diethylenetriaminepentaacetic acid
diethylnitrosamine
diethylpropion hydrochloride
diethylstilbestrol
    d. diphosphate
    d. dipropionate
diethyltoluamide
diethyltryptamine
diff. — differential
difference
    alveolar-arterial carbon dioxide d.
    alveolar-arterial oxygen d.
    arteriovenous carbon dioxide d.
    arteriovenous oxygen d.
    cation-anion d.
    electric potential d.
    mean of consecutive d's
    no significant d.
differential
    d. agglutination titer
    d. count
    d. diagnosis
    d. leukocyte count
    d. leukocyte count automation
    d. medium
    d. renal function test
    d. segments
    d. stain
    d. thermometer
    d. ureteral catheterization test
    d. white blood count
differentiated
differentiation
    cell d.
    cellular d.
    cluster of d.
    d.-specific antigens
    sex d.
    thymus cell d.
differentiator
Diff-Quik
diffraction
    d. grating
    x-ray d.

diffusate
diffuse
- d. abscess
- d. acute inflammation
- d. acute peritonitis
- d. alveolar damage
- d. amyloidosis
- d. aneurysm
- d. arterial ectasia
- d. bronchopneumonia
- d. chronic inflammation
- d. cutaneous mastocytosis
- d. emphysema
- d. enlargement
- d. esophageal spasm
- d. fibrosis
- d. ganglion
- d. glomerulonephritis
- d. glomerulosclerosis
- d. goiter
- d. histiocytic lymphoma
- d. hyperplasia
- d. hypertrophy
- d. idiopathic skeletal hyperostosis
- d. illumination
- d. infiltrative lung disease
- d. inflammation
- d. interstitial fibrosis
- d. interstitial pulmonary disease
- d. intravascular coagulation
- d. large cell lymphoma
- d. lymphatic tissue
- d. meningioma
- d. meningiomatosis
- d. mesangial proliferation
- d. mesothelioma
- d. mixed small and large cell lymphoma
- d. necrosis
- d. neuroendocrine system
- d. nontoxic goiter
- d. peritonitis
- d. phlegmon
- d. pigmented villonodular synovitis
- d. pneumonia
- d. poorly differentiated lymphoma
- d. proliferative glomerulonephritis
- d. pulmonary disease
- d. pyelonephritis
- d. reflection
- d. sclerosing osteomyelitis
- d. septal cirrhosis
- d. small cleaved cell lymphoma
- d. toxic goiter
- d. ulceration
- d. waxy spleen

diffusible
diffusing
- d. capacity for carbon monoxide
- d. capacity of the lungs

diffusion
- d. block
- d. coefficient
- d. current
- facilitated d.
- d. method
- d. potential
- d. shell

diffusivity
difluoromethylornithine
digalen
digastric
- d. lobe
- d. muscle

digenetic
Di George's anomaly
digest
- soybean-casein d.

digestion
- deoxyribonuclease d.
- glycogen d.
- hyaluronidase d.
- sialidase d.
- d. vacuole

digestive
- d. albuminuria
- d. disorder
- d. glycosuria
- d. leukocytosis
- d. system

digit
- check d.
- clubbed d's

digital
- d. cassette recorder
- d. computer
- d. image processing

d. mammography
d. radiography
d. readout
d. subtraction angiography
d.-to-analog converter
d. voltmeter
Digitalis
digitalis
    d. glycosides
    d. unit
digitalization
digitate wart
digitize
digitizer
digitonin
    d. method
    d. reaction
digitoxin
digitoxose
digitus (pl., digiti)
    digiti hippocratici
    d. postminimus
diglyceride
diglycoaldehyde
digoxin
Digramma brauni
dihydric alcohol
dihydrobiopterin
dihydrocodeine
dihydrocoenzyme I
dihydroergotamine mesylate
dihydrofolate
    d. deficiency
    d. dehydrogenase
    d. reductase
dihydrofolic acid
dihydrofolliculin
dihydrol
dihydrolipoamide acetyltransferase
dihydromorphinone hydrochloride
dihydro-orotase
dihydro-orotate
dihydropteridine
    d. reductase
    d. reductase deficiency
dihydropyrimidinase
dihydropyrimidine
dihydropyrimidinuria
dihydrorotenone
dihydrosphingosine
dihydrotachysterol
dihydrotestosterone

dihydroubiquinone
dihydro-uracil dehydrogenase
dihydrouridine
dihydroxy
1,25-dihydroxy vitamin D
dihydroxy vitamin D_3
dihydroxyacetone phosphate
dihydroxyacetonetransferase
dihydroxycholecalciferol
    1,25-d.
    24,25-d.
3,4-dihydroxymandelic acid
4-dihydroxymandelic acid
2,5-dihydroxyphenylacetic acid
3,4-dihydroxyphenylacetic acid
dihydroxyphenylalanine
3,4-dihydroxy-L-phenylalanine decar-
    boxylase
dihydroxypropoxymethylguanine
diiodohydroxyquin
diiodothyronine
diiodotyrosine
di-isobutyl cresolyl ethoxy ethyl di-
    methyl benzyl ammonium
    chloride
di-isobutylphenoxyethoxyethyl di-
    methyl benzyl ammonium
    chloride
diisocyanate
    toluene 2,4-d.
di-isopropylfluoro-phosphatase
diisopropyl phosphofluoridate
Dikaryomycota
dikaryon
dikaryote
diktyoma
dil. — dilute
Dilantin
dilatation
    aneurysmal d.
    peroral d.
    poststenotic d.
    sinusoidal d.
    d. thrombosis
dilatator
dilate
dilated cardiomyopathy
dilation
    cardiac d.
dilator
    balloon d.
    Eder-Puestow d.

Hurst's d.
Maloney d.
Savary-Gilliard d.
Tucker's d.
Dilaudid
DILD — diffuse infiltrative lung
    disease
DILE — drug-induced lupus erythema-
    tosus
diloxanide
diluent
    Isoton d.
dilut. — diluted
dilute
    d. acetic acid
    d. hydrochloric acid
    d. phosphoric acid
    d. whole blood clot lysis
dilution
    d. anemia
    d. coefficient
    doubling d.
    d.-filtration technique
    maximum inhibiting d.
    nitrogen d.
    routine test d.
    serial d.
    d. test
dilutor
    Hem-Aliquanter d.
DIM — divalent ion metabolism
Dimastigamoeba
dimefadane
dimefline hydrochloride
dimefox
dimenhydrinate
dimension
dimer
    thymine d.
dimercaprol
dimercaptopropanol
dimercaptosuccinic acid
dimerization
Dimetane
dimethicone
dimethindene maleate
dimethisoquin hydrochloride
dimethisterone
dimethoate
dimethoxanate hydrochloride
2,5-dimethoxy-4-methylamphetamine
3,4-dimethoxyphenylethylamine

dimethpyrindene
dimethyl
    d. ether
    d. ketone
    d. sulfate
    d. sulfoxide
    xanthine d.
dimethylacetamide
N,N-dimethylacetamide
dimethylallyl diphosphate
p-dimethylaminoazobenzene
p-dimethylaminobenzaldehyde
1-dimethylaminonaphthalene-t-
    sulfonyl chloride
dimethylaminopropionitrile
dimethylbenzanthracene
7,12-dimethylbenz[a]anthracene
dimethylbenzene
5,6-dimethylbenziminazole
dimethylcarbamate
dimethyldichlorovinyl phosphate
O,O-dimethyl O-(2,2-dichlorovinyl)
    phosphate
dimethyldithiocarbamate
    zinc d.
dimethyl ether
dimethylformamide
N,N-dimethylglycine
dimethylguanosine
dimethylhydrazine
dimethylketone
dimethylnitrosamine
5,5-dimethyl-2,4-oxazolidinedione
dimethylphthalate
dimethyl sulfate
dimethyl sulfoxide
dimethylthetin homocysteine methyl-
    transferase
dimethyltriazeno imidazole carbox-
    imide
dimethyltryptamine
diminazene aceturate
dimorphic
    d. anemia
    d. erythrocyte
    d. pathogenic fungi
dimorphism
dimorphous leprosy
dimple
    Fuchs' d's
    postanal d.
dineric interface

dinitrate
    ethylene glycol d.
dinitroaminophenol
dinitrobenzene
3,5-dinitrobenzoic acid
dinitrobutyl phenol
dinitrochlorobenzene
dinitro-o-cresol
dinitro-o-cyclohexyl phenol
dinitrofluorobenzene
dinitrogen
    d. monoxide
    d. tetroxide
dinitro-orthocresol
dinitrophenol
dinitrophenylhydrazine test
dinitrotoluene
Dinobdella ferox
dinormocytosis
dinucleotide
    flavin adenine d.
    nicotinamide-adenine d.
    reduced nicotinamide-
        adenine d.
Dioctophyma renale
dioctyl sodium sulfosuccinate
diode
    d. array spectrophotometry
    varactor d.
    Zener's d.
Diodoquin
Diodrast clearance
diopter
dioxane
dioxathion
dioxide
    carbamino-carbon d.
    carbon d.
    lead d.
    silicon d.
    zirconium d.
dioxin
dioxygenase
    homogentisate d.
    p-hydroxyphenylpyruvate d.
    proline 2-oxoglutarate d.
dioxyline phosphate
DIP — desquamative interstitial
        pneumonia
    desquamative interstitial
        pneumonitis
diisopropyl phosphate

distal interphalangeal
dipalmitoylphosphatidylcholine
dip-coating autoradiography
dipeptidase
    aminoacyl-histidine d.
dipeptide
    d. hydrolase
    d. muramyl
dipeptidyl
    d. aminopeptidase IV
    d. carboxypeptidase
    d. peptidase I
Dipetalonema
    D. perstans
    D. streptocerca
dipetalonemiasis
diphacinone
diphallia
diphasic
    d. meningoencephalitis virus
    d. milk fever virus
    d. wave
diphemanil methylsulfate
diphenadione
diphenhydramine hydrochloride
diphenidol
p-diphenol oxidase
diphenoxylate hydrochloride
diphenyl
diphenylamine chlorarsine
diphenylchlorarsine
diphenylcyanarsine
diphenyldiimide
1,6-diphenyl-1,3,5-hexatriene
diphenylhydantoin
    d.-associated thyroiditis
    d. gingivitis
diphenylmethane dyes
diphenylnitrosamine
2,5-diphenyloxazole
diphenylpyraline hydrochloride
diphosphatase
    nucleoside d.
diphosphate
    adenine d.
    adenosine d.
    cytidine d.
    deoxyadenosine d.
    deoxythymidine d.
    dimethylallyl d.
    fructose d.
    geranyl d.

guanosine d.
inosine d.
isopentenyl d.
uridine d.
diphosphatidylglycerol
diphosphoglycerate
    d. mutase
    d. phosphatase
1,3-diphosphoglycerate
2,3-diphosphoglycerate
diphosphoglyceromutase
diphosphoinositide
diphosphonate
    methylene d.
diphosphonic acid
diphosphopyridine nucleotide
diphosphosulfate
    phosphoadenosine d.
diphtheria
    d. antitoxin
    d. antitoxin unit
    d. bacillus
    laryngotracheal d.
    d. toxin immunization reaction
    d. toxin normal
diphtheria, pertussis, and tetanus
    (vaccine)
diphtheria, tetanus, and pertussis
    (vaccine)
diphtheritic
    d. enteritis
    d. membrane
    d. ulcer
diphtheritica
    otitis d.
diphtheroid
    aerobic d.
    anaerobic d.
    d. bacilli
diphyllobothriasis
Diphyllobothrium latum
diphyllobothrium anemia
dipicolinic acid
dipipanone hydrochloride
DIPJ — distal interphalangeal joint
diplasmatic
diplegia
diploalbuminuria
diplobacillus
diplobacterium
diploblastic
diplochromosome

diplococcemia
Diplococcus
    D. *constellatus*
    D. *magnus*
    D. *morbillorum*
    D. *mucosus*
    D. *paleopneumoniae*
    D. *plagarumbelli*
    D. *pneumoniae*
diplococcus (pl., diplococci)
    d. of Morax-Axenfeld
    d. of Neisser
    Weichselbaum's d.
diploë
Diplogaster
Diplogonoporus
    D. *brauni*
    D. *grandis*
diploic vein
diploid
    d. cell lines
    d. merogony
    d. nucleus
    d. number
diploidy
diplomelituria
diplomyelia
diplon
diplonema
diploneural
diplopia
diplopod
Diplopoda
diplosome
Diplosporium
diplotene
dipolar
    d. ion
    d. structure
dipole moment
dipropyl isocinchomeronate
dipstick
Diptera
dipterous
dipygus parasiticus
Dipylidium caninum
dipyridamole
dipyrone
diquat assay
direct
    d. access
    d. agglutination

d. agglutination pregnancy
d. agglutination pregnancy test
d. agglutination test
d. antiglobulin test
d. bilirubin
d. bilirubin test
d. centrifugal flotation
d. Coombs's technique
d. Coombs's test
d.-coupled amplifier
d. culture
d. current
d. detection
d. fluorescent antibody staining
d. hernia
d. light reflex
d. memory access
d.-reacting bilirubin
d. transport
d. vision spectroscope
directed transfusion
directional selection
directory
direct-reading potentiometer
Dirofilaria
    D. conjunctivae
    D. immitis
    D. repens
    D. tenuis
dirofilariasis
"dirty fingers" pattern
disaccharidase deficiency
disaccharide tolerance test
disaggregated
disappearance
    plasma iron d.
disappearing
    d. bile duct syndrome
    d. bone disease
disc; disk
    articular d.
    blood d.
    d. capacitator
    carbohydrate d's
    degenerated intervertebral d.
    d. diffusion test
    d. dilution susceptibility test
    d. electrophoresis
    embryonic d.
    germ d.
    intercalated d.
    interpubic d.

intervertebral d.
d. kidney
Merkel's tactile d.
discharge
    double d.
    epileptiform d.
    exit d.
    d. frequency
    urethral d.
    urinary d.
disciform keratitis
discitis
disclosing solution
discocyte
discography
    cervical d.
    lumbar d.
discoid lupus erythematosus
discontinuous endothelium
discordance
discordant
discrete
    d. smallpox
    d. subaortic stenosis
    d. variable
discriminant function
discriminator
discussive
discutient
disease, noneponymic (For eponymic
    disease names, *see* Appendix 2)
    ABO (blood group) hemo-
      lytic d.
    abortive viral d.
    accumulation d.
    acute cardiovascular d.
    acute infectious d.
    acute respiratory d.
    adrenal d.
    adult celiac d.
    adult polycystic d.
    alpha chain d.
    alpha heavy-chain d.
    altitude d.
    anti–glomerular basement
      membrane (anti-GBM) anti-
      body d.
    aortoiliac occlusive d.
    arboviral virus d.
    arc-welders' d.
    arterial occlusive d.
    arteriosclerotic cardiovascular d.

arteriosclerotic heart d.
arthropod-borne viral d.
atherosclerotic cardiovascu-
    lar d.
atherosclerotic heart d.
atherosclerotic vascular d.
atopic d.
autoimmune d.
bauxite workers' d.
biliary tract d.
black lung d.
blinding filarial d.
branching glycogen storage d.
broad-beta d.
bronzed d.
bullous d.
caisson d.
caloric d.
carcinoid heart d.
cardiac d.
cardiovascular d.
cardiovascular renal d.
cat-scratch d.
celiac d.
central core d. of muscle
cerebrovascular obstructive d.
ceroid storage d.
chlamydial d.
cholesterol ester storage d.
chronic active liver d.
chronic cold agglutinin d.
chronic granulomatous d.
chronic liver d.
chronic lung d.
chronic obstructive lung d.
chronic obstructive pulmo-
    nary d.
chronic renal d.
circling d.
cold agglutinin d.
cold hemagglutinin d.
collagen d.
collagen-vascular d.
combined immunodefi-
    ciency d.
combined systems d.
communicable d.
congenital nonspherocytic
    hemolytic d.
congestive heart d.
connective-tissue d.
constitutional d.

contagious d.
coronary artery d.
coronary atherosclerotic
    heart d.
coronary heart d.
creeping d.
crystal deposition d.
cystic d. of breast
cystic d. of lung
cystic d. of renal medulla
cysticercus d.
cystine storage d.
cytomegalic inclusion d.
cytomegalovirus d.
debranching glycogen stor-
    age d.
deficiency d.
degenerative joint d.
demyelinating d.
dense-deposit d.
deprivation d.
diffuse infiltrative lung d.
diffuse interstitial pulmo-
    nary d.
disappearing bone d.
diverticular d.
echinococcus d.
endemic d.
endocrine d.
eosinophilic endomyocar-
    dial d.
epidemic d.
epithelial cell d.
extrapyramidal d.
familial juvenile nephronoph-
    thisis–medullary cystic d.
fat deficiency d.
femoropopliteal occlusive d.
fibrocystic d. of the breast
fibrocystic d. of the pancreas
fifth d.
fifth venereal d.
fish-slime d.
flax-dressers' d.
flint d.
floating-beta d.
focal d.
fourth d.
fourth venereal d.
functional d.
gamma chain d.
gamma heavy-chain d.

gannister d.
gastrointestinal d.
gay-related immunodeficiency d.
gestational trophoblastic d.
giant platelet d.
glomerular basement membrane d.
glomerulocystic d.
glucose-6-phosphate dehydrogenase d.
glycogen storage d.
graft-vs.-host d.
granulomatous d.
hand-foot-and-mouth d.
heavy chain d.
α heavy-chain d.
γ heavy-chain d.
μ heavy-chain d.
helminthic d.
hemoglobin C–thalassemia d.
hemoglobin E–thalassemia d.
hemoglobin H d.
hemolytic d. of newborn
hemorrhagic d. of newborn
hepatic veno-occlusive d.
hepatolenticular d.
hepatorenal glycogen storage d.
hereditary d.
heredoconstitutional d.
heredodegenerative d.
herpetic viral d.
herring-worm d.
hidebound d.
hock d.
holoendemic d.
hookworm d.
hyaline membrane d. of newborn
hydatid d., alveolar
hydatid d., unilocular
hydrocephaloid d.
hyperendemic c.
hypertensive arteriosclerotic heart d.
hypertensive cardiovascular d.
hypertensive pulmonary vascular d.
hypertensive vascular d.
hypopigmentation-immunodeficiency d.
I-cell d.

idiopathic d.
immune complex d.
immunodeficiency d's
immunoproliferative small intestine d.
inborn lysosomal d's
inclusion d.
inclusion body d.
inclusion cell d.
incompatible hemolytic blood transfusion d.
infantile celiac d.
infantile polycystic d.
infectious d.
inflammatory bowel d.
inflammatory pelvic d.
inherited d.
intercurrent d.
interstitial d.
interstitial lung d.
interstitial pulmonary d.
iron storage d.
ischemic bowel d.
ischemic heart d.
ischemic leg d.
ischemic limb d.
jumping d.
kinky hair d.
kissing d.
knight's d.
L-chain d.
legionnaires' d.
light-chain d.
linear IgA bullous d.
lipid storage d.
lunger d.
lymphoproliferative d.
lymphoreticular d.
lysosomal storage d.
maple bark d.
maple syrup urine d.
marble bone d.
mast cell d.
medullary cystic d.
metabolic bone d.
microcystic d. of renal medulla
microdrepanocytic d.
micromulticystic renal d.
minimal-change d.
mixed connective tissue d.
molecular d.
motor neuron d.

mucopolysaccharide storage d.
μ heavy-chain d.
multicore d.
myeloproliferative d's
myocardial d.
myopathic glycogen storage d.
neurodegenerative d.
neutral lipid storage d.
newborn hemolytic d.
newborn hemorrhagic d.
nil d.
nodular sclerotic d.
oasthouse urine d.
obstructive airway d.
occupational lung d.
oncogenic virus d.
organic d.
pearl-workers' d.
pelvic inflammatory d.
periodic d.
periodontal d.
peripheral arterial occlusive d.
peripheral arteriosclerotic
    occlusive d.
peripheral vascular d.
persistent viral d.
pickwickian d.
pigeon breeders' d.
polycystic d. of kidneys
polycystic liver d.
polycystic ovary d.
polycystic renal d.
polyendocrine autoimmune d.
poststreptococcal hypersensi-
    tivity d.
primary myocardial d.
pulmonary d.
pulmonary airway d.
pulmonary heart d.
pulmonary thromboembolic d.
pulseless d.
pyramidal d.
quiet hip d.
rat-bite d.
redwater d.
renal cystic d.
respiratory viral d.
restrictive lung d.
restrictive pulmonary d.
retroviral viral d.
rheumatic d.
rheumatic heart d.

rheumatoid d.
rheumatoid heart d.
runt d.
salivary gland d.
sea-blue histiocyte d.
secondary d.
segmental cystic d.
senile hip d.
self-limited d.
septic d.
severe combined immunodefi-
    ciency d.
sexually transmitted d.
sickle cell d.
sickle cell hemoglobin C d.
sickle cell hemoglobin D d.
sickle cell–thalassemia d.
sixth d.
sixth venereal d.
skinbound d.
sphingolipid storage d.
storage d.
storage pool d.
subpleural d.
thalassemia–sickle cell d.
thromboembolic d.
thyrocardiac d.
thyrotoxic heart d.
transfusion-associated graft-
    versus-host d.
transport d.
trophoblastic d.
tsutsugamushi d.
tuberculous respiratory d.
tubulointerstitial d.
unstable hemoglobin d.
upper respiratory d.
uremic medullary cystic d.
urinary tract disease
urogenital d.
vagabonds' d.
venereal d.
veno-occlusive d.
vinyl chloride d.
viral hematodepressive d.
wasting d.
white muscle d.
white spot d.
woolsorters' d.
X-linked lymphoproliferative d.
disequilibrium
    genetic linkage d.
    linkage d.

disfigurative
disgerminoma
DISH — diffuse idiopathic skeletal hy-
        perostosis
dish
       Petri d.
       Stender d.
disinfect
disinfectant
disinfection
disintegration
       d. constant
       radioactive d.
disjunction
disjunctive absorption
disk (see also disc)
diskitis; discitis
diskocyte
diskogram
diskography
       cervical d.
       lumbar d.
dislocation
       anterior complete d.
       closed d.
       complete d.
       complete anterior d.
       complete inferior d.
       complete posterior d.
       complete superior d.
       compound d.
       congenital d.
       fracture d.
       pathologic d.
dismutase
       superoxide d.
dismutation
disodium
       carbenicillin d.
       d. chromoglycate
       d. 3,6-endoxohexahydroph-
         thalate
       d. ethylene bis-(dithiocar-
         bamate)
       d. hydrogen phosphate
disome
disomic
disomy
disopyramide
disorder
       adrenal endocrine d.
       anti-factor d.

       autosomal dominant d.
       autosomal recessive d.
       blood coagulation d.
       circulating antithyromoplas-
         tin d.
       element d.
       functional d.
       gonadal endocrine d.
       immunoproliferative d's
       intestinal flow d.
       ion d.
       lipid transport d.
       lymphoproliferative d's
       lymphoreticular d's
       multi-X-chromosome d.
       myeloproliferative d.
       peristaltic d.
       pituitary endocrine d.
       plasma iodoprotein d.
       thyroidal endocrine d.
       ureteral peristaltic d.
       urogenital d.
       X-linked genetic d.
disorganization
disorientation
       spatial d.
dispermic chimera
dispermy
disperse phase
dispersion
       colloidal d.
       molecular d.
       optical rotary d.
dispersive medium
dispireme
displaceability
displacement
       d. analysis
       anterior d.
       condylar d.
       lateral d.
display
       seven-segment d.
disposable
disposition
disproportion
       cephalopelvic d.
       fiber-type d.
dissect
dissecting
       d. aneurysm
       d. hematoma

dissection
    aortic d.
    axillary d.
    d. tubercle
disseminated
    d. acute lupus erythematosus
    d. candidiasis
    d. condensing osteopathy
    d. cytomegalovirus
    d. encephalomyelitis
    d. foci
    d. gonococcal infection
    d. histoplasmosis
    d. inflammation
    d. intravascular coagulation
    d. lipogranulomatosis
    d. lupus erythematosus
    d. sclerosis
    d. superficial actinic porokeratosis
    d. tuberculosis
    d. zoster
dissemination
    miliary d.
disseminatus
    lupus erythematosus d.
Disse's spaces
dissociation
    albuminocytologic d.
    bacterial d.
    constant d.
    microbic d.
dissolution
dissolve
dissymmetry
distal
    d. anterior closed space
    d. convoluted renal tubule
    d. histidine
    d. ileitis
    d. latency
    d. muscular dystrophy
    d. myopathy
    d. radioulnar joint
    d. tibiofibular joint
    d.-type muscular dystrophy
    d.-type progressive muscular dystrophy
distance
    focal d.
    interelectrode d.
    skin-to-tumor d.

distemper virus
distension; distention
    d. cyst
    d. ulcer
distill
distillate
distillation
    destructive d.
    fractional d.
    molecular d.
    vacuum d.
distilled oil
Distoma
distome
distomiasis
    pulmonary d.
distortion
    barreling d.
distractibility
distribution
    anomalous vascular d.
    binomial d.
    chi-squared d.
    d. coefficient
    d. curve
    dose d.
    F d. (variance from normal distribution)
    frequency d.
    d. function
    gaussian probability d.
    d. leukocytosis
    lognormal d.
    nitrogen d.
    Poisson d.
    d. ratio
    reference d.
    sample d.
    sips d.
    skewed d.
    symmetric d.
    t d. (distribution probability)
disturbance
    consciousness d.
    mental d.
disulfide
    d. bond
    carbon d.
    d. knot
disulfiram assay
disulfoton
disuse atrophy

DIT — diiodotyrosine
dithiazanine iodide
dithioerythritol
dithionite solubility test
dithiothreitol
Dittrich's
        plugs
        stenosis
diuresis (pl., diureses)
diuretic
        cardiac d.
        hemopiesic d.
        loop d.
        mechanical d.
        mercurial d.
        osmotic d.
        thiazide d.
diurnal
diuron
divalent ion metabolism
divarication
divergence
diversion
        antigenic d.
        urinary d.
diverticular
diverticulogram
diverticulitis
        hemorrhagic d.
        obstructive d.
        perforated d.
        urethral d.
diverticuloma
diverticulosis
diverticulum (pl., diverticula)
        cervical d.
        colonic d.
        duodenal d.
        epiphrenic d.
        esophageal d.
        false d.
        hypopharyngeal d.
        intestinal d.
        Meckel's d.
        Pertik's d.
        pharyngoesophageal d.
        d. pressure
        pulsion d.
        traction d.
        true d.
        urethral d.
        ventricular d.
        vesical d.

        Zenker's d.
        Zenker's pulsation d.
divicine
divider
        voltage d.
diving goiter
divinylbenzene
division
        cell d.
        equational d.
        maturation d.
        reduction d.
Dixon's test
dizygotic twins
dizziness
DJD — degenerative joint disease
DK — decay
        diseased kidney
DL — diffusing capacity of the lung
        distolingual
        Donath-Landsteiner (test)
dL, dl — deciliter
DLA — distolabial
D-L Ab — Donath-Landsteiner an-
        tibody
DLAI — distolabioincisal
DLCO — diffusing capacity of the lung
        for carbon monoxide
DLE — discoid lupus erythematosus
        disseminated lupus erythema-
        tosus
D-L hemolysin
DLI — distolinguoincisal
D line
DLO — distolinguo-occlusal
DLP — distolinguopulpal
DM — diabetes mellitus
        diastolic murmur
        dopamine
D.M. — diphenylamine-arsine
        chloride
dm — decimeter
DMA — dimethyladenosine
        direct memory access
DMAB — dimethylaminobenzal-
        dehyde
DMAC — dimethylacetamide
DMAPN — dimethylaminopropioni-
        trile
DMBA — dimethylbenzanthracene
DMCT — dimethylchlortetracycline
DMD — Duchenne's muscular dys-
        trophy

DME — dimethyl ether (of d-tubocurarine)
DMF — dimethylformamide
DMM — dimethylmyleran
DMN — dimethylnitrosamine
DMO — dimethyloxazolidinedione
DMPA — depomedroxyprogesterone acetate
DMPE — 3,4-dimethoxyphenylethylamine
DMPP — dimethylphenylpiperazinium
DMS — dimethylsulfoxide
DMSO — dimethylsulfoxide
DMT — dimethyltryptamine
DN — dextrose-nitrogen (ratio)
    dibucaine number
Dn. — dekanem
dn — decinem
DNA — deoxyribonucleic acid
    DNA adducts
    DNA-Alu I family
    DNA analysis
    B-DNA
    circulating DNA
    DNA-chain terminator
    complementary DNA
    copy DNA
    DNA : D-histone
    DNA-directed DNA polymerase
    DNA-directed RNA polymerase
    DNA : D-virus
    DNA fingerprint
    DNA fingerprinting
    DNA-germ line
    DNA-DNA hybridization
    DNA indices
    DNA intercalators
    DNA library
    DNA ligase
    DNA marker
    DNA nucleotidylexotransferase
    DNA nucleotidyltransferase
    DNA polymerase
    DNA polymorphism
    DNA probe analysis
    DNA rearrangement
    DNA reassociation
    recombinant DNA
    DNA renaturation

    DNA repair
    repetitive DNA
    DNA replication
    DNA-RNA hybridization
    satellite DNA
    DNA sequencing
    single copy DNA
    spacer DNA
    DNA synthesis
    DNA thymine
    DNA topoisomerase
    DNA tumor virus
    DNA virus
    Z-DNA
DNase — deoxyribonuclease
DNase agar
DNase I hypersensitivity
DNB — dinitrobenzene
    Diplomate of the National Board of Medical Examiners
DNC — dinitrocarbanilide
DNCB — dinitrochlorobenzene
DNFB — dinitrofluorobenzene
DNOC — dinitro-orthocresol
DNP — deoxyribonucleoprotein
    dinitrophenol
DNPH — dinitrophenylhydrazine
DNPM — dinitrophenylmorphine
DO — diamine oxidase
    disto-occlusal
D.O. — Doctor of Osteopathy
DOA — dead on arrival
Dobell and O'Connor's iodine solution
dobutamine hydrochloride
DOC — deoxycholate
    deoxycorticosterone
DOCA — deoxycorticosterone acetate
docimasia
    auricular d.
    hepatic d.
    pulmonary d.
docosahexaenoic acid
DOCs — deoxycorticoids
document
documentation
dodecylguanidine acetate
Döderlein's bacillus
DOE — dyspnea on exercise
    dyspnea on exertion

dog
>   d. heartworm
>   d. hookworm
>   d. tapeworm

Döhle-Heller aortitis
Döhle's inclusion bodies
Dold's
>   reaction
>   test

dolichocolon
dolichol phosphate
Dolichos biflorus
dolipore
doll's eye movements
Dolobid
Dolophine
DOM — deaminated-O-methyl
>   metabolite
>   dimethoxymethylamphet-
>   amine
>   2,5-dimethoxy-4-
>   methylamphetamine

DOMA — dihydroxymandelic acid
domain
>   immunoglobulin d's
>   Kringle d.

Dombrock antigens
dominance
>   incomplete d.

dominant
>   d. character
>   d. complement
>   d. complementarity
>   d. gene
>   d. inheritance
>   d. phenotype

dominantly inherited
domiphen bromide
DON — diazo-oxonorleucine
Donath-Landsteiner
>   antibody
>   cold hemolysis
>   phenomenon
>   test

Donnan's potential
Donné's
>   bodies
>   corpuscles
>   test

donor
>   cadaver d.
>   consanguineous d.

>   F d.
>   isogenic d.
>   living d.
>   proton d.
>   universal d.

Donovania granulomatis
Donovan's bodies
L-DOPA — dihydroxyphenylalanine
dopa
>   d. decarboxylase
>   d.-hydroxylase
>   d. reaction

DOPAC — dihydroxyphenyl-acetic
>   acid

dopamine
>   d. hydroxylase
>   d. β-hydroxylase
>   d. monooxygenase
>   d. β-monooxygenase

dopaminergic
dopaquinone
Doppler
>   echocardiography
>   effect
>   unit

Doriden
dormancy
dormant
Dorner stain
Dorothy Reed cells
dorsal
>   d. accessory olivary nucleus
>   d. cutaneous nerve
>   d. digital artery
>   d. digital vein
>   d. displacement
>   d. external arcuate fibers
>   d. fascia
>   d. funiculus
>   d. intermediate sulcus
>   d. lateral nucleus
>   d. lateral sulcus
>   d. longitudinal fasciculus
>   d. median sulcus
>   d. mesentery
>   d. metacarpal vein
>   d. metatarsal artery
>   d. metatarsal vein
>   d. motor nucleus
>   d. nasal artery
>   d. nerve
>   d. nucleus

d. paraflocculus
d. proper fasciculus
d. respiratory group
d. root ganglion
d. spinal nerve root
d. spinocerebellar tract
d. spinothalamic tract
d. subaponeurotic space
d. tegmental nucleus, pons
d. thoracic nerve
d. ventral nucleus
d. vertebra

dorsalis pedis artery
dorsiflex
dorsiflexion
dorsolateral
dorsomedial nucleus
dorsoplantar
dorsum (pl., dorsa)
d. sellae

dosage
d. compensation
gene d.

dose
absorbed d.
d. account
air d.
booster d.
d. calibrator
curative d.
depth d.
d. distribution
effective d.
epilating d.
erythema d.
d. estimate
exit d.
fatal d.
genetically significant d.
infective d.
integral d.
lethal d.
loading d.
maximal permissible d.
mean d.
mean hemolytic d.
mean d. per unit cumulated activity
median effective d.
median fatal d.
median infectious d.
median lethal d.

median tissue culture d.
median tissue culture infective d.
minimal erythema d.
minimal lethal d.
minimal morbidostatic d.
minimum infective d.
minimum lethal d.
normal single d.
organ tolerance d.
radiation d.
radiation absorbed d.
d. rate
d.-reduction factor
d.-response curve
sensitizing d.
skin d.
threshold d.
threshold erythema d.
tissue culture d.
tissue culture infectious d.
tissue culture infective d.
tissue tolerance d.
titrated initial d.
tumor lethal d.

dosimeter
pencil d.
pocket d.
thermoluminescent d.
ultraviolet fluorescent d.

dosimetry
dot
d. blot test
Maurer's d's
Mittendorf's d's
d. product
d. scan
Schüffner's d's
Ziemann's d's

Dothideales
double
d. albuminemia
d. aortic arch
d. artery
d.-beam spectrophotometry
d.-blind
d.-blind experiment
d. cardiac valve orifice
d.-contrast enema
d.-contrast examination
d.-contrast study
d. diffusion test

d. discharge
d. ductus arteriosus
d. helix
d. intussusception
d. kidney
d.-masked experiment
d.-minute chromosome
d. minutes
d. oxalate
d. pneumonia
d.-pole double-throw switch
d.-pole single-throw switch
d.-precision variable
d. refraction
d. renal pelvis
d. stain
d. tertian malaria
d. trisomy
d. ureter
d. uterus
d. vagina
d. vas deferens
doubling
d. dilution
d. time
Douglas's
abscess
cul-de-sac
pouch
Dowex
Downey
cells
-type lymphocyte
downtime
doxepin hydrochloride assay
doxorubicin hydrochloride
doxycycline
doxylamine succinate
Doyen's clamp
DP — dementia praecox
diastolic pressure
distopulpal
DPA — dipropylacetate
DPC — delayed primary closure
DPD — diffuse pulmonary disease
DPDL — diffuse, poorly differentiated
lymphoma
dpdt — double-pole double-throw
(switch)
D-penicillamine
DPG — diphosphoglycerate
displacement placentogram

DPGM — diphosphoglyceromutase
DPGP — diphosphoglycerate phos-
phatase
DPH — diphenylhydantoin
DPL — distopulpolingual
dpm — disintegrations per minute
DPN — diphosphopyridine nucleotide
DPN synthetase
D^u positive
DPP — dimethoxyphenyl penicillin
DPS — dimethylpolysiloxane
dpst — double-pole single-throw
(switch)
DPT — diphtheria, pertussis, and
tetanus
dipropyltryptamine
DPTA — diethylenetriaminepentaacetic acid
DPVNS — diffuse pigmented villonodular synovitis
DQ — developmental quotient
DR — diabetic retinopathy
reaction of degeneration
dr. — drachm
dram
Drabkin's reagent
dracontiasis
dracunculiasis
dracunculosis
Dracunculus medinensis
Dragendorff's
solution
test
dragon worm infection
drain
drainage
anomalous venous d.
drain-trap stomach
Drechslera hawaiiensis
drench hose
Drepanidotaenia lanceolata
drepanocyte
drepanocytemia
drepanocythemia
drepanocytic anemia
drepanocytosis
Drepanospira
Dresbach's anemia
Dreser's formula
dressing
anorectal d.

DRF — dose-reduction factor
drift
    antigenic d.
    genetic d.
    random genetic d.
    ulnar d.
Drinker respirator
drip
    intravenous d.
drive
    tape d.
Drolban
dromostanolone propionate
drop
    hanging d.
    d. heart
    Ir d.
    d.-out necrosis
    voltage d.
droperidol
droplet
    hyaline d's
    d. nuclei
dropper
dropsical
dropsy
    abdominal d.
Drosophila
drowsiness
droxacin sodium
drug
    d. abuse screen
    d. addiction
    antibiotic antitumor d's
    d.-associated hypothyroidism
    d. dependence
    d. desensitization
    generic d.
    d. half-life
    d.-induced dermatitis
    d.-induced hemolysis
    d.-induced hepatitis
    d.-induced nephritis
    d.-induced thrombocytopenia
    d. interaction
    d. interference
    d. monitoring
    oxytocic d's
    radioactive d.
    d.-resistant
    d. screening assay

    sulfa d's
    d. tolerance
drumstick
    d. fingers
    d. spore
drunkenness
drusen
dry
    d. abscess
    d. bronchietasis
    d. catarrh
    d. gangrene
    d. ice
    d. leprosy
    d. objective
    d. pack
    d. pleurisy
drying agent
DS — defined substrate
    dehydroepiandrosterone sulfate
    dextrose-saline
    Down's syndrome
DSA — digital subtraction angiography
DSAP — disseminated superficial actinic porokeratosis
DSC; DSCG — disodium cromoglycate
dsDNA — double-stranded DNA
DSM — dextrose solution mixture
dsRNA — double-stranded RNA
DST — dexamethasone suppression test
DT — delirium tremens
    duration tetany
    dye test
DTBN — di-*t*-butyl nitroxide
DTC; DTBC — *d*-tubocurarine
dTDP — deoxythymidine diphosphate
DTF — detector transfer function
DTH — delayed-type hypersensitivity
DTIC — dacarbazine
    dimethyltriazeno imidazolecarboximide
DTM — dermatophyte test medium
DTMP — deoxythymidine monophosphate
dTMP — thymidine phosphate
DTN — diphtheria toxin normal
DTNB — dithiobisnitrobenzoic acid
DTP — diphtheria, tetanus, and pertussis (vaccine)
    distal tingling on percussion

DTPA — diethylenetriamine-
                pentaacetic acid
DTR — deep tendon reflex
dTTP — thymidine triphosphate
DTZ — diatrizoate
DU — duodenal ulcer
dU — deoxyuridine
du — dial unit
dual
        d.-contrast study
        d.-in-line package
dualism
Duane-Hunt relation
duazomycin
Dubois's abscesses
Duboisia
duboisine
Dubreuilh's melanosis
Duchenne-Landouzy dystrophy
Duchenne's muscular dystrophy
duck embryo vaccine
Ducrey's bacillus
duct
        aberrant d.
        allantoic d.
        alveolar d.
        d. of Arantius
        Bellini's papillary d.
        bile d.
        d. carcinoma
        cochlear d.
        collecting d.
        common excretory d.
        Cuvier's d.
        cystic d.
        d. ectasia
        ejaculatory d.
        endolymphatic d.
        d. of epididymis
        extrahepatic bile d.
        Gartner's d.
        genital d.
        hepatic d.
        intercalated d.
        interlobular bile d.
        lacrimal d.
        lactiferous d.
        lobular d.
        Luschka's d's
        lymphatic d.
        mesonephric d.
        Müller's d.

müllerian d.
nasolacrimal d.
omphalomesenteric d.
pancreatic d.
d. papilloma
paramesonephric d.
parotid d.
periurethral d.
prostatic d.
salivary d.
Santorini's d.
semicircular d.
Stensen's d.
sudoriferous d.
thoracic d.
thymopharyngeal d.
thyroglossal d.
utriculosaccular d.
vitelline d.
vitellointestinal d.
Wharton's d.
Wirsung's d.
wolffian d.
ductal
        d. adenocarcinoma
        d. breast cancer
        d. carcinoma in situ
        d. ectasia
        d. hyperplasia
        d. papillomatosis
ductule
        aberrant d.
ductus (pl., ductus)
        d. arteriosus
        d. deferens
        d. venosus
Duffy's
        antibodies, Fy^a, Fy^b
        antigen
        blood group system
Duke's
        cell counter
        classification
        method of bleeding time
        staging system
        test
dullness
        Gerhardt's d.
        relative hepatic d.
        shifting d.
        tympanitic d.
dumbbell ganglioneuroma

Dumdum fever
dummy variable
dUMP — deoxyuridine monophosphate
dumping syndrome
duod — duodenum
duodenal
    d. atresia
    d. contents
    d. diverticulum
    d. fistula
    d. juice
    d. lumen
    d. mucous membrane
    d. muscularis propria
    d. serosa
    d. smear
    d. submucosa
    d. subserosa
    d. ulcer
duodenectomy
duodenitis
duodenocholangitis
duodenocholecystostomy
duodenocystostomy
duodenoenterostomy
duodenography
    hypotonic d.
duodenohepatic
duodenoileostomy
duodenojejunal recess
duodenojejunostomy
duodenopancreatectomy
duodenorrhaphy
duodenoscopy
duodenostomy
duodenum
duovirus
DU-PAN-2 (tumor marker)
duplex
    d. ileum
    d. kidney
    d. placenta
duplication
    caudal d.
    caudal dipygus d.
    congenital d.
    cranial d.
    d. cyst
    d. deficiency
    facial diprosopus d.
    fetal d.

    monocephalic cranial d.
    trunk d.
duplicity theory
Dupuytren's
    contracture
    fibromatosis
dural terminal filament
dura mater
duration
Dürck's
    granuloma
    nodes
Duret's hemorrhage
Durham's tube
dust
    blood d.
    d. cell
    chromatin d.
    d. corpuscles
    d. mite
    nuclear d.
    organic d.
Dutcher body
dUTP — deoxyuridine triphosphate
Duttonella
Duval's nucleus
Duverney's gland
d.v. — double vibration
DVA — distance visual acuity
D value (decimal reduction time)
DVM — digital voltmeter
DW — distilled water
D5W, D5 & W,
    or D_5W — 5% dextrose in water
D/W — dextrose in water
dwarf
    achondroplastic d.
    d. colony
    constitutional d.
    d. megakaryocyte
    pituitary d.
    primordial d.
    d. tapeworm
dwarfism
    achondroplastic d.
    acromelic d.
    chondrodystrophic d.
    deprivation d.
    Frölich's d.
    Laron d.
    lethal d.
    mesomelic d.

micromelic d.
phocomelic d.
pituitary d.
polydystrophic d.
senile d.
Silver-Russell d.
thanatophoric d.
DX — dextran
DXM — dexamethasone
DXT — deep x-ray therapy
D-xylose
    D-x. absorption test
    D-x. tolerance test
Dy — dysprosium
dyad
dyclonine hydrochloride
dydrogesterone
dye
    acid d.
    acidic d.
    acridine d.
    aminoanthraquinone d's
    aminoketone d.
    amphoteric d.
    aniline d.
    anionic d.
    anthraquinone d.
    Arsenazo III d.
    azin d's
    azine d.
    azo d.
    azocarmine d's
    azoic d.
    basic d.
    d.-binding capacity
    carmine d.
    d.-dilution curve
    cationic d.
    diphenylmethane d.
    d. exclusion test
    d. excretion test
    fluorescent d.
    hydroxyketone d.
    indamine d.
    indigoid d.
    indophenol d.
    ketonimine d's
    lactone d.
    Magon d.
    metachromatic d.
    methine d.
    methylene blue d.

    natural d's
    nitro d.
    nitroso d.
    oxazin d's
    oxazine d.
    phthalocyanine d.
    polymethine d.
    quinoline d.
    rosaniline d's
    salt d.
    stilbene d.
    sulfur d.
    synthetic d's
    d. test
    thiazine d.
    thiazole d.
    triarylmethane d.
    triphenylmethane d.
    vital d.
    xanthene d.
dyed starch method
dyn. — dyne
dynamic
    d. equilibrium
    d. ileus
    d. isomerism
    d. storage allocation
    d. venous plethysmography
    d. viscosity
dynamics
dyne
dynein
dynorphin
dyphylline
Dyrenium
dysalbuminemic hyperthyroxinemia
dysarthria
dysaudia
dysautonomia
    familial d.
dysbarism
dysbasia
dysbetalipoproteinemia
    familial d.
dysbolism
dyscephalia mandibulo-oculofacialis
dyschezia
dyschondrogenesis
dyschondroplasia with hemangiomas
dyschondrosteosis
dyscrasia
    blood d.

lymphatic d.
plasma cell d.
dyscrasic; dyscratic
dysdiadochokinesia
dysdiemorrhysis
dysembryoma
dysemia
dysencephalia splanchnocystica
dysentery
    amebic d.
    bacillary d.
    d. bacilli
    balantidial d.
    bilharzial d.
    catarrhal d.
    ciliary d.
    ciliate d.
    epidemic d.
    flagellate d.
    Flexner's d.
    fulminant d.
    giardiasis d.
    malarial d.
    protozoal d.
    scorbutic d.
    Sonne d.
    spirillar d.
    sporadic d.
    viral d.
dyserythropoiesis
dyserythropoietic congenital anemia
dysesthesia
dysfibrinogenemia
dysfunction
    constitutional hepatic d.
    minimal brain d.
    myocardial d.
    ovarian d.
    papillary muscle d.
    sensorineural d.
    uterine d.
    vasomotor d.
dysfunctional bleeding
dysgammaglobulinemia
dysgenesis
    embryonic testicular d.
    familial gonadal d.
    gonadal d.
    reticular d.
    seminiferous tubule d.
    testicular d.
    XO gonadal d.

    XX gonadal d.
    XY gonadal d.
dysgenetic
dysgerminoma
    ovarian d.
dysglobulinemia
dysglycemia
dysgonic
dysgranulopoiesis
dyshematopoiesis
dyshematopoietic
dyshemopoiesis
dyshemopoietic anemia
dyshesion
dyshesive
dyshidrosis
dyshormonogenesis
dyshormogenic goiter
dyskaryosis
dyskaryotic
dyskeratoma
    warty d.
dyskeratosis
    benign d.
    d. congenita
    hereditary benign intraepithel-
      ial d.
    intraepithelial d.
    isolated d. follicularis
    malignant d.
    warty d.
dyskeratotic
dyskinesia
    tardive d.
    tracheobronchial d.
dyslexia
dyslipoproteinemia
dysmegakaryocytopoiesis
dysmenorrhea
dysmentation
dysmorphia
    mandibulo-oculofacial d.
dysmorphic erythrocyte
dysmorphism
dysmotility
    cilia d.
dysmyelopoietic syndrome
dysosteogenesis
dysostosis
    acrofacial d.
    cleidocranial d.; clidocranial d.
    cleidocranialis d.

craniofacial d.
Crouzon's craniofacial d.
mandibuloacral d.
mandibulofacial d.
metaphyseal d.
d. multiplex
Nager's acrofacial d.
orodigitofacial d.
otomandibular d.
peripheral d.
dysoxidative carbonuria
dyspareunia
dyspepsia
dysphagia
oropharyngeal d.
sideropenic d.
dysphagocytosis
congenital d.
dysphasia
dysphonia
dysphoria
dyspigmentation
dysplasia
acantholytic d.
acquired d.
anhidrotic ectodermal d.
anterofacial d.
anteroposterior d.
asphyxiating thoracic d.
atriodigital d.
basal cell d.
bone d.
bronchopulmonary d.
carpocarpal d.
cellular d.
cemental d.
cerebral d.
cervical d.
chondroectodermal d.
cleidocranial d.; clidocranial d.
congenital thymic d.
craniocarpotarsal d.
craniodiaphyseal d.
craniometaphyseal d.
cystic d.
cystic renal d.
dentin d.
diaphyseal d.
ectodermal d.
ectodermal hereditary d.
d. epiphysealis hemimelica
d. epiphysealis multiplex

d. epiphysealis punctata
epithelial d.
faciodigitogenital d.
familial fibrous d.
fibromuscular d.
fibrous d.
fibrous d. of bone
fibrous familial d.
fibrous monostotic d.
fibrous polyostotic d.
florid osseous d.
hereditary d., ectodermal
hereditary renal-retinal d.
hidrotic ectodermal d.
hyperkeratotic d.
hypohidrotic ectodermal d.
lymphopenic thymic d.
mammary d.
mandibulofacial d.
metaphyseal d.
monostotic fibrous d.
mucoepithelial d.
multiple epiphyseal d.
neuroendocrine d.
nodular d.
oculoauriculovertebral d.
oculodentodigital d.
oculovertebral d.
ophthalmomandibulomelic d.
oropharyngeal d.
osseous d.
pagetoid d.
polyostotic fibrous d.
postradiation d.
precancerous d.
pseudoachondroplastic spondyloepiphyseal d.
renal d.
retinal-renal d.
spondyloepiphyseal d.; spondy-
loepiphysial d.
thoracic d.
thymic d.
urothelial/aplasia d.
ventriculoradial d.
vesical d.
Zenker's d.
dysplastic
d. leukoplakia
d. nevus
d. nevus syndrome

dyspnea
    cardiac d.
    exertional d.
    nocturnal d.
    paroxysmal d.
    paroxysmal nocturnal d.
dyspneic
dyspoiesis
dysprosium
dysproteinemia
dysproteinemic
dysprothrombinemia
dysrhythmia
dyssynergia
    progressive cerebellar d.
dystaxia
dystocia
dystonia
dystonic
dystopia
dystopic
dystrophia
    d. brevicollis
    d. unguium
dystrophic
    d. calcification
    d. calcinosis
dystrophodextrin
dystrophy
    adiposogenital d.

    asphyxiating thoracic d.
    calcific d.
    craniocarpotarsal d.
    distal muscular d.
    Duchenne-Landouzy d.
    Duchenne's muscular d.
    d.-dystocia syndrome
    facioscapulohumeral muscular d.
    granular d.
    hyperplastic d.
    infantile neuroaxonal d.
    Landouzy-Dejerine progressive muscular d.
    lattice d.
    limb-girdle muscular d.
    lipoid d.
    macular d.
    muscular d.
    myotonic d.
    ocular muscle d.
    ophthalmoplegic-type muscular d.
    progressive muscular d.
    thoracic asphyxiant d.
    thoracic-pelvic-phalangeal d.
    vulvar d.
dysuria-pyuria syndrome
dysuric
DZ — dizygous

E

E — cortisone (compound E)
    electric charge
    electron
    emmetropia
    energy
    epinephrine
    erythrocyte
    extraction fraction
    eye
E. — *Entamoeba*
    Escherichia
E_1 — estrone
E_2 — estradiol
E_3 — estriol
E_4 — estetrol

EA — early antigen
    ethacrynic acid
EAC — Ehrlich ascites carcinoma
    erythrocyte, antibody, and complement
    external auditory canal
EACA — epsilon-aminocaproic acid
EAC rosette assay
Eadie-Hofstee equation
EAE — experimental allergic encephalomyelitis
Eagle's
    basal medium
    minimum essential medium
EAHF — eczema, asthma, hay fever

EAHLG — equine antihuman
lymphoblast globulin
EAHLS — equine antihuman
lymphoblast serum
EAM — external auditory meatus
EAN — experimental allergic neuritis
E antigen
EAP — epiallopregnanolone
ear
cauliflower e.
e. culture
external e.
internal e.
e. lobe
e. lobule
middle e.
scroll e.
Earle L fibrosarcoma
Earle's solution
early
e. antigen
e. neonatal death
earth
diatomaceous e.
e. electrode
eastern
e. equine encephalitis
e. equine encephalomyelitis
Eaton agent
EB — epidermolysis bullosa
Epstein-Barr (virus)
estradiol benzoate
Eberthella typhi
Eberth's lines
EBI — elective brain irradiation
emetine bismuth iodide
EBL — estimated blood loss
EBNA — EBV nuclear antigen
Epstein-Barr nuclear an-
tigen
EBNC — Epstein-Barr nasopharyngeal carcinoma
Ebner's gland
Ebola virus
EBRT — electron beam radiation
therapy
Ebstein's
anomaly
malformation
eburnation
EBV — Epstein-Barr virus

EC — electron capture
enteric-coated
Escherichia coli
excitation-contraction
experimental control
extracellular
ECA — ethacrynic acid
ECBO virus — enteric cytopathogenic bovine or-
phan virus
ECBV — effective circulating blood
volume
ECC — extracorporeal circulation
eccentric hypertrophy
eccentrochondroplasia
ecchondroma; ecchondrosis
ecchordosis physaliphora
ecchymoma
ecchymosed
ecchymosis (pl., ecchymoses)
Tardieu's e.
ecchymotic
eccrine
e. acrospiroma
e. carcinoma
e. gland
e. hidrocystoma
e. poroma
e. spiradenoma
e. tumor
ECD — electron capture detector
EC detector
ECDO virus — enteric cytopathogenic
dog orphan virus
ECF — effective capillary flow
eosinophil chemotactic factor
extracellular fluid
ECF-A — eosinophil chemotactic factor of anaphylaxis
ECFV — extracellular fluid volume
ECG — electrocardiogram
ecgonine
Echidnophaga
Echinochasmus perfoliatus
echinococciasis
echinococcosis
e. serological test
unilocular e.
Echinococcus
E. granulosus
E. multilocularis
E. vogeli

echinococcus cyst
echinocyte
echinocytosis
echinoderm
echinomycin
Echinorhynchus
echinosis
Echinostoma
    E. cinetorchis
    E. ilocanum
    E. lindoensis
    E. malayanum
    E. melis
    E. paryphostomum
    E. perfoliatum
    E. revolutum
echinostomiasis
ECHO — enteric cytopathogenic human orphan (virus)
echo
echocardiogram
echocardiography
    contrast e.
    cross-sectional e.
    Doppler e.
echoencephalogram
echoencephalography
echogenic
echogram
echography
echolucent
echo-ophthalmography
echophonocardiography
echothiophate
ECHO virus
    type 1
    type 12
    type 28
echovirus
ECI — electrocerebral inactivity
ECI; ECIB — extracorporeal irradiation of blood
ECIL — extracorporeal irradiation of lymph
ECL — emitter-coupled logic
eclampsia
    puerperal e.
    uremic e.
eclipse
ECLT — euglobulin clot lysis time
ECM — erythema chronicum migrans
    extracellular material

ECMO virus — enteric cytopathogenic monkey orphan virus
ECoG — electrocorticogram
    electrocorticography
ecoid
E. coli — *Escherichia coli*
ecologic niche
ecology
econazole nitrate
Economo's encephalitis
ecosystem
ecotaxis
ecphyma
ECS — extracellular space
ECSO virus — enteric cytopathogenic swine orphan virus
ecstrophy; exstrophy
ECT — euglobulin clot test
ectacolia
ectasia; ectasis
    biliary e.
    e. cordis
    diffuse arterial e.
    ductal e.
    hypostatic e.
    mammary duct e.
    medullary ductal e.
    papillary e.
    renal medullary ductal e.
    senile e.
    sperm duct e.
    vascular e.
    e. ventriculi paradoxa
ectatic aneurysm
ecterograph
ecthyma
    e. contagiosum
    e. gangrenosum
    e. infectiosum
    e. infectiosum virus
ecthymatiform; ecthymiform
ectoantigen
ectoblast
ectocervical smear
ectocervix
ectocolon
ectocyst
ectocytic
ectoderm
ectodermal
    e. defect

e. dysplasia
e. hereditary dysplasia
ectodermatosis
ectodermosis
    e. erosiva pluriorificialis
ectoenzyme
ectoglobular
ectomere
ectomesoblast
ectonuclear
ectoparasite
ectoperitonitis
ectophyte
ectopia
    adrenal e.
    e. cloacae
    e. cordis
    e. lentis
    e. renis
    e. testis
    e. vesicae
ectopic
    e. ACTH syndrome
    e. ACTH-CRF syndrome
    adrenal gland
    e. anus
    e. Cushing's syndrome
    e. decidua
    e. focus
    e. hormone
    e. kidney
    e. myelopoiesis
    e. pregnancy
    e. testis
    e. thyroid
    e. thyroid tissue
    e. tissue
ectoplasm
ectoplast
ectoplastic
ectopy
    ureteral e.
ectosteal
ectostosis
ectothrix infection
ectozoic
ectozoon (pl., ectozoa)
ectromelia
ectromelus
ectrometacarpia
ectropion
ectylurea

ECV — extracellular volume
ECW — extracellular water
eczema
    chronic e.
    e. erythematosum
    e. herpeticum
    e. hypertrophicum
    lichenoid e.
    nummular e.
    e. vaccinatum
    e. verrucosum
    e. vesiculosum
eczematoid dermatitis
eczematous dermatitis
ED — effective dose
    Ehlers-Danlos (syndrome)
    epileptiform discharge
    erythema dose
ED_{50} — median effective dose
edathamil calcium-disodium
eddy current
Edelmann's anemia
edema
    alveolar e.
    angioneurotic e.
    blue e.
    brown e.
    bullous e.
    bullous e. vesicae
    cardiac e.
    cellular e.
    cerebral e.
    circumscribed e.
    congestive e.
    cytotoxic e.
    dependent e.
    facial e.
    heat e.
    hereditary angioneurotic e.
    inflammatory e.
    lymphatic e.
    malignant e.
    e. neonatorum
    noninflammatory e.
    orthostatic e.
    periodic e.
    periorbital e.
    peripheral e.
    pitting e.
    pulmonary e.
    Quincke's e.
    renal e.

scrotal e.
solid e.
systemic e.
vasogenic e.
visceral e.
edematization
edematous pancreatitis
edentulous
Eder-Puestow dilator
edetate
calcium disodium e.
e. disodium
e. sodium
e. trisodium
edetic acid
edge
Compton e.
Edinger-Westphal nucleus
Edlefsen's reagent
Edman reaction
EDP — end-diastolic pressure
EDR — effective direct radiation
electrodermal response
EDRF — endothelial-derived relaxant
factor
edrophonium chloride test
EDS — Ehlers-Danlos syndrome
EDTA — edetic acid
ethylenediaminetetra-
acetate
EDV — end-diastolic volume
Edwardsiella tarda
Edwardsielleae
EDX — electrodiagnosis
EEA — electroencephalic audiometry
E, EA, EAC rosette
EEC — enteropathogenic *Esche-
richia coli*
EEE — eastern equine encephalomy-
elitis
EEE virus — eastern equine encepha-
lomyelitis virus
EEG — electroencephalogram
eelworm
EEME — ethinylestradiol methyl
ether
EER — electroencephalic response
EF — ectopic focus
ejection fraction
encephalitogenic factor
etiologic fraction
EFA — essential fatty acids

EFC — endogenous fecal calcium
EFE — endocardial fibroelastosis
effect
Arias-Stella e.
Auger e.
Bayliss e.
Bohr e.
Compton e.
Crabtree e.
crowding e.
cumulative e.
cytopathic e.
Deelman e.
Doppler e.
Faraday e.
founder e.
Haldane e.
Hamburger e.
Lyon's e.
McCollough e.
oxygen e.
Pasteur e.
photoelectric e.
photographic e.
piezoelectric e.
radiation e's
Somogyi e.
Staub-Traugott e.
Warburg's e.
Whitten e.
Wolff-Chaikoff e.
Zeeman's e.
effective
e. circulating blood volume
e. half-life
median e. dose
e. oxygen transport
e. refractory period
e. renal blood flow
e. renal plasma flow
e. temperature
effectiveness
relative biological e.
effector
allosteric e.
e. cells
e.-to-target ratio
effemination
efferent
e. arteriole
e. ductule
e. lymphatics

e. neuron
e. pathway
e. sacral branch
e. vagus branch
efficiency
geometric e.
photopeak detection e.
visual e.
efflorescence
effuse colony
effusion
chylous e.
e. cytology
hemorrhagic e.
parapneumonic e.
pericardial e.
peritoneal e.
pleural e.
pseudochylous e.
serofibrinous e.
serosanguineous e.
serous e.
synovial fluid e.
EFV — extracellular fluid
volume
EFVC — expiratory flow-volume
curve
EG — esophagogastrectomy
EGCT — extragonadal germ cell
tumor
EGF — epidermal growth factor
EGF-R — epithelial growth factor receptor
egg-base culture media
egg-white lysozyme
egg-yolk agar
EGG — electrogastrogram
EGL — eosinophilic granuloma of
the lung
EGM — electrogram
egobronchophony
egophony
EGOT — erythrocyte glutamic oxaloacetic transaminase
Egyptian splenomegaly
EH — essential hypertension
EHBF — estimated hepatic blood
flow
exercise hyperemia blood
flow

EHC — enterohepatic circulation
essential hypercholester-
olemia
EHDP — ethane hydroxydiphosphate
EHF — exophthalmos-hyperthyroid
factor
EHL — endogenous hyperlipidemia
EHO — extrahepatic obstruction
EHP — excessive heat production
Ehrlich-Heinz granules
Ehrlichia
ehrlichiosis
Ehrlich's
acid hematoxylin stain
aldehyde reaction
anemia
aniline crystal violet stain
ascites carcinoma
diazo reaction
diazo reagent
hemoglobinemic body
inner body
postulate
reaction
reagent
side-chain theory
test
triacid stain
triple stain
unit
EI — enzyme inhibitor
eosinophilic index
E/I — expiration-inspiration ratio
EIA — enzyme immunoassay
EIA interface
Eichhorst's corpuscles
eicosanoid
eicosapentaenoic acid
eicosatrienoic acid
EID — electroimmunodiffusion
eighth cranial nerve
Eikenella corrodens
Eimeria
EIN — esophageal intraepithelial neoplasia
Einarson's stain
einsteinium
Einthoven's
law
triangle
EIP — extensor indicis proprius

Eisenmenger's
    complex
    tetralogy
EIT — erythrocyte iron turnover
ejaculation
ejaculatory duct
ejecta
ejection
    e. fraction
    milk e.
    e. murmur
    e. phase
    e. time
EK — erythrokinase
EKC — epidemic keratoconjunctivitis
EKG — electrocardiogram
EKY — electrokymogram
elaidate
elaidic acid
elastance
elastase
elastic
    e. artery
    e. connective tissue
    e. fiber
    e. fiber stains
    e. lamellae
    e. lamina
    e. membrane
    e. recoil
    e. scattering
    e. skin
    e. tissue
elasticity
elastic lamellae
    external e.l.
    internal e.l.
elastin fiber
elastofibroma dorsi
elastoid degeneration
elastoma
    juvenile e.
    Miescher's e.
elastorrhexis
elastosis
    e. colloidalis conglomerata
    e. perforans serpiginosa
    senile e.
    solar e.
elastotic degeneration
Elavil
elbow

electric
    e. charge
    e. field vector
    e. potential
    e. potential difference
    e. susceptibility
electrical
    e. alternans
    e. artifact
    e. synapse
Electrion system
electrocardiogram
    fetal e.
electrocardiograph
electrocardiography
electrocautery
electrocerebral inactivity
electrochemical cell
electrochemistry
electrocoagulation
electrocorticogram
electrocorticography
electrocystography
electrode
    active e.
    bipolar needle e.
    calomel e.
    carbon dioxide e.
    Clark's e.
    Clark's oxygen e.
    earth e.
    glass e.
    ground e.
    hydrogen e.
    e. impedance
    indicator e.
    indifferent e.
    inert e.
    ion-selective e.
    multiple-point e.
    patch e.
    P_{CO_2} e.
    pH e.
    P_{O_2} e.
    e. potential
    quinhydrone e.
    recording e.
    reference e.
    e. response time
    saturated calomel e.
    e. sensitivity
    Severinghaus e.

silver e.
silver chloride e.
solid state e.
standard hydrogen e.
electrodesiccation
electrodiagnosis
electroencephalogram
electroencephalography
electroendosmosis
electroexcision
electrofluoroscopy
electrogastrogram
electrogastrograph
electrogastrography
electrogenic pump
electrohemostasis
electroimmunoassay
    Laurell e.
electroimmunodiffusion
    single-dimension e.
electrolysis
    Faraday's law of e.
electrolyte
    amphoteric e.
    e. balance and homeostasis
    colloidal e.
    e. imbalance
    protein e.
    serum e.
electrolytic
    e. capacitor
    e. cell
    e. stripping
electromagnet
electromagnetic
    e. flowmeter
    e. radiation
    e. unit
electrometer
electromotive force
electromyogram
electromyograph
electromyography
    single-fiber e.
electron
    e. affinity
    Auger e.
    e. beam
    e. capture
    e. capture detector
    conduction e.
    conversion e.

free e.
e. lens
e. micrograph
e. microprobe
e. microscope
e. microscopy
e. pair bond
e. paramagnetic resonance
e. spin resonance
e. transport chain
e. transport inhibitors
valence e's
e. volt
electron-dense
electronegative
electronegativity
electronic
    e. cell counter
    e. focal spot
    e. voltmeter
electron microscope
    analytical e.m.
    scanning e.m.
    transmission e.m.
electron microscopic
electrooculogram
electrooptical system
electroosmosis
electropathology
electropherogram
electrophile
electrophilic
electrophoresis
    acrylamide gel e.
    agarose gel e.
    alkaline phosphatase isoen-
        zyme e.
    capillary e.
    cellulose acetate e.
    cerebrospinal fluid e.
    citrate agar gel e.
    counter e.
    creatine kinase isoenzyme e.
    disc e.
    field invasion gel e.
    frontal e.
    gel e.
    hemoglobin e.
    high-voltage e.
    immunofixation e.
    isoelectric e.
    isoenzyme e.

lipoprotein e.
moving boundary e.
paper e.
polyacrylamide gel e.
protein e.
pulsed-field gradient gel e.
serum protein e.
starch gel e.
e. test
thin-layer e.
two-dimensional gel e.
zonal e.
electrophoretic mobility
electrophoretogram
electrophysiology
electroporation
electropositive
electroretinogram
electroretinography
electroscission
electroscope
electrospinogram
electrostatic
e. imaging
e. unit
electrosurgery
electrotome
electrotomy
electrotransfer test
electrotropism
eleidin
Elek immunodiffusion test
element
e. disorder
inert e.
kappa-deleting e.
radioactive e's
rare earth e's
symmetry e.
trace e.
transposable e.
elementary
e. body
e. charge
e. granule
e. particle
elements (*see also* Appendix 4, "Table of Elements")
eleoma
elephantiac; elephantiasic; elephantoid

elephantiasis
e. congenita angiomatosa
congenital e.
e. nervosa
e. neuromatosa
nevoid e.
e. nostras
e. scroti
e. telangiectodes
e. vulvae
elephant leg
eleventh cranial nerve
elfin facies
elimination
immune e.
e. reaction
ELISA — enzyme-linked immunosorbent assay
elixophyllin
Elkind recovery
ellipse
ellipsin
ellipsoid
ellipsoidal
elliptical erythrocyte
ellipticinium
elliptocyte
elliptocytosis
hereditary e.
elliptocytotic
Ellis
type 1 glomerulonephritis
type 2 glomerulonephritis
types 1 and 2 nephritis
Ellman reagent
Ellsworth-Howard test
elongation factor
ELT — euglobulin lysis time
El Tor vibrio
ELT-series hematology analyzers
eluant
eluate
eluent
elusive ulcer
elute
elution
elutriation
EM — ejection murmur
electron microscope
electron microscopy
erythrocyte mass
Em — emmetropia

emaciation
emanation
EMB — eosin–methylene blue
     ethambutol
     ethambutol-myambutol
Embadomonas
EMB (eosin–methylene blue) agar
Embden-Meyerhof
    cycle
    pathway
embed
embedding agents
embolectomy
embolemia
embolic
    e. abscess
    e. aneurysm
    e. gangrene
    e. glomerulonephritis
    e. infarct
embolism
    air e.
    amniotic fluid e.
    arterial e.
    atheromatous e.
    bacillary e.
    bland e.
    bone marrow e.
    capillary e.
    cellular e.
    cerebral e.
    cholesterol e.
    coronary e.
    cotton-fiber e.
    hemodynamic fat e.
    hemodynamic gas e.
    hemodynamic pulmonary e.
    hemodynamic system e.
    infective e.
    lipid e.
    lymph e.
    lymphogenous e.
    miliary e.
    obturating e.
    oil e.
    pantaloon e.
    paradoxical e.
    plasmodium e.
    pulmonary e.
    pyemic e.
    retinal e.
    retrograde e.

    riding e.
    saddle e.
    spinal e.
    straddling e.
    systemic e.
    trichinous e.
    tumor e.
    venous e.
embolization
embolomycotic aneurysm
embolus (pl., emboli)
    air e.
    amniotic fluid e.
    atheromatous e.
    bland e.
    bone marrow e.
    fat e.
    foreign body e.
    massive e.
    paradoxical e.
    parasitic e.
    recent e.
    saddle e.
    septic e.
    tumor e.
    valvular tissue e.
embryo
    cylindrical e.
    nodular e.
    stunted e.
embryoblast
embryocardia
embryogenesis
embryoid bodies
embryology
embryoma
    e. of kidney
    renal e.
embryonal
    e. adenoma
    e. carcinoma
    e. carcinosarcoma
    e. cell carcinoma
    e. duct cyst
    e. leukemia
    e. nephroma
    e. rest
    e. rhabdomyosarcoma
    e. teratoma
    e. tumor
embryonate

embryonic
 e. blood vessel
 e. competence
 e. disc
 e. ependymal layer
 e. hematopoiesis
 e. hemoglobin
 e. kidney
 e. mantle layer
 e. marginal layer
 e. sphere
 e. structure
 e. testicular dysgenesis
 e. tumor
embryoniform
embryonization
embryonum
 smegma e.
embryoplastic
 e. odontoma
 e. tumor
embryotoxicity
EMC — electron microscopy
 encephalomyocarditis
EMC (encephalomyocarditis) virus
Emcyt
emedullate
emesis
emetatrophia
emetine
EMF — electromagnetic flowmeter
 electromotive force
 endomyocardial fibrosis
 erythrocyte maturation factor
EMG — electromyogram
 exophthalmos, macroglossia,
  gigantism
EMG syndrome
emigration
 e. of white cells
 e. theory
eminence
 frontal e.
 hypothenar e.
 median e.
 parietal e.
 thenar e.
EMI scanner
emissary vein
emission
 e. line
 nocturnal e.

e. spectroscopy
e. spectrum
thermionic e.
EMIT — enzyme-multiplied immunoassay technique
emitter
 beta e.
 e.-coupled logic
Emmens's S/L test
EMMIA — enzyme modulator–mediated immunoassay
Emmonsia
Emmonsiella
emollient
emperipolesis
emphysema
 alveolar e.
 blue bloater e.
 bullous e.
 centriacinar e.
 centrilobular e.
 chronic pulmonary e.
 compensatory e.
 cutaneous e.
 diffuse e.
 familial e.
 gangrenous e.
 generalized e.
 interstitial e.
 intestinal e.
 irregular e.
 obstructive e.
 panacinar e.
 panlobular e.
 paraseptal e.
 pulmonary e.
 pulmonary interstitial e.
 senile e.
 subcutaneous e.
 surgical e.
 vesicular e.
emphysematous
 e. asthma
 e. bleb
 e. cholecystitis
 e. cystitis
 e. gangrene
 e. phlegmon
 e. vaginitis
empiric
empirical
Empirin

empty sella syndrome
empyema
    e. articuli
    e. benignum
    latent e.
    loculated e.
    e. necessitatis
    nocardial e.
    e. of pericardium
    pneumococcal e.
    pulsating e.
    subdural e.
    tuberculous e.
empyemic
empyocele
emu — electromagnetic unit
emulsify
emulsion
emylcamate
EN — erythema nodosum
ENA — extractable nuclear antigen
enamel
    e. hypoplasia
    mottled e.
enamelogenesis imperfecta
enanthate testosterone
enanthema (pl., enanthemas, enan-
    themata)
enantiobiosis
enantiomer
enantiomerism
enantiomorph
enantiomorphism
encainide
encapsulated hemoglobin
encarditis
encelitis; enceliitis
encephalemia
encephalic; encephalitic
encephalitis (pl., encephalitides)
    allergic e.
    amebic e.
    arboviral e.
    arthropod-borne virus e.
    bacterial e.
    California e.
    Dawson's e.
    eastern equine e.
    herpes e.
    e. herpes simplex
    inclusion e.
    Japanese B e.

    kuru e.
    lethargic e.
    e. lethargica
    limbic e.
    multifocal e.
    postinfectious allergic e.
    post-vaccination allergic e.
    spongiform e.
    St. Louis e.
    subacute sclerosing e.
    toxoplasmic e.
    tuberculous e.
    Venezuelan equine e.
    viral e.
    western e.
    western equine e.
encephalitogenic factor
encephalitozoon
encephalization
encephaloarteriography
encephalocele
encephaloclastic porencephaly
encephalocraniocutaneous lipomatosis
encephalocystocele
encephalogram
encephalography
encephaloid cancer
encephalomalacia
encephalomeningocele
encephalomyelitis
    acute disseminated e.
    allergic e.
    autoimmune e.
    disseminated e.
    eastern equine e.
    experimental allergic e.
    perivenous e.
    postinfectious e.
    postvaccinal e.
    western e.
    western equine e.
encephalomyelopathy
    carcinomatous e.
    infantile necrotizing e.
    necrotizing e.
    paracarcinomatous e.
encephalomyocarditis virus
encephalomyopathy
    mitochondrial e.
    subacute necrotizing e.
encephalon

encephalopathy
    anoxic e.
    bilirubin e.
    hepatic e.
    hypercapnic e.
    hypertensive e.
    hypoglycemic e.
    hypoxic e.
    ischemic e.
    lead e.
    metabolic e.
    portasystemic e.
    subacute necrotizing e.
    subacute spongiform e.
    uremic e.
    Wernicke's e.
encephaloscope
encephaloscopy
encephalotrigeminal angiomatosis
encephalovirus
enchondroma
enchondromatosis
enchondromatous
enchondrosarcoma
enchondrosis
encode
encoder
encoding
en coup de sabre
encrusted cystitis
encysted
    e. calculus
    e. pleurisy
encystment
end — endoreduplication
end
    blunt e.
    cohesive e.
    e.-diastolic pressure
    e.-foot
    e.-plate potential
    e. point
    e.-point measurement
    e. product
    e.-product repression
    e. stage
    e.-stage kidney disease
    e.-stage lung
    e.-systolic pressure
    e.-tidal CO_2 tension
Endamoeba blattae

endangiitis; endangeitis
    e. obliterans
endaortitis
    bacterial e.
endarterectomy
endarteritis
    bacterial e.
    e. deformans
    e. obliterans, obliterating e.
    obliterative e.
    e. proliferans, proliferating e.
end bulb
    Krause's e.b.
endemic
    e. colic
    e. fluorosis
    e. funiculitis
    e. goiter
    e. hemoptysis
    e. hypertrophy
    e. murine typhus
    e. typhus
endergonic reaction
endermosis
ending
    nonencapsulated nerve e.
    primary e's
    Ruffini's e.
    secondary e's
endoamylase
endoangiitis
endoaortitis
endoappendicitis
endoarteritis
endobronchial
    e. tube
    e. tuberculosis
    e. tumor
endocardial
    e. cushion defect
    e. fibroelastosis
    e. sclerosis
endocardiosis
    nonbacterial verrucal e.
endocarditic
endocarditis
    abacterial thrombotic e.
    acute bacterial e.
    acute infective e.
    atypical verrucal e.
    atypical verrucous e.
    bacterial e.

cachectic e.
candidal e.
e. chordalis
constrictive e.
fibroplastic parietal e.
gonococcal e.
infectious e.
infective e.
isolated parietal e.
Libman-Sacks e.
Löffler's e.
Löffler's fibroplastic e.
malignant e.
marantic e.
mural e.
nonbacterial thrombotic e.
nonbacterial verrucous e.
polypous e.
pulmonic e.
rheumatic e.
septic e.
staphylococcal e.
streptococcal e.
subacute bacterial e.
subacute infective e.
terminal e.
thrombotic e.
thrombotic nonbacterial e.
ulcerative c.
valvular e.
vegetative e.
verrucal atypical e.
verrucal nonbacterial e.
verrucous e.
viridans e.
endocardium
endocellular complement
endocervical
    e. canal
    e. connective tissue
    e. epithelium
    e. hyperplasia
    e. mucus
    e. polyp
    e. smear
endocervicitis
endocervix
endochondral ossification
endochondromatous myxoma
endochrome
endocranium

endocrine
    e. adenomatosis
    e. amyloidosis
    e. cells
    e. gland
    e. myopathy
    e. pancreas
    e. polyglandular syndrome
    e. system
endocrinologist
endocrinology
endocrinoma
    multiple e.
endocrinopathy
endocyst
endocystitis
endocyte
endocytosis
    reverse e.
endodeoxyribonuclease
endoderm
endodermal sinus tumor
Endodermophyton
"endo-ecto cytoplasmic" rim
endodiascope
endodiascopy
endodyogeny
endoenteritis
endoenzyme
endoesophagitis
endogastritis
endogenote
endogenous
    e. aneurysm
    e. antigen
    e. antigen–cell-bound antibody reaction
    e. antigen–circulating antibody reaction
    e. antigen–transferred antibody reaction
    e. bacterium
    e. creatinine clearance
    e. fecal calcium
    e. hemosiderosis
    e. hyperglyceridemia
    e. hyperlipemia
    e. hyperlipidemia
    e. infection
    e. pigments and deposits
    e. pyrogen
    e. variable

endoglobular; endoglobar
endointoxication
endolaryngeal
Endolimax nana
endolymph
endolymphatic
    e. duct
    e. hydrops
    e. sac
    e. stromal miosis
endolysis
endometria
endometrial
    e. adenocarcinoma
    e. anaerobic culture
    e. atrophy
    e. brush
    e. cancer
    e. cast
    e. cavity
    e. curettage
    e. cyst
    e. cytology
    e. gestational alteration
    e. gland
    e. hyperplasia
    e. morula
    e. polyp
    e. secretion
    e. smear
    e. stroma
    e. stromal sarcoma
    e. stromatosis
    e. zona basalis
    e. zona functionalis
endometrioid
    e. carcinoma
    e. tumor
endometrioma
endometriosis
    bladder e.
    stromal e.
    tuberculous e.
    urethral e.
    vesical e.
endometritis
    decidual e.
    gonococcal e.
    syncytial e.
    tuberculous e.
endometrium (pl., endometria)
    anovulatory cycle e.

    atrophic e.
    carcinoma of e.
    cyclic alteration e.
    cystic hyperplasia of e.
    estrin-type e.
    inactive e.
    interval e.
    late interval e.
    menopausal e.
    menstrual e.
    postmenopausal e.
    postmenstrual e.
    premenstrual e.
    progestational e.
    proliferative e.
    regenerative e.
    secretory e.
    senile e.
    Swiss cheese e.
endomitosis
endomitotic
Endomyces
    E. albicans
    E. capsulatus
    E. epidermatidis
    E. epidermidis
Endomycetales
endomycosis
endomyocardial
    e. fibroelastosis
    e. fibrosis
    e. sclerosis
endomyocarditis
endomyometritis
endomysial antibodies
endomysium
endoneurium
endonuclear
endonuclease
    restriction e.
endonucleolus
endoparasite
endopeduncular nucleus
endopeptidase
endoperiarteritis
endopericarditis
endoperimyocarditis
endoperitonitis
endoperoxide
    prostaglandin e.
endophlebitis

endophthalmitis
    phacoanaphylactic e.
endophthalmos
endophyte
endophytic retinoblastoma
endoplasm
endoplasmic reticulum
endoplast
endoplastic
endopolyploidy
endoprosthesis
endoradiography
endoreduplication
end-organ damage
endoribonuclease
β-endorphin
endorphin assay
endosalpingiosis
endosalpingitis
endosalpingoma
endoscope
endoscopic
    e. biopsy
    e. retrograde cholangiopancrea-
      tography
    e. retrograde pancreatography
    e. unit
endoscopy
    peroral e.
    transcolonic e.
endosmosis
endosome
endospore
endosporium
endosteitis; endostitis
endosteoma
endosteum
endostoma
endostreptosin
endosulfan
endosymbiont
endosymbiosis
endothelia
endothelial
    e. cancer
    e. capillaries
    e. cells
    e. cyst
    e.-derived relaxant factor
    e. leukocyte
    e. metaplasia
    e. myeloma

    e. phagocyte
    e. pore
    e. sarcoma
endothelioblastoma
endotheliocyte
endotheliocytosis
endothelioid
endotheliolysin
endotheliolytic serum
endothelioma
endotheliomatosis
endotheliomyoma
endotheliosarcoma
endotheliosis
endothelium (pl., endothelia)
    e. anterius corneae
    continuous e.
    e.-derived relaxing factor
    discontinuous e.
    fenestrated e.
    vascular e.
endothermic
endothrix
endotoxemia
endotoxic shock
endotoxicosis
endotoxin
endotracheal
    e. insufflation
    e. intubation
    e. tuberculosis
endotrachelitis
endovasculitis
    hemorrhagic e.
Endoxan
endrin
enema
    barium e.
    double-contrast e.
energetics
    biochemical e.
energometer
energy
    activation e.
    binding e.
    bond e.
    free e.
    kinetic e.
    potential e.
    radiant e.
    e. resolution

e.-rich phosphate
standard free e.
enflagellation
enflurane
ENG — electronystagmography
Engel's alkalimetry
engineering
 biomedical e.
 genetic e.
 human e.
engorged
engorgement
engulfment
 cytologic e.
enhancement
 fluorescence e.
 immunologic e.
enhancer
enkephalin
ENL — erythema nodosum lep-
   roticum
  erythema nodosum leprosum
enlargement
 cardiac e.
 left atrial e.
 left ventricular e.
 nuclear e.
 right atrial e.
 right ventricular e.
enol
enolase
 gamma e.
 neuron-specific e.
enol-keto tautomerism
enostosis
enoyl–coenzyme A hydratase
enpromate
enrichment
 e. broth
 e. medium
ensheathing callus
entamebiasis
Entamoeba
 E. buccalis
 E. buetschlii
 E. coli
 E. gingivalis
 E. hartmanni
 E. histolytica
 E. nana
 E. nipponica
 E. polecki

 E. tetragena
 E. tropicalis
enteramine
enterectasis
enterectomy
enterelcosis
enteric
 e. bacillus
 e. cytopathogenic bovine orphan virus
 e. cytopathogenic human orphan virus
 e. cytopathogenic monkey orphan virus
 e. cytopathogenic swine orphan virus
 e. infection
 e. tularemia
enteric-coated
Enteritidis salmonella — *Salmonella en-*
     teritidis
enteritis
 bovine e.
 choleriform e.
 coccidial e.
 chronic cicatrizing e.
 cryptosporidial e.
 diphtheritic e.
 granulomatous e.
 e. gravis
 e. necroticans
 necrotizing e.
 e. nodularis
 phlegmonous e.
 e. polyposa
 regional e.
 segmental e.
 staphylococcal e.
 viral e.
Enterobacter
 E. aerogenes
 E. agglomerans
 E. alvei
 E. cloacae
 E. gergoviae
 E. hafnia
 E. liquefaciens
 E. sakazakii
 E. subgroup C
Enterobacteriaceae
enterobiasis
enterobiliary
Enterobius vermicularis

enterocele
enterocholecystostomy
enterochromaffin
    e. cells
    e. staining
enterococcal infection
enteroclysis
enterococcemia
enterococcus (pl., enterococci)
enterocolectomy
enterocolitis
    acute necrotizing e.
    bacterial e.
    cicatrizing e.
    fungal e.
    necrotizing e.
    neonatal necrotizing e.
    protozoal e.
    pseudomembranous e.
    regional e.
    viral e.
enterocolostomy
enterocutaneous fistula
enterocyst
enterocystoma
enterocyte
Enterocytozoon bienusi
enteroenteric anastomosis
enteroenterostomy
enterogastritis
enterogastrone
enterogenous
    e. cyanosis
    c. cysts
    e. methemoglobinemia
enteroglucagon
enterogram
enterograph
enterography
enterohemorrhagic
enterohepatitis
enteroinvasive
enterokinase
enterolith
enterolithiasis
enteromegaly; enteromegalia
Enteromonas hominis
enteromycosis
enteronitis
enteropathogenic
    e. *Campylobacter*
    e. *Escherichia coli*

    e. *Salmonella*
    e. *Yersinia*
enteropathy
    gluten-sensitive e.
    protein-losing e.
enteropeptidase
enteroptosis; enteroptosia
enteroptotic
enteroscope
enterostenosis
enterostomal
enterostomy
enterotoxigenic
enterotoxin
enterovaginal fistula
enterovesical fistula
enterovirus
enterozoon (pl., enterozoa)
enthalpy of reaction
enthesitis
enthesopathic
enthesopathy
Entner-Doudoroff pathway
entoblast
entocyte
entoderm
Entoloma lividum
entomology
Entomophthora coronata
entomophthoromycosis
    e. basidiobolae
    e. conidiobolae
entomopox virus
entopic
entoplasm
entoplastic
entozoic
entrapment neuropathy
entropion
entropy
enucleate
enucleated
enucleation
enuresis
Envacor test
env antigen
envelope
    cell e.
    nuclear e.
envenomation
env gene
environment

environmental
    e. gastritis
    e. stress
    e. toxicology
enz. — enzymatic
enzootic
enzymatic; enzymic
    e. adaptation
    e. digestion methods
enzyme
    activating e.
    adaptive e.
    allosteric e.
    amino acid–activating e.
    amylolytic e.
    e. analyzer
    angiotensin I–converting e.
    e. antagonist
    antitumor e's
    e. assay
    e.-assisted immunoassay technique
    e. autoagglutination factor
    autolytic e.
    bacterial e's
    e. balance
    brancher e.
    branching e.
    catheptic e.
    citrate condensing e.
    coagulating e.
    conjugase e.
    constitutive e.
    converting e.
    cryptic e.
    cuprein e's
    cytoplasmic glycolytic e.
    debrancher e.
    debranching e.
    e. deficiency
    e. demonstration methods
    e.-derived neurotoxin
    $1,4\text{-}\alpha$-glucan branching e.
    glycogen branching e.
    glycolytic e.
    hydrolytic e.
    immobilized e.
    e. immunoassay
    inducible e.
    e. induction
    e. inhibition
    inhibitory e.

    inverting e.
    iron e's
    e.-linked antibody test
    e.-linked immunochemistry
    e.-linked immunoelectrotransfer blot
    e.-linked immunosorbent assay
    lipolytic e.
    microsomal e.
    mitochondrial e.
    e. modulator–mediated immunoassay
    e.-multiplied immunoassay technique
    nuclear e.
    proteolytic e.
    receptor-destroying e.
    e. repression
    restriction e's
    serum e.
    steatolytic e.
    terminal addition e.
    e. unit
enzymic fat necrosis
enzymolysis
EO — eosinophil
    ethylene oxide
EOG — electrooculogram; electro-olfactogram
EOM — extraocular movement
eos — eosinophil(s)
eosin
    alcohol-soluble e.
    e. B
    ethyl e.
    hematoxylin and e.
    e. I bluish
    e.–methylene blue agar
    e. stain
    e. Y
    yellowish e.
eosinocyte
eosinopenia
eosinophil; eosinophile
    e. adenoma
    e. cationic protein
    e. chemotactic factor of anaphylaxis
    e. count
    e.-derived neurotoxin
    e. granule
    e. leukocyte infiltrate
    polymorphonuclear e.

e. protein
e. smear
e. stimulation promoter
eosinophilia
hereditary e.
Löffler's e.
persistent e.
pulmonary e.
pulmonary infiltration and e.
reactive e.
simple pulmonary e.
tropical e.
tropical pulmonary e.
eosinophilic
e. adenoma
e. cellulitis
e. cystitis
e. erythroblast
e. exudates
e. fasciitis
e. gastritis
e. gastroenteritis
e. granule
e. granulocyte
e. granulocytosis
e. granuloma
e. hyperplasia
e. inclusions
e. index
e. leukemia
e. leukemoid reaction
e. leukocyte
e. leukocytosis
e. leukopenia
e. lung
e. marrow
e. meningoencephalitis
e. metamyelocyte
e. myelocyte
e. myeloencephalitis
e. neurotoxin
e. normoblast
e. pneumonia
e. promyelocyte
e. prostatitis
eosinophilocytic leukemia
eosinophilopoiesis
eosinophilopoietin
eosinophiluria
eosinotactic
EOT — effective oxygen transport

EP — ectopic pregnancy
electrophoresis
erythrocyte protoporphyrin
erythropoietin
EPA — erythroid potentiating activity
EPC — epilepsia partialis continua
EPEC — enteropathogenic *Escherichia coli*
epencephalon
ependyma
ependymal
e. cells
e. glioma
e. layer
ependymitis
ependymoblastoma
ependymoma
epithelial e.
malignant e.
myxopapillary e.
papillary e.
EPF — exophthalmos-producing factor
ephedrine
ephelis (pl., ephelides)
Epi. — epinephrine
epiallopregnanolone
epiboly; epibole
epicanthus
epicarcinogen
epicardium
epichlorohydrin
epicondyle
epicondylitis
epicranial aponeurosis
epicranius muscle
epicystitis
epidemic
e. curve
e. dysentery
e. hemoglobinuria
hemorrhagic fever e.
e. hepatitis
e. keratoconjunctivitis
e. keratoconjunctivitis virus
e. louse-borne typhus
e. myeloencephalitis
parotitis virus e.
typhus e.
epidemiologist
epidemiology

epidermal
  e. cyst
  e.-dermal nevus
  e. growth factor
  e. inclusion cyst
  e. nevus
  e. reactive dermatitis
epidermalization
epidermic-dermic nevus
epidermidization
  cervical e.
epidermidosis
epidermis (pl., epidermides)
  keratohyalin granule of e.
epidermitis
epidermodysplasia verruciformis
epidermoid
  e. cancer
  e. carcinoma
  e. carcinoma in situ
  e. cyst
  e. inclusion cyst
  e. metaplasia
  e. tumor
epidermoidoma
epidermolysin
epidermolysis
  e. bullosa
  e. bullosa dystrophica
  e. bullosa lethalis
  e. bullosa simplex
epidermolytic hyperkeratosis
epidermophytid
Epidermophyton
  E. floccosum
  E. inguinale
  E. rubrum
epidermophytosis
epidermosis
epidermotropism
epididymal
  e. atresia
  e. cyst
  c. fluid
  e. hamartoma
  e. ligament
  e. lumen
  e. spermatocele
epididymectomy
epididymis (pl., epididymides)
epididymitis
  gonococcal e.

  e. nodosa
  nonspecific e.
epididymography
epididymo-orchitis
epididymovesiculography
epidophyllotoxin
epidural
  e. abscess
  e. hematoma
  e. reactive dermatitis
  e. space
epidurography
epigastric
  e. artery
  e. hernia
  e. lymph node
epigastrius parasiticus
epigenesis
epigenetic carcinogen
epigenotype
epiglottic
  e. cartilage
  e. mucus
epiglottiditis; epiglottitis
  bacterial e.
epiglottis
epignathus
epihyal bone
epilating dose
epilepidoma
epilepsia partialis continua
epilepsy
  familial myoclonic e.
  focal e.
  focal cortical e.
  grand mal e.
  jacksonian e.
  minor e.
  myoclonic e.
  petit mal e.
  post-traumatic e.
  psychomotor e.
  rolandic e.
  temporal lobe e.
  uncinate e.
epileptiform discharge
epileptogenesis
epileptogenic zone
epiloia
epimastigote
epimer
epimerase

epimerization
epimorphic regeneration
epimorphosis
epimysium
epinephrine
    e. and norepinephrine assay
    e. glycosuria
    e.-norepinephrine ratio
epineurium
epiphenotype
epiphrenic diverticulum
epiphyseal; epiphysial
    e. arrest
    e. aseptic necrosis
    e. giant cell tumor
    e. plate
epiphysis (pl., epiphyses)
    stippled e.
epiphysitis
epiphyte
epipodophyllotoxin
epirubicin
episcleritis
    rheumatoid e.
episode
    transient cerebral ischemic e.
    transient ischemic e.
episomal
episome
epispadias
epistasis; epistaxy
epistatic
epistaxis; epistaxy
epitestosterone
epith. — epithelium
epithalamus
epithalaxia
epithelial   "EPis"
    e. basement membrane
    e. cancer
    e. cast
    e. cell disease
    e. cells
    e. cell urinary cast
    e. cyst
    c. dysplasia
    e. ependymoma
    e. hyperplasia
    e. inclusion cyst
    e. interferon
    e. membrane antigen
    e. neoplasm

    e. nest
    e. pearl
    e. pigment
    e. rest
    e. structural antigen
    e. thymic-activating factor
    e. thymoma
    e. tumor
    e.-type mesothelium
epithelialization
epithelialize
epithelioceptor
epitheliocyte
epithelioid
    e. cell
    e. cell melanoma
    e. cell nevus
    e. hemangioendothelioma
    e. leiomyoma
    e. leiomyosarcoma
    e. nevus
    e. sarcoma
    e.-type macrophage
epitheliolytic
epithelioma
    e. adamantinum
    e. adenoides cysticum
    basal cell e.
    benign e.
    Borst-Jadassohn intraepidermal
      basal cell e.
    calcifying e. of Malherbe
    chorionic e.
    cylindrical e.
    e. cuniculatum
    Ferguson-Smith e.
    intraepithelial e.
    Malherbe's calcifying e.
    malignant e.
    multiple self-healing squa-
      mous e.
    sebaceous e.
    suprarenal e.
epitheliomatous
epitheliopathy
epitheliosis
epitheliotoxin
epithelium (pl., epithelia)
    Barrett's e.
    bronchial e.
    cardiac e.
    ciliated e.

coelomic e.
colonic e.
columnar e.
endocervical e.
exocervical e.
germinal e.
glandular e.
oral e.
seminiferous e.
squamous e.
thymic e.
tubal e.
epithermal neutron
epitope
epitrochlear lymph node
epituberculosis
epituberculous infiltration
epitympanum
epizootic
eponychium
eponym(s) (*see also* Appendix 2, "Eponymic Diseases and Syndromes")
epoöphoron
epoxide
    heptachlor e.
epoxy resin
EPP — end-plate potential
    equal pressure point
    erythropoietic protoporphyria
EPR — electron paramagnetic resonance
    electrophrenic respiration
    estradiol production rate
EPS — exophthalmos-producing substance
epsilon
    e. acid
    e.-aminocaproic acid
    e. staphylolysin
Epstein-Barr
    nasopharyngeal carcinoma
    nuclear antigen
    virus
    virus antibody assay
    virus culture
    virus serology
epulis (pl., epulides)
    congenital e.
    e. fibromatosa
    e. fissurata

giant cell e.
e. gigantocellularis
e. granulomatosa
pigmented e.
epulofibroma
eq. — equivalent
equal pressure point
Equanil
equation
    alveolar air e.
    alveolar ventilation e.
    Bohr e.
    Botzmann's e.
    chemical e.
    Eadie-Hofstee e.
    Fick's e.
    Gompertz e.
    Hanes e.
    Hardy-Weinberg e.
    Hasselbalch's e.
    Henderson-Hasselbalch e.
    Hill e.
    Hufner's e.
    linear e.
    Lineweaver-Burk e.
    Michaelis-Menten e.
    Nernst e.
    Scatchard e.
    van der Waals e.
equational division
equatorial plate
equilibration
equilibrium
    chemical e.
    e. constant
    e. dialysis
    dynamic e.
    oxygen e.
    physiologic e.
    radioactive e.
    secular e.
    sedimentation e.
    thermal e.
    thermodynamic e.
    transient e.
equine
    e. antihuman lymphoblast globulin
    e. antihuman lymphoblast serum
    e. encephalomyelitis virus

e. gonadotropin unit
e. rhinopneumonitis
equine encephalitis
eastern e.e.
Venezuelan e.e.
western e.e.
equinus
equipotential line
equivalence
e. point
e. relation
e. zone
equivalent
age e.
Joule's e.
lethal e.
nitrogen e.
toxic e.
ER — ejection rate
endoplasmic reticulum
estrogen receptors
Er — erbium
ERA — evoked response audiometry
Eranko's fluorescence stain
erase
Erb's
palsy
point
waves
erb-A oncogene
erb-B oncogene
ERBF — effective renal blood flow
erbium
ERC — erythropoietin-responsive cell
ERCP — endoscopic retrograde cholangiopancreatography
Erdheim
rest
tumor
erectile
e. bodies
e. myxoma
erection
penile e.
erector muscle of spine
ERG — electroretinogram
erg
ergastoplasm
ergastoplasmic
ergocalciferol
ergoloid mesylates
ergometer
ergonovine maleate

ergosterol
ergot
ergotamine tartrate
ergothioneine
ergotism
ergotoxine
Erlenmeyer's flask
erode
E (erythrocyte) rosette
E r. assay
E r. test
erosion
erosive
e. adenomatosis of nipple
e. aneurysm
e. esophagitis
e. gastritis
e. inflammation
ERP — effective refractory period
equine rhinopneumonitis
ERPF — effective renal plasma flow
error
coincidence e.
machine e.
probable e.
random e.
e. rate
standard e.
standard e. of the mean
systematic e.
Type I e.
Type II e.
eructation
eruption
bullous e.
creeping e.
Kaposi's varicelliform e.
macular e.
maculopapular e.
photoeczematous e.
polymorphic light e.
polymorphous e.
varicelliform e.
eruptive keratoacanthoma
ERV — expiratory reserve volume
Erwinia
E. *amylovora*
E. *herbicola*
Erwinieae
erysipelas
erysipeloid

Erysipelothrix
 E. *insidiosa*
 E. *rhusiopathiae*
erythema
 e. ab igne
 e. annulare centrifugum
 e. chronicum migrans
 e. dose
 e. elevatum diutinum
 e. exfoliativa
 e. figuratum
 e. gyratum
 e. induratum
 e. infectiosum
 e. keratodes
 e. marginatum rheumaticum
 e. multiforme
 e. multiforme bullosum
 e. multiforme exudativum
 necrolytic migratory e.
 e. neonatorum
 e. nodosum
 e. nodosum leprosum
 Osler's e.
 palmar e.
 e. pernio
 e. perstans
 e.-producing rays
 e. streptogenes
 toxic e.
erythematosum
 anetoderma e.
erythematosus
 acute disseminated lupus e.
 discoid lupus e.
 lupus e.
 systemic lupus e.
erythematous dermatitis
erythrasma
 scrotal e.
erythremia
erythremic myelosis
erythritol
erythrityl tetranitrate
Erythrobacillus
Erythobacter longus
erythroblast
 acidophilic e.
 basophilic e.
 definitive e.
 eosinophilic e.
 intermediate e.

 orthochromatic e.
 oxyphilic e.
 polychromatic e.
 primitive e.
erythroblastemia
erythroblastic
 e. anemia
 e. island
 e. multinuclearity
erythroblastoma
erythroblastomatosis
erythroblastopenia
 transient e.
erythroblastosis
 e. fetalis
 fetal e.
 e. neonatorum
erythroblastotic
erythrocatalysis
erythrochromia
erythroclasis
erythroclast
erythroclastic
erythrocuprein
erythrocytapheresis
erythrocyte
 achromic e.
 anisocytic e.
 e. antigen
 basophilic e.
 contracted e.
 dimorphic e.
 dysmorphic e.
 elliptical e.
 e. fragility
 e. fragility test
 fragmented e.
 globulin-coated e.
 e. glutamic oxaloacetic transaminase
 hemolyzed e.
 e. hexokinase deficiency
 hydrated e.
 hyperchromic e.
 hypochromic e.
 immunoglobulin-coated e.
 e. index
 leukocyte-poor e.
 macrocytic e.
 e. mass
 e. maturation factor
 e. membrane

microcytic e.
e. multinuclearity
non-nucleated e.
normochromic e.
normocytic e.
nucleated e.
orthochromatic e.
packed e's
e.-phosphate buffer system
polychromatic e.
e. porphyrin
e. protoporphyrin
e. rosette test
e. sedimentation
e. sedimentation rate
e.-sensitizing substance
sheep e.
spherical e.
spheroid e.
spiculated e.
tear-shaped e.
e. vacuole
e. zinc protoporphyrin
erythrocythemia
erythrocytic
e. blood cell
e. capillaries
e. marrow
e. series
erythrocytoblast
erythrocytolysin
erythrocytolysis
erythrocytometer
erythrocytopenia
erythrocytophagy
erythrocytopoiesis
erythrocytorrhexis
erythrocytoschisis
erythrocytosis
absolute e.
leukemic e.
e. megalosplenica
relative e.
stress e.
erythrocyturia
erythrodegenerative
erythroderma
exfoliative e.
e. foliativa
Sézary's e.
erythrodextrin
erythrodontia

erythrodysesthesia syndrome
erythrogenesis imperfecta
erythrogenic toxin
erythrogonium (pl., erythrogonia)
erythrohepatic
e. porphyria
e. protoporphyria
erythroid
e. aplasia
e. cell
e. hyperplasia
e. hypoplasia
e.-potentiating activity
erythrokatalysis
erythrokeratodermia
e. variabilis
erythrokinase
erythrokinetics
erythrokinetic studies
erythroleukemia
acute e.
erythroleukosis
erythroleukothrombocythemia
erythrolysin
erythrolysis
erythromelia
erythromycin
erythromyeloblastic leukemia
erythron
erythroneocytosis
erythronoclastic
erythronormoblastic anemia
erythropenia
erythrophage
erythrophagia
erythrophagocytic
erythrophagocytosis
erythrophil
erythrophilic
erythroplakia
erythroplasia
Queyrat's e.
erythropoiesis
extramedullary e.
ineffective e.
megaloblastic e.
e.-stimulating factor
erythropoietic
e. hormone
e. porphyria
e. protoporphyria
e.-stimulating factor

e. tissue
e. uroporphyria
erythropoietin
recombinant e.
e.-responsive cell
erythropyknosis
erythrorrhexis
erythrose
e. isomerase
e. 4-phosphate
erythrosedimentation
erythrosin B
erythrostasis
erythruria
ES — emission spectrometry
endoscopic sphincterotomy
Es. — *einsteinium*
ESB — electrical stimulation to brain
Esbach's reagent
escalator
mucociliary e.
escape
e. beats
junctional e.
nodal e.
vagal e.
ventricular e.
Esch. — *Escherichia*
eschar
Escherichia
E. aerogenes
E. alkalescens
E. aurescens
E. coli
E. dispar
E. dispar var. ceylonensis
E. dispar var. madampensis
E. fergusonii
E. freundii
E. intermedia
E. vulneris
Escherichieae
Escherich's bacillus
esculin hydrolysis test
ESF — erythropoietic-stimulating
factor
ESL — end-systolic length
ESM — ejection systolic murmur
eso — esophagoscopy
esophagus
esoethmoiditis
esogastritis

esophagalgia
esophagastrostomy
esophageal
e. achalasia
e. adventitia
e. apudoma
e. artery
e. atresia
e. axis
e. branch
e. cancer
e. contraction ring
e. diverticulum
e. gland
e. hernia
e. intraepithelial neoplasia
e. intubation
e. lumen
e. manometry
e. mucous membrane
e. mucus
e. muscularis propria
e. plexus
e. smear
e. sphincter
e. submucosa
e. tumors
e. varices
e. vein
e. web
esophagectasis; esophagectasia
esophagectomy
esophagitis
candidal e.
corrosive e.
e. dissecans superficialis
erosive e.
herpetic e.
infectious e.
monilial e.
peptic e.
reflux e.
ulcerative e.
uremic e.
esophagobronchial
esophagocele
esophagocologastrostomy
esophagocoloplasty
esophagoduodenostomy
esophagodynia
esophagoenterostomy
esophagoesophagostomy

esophagofundopexy
esophagogastrectomy
esophagogastric anastomosis
esophagogastroanastomosis
esophagogastroduodenoscopy
esophagogastroplasty
esophagogastroscopy
esophagogastrostomy
esophagogram
esophagography
esophagojejunogastrostomy
esophagojejunoplasty
esophagojejunostomy
esophagolaryngectomy
esophagology
esophagomalacia
esophagomycosis
esophagomyotomy
esophagopharyngoscopy
esophagopharynx
exophagoplasty
esophagoplication
esophagoptosis; esophagoptosia
esophagosalivary reflex
esophagoscopy
    fiberoptic e.
esophagostenosis
esophagostomy
esophagotomy
esophagotracheal
esophagram
    barium e.
esophagus (pl., esophagi)
    Barrett's e.
esosphenoiditis
esotoxin
ESP — end-systolic pressure
    eosinophil stimulation promoter
espundia
ESR — electron spin resonance
    erythrocyte sedimentation rate
esr — electron spin resonance
ESS — erythrocyte-sensitizing substance
essential
    e. albuminuria
    e. asthma
    e. atrophy
    e. fatty acid
    e. fructosuria

    e. hematuria
    e. hypercholesterolemia
    e. hyperlipemia
    e. hypertension
    e. oil
    e. pentosuria
    e. telangiectasia
    e. thrombocythemia
    e. thrombocytopenia
established cell line
ester
    cholesteryl e. hydrolase
    hexosephosphoric e.
    indoxyl carbonic acid e.
    phorbol e.
esterase
    naphthol ASP chloroacetate e.
    d-naphthyl acetate e.
    d-naphthyl butyrate e.
    e. test
esterification
esterol
estetrol
esthesioneuroblastoma
esthesioneurocytoma
esthiomene
esthiomenous
estimate
    biased e.
    dose e.
    interval e.
    median unbiased e.
    point e.
    pooled e.
    standard error of e.
    unbiased e.
estimated
    e. blood loss
    e. hepatic blood flow
Estlander flap
estracyt
estradiol
    e. benzoate
    e. benzoate unit
    e. production rate
    e. receptor
estramustine
Estren-Dameshek
    anemia
    aplasia
    familial aplasia
estrin-type endometrium

estriol
      conjugated e.
      free e.
      serum e.
      total e.
      unconjugated e.
      urinary e.
estrogen
      exogenous e.
      e.-producing tumor
      e. receptor
      e. withdrawal bleeding
estrogenic
      e. hormone activity
      e. steroids
estrone unit
estrophilin
estrous cycle
e.s.u. — electrostatic unit
ESV — end-systolic volume
ET — effective temperature
      endotracheal
      essential thrombocythemia
      etiology
      eustachian tube
Et — ethyl
ETA — ethionamide
ETAF — epithelial thymic-activating
          factor
état
      é. mamelonné
      é. marbré
ETF — eustachian tube function
ETH — elixir of terpin hydrate
ethacrynic acid
ethambutol
ethamivan
ethane
ethanedial
ethanoic acid
ethanol
      acidified e.
      e. gelation test
      e. level
ethanolamine
ethanolaminephosphate cytidylyltrans-
    ferase
ethanolaminephosphotransferase
ETH/C — elixir of terpin hydrate
          with codeine
ethchlorvynol assay
ethene

ether
      alkyl phenol polyglycol e.
      dichloroethyl e.
      dimethyl e.
      ethyl e.
      petroleum e.
      propylene glycol mono-
        methyl e.
      e. storage
      vinyl e.
ethidium bromide
ethinamate
ethinyl estradiol
ethion
ethionamide
ethionine
ethisterone
ethmoid
      e. antrum
      e. bone
      e. sinus
ethmoidal
      e. artery
      e. bulla
      e. labyrinth
ethmoidectomy
ethmoiditis
ethmoidomaxillary suture
ethoheptazine
ethohexadiol
ethopropazine
ethosuximide assay
ethotoin
ethoxazene hydrochloride
ethoxzolamide
ethyl
      e. acetate
      e. alcohol
      e. alcohol poisoning
      e. aminobenzoate
      e. benzene
      e. biscoumacetate
      e. bromide
      e. butyl propanediol
      e. carbamate
      e. chloride
      e. cyanide
      e. di-(p-chlorophenyl) gly-
        collate
      e. dipropylthiocarbamate
      e. eosin
      e. ether

e. formate
e. green
e. hexanediol
e. hydrocupreine hydrochloride test
e. iodide
e. iodophenylundecylate
e. mercaptan
e. mercaptoethyl diethyl thiophosphate
e. mercury chloride
e. mercury phosphate
e. nitrate
e. nitrophenyl benzene thiophosphate
e. nitrophenyl thiobenzene
e. orange
e. phosphate
ethylamine
ethyl-benzyl-nitrosamine
ethylene
e. chlorobromide
e. chlorohydrin
e. dibromide
e. dichloride
e. glycol
e. glycol dinitrate
e. oxide
e. poisoning
ethylenediamine
ethylenediaminetetraacetic acid
ethylenimine
ethylidene chloride
N-(ethylmercuri)-p-toluenesulfonanilide
ethylmethacrylate
ethylmorphine hydrochloride
ethyne
etiocholanolone
etiocobalamin
etiol. — etiology
etiologic
e. agent
e. fraction
etiology
genetic e.
pyrexia of unknown e.
unknown e.
ETKM — every test known to mankind
ETM — erythromycin
ETOH — ethyl alcohol

etoposide
etoprine
ETOX — ethylene oxide
ETP — eustachian tube pressure
ETT — extrathyroidal thyroxine
EU — Ehrlich unit
enzyme unit
Eu — europium
EUA — examination under anesthesia
eubacteria
Eubacteriales
Eubacterium
E. aerofaciens
E. alactolyticum
E. contortum
E. endocarditis
E. lentum
E. limosum
E. parvum
E. rectale
E. ventriosum
eucalyptol
eucalyptus oil
eucapnia
eucaryote
eucaryotic
eucatropine hydrochloride
eucholia
euchromatic
euchromatin
eudermol
eugenol
Euglena gracilis
euglenoid movement
euglobulin
e. clot lysis
e. clot lysis time
e. clot test
e. lysis test
e. lysis time
euglycemia
euglycemic
eugonic
eukaryon
eukaryosis
eukaryote
eukaryotic
eumelanin
Eumycetes
Eumycota

eumycotic
  e. mutation
  e. mycetoma
eunuch
eunuchoidism
euparal
euplastic lymph
euploid
euploidy
Euproctis chrysorrhoea
European
  blastomycosis
  hookworm
  rat flea
europium
Eurotium malignum
eurythermal
Eusimulium
eustachianography
eustachian tube
Eustrongylus
eutectic temperature
euthanasia
euthyroid
euthyroidism
eutopic hormone
Eutriatoma
Eutrombicula alfreddugesi
eutrophic
EV — extravascular
eV; ev — electron volt
evacuation
  e. hospital
  e. procedures
evagination
Evans blue
Evans's staging system
evaporation
eventration of diaphragm
eversion
evil
  king's e.
evisceration
EVM — electronic voltmeter
evoked potential
  brain stem auditory e.p.
  scalp-recorded somatosensory e.p.
  somatosensory e.p.
  spinal somatosensory e.p.
  visual e.p.
evolution

Ewart's sign
E wave
EWB — estrogen withdrawal bleeding
Ewingella
Ewing's
  sarcoma
  tumor
EWL — egg-white lysozyme
ex — excision
  exophthalmos
exacerbation
examination
  cytologic e.
  double-contrast e.
  duodenal contents e.
  full blood e.
  gastric residue e.
  Papanicolaou e.
  pericardial fluid e.
  peritoneal fluid e.
  pleural fluid e.
  postmortem e.
  semen e.
  slit-lamp e.
  sputum e.
  synovial fluid e.
exanthem
  Boston e.
  e. subitum
exanthematous inflammation
EXBF — exercise hyperemia blood flow
exc — excision
excavation
excavatum
excess
  androgen e.
  base e.
  catecholamine e.
  mineral e.
  negative base e.
excessive
  e. cornification
  e. fatigue
  e. heat production
  e. lacrimation
  e. sweating
  e. tearing
  e. weakness
  e. weeping
  e. weight gain
  e. weight loss

exchange
    e. pairing
    plasma e.
    e. transfusion
exchangeable mass
excipient
excision
    marginal e.
    radical e.
    wide e.
excisional biopsy
excitable
    e. cell
    e. gap
    e. membrane
excitation spectrum
excited skin syndrome
exciter filter
excitotoxin
exclusion
    allelic e.
    isotypic e.
excoriation
excrescence
    Lambl's e's
excretion
    fractional sodium e.
    pseudouridine e.
excretory
    e. gland
    e. urogram
excystation
execute
execution time
exemia
exenteration
exenteritis
exercise hyperemia
exeresis
exergonic reaction
exertional dyspnea
exfoliatin
exfoliation
exfoliative
    e. cytodiagnosis
    e. cytologic alteration
    e. cytology
    e. dermatitis
    e. erythroderma
    e. gastritis
    e. psoriasis
exhalation

exhaust
    slot e.
exhaustion
    e. atrophy
    heat e.
existence proof
exit
    e. access
    e. discharge
    e. dose
exoantigen test
exocellular
exocelomic
    e. cavity
    e. membrane
exocervical
    e. connective tissue
    e. epithelium
exocervix
exocrine
    e. gland
    e. pancreas
exocytosis
exodeoxyribonuclease
exodus
exoenzyme
exoerythrocytic plasmodium
exogenote
exogenous
    e. aneurysm
    e. anticoagulant coagulation
    e. antigen
    e. antigen–cell-bound antibody reaction
    e. antigen–circulating antibody reaction
    e. bacterium
    e. creatinine clearance
    e. estrogen
    e. hemochromatosis
    e. hemosiderosis
    e. hyperglyceridemia
    e. hyperlipemia
    e. infection
    e. pigments and deposits
    e. pigmentation
    e. variable
exon
exonuclease
exopeptidase
Exophiala
    E. jeanselmei

E. *mycetoma*
E. werneckii
exophthalmic
    e. gigantism
    e. goiter
exophthalmos
    e. hyperthyroid factor
    e.-producing factor
    e.-producing substance
exophyte
exophytic
    e. growth
    e. retinoblastoma
exoribonuclease
exosmosis
exostosis (pl., exostoses)
    bone e.
    e. bursata
    e. cartilaginea
    cartilaginous e.
    chondromatous e.
    diaphyseal juxtaepiphyseal e.
    hereditary multiple exostoses
    ivory e.
    multiple e.
    osteocartilaginous e.
    solitary osteocartilaginous e.
    subungual e.
exothermic
exotoxin
    bacterial e's
    clostridial e.
    corynebacterial e.
    streptococcal pyrogenic e.
exotropia
"expanded rubella syndrome"
expander
    plasma volume e.
expansion
    periurethral e.
expectancy wave
expectorate
expectoration
    prune juice e.
experiment
    control e.
    double-blind e.
    double-masked e.
experimental
    e. allergic encephalomyelitis
    e. allergic neuritis
    e. pathology

expiration
expiratory reserve volume
explode
exploratory
    e. biopsy
    e. surgery
explosion
explosion-proof
explosive
    e. limits
    e. material
exponent
exponential
    e. decay
    e. function
    e. phase
exposure
expression
    Langmuir e.
    e. vector
expressivity
exsanguinate
exsanguination
exsanguine
exsiccant
exsiccate
exsiccation
exstrophy
    e. of bladder
    e. of cloaca
ext. — exterior
    external
    extract
Extended Binary Coded Decimal Interchange Code
extender
    artificial plasma e.
extension
extensor
    e. carpi radialis brevis muscle
    e. carpi radialis longus muscle
    e. carpi ulnaris muscle
    e. digiti minimi muscle
    e. digitorum muscle
    e. hallucis brevis muscle
    e. hallucis longus muscle
    e. plantar reflex
    e. pollicis brevis muscle
    e. pollicis longus muscle
external
    e. arcuate fibers
    e. auditory canal

e. auditory meatus
e. capsule
e. carotid artery
e. carotid nerve
e. ear
e. elastic lamellae
e. endometriosis
e. fistula
e. genitalia
e. hemorrhoids
e. hydrocephalus
e. iliac artery
e. iliac vein
e. inguinal ring
e. jugular vein
e. limiting membrane
e. maxillary artery
e. medullary lamina
e. nasal branch
e. os
e. pudendal artery
e. pudendal vein
e. storage
e. terminal filament
externalia
exteroceptor
exterofection
exterofective
exterogestate
extinction coefficient
extinguishing
extirpation
Exton's reagent
extra-abdominal desmoid
extra-adrenal paraganglioma
extracapillary glomerulonephritis
extracapsular ankylosis
extracellular
e. aggregate alteration lipid
e. alteration
e. background material alteration
e. cholesterolosis
e. fiber
e. fibril alteration
e. fluid volume
e. granule
e. ground substance
e. lipid aggregate
e. macromolecular aggregate
e. material
e. matrix
e. matrix alteration
e. parasite
e. plasma
e. sap
e. sauce
e. structural alteration
e. vacuole
e. volume
e. water
extracerebral
extrachromosomal inheritance
extracorporeal
e. dialysis
e. heart
extracorpuscular
extract
adipose tissue e.
adrenocortical e.
anterior pituitary e.
ceanothus e.
parathyroid e.
pollen e.
whole ragweed e.
extractable nuclear antigen
extraction
Baker's pyridine e.
e. coefficient
countercurrent e.
e. fraction
solvent e.
extracystic
extraembryonic mesoblast
extrafective
extrafusal fibers
extraglomerular mesangium
extragonadal germ cell cancer
extrahepatic
e. biliary atresia
e. bile duct
e. cholestasis
e. obstruction
extrahypothalamic
extrainguinal
extralymphatic
extramammary Paget's disease
extramedullary
e. erythropoiesis
e. hematopoiesis
e. leukemia
e. megakaryocytopoiesis
e. myeloid cell tumor

e. myeloid tumor
e. myelopoiesis
extranodal lymphoma
extranuclear
extraocular muscle
extraosseous
    e. ameloblastoma
    e. osteosarcoma
extrapancreatic
extraparotid lymph glands
extrapolation
extraprostatitis
extrapulmonary tuberculosis
extrapyramidal tract
extrarenal azotemia
extraskeletal
    e. chondroma
    e. osteosarcoma
extrasystole
extrathoracic
extrauterine pregnancy
extravasate
extravasation
    bile e.
    blood e.
    e. cyst
    e. feces
    e. gas
    mucus e.
    punctiform e.
extravascular hemolysis
extreme capsule
extremital
extremity
    lower e.
    upper e.
extrinsic
    e. allergic alveolitis
    e. factor
    e. hemolysis
    e. ocular muscle
    e. pathway
    e. semiconduction
    e. tongue muscle
extrude
extrusion
exuberant
    e. granulation
    e. granuloma

exudate
    acute inflammatory e.
    eosinophilic e's
    inflammatory e.
    mucopurulent e.
    peritoneal e's
    pleural e.
exudation
    e. cell
    e. corpuscle
    e. cyst
exudative
    e. arthritis
    e. bronchiolitis
    e. glomerulonephritis
    e. granulomatous inflammation
    e. inflammation
exude
exulcerans
exuviae
exuviation
ex vivo (outside the living body; denoting surgical removal, repair, and return of an organ)
eye
    e. appendages
    crab e.
    e. field, frontal, occipital
    e. tumor
    e. tumor localization
    e. worm
eyeball
    tunica fibrosa of e.
    tunica interna of e.
    tunica vasculosa of e.
eyebrow
eyelash
eyelid
    third e.
eyepiece
    comparison e.
    compensated e.
    high eyepoint e.
    huygenian e.
    negative e.
    Ramsden's e.
    widefield e.
eyepoint

F— Fahrenheit
  farad
  feces
  female
  field of vision
  fluorine
  foramen
  force
  formula
  French (catheter size)
  gilbert (unit of magnetomotive force)
  hydrocortisone (compound F)
F. — *Filaria*
  Fusiformis
F₁ — first filial generation
F₂ — second filial generation
FA — fatty acid
  femoral artery
  fluorescent antibody
  free acid
FAB — formalin ammonium bromide
  fragment antigen binding
  French, American, British Leukemia Classification
FAB fragments
Faber's anemia
fabism; favism
FABP — fatty acid–binding protein
Fabricius
  bursa of F.
face
  adenoid f.
  hippocratic f.
  f. presentation
facial
  f. artery
  f. bones
  f. diprosopus duplication
  f. edema
  f. hemiatrophy
  f. lymph node
  f. muscle
  f. myiasis
  f. nerve
  f. palsy
  f. prosthesis
  f. trophoneurosis
  f. vein
facies
  adenoid f.

  cherubic f.
  cushingoid f.
  elfin f.
  f. hepatica
  f. hippocratica
  hurloid f.
  leonine f.
  leprechaun f.
  moon f.
  Parkinson's f.
  Potter's f.
  scaphoid f.
facilitated diffusion
faciodigitogenital dysplasia
facioscapulohumeral muscular dystrophy
FACS — fluorescence-activated cell sorting
facteur thymique serique
factitia
  thyrotoxicosis f.
factitial panniculitis
factitious
  f. dermatitis
  f. hyperthyroidism
  f. hypoglycemia
  f. melanin
  f. urticaria
factor
  f. A
  accelerator f.
  acetate replacement f.
  adrenal weight f.
  adrenocorticotropic hormone–releasing f.
  albumin-agglutinating f.
  aldosterone-stimulating f.
  allogeneic effect f.
  amplification f.
  anabolism-promoting f.
  angiogenesis f.
  animal protein f.
  antichromotrichia f.
  antiacrodynia f.
  antigen-specific helper f.
  antigen-specific suppressor f.
  antihemophilic f.
  antihemophilic f. A
  antihemophilic f. B
  antiheparin f.

antinuclear f.
antipernicious anemia f.
autocrine growth f.
autocrine motility f.
automated motility f's
f. B
basophil chemotactic f.
B-cell growth f. I, II
B-cell-stimulating f.
blastogenic f.
blood f.
B-lymphocyte stimulatory f's
C3 Nef (C3 nephritic) f.
CAMP (cyclophosphamide, Adriamycin, methotrexate, procarbazine) f.
certainty f.
chemotactic f.
Christmas f.
chromotrichial f.
citrovorum f.
clearing f's
clone-inhibiting f.
cloning inhibitor f.
clotting f.
coagulation f.
coagulation f's I, II, III, IV, V, VII, VIII, IX, X, XI, XII, XIII
cobra venom f.
coding f.
coenzyme f.
colony-stimulating f.
complement chemotactic f.
conglutinogen-activating f.
cord f.
corticotropin-releasing f.
cryoprecipitated antihemophilic f.
crystal-induced chemotactic f.
cytotoxic T-lymphocyte differentiation f.
f. D
decay antibody-accelerating f.
deficiency f.
f. deficiency anemia
deficiency f's I, II, V, VII, VIII, IX, X, XI
f. D, H, I deficiency
dose-reduction f.
f. E
elongation f.

encephalitogenic f.
endothelial-derived relaxant f.
endothelium-derived relaxing f.
eosinophil chemotactic f.
epidermal growth f.
epithelial thymic-activating f.
erythrocyte maturation f.
erythropoietic stimulating f.
exophthalmos-hyperthyroid f.
exophthalmos-producing f.
extrinsic f.
F. f
fertility f.
fibrin-stabilizing f.
Fitzgerald f.
Fitzgerald-Williams-Flaujeac f.
Flaujeac f.
Fletcher's f.
follicle-stimulating hormone–releasing f.
G f.
g f.
genetic f.
glass f.
glycotropic f.
f. Gm
gonadotropin-releasing f.
granulocyte colony–stimulating f.
granulocyte-macrophage colony–stimulating f.
growth f.
growth hormone–releasing f.
growth inhibitory f.
H f.
Hageman f.
hematopoietic growth f.
hepatocyte-stimulating f.
high-molecular-weight neutrophil chemotactic f.
histamine-releasing f.
human antihemophilic f.
humoral thymic f.
hydrazine-sensitive f.
hyperglycemic-glycogenolytic f.
hypothalamic corticotropin-releasing f.
I f.
f. I (fibrinogen)
f. II (prothrombin)
f. III (thromboplastin)

f. IV (calcium)
f. V (proaccelerin)
f. VI (accelerin)
f. VII (pro-serum prothrombin-converting activity)
f. VIII
f. VIII antibody stain
f. VIII antigen
f. VIII (antihemophilic factor)
f. VIII:C
f. VIII concentrate
f. VIII–crossed immunoelectrophoresis
f. VIII inhibitor
f. VIII R
f. VIII–related antigen test
f. IX (Christmas factor, plasma thromboplastin component)
f. IX complex
f. X (Stuart factor)
f. XI (plasma thromboplastin antecedent)
f. XII (Hageman factor)
f. XIII (fibrin-stabilizing factor)
immunoglobulin-binding f.
inhibiting f.
initiation f.
insulin f.
insulin-like growth f.
intermediate lobe inhibiting f.
intrinsic f.
kappa f.
labile f.
Lactobacillus bulgaricus f.
Laki-Lorand f.
LE f.
leukocyte inhibitory f.
leukocytosis-promoting f.
leukopenic f.
L-L f.
load f.
luteinizing hormone–releasing f.
lymph node permeability f.
lymphocyte-activating f.
lymphocyte blastogenic f.
lymphocyte mitogenic f.
lymphocyte-transforming f.
lymphocytosis-promoting f.
macrophage-activating f.
macrophage agglutination f.
macrophage chemotactic f.
macrophage colony–stimulating f.
macrophage-derived growth f.
macrophage fusion f.
macrophage growth f.
macrophage-inhibiting f.
macrophage migration inhibition f.
maturation f.
melanocyte-stimulating hormone–inhibiting f.
melanocyte-stimulating hormone–releasing f.
migration-inhibiting f.
migratory inhibiting f.
mitogenic f.
müllerian inhibitory f.
multicolony-stimulating f.
myocardial depressant f.
natriuretic f.
necrotizing f.
nephritic f.
nerve growth f.
neutrophil chemotactic f.
osteoclast-activating f.
Ovenstone f.
P f.
Passovoy f.
P-cell growth f.
plasma coagulation f.
plasma immune f.
plasma labile f.
plasma thromboplastin f.
plasma thromboplastin f. B
plasma f. X
plasmin prothrombin conversion f.
platelet f.
platelet f. 3
platelet-activating f.
platelet-aggregating f.
platelet coagulation f.
platelet-derived growth f.
platelet tissue f.
polymorphonuclear neutrophil chemotactic f.
prognostic f.
prolactin-inhibiting f.
prolactin-releasing f.
proliferation inhibitor f.
properdin f. A
properdin f. B

properdin f. D
prothrombin conversion f.
prothrombokinase f.
Prower f.
pseudosarcomatous f.
R f.
recognition f.
relative risk f.
releasing f.
renal erythropoietic f.
resectability f.
resistance f.
resistance-inducing f.
resistance transfer f.
Rhesus f.
rheumatic f.
rheumatoid f.
rheumatoid arthritis f.
rho f.
ripple f.
risk f.
S f.
sarcoma growth f.
secretor f.
serum prothrombin conversion accelerator f.
Simon's septic f.
skin-reactive f.
somatotropin-releasing f.
SPCA (serum prothrombin conversion accelerator) f.
specific macrophage-arming f.
spreading f.
stable f.
Stuart f.; Stuart-Prower f.
sulfation f.
T f.
T-cell growth f.
T-cell–replacing f.
termination f.
thymic f.
thymic humoral f.
thymic lymphopoietic f.
thymic replacing f.
thymus-replacing f.
thyroid-stimulating hormone–releasing f.
thyrotropin-releasing f.
tissue f.
tissue-coding f.
tissue-damaging f.
trans-acting f.

transfer f.
transforming f.
transforming growth f.
translocation f.
tumor angiogenic f.
tumor necrosis f.
undegraded insulin f.
V f.
Va f.
vitamin K–dependent f.
von Willebrand's f.
W f.
Williams' f.
Wills f.
X f.
Xa f.
f. Xa inhibitor
factorial
facultative
    f. anaerobe
    f. autotroph
    f. bacterium
    f. heterochromatin
    f. organisms
    f. parasite
FAD — flavin adenine dinucleotide
FADF — fluorescent antibody dark-field
Fahey method
Fahr. — Fahrenheit
Fahrenheit
    temperature scale
    thermometer
FAIDS — feline AIDS
failure
    acute renal f.
    f. of all vital forces
    baroreflex f.
    cardiac f.
    chronic renal f.
    circulatory f.
    congestive cardiac f.
    congestive heart f.
    gonadal f.
    heart f.
    left ventricular f.
    peripheral circulatory f.
    pituitary f.
    pituitary gonadotropic f.
    postpartum renal f.
    f. rate
    renal f.
    respiratory f.

fainting
faintness
Fajans-Conn criteria
falciform ligament
falcine meningioma
falciparum
    f. fever
    f. malaria
Falcon assay
falcular
fallopian tube
    f.t. ampulla
    f.t. fimbria
    f.t. infundibulum
    f.t. isthmus
    f.t. lumen
    f.t. lymphatics
    f.t. secretion
    f.t. tumor
Fallopius's aqueduct
Fallot
    tetralogy of F.
false
    f. agglutination
    f. albuminuria
    f. anemia
    f. aneurysm
    f. cast
    f. cyanosis
    f. cyst
    f. dextrocardia
    f. diverticulum
    f. hematuria
    f. hypertrophy
    f. membrane
    f. mole
    f.-negative reaction
    f.-neuroma
    f.-positive reaction
falx (pl., falces)
    f. cerebelli
    f. cerebri
    f. inguinalis
    f. meningioma
familial
    f. amyloid polyneuropathy
    f. benign pemphigus
    f. cancer
    f. carcinoma
    f. cardiomyopathy
    f. cerebellar ataxia
    f. cystinuria

    f. dysalbuminemic hyperthyrox-
       inemia
    f. dysautonomia
    f. dysbetalipoproteinemia
    f. endocrine adenomatosis
    f. erythroblastic anemia
    f. erythrophagocytic lymphohis-
       tiocytosis
    f. fibrous dysplasia
    f. goiter
    f. gonadal dysgenesis
    f. hemolytic anemia
    f. hereditary pancreatitis
    f. hyperalphalipoproteinemia
    f. hyperbetalipoproteinemia
    f. hypercholesterolemia
    f. hyperglucagonemia
    f. hyperlipoproteinemia
    f. hypertriglyceridemia
    f. hypobetalipoproteinemia
    f. hypocalciuric hypercalcemia
    f. hypophosphatemia
    f. hypoplastic anemia
    f. intestinal polyposis
    f. juvenile nephronophthisis–
       medullary cystic disease
       complex
    f. Mediterranean fever
    f. megaloblastic anemia
    f. microcytic anemia
    f. myoclonic epilepsy
    f. nephritis
    f. nephronophthisis
    f. nephrosis
    f. nonhemolytic jaundice
    f. paroxysmal rhabdomyolysis
    f. periodic paralysis
    f. polycythemia
    f. polyposis syndromes
    f. primary systemic amyloidosis
    f. pyridoxine-responsive
       anemia
    f. recessive abetalipopro-
       teinemia
    f. recurrent cholestasis
    f. splenic anemia
    f. testotoxicosis
family
    integrin f.
    systematic f.
FAMMM — familial atypical
        mole–malignant
        melanoma

FAN — fuchsin, amido black, and naphthol yellow
FANA — fluorescent antinuclear antibody (test)
Fañana's cell
Fanconi's
    anemia
    pancytopenia
F and R — force and rhythm (of pulse)
Fannia
    F. canicularis
    F. scalaris
f antigen
farad
faraday
Faraday's
    constant
    effect
    law of electrolysis
faradic shock
Farber's lipogranulomatosis
farcy
farmer's
    f. lung
    f. skin
farnesyl-pyrophosphate synthetase
Farrant's
    medium
    mounting fluid
Farr test
fascia (pl., fasciae)
    antebrachial f.
    axillary f.
    brachial f.
    cervical f.
    clavipectoral f.
    clitoridal f.
    cremasteric f.
    crural f.
    dorsal f.
    Gerota's f.
    f. lata
    masseter f.
    nuchal f.
    f. occludens
    orbit f.
    parotid f.
    pectoral f.
    pelvic f.
    penile f.
    perirenal f.
    renal f.
    superficial f.
    temporal f.
    thoracolumbar f.
    transversalis f.
    urogenital diaphragmatic f.
fasciagram
fasciagraphy
fascial
    f. breast
    f. fibrosarcoma
    f. lymphosarcoma
    f. space
fascicle
fascicular
    f. lymphosarcoma
    f. sarcoma
fasciculate bladder
fasciculation potential
fasciculus (pl., fasciculi)
    f. arcuatus
    f. cingulate
    f. cuneatus
    dorsal proper f.
    frontotemporal f.
    f. gracilis
    inferior fronto-occipital f.
    inferior longitudinal f.
    f. interfascicularis
    lateral proper f.
    lenticular f.
    longitudinal f.
    medial longitudinal f.
    f. of middle cerebellar peduncle (deep, inferior, superior)
    perforating f.
    perpendicular f.
    subthalamic f.
    sulcomarginal f.
    superior fronto-occipital f.
    superior longitudinal f.
    temporo-occipital f.
    thalamic f.
    uncinate f.
    ventral proper f.
    vertical occipital f.
fasciectomy
fasciitis
    cranial f.
    eosinophilic f.
    infiltrative f.
    intravascular f.

necrotizing f.
nodular f.
parosteal f.
proliferative f.
pseudosarcomatous f.
fasciofacial anastomosis
Fasciola
  F. *gigantica*
  F. *hepatica*
fasciolar gyrus
fascioliasis
Fascioloides magna
fasciolopsiasis
Fasciolopsis buski
fascitis
FASEB — Federation of American
      Societies for
      Experimental Biology
fast
  acid f.
  f. channel
  f. green
  f. hemoglobin
  low-voltage f.
  f. smear
  f. twitch
  f. yellow
fastidious
fastigiobulbar projection
fasting blood sugar
fastness
FAT — fluorescent antibody test
fat
  f. absorption
  f. absorption studies
  f. absorption test
  f. assay
  brown f.
  f. cells
  f. depot
  f. embolism
  f. embolus
  fecal f.
  f.-free
  f.-induced hyperlipidemia
  f. necrosis
  f.-soluble vitamins
  f. staining
  subcutaneous f.
  f. tide
  total body f.
  yellow f.

fatal dose
fatality rate
FA (fluorescent antibody) technique
fat-free
  f.-f. dry weight
  f.-f. mass
  f.-f wet weight
fatigue
fat-mobilizing
  f.-m. hormone
  f.-m. substance
fatty
  f. acid assays
  f. ascites
  f. atrophy
  f. cast
  f. cirrhosis
  f. cyst
  f. degeneration
  f. deposition
  f. heart
  f. infiltration
  f. kidney
  f. liver
  f. metamorphosis
  f. nutritional cirrhosis
  f. oil
  f. phanerosis
  f. streaks
  f. tissue
  f. tumor
  f. urinary cast
fatty acid
  f.a. deficiency
  essential f.a.
  free f.a.
  monounsaturated f.a's
  n-3 f.a's
  nonesterified f.a.
  ω-3 f. a.'s; omega-3 f.a's
  ω-6 f. a's; omega-6 f.a's
  f.a. oxidation
  f.a. profile
  saturated f.a's
  f.a. synthesis
  unesterified f.a.
  unsaturated f.a's
fauces (pl. of faux)
faucial
  f. arch
  f. pillar
faucitis

faulty union
faun tail nevus
Faust zinc sulfate flotation procedure
FAV — feline ataxia virus
favid
favism
favosa
     trichomyosis f.
favus
FB — foreign body
FBE — full blood examination
     full body examination
F body
FBP — femoral blood pressure
     fibrinogen breakdown
        products
FBS — fasting blood sugar
     fetal bovine serum
Fc (fragment crystallizable) receptor,
   region
FCA — ferritin-conjugated antibodies
FCC — follicular center cells
F$^+$ cell
FD — fatal dose
     focal distance
     forceps delivery
FD$_{50}$ — median fatal dose
FDA — Food and Drug Adminis-
        tration
     frontodextra anterior
F distribution
FDNB — fluorodinitrobenzene
     fluoro-2,4-dinitrobenzene
F (plasmid) donor
FDP — fibrin degradation product
     fibrin/fibrinogen degradation
        product
     flexor digitorum profundus
     frontodextra posterior
     fructose 1,6-diphosphate
FDS — flexor digitorum superficialis
FDT — frontodextra transversa
F-duction
Fe — iron
feathery degeneration
febrile
     f. agglutination test
     f. agglutinins
     f. albuminuria
     f. antigen
     f. nodular panniculitis

     f. nonhemolytic transfusion re-
        action
     f. urine
FEC — free erythrocyte coropor-
        phyrin
fecal
     f. abscess
     f. fat
     f. fat quantitation
     f. fistula
     f. impaction
     f. incontinence
     f. marker
     f. tumor
     f. urobilinogen
     f. vomitus
fecalith
fecaloma
fecaluria
feces
     extravasation f.
     impacted f.
FECG — fetal electrocardiogram
FECP — free erythrocyte coropor-
        phyria
FECU — Factor VIII correctional
        unit
FECV — functional extracellular fluid
        volume
Federation of American Societies for
   Experimental Biology
feedback
     f. inhibition mutation
     f. loop
FEF — forced expiratory flow
Fehleisen's streptococcus
Fehling's
     solution
     test
FEKG — fetal electrocardiogram
FEL — familial erythrophagocytic
        lymphohistiocytosis
feline ataxia virus
Felix-Weil reaction
felon
Felton phenomenon
FeLV — feline leukemia virus
female
     f. carrier
     f. genital fluids
     f. genitalia
     f. genital spaces

f. genital tract cytologic smear
f. hormones
f. pseudohermaphroditism
f. sex chromatin pattern
f. urethra
feminization
f. syndrome, adrenal
testicular f.
feminizing tumor
Femogen
femoral
f. artery
f. canal
f. circumflex vein
f. cutaneous vein
f. hernia
f. lymph node
f. nerve
f. puncture
f. vein
femorocele
femoroiliac
femoropopliteal occlusive disease
femorotibial
femtoliter
femtocurie
femtometer
femtomole
femur (pl., femora)
FeNa — fractional sodium excretion
fenac
fenestra (pl., fenestrae)
alveolar f.
f. cochleae
f. vestibuli
fenestrated
f. capillaries
f. endothelium
fenestration
atrophic f.
fenfluramine
fennel oil
fenoprofen calcium
fentanyl citrate
Fenton reaction
Fenwick-Hunner ulcer
FEP or FEPP — free erythrocyte proto-
                porphyrin
Ferguson-Smith epithelioma
ferment
fermentation
mannitol f.

mixed acid f.
f. test
fermenter
glucose f's
fermi
fermium
Fernandez reaction
Fernbach flask
ferning
fern test
Ferrata's cell
ferredoxin
Ferribacterium
ferric
f. chloride
f. chloride reaction
f. chloride test
f. ferricyanide reduction test
f. ferrocyanide
f. fructose
f. hydroxide
f. oxide
ferricyanide
ferrous f.
ferriheme
ferrihemoglobin
ferrimagnetic
ferrite
ferritin
cationized f.
f.-coupled antibodies
f.-conjugated antibodies
ferrocalcinosis
ferrocalcinotic deposition
ferrochelatase
ferrocholinate
ferrocyanide
ferric f.
potassium f.
ferroflocculation
ferroheme
ferrohemoglobin
ferrokinetic study
ferromagnetic
ferroprotein
ferrous
f. carbonate
f. chloride
f. citrate
f. citrate Fe 59
f. ferricyanide
f. fumarate

f. gluconate
f. sulfate
ferroxidase
ferrozine
ferruginous
    f. bodies
    f. micelles
fertile eunuch syndrome
fertility
    f. factor
    f. inhibition
fertilization
fervescence
FES — flame emission spectroscopy
    forced expiratory spirogram
fester
festinating gait
festooning
FET — forced expiratory time
fetal
    f. abnormality
    f. adenoma
    f. adrenal cortex
    f. alcohol syndrome
    f. antigen
    f. bovine serum
    f. death
    f. death rate
    f. duplication
    f. electrocardiogram
    f. erythroblastosis
    f. face syndrome
    f. fat cell lipoma
    f. fluids
    f. hematopoiesis
    f. hemoglobin
    f. hemoglobin test
    f. hydantoin syndrome
    f. implantation site
    f. lipoma
    f. lobulation
    f. membrane
    f. pupillary membrane
    f. rhabdomyosarcomatous neph-
      roblastoma
    f. spaces
    f. surface
    f. testis
    f. testosterone
    f. toxoplasmosis
    f. transfusion
    f. trimethadione syndrome

f. urachus
f. urine
f. zone
FETI — fluorescence excitation trans-
    fer immunoassay
fetid rhinitis
fetoglobulin
α-fetoglobulin
fetography
fetoplacental anasarca
fetoprotein
α-fetoprotein
α_1-fetoprotein
β-fetoprotein
γ-fetoprotein
fetor
    f. hepaticus
    f. oris
fetoscopy
fetotoxicity
FETS — forced expiratory time, in
      seconds
fetus
    f. acardiacus
    f. amorphus
    f. compressus
    dead retained f.
    f. in fetu
    harlequin f.
    macerated f.
    f. papyraceus
    parasitic f.
    stunted f.
Feulgen's
    reaction
    stain
    test
FEV — forced expiratory volume
FEV_1 — forced expiratory volume in
      1 second
fever
    abortus f.
    aestivoautumnal f.
    African tick-borne f.
    aphthous f.
    black f.
    blackwater f.
    f. blister
    boutonneuse f.
    breakbone f.
    Bullis f.
    Bwamba f.

cat-bite f.
chikungunya f.
childbed f.
Colorado tick f.
dandy f.
death f.
dengue f.
Dumdum f.
falciparum f.
familial Mediterranean f.
Fort Bragg f.
glandular f.
Haverhill f.
hematuric bilious f.
hemoglobinuric f.
hemorrhagic f.
intermittent malarial f.
jungle f.
Katayama's f.
Lassa f.
malarial f.
malignant tertian f.
Malta f.
Marburg f.
marsh f.
Mediterranean f.
metal fume f.
mountain f.
Murchison-Pel-Ebstein f.
Omsk hemorrhagic f.
O'nyong-nyong f.
Oroya f.
paludal f.
pappataci f.
paratyphoid f.
parrot f.
Pel-Ebstein f.
pharyngoconjunctival f.
phlebotomus f.
Pontiac f.
pyrogenic f.
Q f.
quartan f.
quotidian f.
rabbit f.
rat-bite f.
recrudescent f.
relapsing f.
remittent malarial f.
rheumatic f.
Rift Valley f.
Rocky Mountain spotted f.

sandfly f.
San Joaquin f.; San Joaquin
    Valley f.
scarlet f.
septic f.
South American hemor-
    rhagic f.
spotted f.
swamp f.
syphilitic f.
tertian f.
tick f.
trench f.
tsutsugamushi f.
typhoid f.
typhus f.
f. of undetermined origin
f. of unknown origin
undulant f.
uveoparotid f.
valley f.
vivax f.
West Nile f.
Wolhynia f.
yellow f.
feverish urine
Fevold test
FF — fat free
    fecal frequency
    filtration fraction
FFA — free fatty acid
F factor
FFDW — fat-free dry weight
FFM — fat-free mass
FFP — fresh frozen plasma
FFWW — fat-free wet weight
FG — fibrinogen
FGD — fatal granulomatous disease
FGT (female genital tract) cytologic
    smear
FHR — fetal heart rate
FHS — fetal heart sound
FHT — fetal heart
    fetal heart tones
FI — fever caused by infection
    fibrinogen
    forced inspiration
FIA — fluorescent immunoassay
fib. — fibrillation
    fibrinogen
fiber
    A delta f's

amygdalofugal f's
anterior external arcuate f's
arcuate f's
argyrophilic f's
association f's
association nerve f's
bag f.
cerebellovestibular f's
chain f.
collagenous f's
corticostriate f's
f. density
dorsal external arcuate f's
elastic f's
external arcuate f's
fusimotor f's
geniculostriate f's
internal arcuate f's
intersegmental f's
intrasegmental f's
long arcuate f's
long association f's
macular f's
muscle f's, type I
muscle f's, type II
nigrostriate f's
nuclear bag f.
nuclear chain f.
occipitopontine f's
oxytalan f.
pallidofugal f's
parallel f's
posterior external arcuate f's
Purkinje's f's
ragged red f's
Reissner's f.
retinothalamic projection f's
ring f's
Rosenthal's f's
Sharpey's perforating f's
somatic f's
somatic efferent f's
f. spectrum
striatonigral f's
terminal conducting f's of Purkinje
Tomes' f's
"U" f's
ventral external arcuate f's
visceral f's (afferent, efferent)
wavy f's
fibercolonoscope

fibergastroscope
fiberoptic esophagoscopy
fiberscope
fibremia
fibril
    collagen f's
    fibroglia nerve f.
    muscular f.
fibrillar
    f. astrocyte
    f. collagen
fibrillary
    f. astrocyte
    f. astrocytoma
fibrillated
fibrillation
    atrial f.
    auricular f.
    cardiac f.
    muscular f.
    ventricular f.
fibrin
    f. body
    f. breakdown products
    f. calculus
    f. clots
    f. degradation product
    f. degradation products method
    f.-fibrinogen degradation
        product
    gluten f.
    f. monomer
    myosin f.
    f. plate lysis
    reptilase f.
    f.-stabilizing factor test
    f. staining
    stroma f.
    f. thrombus
    f. titer
    f. titer test
fibrinase
fibrinocellular
fibrinogen
    f. breakdown products
    f. deficiency
    f. I-125
    f. method
    f. split products
    f. test
    f. titer test
fibrinogenase

fibrinogenemia
fibrinogen-fibrin conversion syndrome
fibrinogenic; fibrinogenous
fibrinogenolysis
fibrinogenopenia
fibrinogenous
fibrinoid
    f. degeneration
    f. necrosis
    f. necrotizing inflammation
fibrinokinase
fibrinolamellar
fibrinolysin
    f. coagulation
    seminal f.
    streptococcal f.
fibrinolysis
    primary f.
fibrinolysokinase
fibrinolytic
    f. hemorrhage
    f. inhibitor
    f. purpura
    f. split products
    f. system
fibrinonectin
fibrinopenia
fibrinopeptide A
fibrinopeptide B
fibrinoplastin
fibrinoplatelet
fibrinopurulent inflammation
fibrinoscopy
fibrinous
    f. acute lobar pneumonia
    f. acute pleuritis
    f. adhesion
    f. bronchitis
    f. cast
    f. degeneration
    f. exudation
    f. inflammation
    f. lymph
    f. pericarditis
    f. peritonitis
    f. pleurisy
    f. pleuritis
    f. polyp
fibrinuria
fibroadenia
fibroadenoma
    f. of breast

    giant f.
    intracanalicular f.
    juvenile f.
    pericanalicular f.
fibroadenosis
fibroadipose tissue
fibroameloblastic
    f. dentinoma
    f. odontoma
fibroblast
    chick embryo f.
    f. interferon
    pericryptal f's
fibroblastic
    f. meningioma
    f. osteosarcoma
    f. parietal endocarditis
fibroblastoma
    perineural f.
fibrocalcific nodule
fibrocarcinoma
fibrocartilage
    degenerated intervertebral f.
    intervertebral f.
    f. matrix alteration
fibrocartilaginous annulus
fibrocaseous
    f. inflammation
    f. peritonitis
    f. tuberculosis
fibrocellular
fibrochondritis
fibrochondroma
fibrocongestive
    f. hypertrophy
    f. splenomegaly
fibrocyst
fibrocystic
    f. disease of breast
    f. mastitis
    f. mastopathy
fibrocystoma
fibrocyte
fibrocytogenesis
fibrodysplasia ossificans progressiva
fibroelastic
    f. cartilage
    f. hyperplasia
    f. membrane
fibroelastoma
    papillary f.

fibroelastosis
    endocardial f.
    endomyocardial f.
fibroenchondroma
fibroepithelial
    f. interferon
    f. papilloma
    f. polyp
fibroepithelioma
    Pinkus' f.
    premalignant f.
fibrofolliculoma
fibrogenesis imperfecta ossium
fibroglioma
fibrohistiocytic tumor
fibrohistiocytoma
fibroid
    f. adenoma
    f. inflammation
    f. lung
    f. tumor
    f. uterus
fibroidectomy
fibroin
fibrokeratoma
fibrolamellar
    f. hepatocellular carcinoma
    f. hepatoma
fibroleiomyoma
fibrolipoma
fibrolipomatous
fibroliposarcoma
fibrolytic inhibitor
fibroma
    acanthomatous ameloblastic f.
    ameloblastic f.
    aponeurotic f.
    f. cavernosum
    cementifying f.
    cemento-ossifying f.
    chondromyxoid f.
    concentric f.
    cordal f.
    f. cutis
    cystic f.
    desmoplastic f.
    f. durum
    giant cell f.
    intracanalicular f.
    intracellular f.
    irritation f.
    juvenile active ossifying f.

    juvenile nasopharyngeal f.
    medullary f.
    f. molle
    f. molle gravidarum
    f. mucinosum
    myxoid f.
    f. myxomatodes
    nasopharyngeal f.
    nonossifying f.
    nonosteogenic f.
    odontogenic f.
    ossifying f.
    osteogenic f.
    parasitic f.
    paratesticular f.
    periosteal f.
    peripheral odontogenic f.
    periungual f.
    pleural f.
    rabbit f.
    recurring digital f's
    renal medullary f.
    f. sarcomatosum
    senile f.
    Shope f.
    subungual f.
    telangiectatic f.
    f. thecocellulare xantho-
      matodes
    f. xanthoma
fibromatogenic
fibromatoid
fibromatosis
    abdominal f.
    aggressive infantile f.
    f. colli
    congenital generalized f.
    desmoid f.
    Dupuytren's f.
    infantile digital f.
    juvenile aponeurotic f.
    juvenile hyalin f.
    juvenile palmoplantar f.
    musculoaponeurotic f.
    palmar f.
    penile f.
    plantar f.
    pseudosarcomatous f.
    retroperitoneal f.
    subcutaneous pseudosarco-
      matous f.
fibromatous

fibromectomy
fibromembranous
fibromuscular
    f. dysplasia
    f. hyperplasia
fibromyalgia
fibromyomatous hamartoma
fibromyoma uteri
fibromyomectomy
fibromyositis
    nodular f.
fibromyxoid tumor
fibromyxolipoma
fibromyxoma
fibromyxosarcoma
fibronectin
    plasma f.
fibroneuroma
fibronuclear
fibro-odontoma
    ameloblastic f.
fibro-osseous
fibro-osteoma
fibropapilloma
fibroplasia
    retrolental f.
fibroplastic
    f. osteosarcoma
    f. parietal endocarditis
fibropolypus
fibropurulent
fibrosa
    periosteitis f.
fibrosarcoma
    ameloblastic f.
    chordal f.
    Earle L f.
    fascial f.
    infantile f.
    laryngeal f.
    medullary f.
    odontogenic f.
    paratesticular f.
    perineural f.
    periosteal f.
    pharyngeal f.
fibrosarcomaneuroblastoma
fibrosclerosis
    multifocal f.
fibrose
fibroserous
fibrosiderotic nodule

fibrosing
    f. adenomatosis
    f. adenosis
    f. alveolitis
fibrosis
    condensation f.
    congenital hepatic f.
    cortical stroma f.
    cystic f.
    diffuse f.
    diffuse interstitial f.
    endomyocardial f.
    focal f.
    hepatic f.
    idiopathic pulmonary f.
    idiopathic retroperitoneal f.
    interstitial f.
    liver f.
    mediastinal f.
    multifocal f.
    neoplastic f.
    nodular f.
    nodular subepidermal f.
    pericentral f.
    perimuscular f.
    pipestem f.
    progressive massive f.
    proliferative f.
    pulmonary f.
    replacement f.
    retroperitoneal f.
    septal f.
    subadventitial f.
    subepidermal f.
    Symmers' clay pipestem f.;
        Symmers' f.
fibrositis
fibrothecoma
fibrothorax
fibrotic inflammation
fibrous
    f. adhesion
    f. ankylosis
    f. astrocyte
    f. astrocytoma
    f. body
    f. cavernitis
    f. cortical defect
    f. degeneration
    f. dysplasia
    f. dysplasia of bone
    f. familial dysplasia

f. goiter
f. hamartoma of infancy
f. histiocytoma
f. hypertrophic pachymeningitis
f. joint
f. layer
f. long-spacing collagen
f. meningioma
f. mesothelioma
f. monostotic dysplasia
f. nodule
f. nuclear lamina
f. obliteration
f. osteoma
f. polyp
f. proteins
f. pseudotumor
f. replacement
f. tendon sheath
f. thyroiditis
f. tissue
f. tubercle
f. union
f. xanthoma
fibrovascular
fibroxanthoma
atypical f.
fibroxanthosarcoma
fibula
fibular
Fichera's treatment
ficin
Fick's
bacillus
equation
law
principle
Ficoll-Hypaque
separation
technique
FID — flame ionization detector
Fiedler's myocarditis
field
depth of f.
f. effect transistor
eye f., frontal, occipital
high-power f.
low-power f.
low-voltage f.
magnetic f.
f. method

f. of microscope
oil immersion f.
red blood cells per high-
power f.
f. of view
white blood cells per high-
power f.
Field's rapid stain
FIF — forced inspiratory flow
fifth
f. cranial nerve
"f. disease" virus
f. metacarpal
f. metatarsal
FIGE — field inversion gel electrophoresis
FIGLU — formiminoglutamic acid
FIGLU (formiminoglutamic acid) test
FIGO — International Federation of
Gynecology and Obstetrics
FIGO classification of staging
figure
flame f.
mitotic f.
myelin f's
fig wart
filament
actin f.
desmin f's
dural terminal f.
external terminal f.
giant f's
glial f's
intermediate f's
internal terminal f.
keratin f's
lymphatic anchoring f's
muscle f.
myosin f.
f.-nonfilament count
pial terminal f.
polar injecting f.
prekeratin f's
filamented
f. neutrophil
f. polymorphonuclear leu-
kocyte
filamentous
f. fungus
f. mass
f. substance
filamin

Filaria
  F. *bancrofti*
  F. *conjunctivae*
  F. *demarquayi*
  F. *hominis oris*
  F. *juncea*
  F. *labialis*
  F. *lentis*
  F. *loa*
  F. *lymphatica*
  F. *medinensis*
  F. *ozzardi*
  F. *palpebralis*
  F. *philippinensis*
  F. *sanguinis*
  F. *tucumana*
  F. *volvulus*
filaria (pl., filariae)
filarial
  f. arthritis
  f. funiculitis
  f. infection
filariasis
  bancroftian f.
  Bancroft's f.
  Brug's f.
  chronic f.
  Malayan f.
  occult f.
  onchocerciasis-type f.
  Ozzard's f.
  persistent f.
  f. serological test
  zoonotic f.
filaricide
filariform larvae
Filarioidea
file
  periodontal f.
filiform
  f. hyperkeratosis
  f. papillae
  f. wart
filix mas
filling
  f. defect
  f. gallop
  f. rumble
film
  f. density calibration
  fixed blood f.
  gelatin f.

spot f.
f.-stripping autoradi-
    ography
sulfa f.
x-ray f.
Filobasidiella
  F. *bacillisporus*
  F. *neoformans*
filter
  bacterial f.
  barrier f.
  Berkefeld f.
  blocking f.
  f. capacitor
  Centriflo f.
  Chamberland f.
  collodion f.
  exciter f.
  gelatin f.
  Gelman f.
  glass fiber f.
  HEPA (high-efficiency particu-
      late air) f.
  heparin-treated f.
  high-pass f.
  f. hybridization
  inherent f.
  interference f.
  line f.
  low-pass f.
  membrane f.
  microaggregate f.
  Millipore f.
  Nucleopore f.
  f. paper microscopic test
  f. photometer
  Seitz f.
  Selas f.
  Wratten f.
filterable virus
filtering
filtrate
  tuberculin f.
filtration
  f. barrier
  f. fraction
  gel f.
  glomerular f.
  f. slits
filum terminale (pl., fila terminalia)
  f.t. externum
  f.t. internum

fimbria
>   hippocampal f.
fimbriated
fimbrin
fimbriodentate sulcus
fine-needle biopsy
fine structure
finger
>   clubbed f.
>   dead f's
>   drumstick f's
>   hippocratic f's
>   mallet f.
>   rudimentary f.
>   sausage f's
>   spade f's
>   waxy f's
>   webbed f's
>   zinc f.
"fingeroma"
fingerprint
>   DNA f.
fingerprinting
>   DNA f.
finite
Fink-Heimer stain
Finn chamber test
Finney's gastroenterostomy
Finsen's
>   bath
>   lamp
fire
>   f. ant
>   Saint Anthony's f.
first
>   f. arch syndrome
>   f. branchial arch
>   f. cranial nerve
>   f.-degree burn
>   f.-degree frostbite
>   f.-degree heart block
>   f.-degree radiation injury
>   f. division, fifth cranial nerve
>   f. division, trigeminal nerve
>   f. filial generation
>   f. metacarpal
>   f. metatarsal
>   f.-order reaction
>   f. pharyngeal pouch
>   f.-set graft rejection
>   f. trimester pregnancy
Fischer projection formula

fish
>   f.-mouth stenosis
>   f. skin
>   f. tapeworm
>   f. tapeworm anemia
Fishberg's concentration test
Fisher autocytometer
Fisher-Race
>   system
>   theory
Fisher's
>   exact test
>   procedure
Fishman-Lerner unit
fission
>   binary f.
>   f. fungus
>   multiple f.
>   f. product
fissural
>   f. angioma
>   f. cyst
fissure
>   f. in ano
>   ansaparamedian f.
>   calcarine f.
>   centrolingual f.
>   cerebellar f.
>   hippocampal f.
>   horizontal f.
>   inferior orbital f.
>   interhemispheric f.
>   interlobar f.
>   intrabiventral f.
>   intraculminate f.
>   intrapyramidal f.
>   lateral cerebral f.
>   longitudinal cerebral f.
>   parieto-occipital f.
>   postcentral f.
>   posterolateral f.
>   postlingual f.
>   postlunate f.
>   postnodular f.
>   prebiventral f.
>   precentral f.
>   preculminate f.
>   prepyramidal f.
>   primary f.
>   Rolando's f.
>   Santorini's f.
>   secondary f.

superior posterior f.
f. of Sylvius
ventral medial f.
ventral median f.
fissured nucleus
fisting
fistula (pl., fistulae; fistulas)
  abdominal f.
  amphibolic f.; amphibolous f.
  anal f.
  f. in ano
  arteriovenous f.
  biliary f.
  f. bimucosa
  blind f.
  branchial f.
  bronchoesophageal f.
  bronchopleural f.
  carotid-cavernous f.
  cervical f.
  cholecystoduodenal f.
  chylous f.
  coccygeal f.
  colocutaneous f.
  coloileal f.
  colonic f.
  colovaginal f.
  colovesical f.
  complete f.
  cutaneous f.
  duodenal f.
  enterocutaneous f.
  enterovaginal f.
  enterovesical f.
  external f.
  fecal f.
  gastric f.
  gastrocolic f.
  gastrocutaneous f.
  gastroduodenal f.
  gastrointestinal f.
  genitourinary f.
  hepatic f.
  hepatopleural f.
  horseshoe f.
  incomplete f.
  inflammatory f.
  internal f.
  lacteal f.
  laryngoesophageal f.
  mammary f.
  metroperitoneal f.

  parietal f.
  perineovaginal f.
  pharyngocutaneous f.
  pilonidal f.
  pulmonary f.
  pulmonary arteriovenous f.
  rectolabial f.
  rectourethral f.
  rectovaginal f.
  rectovesical f.
  rectovestibular f.
  rectovulvar f.
  salivary f.
  sigmoidovesical f.
  spermatic f.
  stercoral f.
  thoracic f.
  thoracic duct f.
  thyroglossal f.
  tracheobiliary f.
  tracheoesophageal f.
  umbilical f.
  urachal f.
  urachal-vesical f.
  ureteral vasocutaneous f.
  ureterocutaneous f.
  ureterovaginal f.
  urethrovaginal f.
  urinary f.
  urogenital f.
  uteroperitoneal f.
  vasocutaneous f.
  vesical f.
  vesicocolic f.
  vesicocutaneous f.
  vesicointestinal f.
  vesicoumbilical f.
  vesicouterine f.
  vesicovaginal f.
  vesicovaginorectal f.
fistulation; fistulization
fistulous
fit
  running f.
FITC — fluorescein isothiocyanate
Fite's method
fitness
"fitter" cell theory
fitting
  curve f.
Fitzgerald factor
Fitzgerald-Williams-Flaujeac factor

FIV₁ — forced inspiratory volume in
        1 second
fixation
    alcohol f.
    f. artifact
    autotrophic f.
    carbon dioxide f.
    complement f.
    nitrogen f.
    secondary f.
fixative
    acetone f.
    aldehyde f's
    Altmann's f.
    Bouin's f.
    Bouin's picroformol-acetic f.
    Brasil's f.
    Carnoy's f.
    Champy's f.
    coating f.
    Flemming's f.
    formaldehyde f.
    formol-calcium f.
    formol-Müller f.
    formol-saline f.
    formol-Zenker f.
    glutaraldehyde f.
    Golgi's osmiobichromate f.
    Heidenhain's Susa f.
    Helly's f.
    Hermann's f.
    Kaiserling's f.
    lead f's
    Luft's potassium permanga-
      nate f.
    Marchi's f.
    Maximow's f.
    mercuric f.
    methanol f.
    Müller's f.
    neutral buffered formalin f.
    Newcomer's f.
    Orth's f.
    osmic acid f.
    Park-Williams f.
    picroformol f.
    Regaud's f.
    Saccomanno's f.
    Thomas's f.
    Zenker-formol f.
    Zenker's f.

fixed
    f. blood film
    f. oil
    f.-point variable
    f. sediment method
    f. virus
FJN — familial juvenile nephro-
      nophthisis
FJN-MCD — familial juvenile
      nephronophthisis–
      medullary
      cystic disease
fl. — femtoliter
    fluid
FLA — left frontoanterior
flaccid
flaccidity
flagella
flagellar antigen
Flagellata
flagellate
    f. dysentery
    intestinal f's
flagellin
flagellum (pl., flagella)
    sperm f.
"flag sign"
Flagyl
flail limb
flame
    f. background
    capillary f's
    f. cell
    f. emission spectrophotometry
    f. emission spectroscopy
    f. figure
    f. intensity zones
    f. ionization detector
    manometric f.
    f. nevus
    f. photometer
    f. photometry
flammability
flammable
flank mass
flap
    Abbé-Estlander f.
    Bakamjian deltopectoral f.
    bicoronal f.
    bilobed f.
    bipedicle f.
    buccal cheek f.

cervical f.
coronal f.
deltopectoral f.
Estlander f.
forehead f.
galeal perichondrial f.
galeal pericranial f.
Gillies's f.
Karapandzic f.
latissimus dorsi muscle f.
mucoperiosteal f.
myocutaneous f.
nasolabial f.
osteomucoperiosteal f.
palatal f.
pectoralis major myocutaneous f.
platysma musculocutaneous f.
rotation f.
septal mucoperichondrial f.
sternocleidomastoid musculocutaneous f.
sternohyoid f.
transverse rectus abdominis muscle f.
transverse rectus abdominis myocutaneous f.
trapezius musculocutaneous f.
trapezius myocutaneous f.
trapezius osteomusculocutaneous spinal f.
visor f.
Wookey skin f.

flashcard
flash-point temperature
flask
f. culture
Dewar's f.
Erlenmeyer's f.
Fernbach's f.
Florence's f.
vacuum f.
volumetric f.
flat
f. condyloma
f.-field objective
f. substrate method
f. wart
flatulence
flatus
flatworm
Flaujeac factor

flaval ligament
flavianic acid
flavin
f.-adenine dinucleotide
f. mononucleotide
f. mono-oxygenase
flavivirus
Flavobacterium meningosepticum
flavoenzyme
flavoprotein
flaxseed oil
fld. — fluid
fl.dr. — fluid dram
flea
American rat f.
f.-bitten kidney
dog f.
European rat f.
human f.
Indian rat f.
flecainide
Flechsig's tract
fleckmilz
Fleitmann's test
Flemming's
fixative
triple stain
flesh
proud f.
fleshy
f. mole
f. polyp
Fletcher's
factor
medium
fleurette
flexible
flexion
Flexner's
bacillus
dysentery
Flexner-Strong bacillus
Flexner-Wintersteiner rosette
flexor
f. carpi radialis muscle
f. carpi ulnaris muscle
f. digiti minimi brevis muscle
f. digitorum longus muscle
f. digitorum muscle
f. digitorum pedis longus muscle
f. hallucis brevis muscle

f. hallucis longus muscle
f. plantar reflex
f. pollicis brevis muscle
f. pollicis longus muscle

flexure; flexura
hepatic f.
left colic f.
right colic f.
splenic f.

flint glass

floating
"f. beta" lipoprotein
f. organ
f.-point variable

floc. — flocculation
floccose
flocculable
floccular degeneration
flocculate
flocculation
cephalin f.
cephalin-cholesterol f.
limit f.
Ramon f.
f. reaction
f. test
thymol f.

floccule
toxoid-antitoxin f.

flocculence
flocculent
flocculonodular lobe
flocculoreaction
flocculus (pl., flocculi)

floppy
f. infant
f. valve syndrome

flora
intestinal f.

florantyrone

Florence
flask
test

Florence's crystals
Florentine iris
Florey unit
florid oral papillomatosis
Florisil

flotation
f. bath
centrifugal f.
direct centrifugal f.

f. rate
f. techniques

flow
abnormal f.
f. birefringence
blood f.
cerebral blood f.
f. chart
coronary blood f.
f. cytometry
f. cytophotometry
effective renal blood f.
effective renal plasma f.
estimated hepatic blood f.
exercise hyperemia blood f.
gene f.
hepatic blood f.
high f.
f. meter
pulmonary blood f.
f. rate
reactive hyperemia blood f.
renal plasma f.
splanchnic blood f.
uterine blood f.
f.-volume curve

flowing hyperostosis

flowmeter
electromagnetic f.

floxuridine
fl.oz. — fluid ounce
FLP — left frontoposterior
FLS — fibrous long-spacing (collagen)
FLSA — follicular lymphosarcoma
FLT — left frontotransverse
flu — influenza
fluctuation
flucytosine
fludarabine monophosphate
fludorex
fludrocortisone

fluid
f. alteration
amniotic f.
ascitic f.
f. balance
f. balance and homeostasis
Bensley's osmic dichromate f.
body f's
Bouin's f.
Callison's f.
cerebrospinal f.
Ciaccio's f.

Clarke's f.
cutaneous f.
De Castro's f.
dentinal f.
epididymal f.
extracellular f.
Farrant's mounting f.
female genital f.
fetal f.
gastric f.
Gendre's f.
Helly's f.
interstitial f.
intracellular f.
joint f.
left pleural f.
male genital f.
mammary f.
menstrual f.
f. mosaic model
Orth's f.
pancreatic f.
pericardial f.
peritoneal f.
Pitfield's f.
placental f.
pleural f.
Reese-Ecker f.
respiratory tract f.
f. retention
seminal f.
seminal vesicle f.
serous f.
spinal f.
subretinal f.
synovial f.
f. thioglycollate
tubular f.
urinary tract f.
ventricular f.
f. volume
Zenker's f.

fluke

blood f.
cat liver f.
Chinese liver f.
giant intestinal f.
giant liver f.
intestinal f's
lancet f.
liver f.
lung f.

Manson's blood f.
oriental blood f.
oriental lung f.
sheep liver f.
vesical blood f.
Yokogawa's f.
flumethiazide
fluocinolone
fluoracetate
fluor albus
fluorescein
f. isothiocyanate
f. mercuric acetate
f. sodium
fluorescence
f.-activated cell sorter
f. correlation immunoassay
f. enhancement
f. excitation transfer immunoassay
f. immunoassay
f. microscopy
f. polarization immunoassay
f. protection immunoassay
f. quenching
relative f.
resonance f.
f. spectrum
fluorescent
f. antibody
f. antibody darkfield
f. antibody technique
f. antibody test
f. antinuclear antibody
f. antinuclear antibody test
f.-auramine-rhodamine stain
f. dye
f. immunoassay
f. material
f. microscope
f. rays
f. spot test
f. stain
f. staining
f. treponemal antibody
f. treponemal antibody–absorption test
fluorescin
fluoride
hydrogen f.
magnesium f.
f. number

fluorine
fluorite objective
fluoroacetamide
fluoroacetate
    f. assay
    sodium f.
fluoroacetic fluid
fluorocarbon assay
fluorochrome stain
fluorochroming
fluorocortisone test
fluorocyte
5-fluorocytosine
fluorodeoxyuridine
fluorodinitrobenzene
1-fluoro-2,4-dinitrobenzene
fluorography
fluoroimmunoassay
    time-resolved f.
fluoroimmunometric method
fluorometer
fluorometholone
fluorometry
fluoroscope
fluoroscopy
    biplane f.
fluorosilicate
    sodium f.
fluorosis
    dental f.
    endemic f.
fluorouracil
fluosilicate salt
Fluosol
fluoxetine
fluoxymesterone
fluphenazine
    f. enanthate
    f. hydrochloride
fluprednisolone
flurandrenolone
flurazepam hydrochloride
flurocitabine
flush
    carcinoid f.
flutamide
flutter
    atrial f.
    ventricular f.
flux
    luminous f.
    magnetic f.

fly
    black f.
    bluebottle f.
    bot f.
    deer f.
    fruit f.
    horse f.
    house f.
    larva f.
    stable f.
    tsetse f.
    warble f.
FM — flowmeter
Fm — fermium
fm — femtometer
FMF — familial Mediterranean fever
FMN — flavin mononucleotide
fmol — femtomole
FMS — fat-mobilizing substance
fms oncogene
FN — false-negative
FNTC — fine-needle transhepatic
        cholangiography
FO — foramen ovale
    fronto-occipital
foam
    f. cell
    f. stability test
FOAVF — failure of all vital forces
focal
    f. amyloidosis
    f. appendicitis
    f. atrophy
    f. bronchopneumonia
    f. calcification
    f. cortical epilepsy
    f. dermal hypoplasia
    f. dermal hypoplasia syndrome
    f. distance
    f. embolic glomerulonephritis
    f. epilepsy
    f. fibrosis
    f.-film distance
    f. glomerulonephritis
    f. granulomatous inflammation
    f. hyperplasia
    f. hypertrophy
    f. infarct
    f. infection
    f. length
    f. lymphocytic thyroiditis
    f. necrosis

f. necrotizing glomerulonephritis
f. nephritis
f. nodular hyperplasia
f. plane
f. plane tomography
f. pneumonia
f. proliferative glomerulonephritis
f. sclerosing glomerulopathy
f. sclerosing osteomyelitis
f. segmental glomerulosclerosis
f. ulcer
f. zone
focus (pl., foci)
conjugate f.
depth of f.
ectopic f.
Ghon's f.
linear f.
low-voltage f.
principal f.
Simon's f.
focused grid
focusing
isoelectric f.
fodrin
foil
air f.
folacin
folate
f. deficiency
f. deficiency anemia
f. polyglutamate
red cell f.
f. reductase
whole-blood f.
fold
aryepiglottic f.
circular f. of intestine
epicanthal f.; epicanthine f.
giant gastric f's
ileocecal f.
labioscrotal f.
urethral f's
urogenital f's
folded
f. cell
f.-cell index
f.-lung syndrome
f. nucleus
foliate papillae

folic
f. acid
f. acid analog
f. acid anemia
f. acid deficiency
Folin-Ciocalteu reagent
folinic acid
Folin-Looney test
Folin's test
Folin-Wu (method)
folium (pl., folia)
f. cerebelli
follicle
atretic f.
cyst f.
cystic ovarian f.
graafian f.
hair f.
f. hormone
lenticular f's
lymphatic f.
lymphoid f.
malpighian f.
mature ovarian f.
f. mite
nabothian f.
ovarian f.
splenic lymphatic f.
f.-stimulating hormone assay
f.-stimulating hormone–releasing hormone
thyroid f.
follicular
f. abscess
f. adenocarcinoma
f. adenoma
f. ameloblastoma
f. and papillary adenocarcinoma
f. atresia
f. bronchiectasis
f. carcinoma
f. cells
f. center
f. center cells
f. cervicitis
f. cholecystitis
f. cleaved cell lymphoma
f. conjunctivitis
f. cyst
f. cystitis
f. dermatitis

f. gastritis
f. gland
f. goiter
f. hyperkeratosis
f. hyperplasia
f. inflammation
f. infundibulum tumor
f. keratosis, inverted
f. lymphoma
f. lymphosarcoma
f. mixed small cleaved and
    large cell lymphoma
f. mucinosis
f. nodule
f. pharyngitis
f. predominantly large cell
    lymphoma
f. predominantly small cleaved
    cell lymphoma
f. salpingitis
f. ulcer
f. urethritis

follicularis
keratosis f.
ureteritis f.

folliculitis
f. abscedens et suffodiens
f. decalvans
granulomatous f.
f. keloidalis
multifocal f.
f. ulerythematosa reticulata

folliculoma lipidique
folliculosis
folliculostatin
folliculus (pl., folliculi)
fomite
Fonio's solution
Fonsecaea
F. *compactum*
F. *dermatitidis*
F. *jeanselmei*
F. *pedrosoi*
Fontana-Masson staining method
Fontana's
space
stain
fontanelle; fontanel
food
f. deprivation
f. intolerance
f. poisoning

Food and Drug Administration
foodball
foot
f.-and-mouth disease virus,
    types A, B, C
athlete's f.
end-f.
Madura f.
Morand's f.
mossy f.
pericapillary end-f.
f. process
sandal f.
trench f.
footprinting
Foot's
reticulin impregnation stain
reticulin method
foramen (pl., foramina)
Bochdalek's f.
cecum f.
interventricular f.
intervertebral f.
jugular f.
f. lacerum
Luschka's f.
Magendie's f.
f. magnum
Monro f.
obturator f.
optic f.
f. ovale
patent f. ovale
primary interventricular f.
f. primum
f. rotundum
f. spinosum
f. spongiosum
stylomastoid f.
f. venae cavae
Winslow's epiploic f.
zygomaticofacial f.
zygomaticotemporal f.
force
centrifugal f.
centripetal f.
electromotive f.
relative centrifugal f.
van der Waals f's
forced
f. expiratory flow
f. expiratory spirogram

f. expiratory volume
f. inspiration in 1 second
f. vital capacity
forceps
Fordyce's
    angiokeratoma
    granules
    spots
forearm
forefinger
foregut
forehead
    olympian f.
foreign
    f. body
    f. body aspiration
    f. body embolus
    f. body giant cell
    f. body granuloma
    f. body reaction
    f. body salpingitis
    f. body tumorigenesis
    f. material deposition
Forel's commissure
forensic
    f. medicine
    f. testing
    f. toxicology
foreskin
forespore
forest yaws
fork
    replication f.
form
    appliqué f.
    band f.
    f. birefringence
    cell wall–deficient bacterial f's
    involution f.
    spore f.
Formad's kidney
formaldehyde
    f. dehydrogenase
    f. fixative
    f.-induced fluorescence method
    f. solution
formalin
    alcoholic f.
    f. ammonium bromide
    B-5 sodium acetate-sublimate f.
    buffered neutral f.
    calcium acetate f.

f. cystitis
f.-ether sedimentation method
f.–ethyl acetate procedure
f. pigment
sodium acetate f.
f.–zinc sulfate flotation pro-
    cedure
formamidase
formamide
formamidoxin
format
formate
    f. dehydrogenase
    methyl f.
formation
    antigenic antibody lattice f.
    bleb f.
    ketone body f.
    localized plaque f.
    mesencephalic reticular f.
    rouleaux f.
    standard enthalpy of f.
    syncytium f.
formazan test
forme
    f. fruste (pl., formes frustes)
    f. tardive
formic
    f. acid
    f. aldehyde
formication
N-formiminoglutamic acid
S-formiminotetrahydrofolate cyclo-
    deaminase
formiminotransferase deficiency
formol (formaldehyde solution)
    f. ammonium bromide solution
    f.-calcium fixative
    f.-gel test
    f.-Müller fixative
    f.-saline fixative
    f.-Zenker fixative
formula (pl., formulae; formulas)
    Arneth's f.
    Christison's f.
    Dreser's f.
    Fischer's projection f.
    Häser's f.
    Haworth f.
    Long's f.
    Ranke's f.
    Reuss's f.

Runeberg's f.
f. translation
Trapp's f.
Van Slyke's f.
formulary
formulation
    working f. of National Cancer
      Institute
    working f. of non-Hodgkin's
      lymphomas for clinical usage
N_5-formyl FH_4
formylkynurenine
formyl-leurosine
N-formyl methionine
formyl-methionyl-leucyl-phenylalanine
formyltetrahydrofolate
    f. deformylase
    f. synthetase
formyltransferase
fornix (pl., fornices)
    f. of cerebrum
    conjunctival f.
    lateral f.
    f. of vagina
Forssman
    antibody
    antigen
Fort Bragg fever
FORTRAN — formula translation
forward
    f. bias
    f. mutation
foscarnet
fosfomycin
Foshay test
fossa (pl., fossae)
    anterior f.
    cranial f.
    cubital f.
    ischiorectal f.
    lacrimal f.
    middle f.
    nasal f.
    oval f. of heart
    pituitary f.
    posterior f.
    pterygoid f.
    pyriform f.
    rhomboid f.
    Rosenmüller's f.
    subhepatic f.
    subphrenic f.

temporal f.
tonsillar f.
Treitz's f.
Fouchet's
    reagent
    stain
    test
founder effect
fourchette
Fourier analysis
Fourneau 309
Fournier's gangrene
fourth
    f. branchial arch
    f. cranial nerve
    f. cranial nerve nucleus
    f.-degree burn
    f.-degree frostbite
    f.-degree radiation injury
    f. metacarpal
    f. metatarsal
    f. metatarsophalangeal joint
    f. pharyngeal pouch
    f. ventricle
fovea centralis
foveate
foveated chest
foveola (pl., foveolae)
Fowler's solution
FP — false-positive
    freezing point
    frontoparietal
    frozen plasma
FPA — fluorophenylalanine
FPC — fish protein concentrate
FPIA — fluorescence polarization im-
      munoassay
F pilus (pl., pili)
F plasmid
FPM — filter paper microscopic (test)
FPN reagent
FR — Fisher-Race (notation)
    flocculation reaction
    flow rate
Fr — francium
    French (catheter gauge)
fract. — fracture
fraction
    amorphous f. of adrenal cortex
    blood plasma f's
    branching f.
    etiologic f.

extraction f.
filtration f.
freeze f.
growth f.
heparin-precipitable f.
mole f.
plasma protein f.
saponifiable f.
fractional
    f. distillation
    f. sodium excretion
    f. uptake of carbon monoxide
    f. urinalysis
fractionated alkaline phosphatase
fractionation
fractography
fracture
    chip f.
    closed f.
    comminuted f.
    compound f.
    compound comminuted f.
    compound multiple f's
    compressed f.
    depressed f.
    f.-dislocation
    greenstick f.
    impacted f.
    incomplete f.
    linear f.
    milkman's f.
    nonunion f.
    oblique f.
    pathologic f.
    simple f.
    spiral f.
    stellate f.
    transverse f.
    ununited f.
frag. — fragility
fragellin
fragile X syndrome
fragilitas
    f. ossium
    f. sanguinis
fragility
    f. of blood
    capillary f.
    erythrocyte f.
    mechanical f.
    osmotic f.

    red cell f.
    f. test
fragilograph
fragilocyte
fragilocytosis
fragment
    FAB (fragment, antigen-binding) f's
    F(ab)$_2$ f.
    Fc f.
    Klenow's f.
    restriction f.
    retained placental f.
    Spengler's f.
    urinary gonadotropin f.
fragmentation
    f. myocarditis
    f. of myocardium
fragmented erythrocyte
fragmentography
    mass f.
frambesia
frame
    reading f.
frameshift mutation
framework
    f. region
    scleral f.
    uveal f.
Francis's skin test
Francisella
    F. (Pasteurella) tularensis
    F. tularensis
francium
Frank-Starling
    curve
    mechanism
    relation
Fraser-Lendrum stain for fibrin
fraternal twins
FRC — frozen red cells
    functional reserve capacity
    functional residual capacity
freckle
    Hutchinson's melanotic f.
    melanotic f.
Freda test
Fredrickson's
    dyslipoproteinemia classification
    phenotype

free
  f. acid
  f. catecholamine fractionation
  f. electron
  f. energy
  f. erythrocyte coproporphyria
  f. erythrocyte coproporphyrin
  f. erythrocyte porphyrin
  f. erythrocyte protoporphyrin
  f. estriol
  fat f.
  f. fatty acids
  f. radicals
  f. thyroxine index
  f. T_4 ratio
  f. triiodothyronine index
  f. (unbound) thyroxine
  f. water clearance
freedom
  degrees of f.
freeze
  f.-clamp
  f.-cleave method
  f.-drying
  f.-etch method
  f.-fracture
  f.-fracture-etch method
  f.-substitution
freezing
  f. injury
  f. microtome
  f. point
  f. point depression osmometer
Frei-Hoffman reaction
Frei's
  antigen
  test
French, American, British Leukemia
  Classification
frenulum (pl., frenula)
  f. clitoridis
  f. labii inferioris
  f. labii superioris
  f. linguae
frequency
  f. counter
  critical flicker f.
  critical fusion f.
  crossover f.
  cutoff f.
  discharge f.
  f. distribution

  gene f.
  high f.
  mean dominant f.
  medium f.
  f. polygon
  recombination f.
  relative f.
  urinary f.
Frerich's theory
Fresnel
  fringe
  zone plate
Freund's
  adjuvant
  anomaly
  incomplete adjuvant
  reaction
friability
friable
friction
  pericardial f. rub
  pleural f. rub
Friedländer's
  bacillus
  pneumobacillus
  pneumonia
  stain for capsules
Friedman's test
Friedreich's ataxia
frigidity
frigorism
fringe
  Fresnel f.
Frisch bacillus
frog test
Fröhlich's dwarfism
Frohn's reagent
frons cranii
frontal
  f. bone
  f. electrophoresis
  f. gyrus
  f. horn, lateral ventricle
  f. lobe
  f. nerve
  f. pole
  f. process
  f. region, subdural space
  f. sinus
  f. sulcus
  f. suture
frontalis

front-end processor
frontoethmoid sinus
frontomalar
frontomarginal sulcus
frontomaxillary
frontonasal
fronto-occipital fasciculus
frontoparietal operculum
frontopolar
frontopontine
frontotemporal fasciculus
frontothalamic
Froriep's induration
frostbite
      fourth-degree f.
      second-degree f.
      third-degree f.
frosted
      f. heart
      f. liver
frozen
      f. blood
      f. pelvis
      f. plasma
      f. red blood cells
      f. red cells
      f. section
      f. section method
FRP — functional refractory period
FRS — furosemide
fructan
fructofuranose
β-fructofuranosidase
fructokinase
fructopyranose
fructosamine
fructose
      f. aldolase
      f. biphosphate aldolase
      f.-1,6-diphosphatase
      f.-1,6-diphosphate aldolase
      ferric f.
      f. intolerance test
      f. 1-phosphate aldolase
fructosemia
fructosuria
      essential f.
fructosyl
fruit fly
Frye test
FS — full scale (IQ)
      function study

FSA — fetal sialoglycoprotein
      fetal sulfoglycoprotein antigen
FSBA — fluorosulfonylbenzoyladenosine
FSD — focal skin distance
FSF — fibrin-stabilizing factor
FSH — follicle-stimulating hormone
FSH-RH — follicle-stimulating hormone–releasing hormone
FSP — fibrinogen split products
      fibrinolytic split products
FSR — fusiform skin revision
FT — false transmitter
      fibrous tissue
FT_4 — free (unbound) thyroxine
FTA — fluorescent treponemal antibody
FTA-ABS — fluorescent treponemal antibody absorption test
F thalassemia
FTI — free thyroxine index
FT_3I — free triiodothyronine index
FU — fecal urobilinogen
      fluorouracil
fuchsin
      acid f.
      aldehyde f.
      aniline f.
      basic f.
      f. bodies
      carbol f.
      diamond f.
      new f.
fuchsinophil
      f. cell
      f. granule
      f. reaction
fuchsinophilia
fuchsinophilic
Fuchs-Rosenthal chamber
Fuchs's
      adenoma
      dimple
L-fucose
fucosidase
fucosidosis
fucosylglycopeptide
fucosyltransferase
FUDR — fluorodeoxyuridine
fugacity

fugitive swelling
Fuhrman's grading system
Fujiwara reaction
fulguration
full
    f. blood examination
    f.-thickness burn
    f.-wave rectifier
    f.-width half-maximum
fulminant
    f. dysentery
    f. hepatitis
fulminating anoxia
fumagillin
fumarase
fumarate hydratase
fumaric acid
fumaricaciduria
fumarylacetoacetase
fumarylacetoacetate
fume hood
fumigation
fuming nitric acid
functio laesa (loss of function)
function
    autocorrelation f.
    B-cell f.
    Boolean f.
    continuous f.
    density f.
    detector transfer f.
    discriminant f.
    distribution f.
    exponential f.
    line-spread f.
    liver f.
    luteal f.
    modulation transfer f.
    pulmonary f.
    split renal f.
    step f.
    T-cell f.
    transfer f.
    ventricular f.
functional
    f. adenoma
    f. aerobic impairment
    f. affinity
    f. albuminuria
    f. bleeding
    f. death
    f. disorder

    f. group
    f. group isomerism
    f. hypertrophy
    f. hypoglycemia
    f. pathology
    f. proteinuria
    f. residual capacity
    f. tumor
functionally patent foramen ovale
functioning tumor
fundal gastritis
fundoesophageal bypass
fundoplication
fundus (pl., fundi)
funduscopy
fundusectomy
fungal
    f. antibody screen
    f. brain
    f. cystitis
    f. enterocolitis
    f. infection
    f. meningitis
    f. pericarditis
    f. pneumonia
    f. smear
    f. spore
    f. staining
    f. thyroiditis
    f. toxin
    f. vasculitis
fungating
    f. sore
    f. tumor
fungemia
fungemic
fungicidal
fungicide
fungiform papillae
Fungi Imperfecti
Fungizone
fungoid
fungoma
fungosity
fungus (pl., fungi)
    aflatoxin-producing f.
    ascopore-forming f.
    f. balls
    f. culture
    cutaneous f.
    dermatiaceous fungi
    dimorphic pathogenic fungi

filamentous f.
fission f.
gamma f.
mosaic f.
mycelial f.
opportunistic f.
pathogenic f.
subcutaneous f.
systemic f.
yeast f.
funicular/encysted hydrocele
funiculitis
    endemic f.
    filarial f.
funiculus (pl., funiculi)
    cerebellar f.
    lateral f.
funiform
funisitis
funnel
    f. breast
    f. chest
    mitral f.
    separatory f.
FUO — fever of undetermined origin
    fever of unknown origin
FUR — fluorouracil riboside
furan
furanose
furanoside
furazolidone
furcal
furcate
furfural reagent
furfuraldehyde
furfurol reaction
furosemide
Furoxone
furuncle
furunculosis
fusariomycosis
Fusarium
    F. javanicum
    F. moniliforme
    F. oxysporum
    F. roseum
    F. solanae
    F. sporotrichoides
fuse alarm
fuseau (pl., fuseaux)
fused kidney
fusible calculus
Fusidium terricola

fusiform
    f. aneurysm
    f. bacillus
    f. bronchiectasis
    f. cell
    f. gyrus
    f. skin revision
Fusiformis necrophorus
fusimotor
    f. axons
    f. fibers
    f. neurons
fusion
    f. area
    cell f.
    centric f.
    protoplast f.
    splenogonadal f.
    whole-arm f.
Fusobacterium
    F. aquatile
    F. fusiforme
    F. glutinosum
    F. gonidiaformans
    F. mortiferum
    F. naviforme
    F. necrophorum
    F. nucleatum
    F. plauti-vincentii
    F. plauti
    F. prausnitzii
    F. russii
    F. symbiosum
    F. varium
fusocellular
fusospirillary
fusospirillosis
fusospirochetal
fusospirochetosis
fusostreptococcosis
fustic
FV — fluid volume
FVC — forced vital capacity
FVL — femoral vein ligation
FW — Felix-Weil (reaction)
    Folin-Wu (method)
F wave
FWHM — full-width half-maximum
FWR — Felix-Weil reaction
Fy
    antibody
    antigen
FZ — focal zone

G — gauss
  giga
  gingival
  glucose
  gonidial (colony)
  gravida
  gravitational constant
  Greek
g — gram
g — force (the pull of
  gravity)
GA — gastric analysis
  general anesthesia
  gestational age
  gingivoaxial
  glucuronic acid
  gut-associated
Ga — gallium
GABA — gamma-aminobutyric acid
GABAergic
GABA receptors
GAD — glutamic acid decarboxylase
Gaddum and Schild test
gadfly
gadolinium
Gadus
Gaffky
  scale
  table
Gaffkya tetragena
GAG — glycosaminoglycan
gag
  g. antigen
  g. gene
  g. reflex
gage
gait
  athetotic g.
  choreic g.
  g. disturbance
  dystonic g.
  festinating g.
  reeling g.
  shuffling g.
  spastic g.
  staggering g.
  steppage g.
  Trendelenburg's g.
  g. unsteadiness
  waddling g.

gal. — gallon
galactan
galactic
galactin
galactitol
galactoblast
galactocele
galactocerebroside
  g. accumulation
  g. galactosidase
  g. β-galactosidase
galactography
galactokinase deficiency
galactolipid; galactolipin
galactonolactone dehydrogenase
galactophoritis
galactopoietic hormone
galactorrhea
galactosamine
galactose
  g. breath test
  g. dehydrogenase
  g.-1-phosphate uridyltrans-
    ferase
  g. tolerance test
galactosemia
galactosialidosis
α-galactosidase
β-galactosidase
  cerebroside β-g.
  β-g. deficiency
  galactocerebroside β-g.
galactoside
galactosuria
galactosyl
galactosylceramidase
galactosylceramide galactosylhydrolase
galactosyl sulfatide
galactosyltransferase isoenzyme II
galactowaldenase
galacturia
galea aponeurotica
galeal
  g. perichondrial flap
  g. pericranial flap
Galeati's gland
galenic
Galen's
  great cerebral vein
  ventricle

Galerina
G. *autumnalis*
G. *marginata*
G. *venerata*
gall
gallamine triethiodide
gallbladder
gangrenous g.
g. hydrops
porcelain g.
sandpaper g.
strawberry g.
Gall body
Gallego's differentiating solution
gallein
Galli-Mainini toad test
gallinatum
pectus g.
gallium
g.-67
g. citrate
g. scan
g. scanning
gallocyanin; gallocyanine
Gallogen
gallop
atrial g.
filling g.
presystolic g.
protodiastolic g.
rhythm g.
gallstone
cholesterol g.
g. ileus
g. pigment
gal-1-p—galactose-1-phosphate
GALT — gut-associated lymphoid
tissue
GaLV — gibbon ape lymphosarcoma
virus
Galv. — galvanic
galvanic
g. cell
g. skin response
galvanism
galvanization
galvanochemical
galvanometer
Gamastan
Gambian trypanosomiasis
gamboge
gamete

gametic chromosome
gametocide
gametocyte
gametocytemia
gametogenesis
gametogony
gametoid theory
gamma
g.-aminobutyric acid
g. benzene hexachloride
g. camera
g.-carboxyglutamic acid
g. cells
g.-chain disease
g. delta beta-thalassemia
g. enolase
g. globulin
g. glutamyl carboxypeptidase
g.-glutamyl-cysteine synthetase
g. glutamyl transferase
g. granules
g. heavy-chain disease
g. hemolysis
g. interferon
g.-lactone
g. metachromasia
g.-pipradol
g. radiation
g. ray
g.-ray spectrum
g. spectrometer
g. spectrometry
g. staphylolysin
g. streptococcus
g. thalassemia
g.-well counter
Gammagard
gammaglobulin
human g.
gammaglobulinopathy
gamma glutamyl transferase
gammagram
gammagraphic
gamma-lactone
gammaphoto
gamma-ray spectrum
gamma-well counter
gammopathy
benign monoclonal g.
biclonal g.
monoclonal g.
polyclonal g.

Gamna-Favre bodies
Gamulin Rh
ganciclovir
Gandy-Gamna
    bodies
    nodules
ganglia
gangliitis
ganglioblast
gangliocyte
gangliocytoma
ganglioglioma
ganglioglioneuroma
ganglioma
ganglion (pl., ganglia)
    accessory g.
    Acrel's g.
    aorticorenal g.
    autonomic g.
    basal g.
    g. blocker
    cardiac g.
    celiac g.
    cell g.
    cell layer g.
    g. cells
    ciliary g.
    Corti's g.
    g. cyst
    diffuse g.
    dorsal root g.
    gasserian g.
    geniculate g.
    inferior cervical g.
    inferior glossopharyngeal
        nerve g.
    inferior mesenteric g.
    inferior ninth cranial nerve g.
    inferior vagus nerve g.
    jugular g.
    jugular glossopharyngeal
        nerve g.
    jugular tenth cranial nerve g.
    jugular vagus nerve g.
    mesenteric g., superior
    middle cervical g.
    nodose g.
    nodose tenth cranial nerve g.
    nodose vagus nerve g.
    otic g.
    periosteal g.

    petrous glossopharyngeal
        nerve g.
    pterygopalatine g.
    Scarpa's g.
    semilunar g.
    sphenopalatine g.
    spinal g.
    spiral g.
    stellate g.
    submaxillary g.
    superior cervical g.
    superior glossopharyngeal
        nerve g.
    superior ninth cranial nerve g.
    superior vagus nerve g.
    g. of sympathetic trunk
    thoracic sympathetic g.
    trigeminal g.
    trigeminal motor root g.
    trigeminal sensory root g.
    Troisier's g.
    vestibular g.
ganglioneuroblastoma
ganglioneurofibroma
ganglioneuroma
    adrenal g.
    dumbbell g.
ganglioneuromatosis
ganglionic
    g. blocking agent
    g. glioma
ganglionitis
ganglionopathy
ganglionostomy
ganglioside GM_1
gangliosidosis (pl., gangliosidoses)
    generalized g.
    GM_1 g.
    GM_2 g.
gangosa
gangrene
    arteriosclerotic g.
    cold g.
    diabetic g.
    dry g.
    embolic g.
    emphysematous g.
    Fournier's g.
    gas g.
    hemorrhagic g.
    hot g.
    Meleny's g.

moist g.
presenile spontaneous g.
progressive bacterial synergistic g.
pulp g.
scrotal g.
static g.
symmetrical g.
thrombotic g.
trophic g.
venous g.
wet g.
white g.

gangrenous
g. appendicitis
g. cholecystitis
g. emphysema
g. gallbladder
g. granulomatous inflammation
g. inflammation
g. necrosis
g. pharyngitis
g. pneumonia
g. stomatitis

gap
anion g.
auscultatory g.
chromatid g.
excitable g.
isochromatid g.
g. junction
osmolar g.

GAPD or
GAPDH — glyceraldehyde phosphate dehydrogenase

Garamycin
Gardnerella vaginalis
Gardos's phenomenon
gargantuan mastitis
gargoylism
garlic breath
Garré's
osteitis
sclerosing osteomyelitis
Gärtner's
bacillus
duct
duct cyst

gas
g. abscess
g. amplification
arsine g.
arterial blood g's

blood g's
g. bubble
carrier g.
g. chromatograph
g. chromatography
g. chromatography–mass spectrometry
combustible g.
g. constant
g. cyst
g. embolism
extravasation g.
g. gangrene
hemolytic g.
hepatic portal venous g.
g.-liquid chromatography
mustard g.
oxidizing g.
g. peritonitis
g. phlegmon
g. retention
g.-solid chromatography
g. sterilizer
g. storage limits
g. thermometer
water g.

gaseous
gasoline
gasometric ninhydrin procedure
gasometry
gasserian ganglion
gaster
Gasteromycetes
Gasterophilus
gastradenitis
gastratrophia
gastrectasis; gastrectasia
gastrectomy

gastric
g. acid
g. adenocarcinoma
g. adenoma
g. algid malaria
g. analysis
g. antrum
g. argentaffin cell
g. artery
g. aspirate cell count
g. aspiration
g. atrophy
g. branch, vagus nerve
g. calculus

g. carcinoma
g. cardia
g. cardiac gland
g. corpus
g. emptying half-time
g. emptying time
g. fistula
g. fluid
g. foveolae
g. function tests
g. fundal gland
g. fundus
g. glands
g. inhibitory polypeptide
g. juice
g. lavage
g. leukemia
g. lipase
g. lumen
g. lymph node
g. mucosa
g. mucosal barrier
g. mucous membrane
g. myiasis
g. parietal cell
g. parietography
g. pits
g. polyp
g. pyloric gland
g. resection
g. residue examination
g. rugae
g. secretion
g. serosa
g. smear
g. submucosa
g. subserosa
g. transposition
g. ulcer
g. ulcer, perforated
g. vein
g. volvulus
g. vomitus
g. washing
g. zymogenic cell
gastricsin
gastrin
    g.-calcium infusion stimulation test
    g.-protein meal stimulation test
    g.-protein stimulation test

g.-releasing peptide
g.-secretin stimulation test
gastrinoma
gastritis
    acute g.
    acute hemorrhagic erosive g.
    antral g.
    atrophic g.
    atrophic chronic g.
    autoimmune g.
    Campylobacter g.
    catarrhal g.
    chronic atrophic g.
    chronic cystic g.
    chronic follicular g.
    chronic hypertrophic g.
    chronic superficial g.
    corrosive g.
    cystic g.
    environmental g.
    eosinophilic g.
    erosive g.
    exfoliative g.
    follicular g.
    fundal g.
    giant hypertrophic g.
    granulomatous g.
    hemorrhagic g.
    hypersecretory g.
    hypertrophic g.
    interstitial g.
    phlegmonous g.
    polypous g.
    pseudomembranous g.
    radiation g.
    sclerotic g.
    syphilitic g.
    type A (fundal) g.
    type B (antral) g.
gastroadenitis
gastroccult test
gastrocele
gastrocnemius muscle
gastrocolic
    g. fistula
    g. ligament
    g. omentum
gastrocolitis
gastrocoloptosis
gastrocolostomy
gastrocutaneous fistula
gastrodiaphanoscopy

gastrodiaphany
gastrodisciasis
Gastrodiscoides hominis
Gastrodiscus hominis
gastroduodenal fistula
gastroduodenectomy
gastroduodenitis
gastroduodenoscopy
gastroduodenostomy
gastroenteralgia
gastroenteric
gastroenteritis
    eosinophilic g.
    uremic g.
    viral g.
gastroenteroanastomosis
gastroenterocolitis
gastroenterocolostomy
gastroenterologist
gastroenterology
gastroenteropancreatic endocrine
  system
gastroenteropathy
    allergic g.
    hemorrhagic g.
    protein-losing g.
gastroenteroplasty
gastroenteroptosis
gastroenterostomy
    Balfour's g.
    Billroth's g.
    Braun and Jaboulay's g.
    Curvoisier's g.
    Finney's g.
    Heineke and Mikulicz g.
    Hofmeister's g.
    Polya's g.
    Roux's g.
    Schoemaker's g.
    Von Haberer's g.
    Wölfler's g.
gastroenterotomy
gastroepiploic
    g. artery
    g. gland
gastroesophageal junction
gastroesophagitis
gastroesophagostomy
gastrofiberscope
gastrogastrostomy
gastrogavage
gastrogenic

Gastrografin
gastrograph
gastrohepatic omentum
gastrohypertonic
gastroileac
gastroileitis
gastrointestinal
    g. adsorbent
    g. bleeding
    g. blood loss test
    g. contents
    g. disease
    g. fistula
    g. fluids
    g. hemorrhage
    g. hormone
    g. intubation
    g. motility study
    g. protein loss test
    g. series
    g. spaces
    g. tract
    g. tuberculosis
Gastrointestinal Tumor Study Group
gastrojejunal fistula
gastrojejunocolic
gastrojejunoesophagostomy
gastrojejunostomy
gastrokinesograph
gastrokinesography
gastrolienal
gastrolith
gastrolithiasis
gastrolysis
gastromalacia
gastromegaly
gastrometry
gastromycosis
gastromyotomy
gastromyxorrhea
gastropancreatitis
gastroparalysis
gastroparesis
gastropathy
    hypersecretory g.
gastroperitonitis
gastropexy
gastropharyngostomy
gastrophrenic ligament
gastrophthisis
gastroptosis; gastroptosia
gastropylorectomy

gastropyloric
gastrorrhagia
gastrorrhexis
gastroschisis
gastroscope
     fiberoptic g.
gastroscopic
gastroscopy
gastrosia fungosa
gastrosplenic ligament
gastrostaxis
gastrostenosis
gastrostogavage
gastrostolavage
gastrostoma
gastrostomy
     Janeway's g.
     Stamm g.
gastrotomy
gastrotonometer
gastrotonometry
gastrula
gastrulation
gate
     circuit g.
gated channel
gating
Gaucher's
     cell
     type of histiocyte
gauge
     vacuum g.
gauss
gaussian
     g. curve
     g. probability distribution
gavage
Gay-Lussac's law
Gay's gland
gaze
     conjugate g.
GB — gallbladder
GBA — ganglionic blocking agent
     gingivobuccoaxial
G-banding stain
GBG — glycine-rich beta-
     glycoprotein
GBH — graphite-benzalkonium-
     heparin
GBIA — Guthrie bacterial inhibition
     assay

GBM — glomerular basement mem-
     brane
GC — ganglion cells
     gas chromatography
     glucocorticoid
     gonococcus
     gonorrhea
     gonorrhea culture
     granular casts
     guanine cytosine
Gc — globulin
g-cal — gram-calorie
g-cm — gram-centimeter
GC-MS — gas chromatography–mass
     spectrometry
GC value
GCSF — granulocyte colony–stimulat-
     ing factor
Gd — gadolinium
GDA — germine diacetate
GDH — glutamic acid dehydrogenase
     glycerophosphate dehydro-
     genase
GDP — guanosine diphosphate
GDP-D-mannose
GDP-L-fucose
GE — gastroenterostomy
G/E — granulocyte-erythroid ratio
Ge — germanium
Gegenbaur's cell
Geiger counter
Geiger-Müller counter
gel
     aluminum hydroxide g.
     denaturing g's
     g. electrophoresis
     g.-filtration chromatography
     hydrophilic g.
     hydrophobic g.
     g.-permeation chromatography
     silica g.
gelatin
     g. film
     g. filter
     g. slide adhesive
     g. strips
     zinc g.
gelatinous
     g. acute inflammation
     g. acute pneumonia
     g. adenocarcinoma
     g. ascites

g. atrophy
g. carcinoma
g. infiltration
g. inflammation
g. marker
g. polyp
gelation
Gell and Coombs classification
Gelman filter
gelosis
gelsemine
gelsolin
gemästete
gem-diol
gemellus muscle
geminal
geminate
gemistocyte
gemistocytic
    g. astrocyte
    g. astrocytoma
    g. tumor
gemma
gemmangioma
gemmation
gemmule
    Hoboken's g's
Gendre's fluid
gene
    allelic g's
    amorphic g.
    g. amplification
    autosomal g.
    g. bank
    betaglobin g.
    g. cloning
    g. code
    codominant g's
    complementary g's
    cumulative g.
    g. deletions
    depressed g.
    g. derepression
    dominant g.
    g. dosage
    env g.
    g. flow
    g. frequency
    gag (group-specific antigen) g.
    globin g's
    H g.
    hemizygous g's

heterozygous g.
histocompatibility g.
holandric g's
hologynic g's
Ig g. arrangement
Ig g. assembly
immunoblastic g's
immunoglobulin g's
Ir (immune response) g's
Is (immune suppressor) g's
jumping g.
lethal g.
Lewis g.
g. library
major g.
g. mapping
mobile g's
modifying g's
mutant g.
nonstructural g's
onc g.
oncogenic g.
operator g.
pleiotropic g.
pol g.
g. pool
g. product
g. rearrangement
recessive g.
reciprocal g's
regulator g.
regulatory g.
repressed g.
repressor g.
secretor g.
sex-limited g.
sex-linked g.
g. splicing
split g.
src g.
structural g.
sublethal g.
supplementary g's
suppressor g.
syntenic g's
tat g.
transactivating g.
tumor suppressor g's
wild-type g.
X-linked g.
Y-linked g.
genera (pl. of genus)

general
    g. gonadotropic activity
    g. paresis
    g. pathology
    g. peritonitis
    g. radiation
    g. tuberculosis
generalization
generalized
    g. anaphylaxis
    g. cortical hyperostosis
    g. emphysema
    g. eruptive histiocytoma
    g. gangliosidosis
    g. pustular psoriasis of Zambusch
    g. Sanarelli-Shwartzman reaction
    g. Shwartzman reaction
    g. transduction
    g. xanthelasma
generation
    alternation of g's
    first filial g.
    parental g.
    second filial g.
    spontaneous g.
    g. time
generative
generator
    aerosol g.
    diazomethane g.
    pattern g.
    random number g.
generic
    g. drug
    g. name
genesis
genesistasis
genestatic
genetic
    g. abnormality
    g. abnormality analysis
    g. adaptation
    g. anemia
    g. balance
    g. code
    g. counseling
    g. drift
    g. engineering
    g. etiology
    g. factor

"g. fingerprint"
    g. heterogeneity
    g. immunity
    g. linkage analysis
    g. linkage disequilibrium
    g. map
    g. mapping
    g. markers
    g. mutation
    g. regulation
    g. screening
    g. susceptibility
genetically significant dose
genetics
    bacterial g.
    bacteriophage g.
    behavioral g.
    biochemical g.
    clinical g.
    developmental g.
    immunogenetic g.
    mathematical g.
    medical g.
    mendelian g.
    molecular g.
    onc g.
    phage g.
    population g.
    reverse g.
    somatic cell g.
genicular artery
geniculate
    g. bodies
    g. ganglion
    g. neuralgia
geniculocalcarine tract
geniculostriate fibers
geniculotemporal tract
geniculum (pl., genicula)
genin
genioglossus muscle
geniohyoid
genital
    g. anlagen
    g. aphthosis
    g. culture
    g. dermatosis
    g. disorder
    g. duct
    g. fluids
    g. gland
    g. herpes simplex

g. ridge
g. spaces
g. syphilis
g. tract
g. tubercle
g. tuberculosis
g. ulcer
g. wart
genitalia
    ambiguous external g.
    external g.
genitocrural
genitofemoral nerve
genitography
genitourinary
g. fistula
g. leukemia
g. myiasis
g. schistosomiasis
g. tract
Gennari's line
genoblast
genocopy
genodermatosis
genome
genomic
g. clone
g. DNA clones
genotoxic carcinogen
genotype
genotypic
gentamicin sulfate
gentian
g. aniline water
g. violet
gentianophil; gentianophile
gentianophilous
gentianophobic
gentiobiase
gentisate oxygenase
genu (pl., genua)
g. corpus callosum
g. internal capsule
g. recurvatum
g. valgum
g. varum
genus (pl., genera)
Geodermatophilus
geographic
g. pathology
g. tongue

geometric
g. efficiency
g. isomerism
g. mean
g. optics
geophagia
geophilic
geotrichosis
Geotrichum
    G. candidum
    G. immite
geotropism
GEP (gastroenteropancreatic) endocrine system
Geraghty's test
geranyl diphosphate
Gerbich blood group system
Gerbich-negative red cell
Gerbode defect
Gerhardt's
    dullness
    ferric chloride test
    reaction
    test
    test for acetoacetic acid
    test for urobilin in the urine
geriatric
geriatrician
geriatrics
germ
g. cell
g. cell aplasia
g. cell hypoplasia
g. cell–stromal–sex cord tumor
g. cell–stromal tumor
g. cell tumor
g.-free
g. layers
g. line theory
g. tube
g. tube test
germanin
germanium
German measles
germicidal
germicide
germinal
g. aplasia
g. center
g. center of lymph node
g. epithelial inclusion cyst
g. epithelium

g. inclusion cyst
g. vesicle
germinoblast
germinoma
mediastinal g.
pineal g.
testicular g.
germogen
geroderma osteodysplastica
geromarasmus
gerontologist
gerontology
Gerota's fascia
gerüstmark
gestagen
gestation
gestational
g. age
g. alteration
g. choriocarcinoma
g. diabetes
g. proteinuria
g. trophoblastic neoplasia
g. tumor
gestosis
GET — gastric emptying time
GET1/2 — gastric emptying half-time
GeV — giga electron volt
GF — gastric fluid
germ-free
gluten-free
G factor
GFAP — glial fibrillary acidic protein
GFR — glomerular filtration rate
GG — gamma globulin
GGA — general gonadotropic
activity
GGG — gummi guttae gambiae
(gamboge)
GG or S — glands, goiter, or stiffness
(the neck)
GGT — gamma-glutamyltransferase
glutamyltransferase
GGTP — gamma-glutamyl transpep-
tidase
GH — growth hormone
GHD — growth hormone deficiency
Ghon's
complex
focus
primary lesion
tubercle

Ghon-Sachs bacillus
ghost
blood g.
g. cell
g. corpuscle
ghoul hand
GH-RF — growth hormone–releasing
factor
GH-RH — growth hormone–
releasing hormone
GH-RIH — growth hormone
release–inhibiting
hormone
GHz — gigahertz
GI — gastrointestinal
globin insulin
giant
g. baby
g. blue nevus
g. cell
g. cell aortitis
g. cell arteritis
g. cell carcinoma
g. cell carcinoma of thyroid
gland
g. cell cystitis
g. cell epulis
g. cell fibroma
g. cell granuloma
g. cell hepatitis
g. cell myeloma
g. cell myocarditis
g. cell pneumonia
g. cell reaction
g. cell reparative granuloma
g. cell sarcoma
g. cell thyroiditis
g. cell tumor
g. cell tumor of bone
g. cell tumor of lung
g. cell tumor of tendon sheath
g. colon
g. condyloma
g. condyloma of Buschke-
Lowenstein
g. fibroadenoma
g. follicle lymphoma
g. follicular hyperplasia
g. follicular lymphoblastoma
g. follicular lymphoma
foreign body g. cells
g. gastric folds
g. hairy nevus

g. hives
g. hypertrophic gastritis
g. hypertrophy of gastric mucosa
g. intestinal fluke
g. intracanalicular fibroadenoma
g. keratoacanthoma
Langhans' g. cells
g. liver fluke
malignant g. cell tumor of soft parts
g. melanosome
multinucleated g. cells
g. neutrophil
g. neutrophilia
osteoclastic g. cells
g. osteoid osteoma
g. pigmented nevus
g. platelets
g. rugal hypertrophy
syncytial g. cells
Touton g. cells
tumor g. cell
g. urticaria
Warthin-Finkeldey g. cells
giantism
Giardia
    G. *intestinalis*
    G. *lamblia*
giardial cyst
giardiasis dysentery
Gibberella fujikuroi
gibbon ape lymphosarcoma virus
Gibbs-Donnan law
Gibson-Cooke sweat test
Gibson's vestibule
Giemsa
    chromosome banding stain
    stain
Gierke's corpuscles
giga electron volt
gigahertz
gigantism
    acromegalic g.
    exophthalmic g.
    exophthalmos g.
    hyperpituitary g.
    macroglossia g.
    pituitary g.
gigantocellular
gigantomastia

GIGO — garbage in, garbage out
gigohm
GIK — glucose, insulin, and potassium
gilbert (unit of magnetomotive force)
Gilchrist's mycosis
gill-arch skeleton
Gillies' flap
GIM — gonadotropin-inhibitory material
Gimenez stain
gingiva
gingival
    g. epithelial attachment
    g. glands
    g. hemorrhage
    g. hyperplasia
    g. hypertrophy
    g. lamina propria
    g. mucous membrane
gingivitis
    acute necrotizing ulcerative g.
    diphenylhydantoin g.
    gonococcal g.
    hypertrophic g.
    necrotizing ulcerative g.
    papillary g.
    scorbutic g.
gingivoglossitis
gingivolabial
gingivosis
gingivostomatitis
    g. herpes
    herpetic g.
    necrotizing ulcerative g.
GIP — gastric inhibitory polypeptide
Girard's reagent
girdle
    pelvic g.
GIS — gastrointestinal system
GI series — gastrointestinal series
GIT — gastrointestinal tract
gitalin
gitaloxin
gitoxin
GITT — glucose-insulin tolerance test
gitter cell
gitterzelle
GK — glycerol kinase
GL — greatest length
Gl — glucinium

gl — gill
    gland
GL 54 — athomin
GLA — gingivolinguoaxial
glabella
glabelloalveolar line
glabellomeatal line
glabrosa
glabrous skin
glacial acetic acid
gladiomanubrial
gland
        absorbent g.
        accessory g.
        acinar g.
        acinotubular g.
        acinous g.
        adrenal g.
        Albarrán's g.
        alveolar g.
        apocrine g.
        areolar g's
        arytenoid g's
        Avicenna's g.
        axillary g's
        Bartholin's g.
        Bowman's g's
        Bruch's g's
        Brunner's g's
        buccal g's
        bulbocavernous g.
        bulbourethral g.
        celiac g's
        ceruminous g's
        cervical g's
        Ciacco's g's
        ciliary g's
        colonic g's
        conglobate g.
        Cowper's g.
        cutaneous g's
        cytogenic g.
        ductless g.
        duodenal g's
        Duverney's g's
        Ebner's g.
        eccrine g.
        endocrine g's
        endoepithelial g.
        esophageal g's
        excretory g.
        exocrine g.

        follicular g's
        Galeati's g.
        gastric g's
        gastroepiploic g's
        Gay's g's
        genital g.
        gingival g's
        globate g.
        glossopalatine g's
        gustatory g's
        guttural g.
        haversian g's
        hematopoietic g's
        hemolymph g's
        hepatic g's
        heterocrine g's
        interscapular g.
        intraepithelial g.
        intramuscular g's of tongue
        jugular g.
        lacrimal g.
        laryngeal g's
        lenticular g's
        lingual g's
        Littre's g.
        lymph g's
        lymphatic g.
        mammary g.
        meibomian g's
        merocrine g.
        mesenteric g's
        minor vestibular g.
        Moll's g.
        mucous g's
        myometrial g.
        Naboth's g's
        nasal g's
        nasopharyngeal g.
        nasopharyngeal pituitary g.
        oxyntic g's
        palatine g's
        palpebral g's
        pancreaticosplenic g's
        parathyroid g.
        paraurethral g.
        parotid g.
        pharyngeal g's
        Philip's g's
        pineal g.
        pituitary g.
        Poirier's g's
        prostate g.

prostatic g.
pyloric g's
racemose g's
saccular g.
salivary g.
sentinel g.
seromucous g.
serous g.
Sigmund's g's
Skene's g.
Stahr's g.
subauricular g's
sublingual g.
submandibular g.
submaxillary g.
suprarenal g.
thymus g.
thyroid g.
tubuloalveolar g.
urethral g.
vaginal g.
vestibular g.
Virchow's g.
Waldeyer's g's
Weber's g's
g. of Zeis
glanders bacillus
glandula
glandular
g. atypia
g. cancer
g. carcinoma
g. cystitis
g. epithelium
g. fever
g. hyperplasia
g. mastitis
g. metaplasia
g. neoplasm
g. pharyngitis
g. tularemia
g. ureteritis
glandularis
g. proliferans cholecystitis
pyelitis g.
ureteritis g.
glans (pl., glandes)
g. clitoridis
g. penis
Glanzmann-Naegeli thrombasthenia
Glanzmann's thrombasthenia

glass
g.-bead retention method
g. body
borosilicate g.
g.-ceramic
cover g.
g. electrode
g. factor
g. fiber filter
flint g.
ground g.
heat-resistant g.
low-actinic g.
optical g.
Wood's g.
glassy
g. cell carcinoma
g. membrane
glaucarubin
glaucoma
angle closure g.
congenital g.
infantile g.
open angle g.
phacolytic g.
primary g.
secondary g.
glaucomatous cataract
glaucosuria
GLC — gas-liquid chromatography
Gleason II adenocarcinoma
Gleason's
score
tumor grade
Glenner-Lillie stain
glenoid cavity
Glenospora graphii
Glenosporella loboi
Gley's cells
glia
ameboid g.
Bergmann's g.
cytoplasmic g.
fibrillary g.
plasmic g.
gliadin
glial
g. fibrillary acidic protein
g. filaments
g. nodules
glioblast

glioblastoma
    g. cell lines
    g. multiforme
Gliocladium
gliocytoma
glioma
    astrocytic g.
    ependymal g.
    ganglionic g.
    malignant g.
    mixed g.
    nasal g.
    optic g.
    subependymal g.
    telangiectatic g.
gliomatosis
    cerebral g.
    g. cerebri
glioneuroma
gliophagia
gliosarcoma
gliosis
    anisomorphic g.
    isomorphic g.
    g. uteri
gliosome
gliotic
gliotoxin
glissonitis
Glisson's
    capsule
    cirrhosis
"glitter cells"
Gln — glutamine
GLNS — gay lymph node syndrome
glob. — globulin
global glomerulonephritis
globatic gland
globe cell anemia
Globidium
globin
    g. genes
    g. insulin
globinometer
globoid cell leukodystrophy
globose
globoside
globular
    g.-fibrous transformation
    g. leukocyte
    g. protein
    g. sputum

    g. thrombus
    g. value
globule
    hyaline g.
globuliferous phagocyte
globulin
    α g's
    α_1 g's
    α_2 g's
    AC (accelerator) g.
    accelerator g.
    antidiphtheritic g.
    antihemophilic g.
    antihemophilic g. A
    antihemophilic g. B
    antihuman g.
    antilymphocyte g.
    antilymphocytic g.
    antimacrophage g.
    antithymocyte g.
    beta g's
    β_{1A}-g.
    β_{1C}-g.
    β_{1E}-g.
    β_{1F}-g.
    bovine gamma g.
    g.-coated erythrocyte
    complex g.
    corticosteroid-binding g.
    cortisol-binding g.
    equine antihuman lympho-
      blast g.
    gamma g's
    Gc-g.
    hepatitis B immune g.
    horse antihuman thymus g.
    human rabies immune g.
    hyperimmune g.
    immune g.
    immune serum g.
    intravenous immune g.
    milk fat g.
    plasma accelerator g.
    rabies immune g.
    $Rh_0(D)$ immune g.
    serum g.
    serum accelerator g.
    sex hormone–binding g.
    testosterone-estradiol–
      binding g.
    thyroxine-binding g.
    unbound thyroxine–binding g.

vaccinia-immune g.
g. X
zoster immune g.
globulinuria
globulomaxillary cyst
globus (pl., globi)
    g. hystericus
    g. pallidus
glomangioma
glomangiomatous osseous malformation syndrome
glomangiosis
    pulmonary g.
glomera aortica
glomerular
    g. basal lamina
    g. basement membrane antibody
    g. basement membrane disease
    g. capillary basement membrane
    g. capillary endothelium
    g. crescents
    g. cyst
    g. filtration
    g. filtration rate
    g. lipoid nephrosis
    g. mesangium
    g. nephritis
    g. pedicel
    g. pores
    g. proteinuria
    g. sclerosis
    g. tuft
    g. urinary pole
    g. vascular pole
glomerulitis
    necrotizing g.
glomerulocystic disease
glomeruloid
glomerulonephritis
    acute g.
    acute crescentic g.
    acute exudative g.
    acute hemorrhagic g.
    acute poststreptococcal g.
    antibasement membrane g.
    antiglomerular basement membrane g.
    autoimmune g.
    Berger's focal g.
    chronic g.

chronic membranous g.
diffuse g.
Ellis type 1 g.
Ellis type 2 g.
embolic g.
extracapillary g.
exudative g.
focal g.
focal capillary g.
focal embolic g.
focal necrotizing g.
focal proliferative g.
global g.
hemorrhagic g.
Heymann's g.
hypocomplementemic g.
idiopathic g.
IgA g.
immune complex g.
induced g.
lobular g.
local g.
malignant g.
membranoproliferative g.
membranous g.
membranous-proliferative g.
mesangial lupus g.
mesangial proliferative g.
mesangiocapillary g.
necrotizing g.
nonstreptococcal g.
postinfectious g.
poststreptococcal g.
proliferative g.
rapidly progressive g.
segmental g.
subacute g.
glomerulopathy
    crescentic g.
    diabetic g.
    focal sclerosing g.
    immune complex g.
    proliferative g.
glomerulosclerosis
    cirrhotic g.
    diabetic g.
    diffuse g.
    focal segmental g.
    intercapillary g.
    malignant focal g.
    nodular g.

obliterative g.
progressive g.
glomerulus (pl., glomeruli)
    pronephric g.
    synaptic g.
glomus (pl., glomera)
    g. caroticum
    g. coccygeum
    g. intravagale
    g. jugulare
    g. jugulare tumor
    g. tumor
    g. tympanicum
glossa
glosssal
glossectomy
Glossina
    G. *fuscipes*
    G. *swynnertoni*
    G. *tachinoides*
glossitis
    atrophic g.
    Hunter's g.
    median rhomboid g.
glossohyal
glossopalatine
    g. arch
    g. glands
glossopharyngeal
    g. nerve
    g. neuralgia
    g. nucleus
glossopharyngeum
glossotomy
glottal
glottis (pl., glottides)
glow modular tube
Glu — glutamic acid
    glutamine
glu. or gluc. — glucose
glucagon
    immunoreactive g.
    g. test
glucagonoma
glucan
    α-g.
    g. branching enzyme
    α-g.-branching glycosyltrans-
      ferase
α-1-4-glucan-4-glucanohydrolase
α-1-4-glucanglucohydrolase
glucaric acid
glucatonia

glucemia
glucide
glucitol
glucoamylase
glucocerebrosidase deficiency
glucocerebroside
glucocorticoid
    g.-secreting adenoma
    g.-suppressive hyperaldoste-
      ronism
    g. suppression test
glucocorticosteroid
Gluco-Ferrum
glucofuranose
glucogenesis
glucogenic amino acid
glucohemia
glucokinase
gluconate
    calcium g.
    6-P-g. dehydrogenase
    ferrous g.
gluconeogenesis
gluconeogenetic
gluconolactonase
glucopenia
glucoproteinase
glucopyranose
glucosamine
    acetyl g.
glucosan transglucosylase
glucosazone
glucose
    blood g.
    buffered desoxycholate g.
    D-g. ceramide
    cerebral metabolic rate of g.
    g.-cysteine agar
    g. dehydrogenase
    g. fermenters
    g.-galactose malabsorption
    g. insulin tolerance test
    g. metabolism
    g. monophosphate synthetase
    g. nitrogen (ratio)
    g. oxidase
    g. oxidase method
    g. oxidase paper strip test
    g. oxidizer
    g.-1-phosphatase
    g.-6-phosphatase
    g.-1-phosphate

g.-6-phosphate
g.-6-phosphate dehydrogenase
g.-phosphate dehydrogenase deficiency
g.-phosphate dehydrogenase deficiency anemia
g.-phosphate dehydrogenase screen
g.-1-phosphate phosphodismutase
g.-6-phosphate translocase
g.-1-phosphate uridylyltransferase
g.-phosphomutase
renal threshold for g.
g. tolerance
g. tolerance test
g. transport system
UDP-g.
UDP-g.-glycogen glucosyltransferase
urinary g.
glucosephosphate isomerase
g.i. assay
g.i. deficiency
α-glucosidase
α-1,3-g.
β-glucosidase
cerebroside β-g.
glucoside
glucosulfone sodium
glucosuria
renal g.
glucosyl
glucosylceramidase assay
glucosylceramide lipidosis
glucosyltransferase
glucurolactone
glucuronate reductase
glucuronic acid
glucuronidase
beta g.
glucuronide
androstanediol g.
bilirubin g.
glucuronolactone reductase
glucuronosyltransferase
UDP-bilirubin g.
glucuronyl-transferase deficiency
Gluge's corpuscles
glutamate
arginine g.

g. decarboxylase
g. dehydrogenase
g. formiminotransferase deficiency
monosodium g.
g. oxaloacetate transaminase
g.-pyruvate transaminase
g. semialdehyde
g.-γ-semialdehyde
glutamic
g. acid decarboxylase
g.-oxaloacetic transaminase
g.-pyruvic transaminase
g. γ-semialdehyde
glutaminase
glutamine
g.-fructose-6-phosphate aminotransferase
g.-ketoacid aminotransferase
g. phenylacetyltransferase
g. synthetase
glutaminyl
g.-peptide-glutamyltransferase
g.-peptide-δ-glutamyltransferase
glutamyl
γ-g. cysteine synthetase
α-g. transferase
γ-g. transferase
g. transfer cycle
γ-g. transpeptidase
γ-glutamylcysteine
glutaral
glutaraldehyde fixative
glutaric acid
D-g.a.
glutaryl–CoA synthetase
glutathione
g.-homocystine transhydrogenase
oxidized g.
g. peroxidase
reduced g.
g. reductase
g. reductase deficiency
g. stability test
g. synthetase
g. thiolesterase
glutathionemia
glutathionuria
gluteal
g. artery
g. flap

g. nerve
g. region
g. sulcus
g. vein
gluten
g. enteropathy
g.-free
g.-sensitive enteropathy
glutenin
glutethimide assay
gluteus maximus muscle
gluteus medius muscle
gluteus minimus muscle
glutin
glutinous
glutitis
Gly — glycine
glycan
glycemia
glyceraldehyde
g.-3-P-dehydrogenase
g. phosphate
g.-3-phosphate
g.-phosphate dehydrogenase
glycerate
g. dehydrogenase
g. kinase
g. phosphomutase
glyceric acid
L-glycericaciduria
glyceride
glycerin
g. blood serum
g. method
glycerinated lymph
glycerite
glyceroboric acid
glycerol
g. dehydrogenase
g. gelatin medium
g. kinase
g.-3-phosphate dehydrogenase
glycerolization
glycerolize
glyceroluria
glycerone
glycerophosphatase
glycerophosphate
glycerophosphatide
glycerophosphorylcholine diesterase
glyceryl
g. ether lipids

g. guaiacolate
g. monostearate
g. triacetate
g. trinitrate
g. trioleate
g. tripalmitate
glycinamide ribonucleotide
glycine
g. acyltransferase
g. amidinotransferase
g.-arginine reaction
g. formiminotransferase
g. metabolism
g.-rich beta-glycoprotein
glycinemia
glycinuria
Glyciphagus
G. *buski*
G. *domesticus*
glycoaldehyde
glycobiarsol
glycocalyx
glycochenodeoxycholate
glycochenodeoxycholic acid
glycocholate
glycocholic acid
glycoconjugate
glycodeoxycholic acid
glycogen
g. acanthosis
accumulation of g.
g. branching enzyme
cytoplasmic g.
g. digestion
hepatic g.
g. infiltration
g. phosphorylase
g. staining
g. storage disease
g. storage test
g. starch synthase
g. synthase
g. synthesis
tissue g.
glycogenase
glycogenesis
glycogenic
glycogenolysis
glycogenolytic
glycogenosis
brancher g.

hepatophosphorylase deficiency g.
hepatorenal g.
hepatorenal glucose-6-phosphatase deficiency g.
idiopathic generalized g.
myophosphorylase deficiency g.
glycoglycinuria
glycohemoglobin
glycol
    ethylene g.
    g. methacrylate
    polyethylene g.
glycolaldehyde
glycolaldehydetransferase
glycolate oxidase
glycolic
    g. acid
    g. aciduria
glycolipid
    g. lipidosis
    g. staining
glycolithocholic acid
glycolysis
    anaerobic g.
glycolytic enzyme
glycone
glyconeogenesis
glycopenia
glycopeptide
glycophorin
glycoprotein
    acid g.
    α_1-acid g.
    g. adenoma
    alpha acid g.
    g. hormone
    g. Mac-1
    membrane g., P-170
    g. P 150, 95
    prostate-specific g.
    g. staining
    submaxillary g.
    transmembrane g.
glycoptyalism
glycopyrrolate
glycopyrronium bromide
glycorrhachia
glycorrhea
glycosaminoglycan
glycosaminolipid
glycosialia
glycosidase

glycoside
    cardiac g.
    cyanophoric g.
    digitalis g's
    g. hydrolase
    sterol g.
glycosphingolipid
glycosulfatase
glycosuria
    alimentary g.
    benign g.
    digestive g.
    epinephrine g.
    normoglycemic g.
    pathologic g.
    phlorhidzin or phloridzin g.
    renal g.
    toxic g.
glycosuric melituria
glycosylated hemoglobin test
glycosylation
    nonenzymatic g.
glycosyl ceramide
glycosyltransferase
    α-glucan-branching g.
glycotropic factor
glycuresis
glycuronuria
glycyl
    g.-glycine dipeptidase
    g.-leucine dipeptidase
glycyltryptophan test
Glycyphagus domesticus
glyodin
glyoxalase
glyoxylate reductase
glyoxylic acid–induced fluorescence technique
GM — gastric mucosa
    geometric mean
    grand multiparity
G/M — granulocyte/macrophage
Gm — gamma
Gm (gamma marker) allotype
gm — gram
g-m — gram-meter
GMA — glyceryl methacrylate
GM-CSA — granulocyte-macrophage colony–stimulating activity
GM-CSF — granulocyte-macrophage colony–stimulating factor

Gmelin's test
GMP — guanosine monophosphate
      3′,5′-guanosine monophos-
        phate
      guanosine phosphate
GMS — Gomori's methenamine-
      silver stain
GMT — geometric mean titer
GMW — gram-molecular weight
GN — glomerulonephritis
      glucose nitrogen (ratio)
      gram-negative
Gnathostoma
      G. *hispidum*
      G. *spinigerum*
gnathostomiasis
GN (gram-negative) broth
GNID — gram-negative intracellular
      diplococci
gnotobiota
gnotobiote
gnotobiotic
gnotobiotics
gnotophoresis
GnRH — gonadotropin-releasing
      hormone
goblet cell
Godwin tumor
GOE — gas, oxygen, and ether
Gofman test
goiter
      aberrant g.
      acute g.
      adenomatous g.
      amyloid g.
      colloid g.
      congenital g.
      cystic g.
      diffuse nontoxic g.
      diffuse toxic g.
      diving g.
      dyshormonogenic g.
      endemic g.
      exophthalmic g.
      familial g.
      fibrous g.
      follicular g.
      hyperplastic g.
      intrathoracic g.
      lingual g.
      lymphadenoid g.
      microfollicular g.
      multinodular g.

      multiple colloid g.
      nodular g.
      nodular colloid g.
      nodular hyperplastic g.
      nonendemic g.
      nontoxic nodular g.
      parenchymatous g.
      plunging g.
      retrosternal g.
      simple g.
      sporadic diffuse g.
      sporadic nodular g.
      sporadic simple g.
      substernal g.
      suffocative g.
      thoracic g.
      toxic g.
      toxic multinodular g.
      toxic nodular g.
      wandering g.
goitrous
gold
      g.-198
      g. chloride
      g. chloride reagent
      colloidal g.
      radioactive g.
      g. sodium thiomalate
      g. sol test
      g. therapy
      g. thioglucose
      g. toning
Goldblatt's
      hypertension
      kidney
"golden" pneumonia
Goldie-Coldman hypothesis
Goldstein rays
Golgi-Mazzoni corpuscle
Golgi's
      alteration
      cavity alteration
      complex
      corpuscle
      cycle
      membrane alteration
      neuron
      organ
      osmiobichromate fixative
      stain
      vacuole alteration
      vesicle alteration

Goll's tract
Gomori-Jones periodic acid–methenamine silver stain
Gomori's
    aldehyde fuchsin stain
    chrome alum hematoxylin-phloxine stain
    methenamine silver stain
    method for chromaffin
    nonspecific acid phosphatase stain
    nonspecific alkaline phosphatase stain
    one-step trichrome stain
    silver impregnation stain
    trichrome stain
gompertzian growth
Gompertz's equation
gonad
    indifferent g.
    streaked g.
gonadal
    g. agenesis
    g. aplasia
    g. dysgenesis
    g. endocrine disorder
    g. failure
    g. leukemia
    g. shield
    g. streak
    g. stroma
    g. stromal tumor
gonadectomy
gonadoblastoma
gonadoma
gonadotrope adenoma
gonadotropic hormone
    g.h.–releasing hormone
gonadotropin
    chorionic g.
    g. deficiency
    human chorionic g.
    human menopausal g.
    human pituitary g.
    g.-inhibitory material
    menopausal g.
    pituitary g.
    pregnant mare serum g.
    g.-producing adenoma
    g.-releasing agent
    g.-releasing factor
    g.-releasing hormone

    total urinary g.
    urinary chorionic g.
gonarthritis
gonatagra
gonatocele
gonecystolith
Gongylonema pulchrum
gongylonemiasis
gonidial
gonioma
gonion (pl., gonia)
gonitis
gonocele
gonococcal
    g. arthritis
    g. arthritis-dermatitis syndrome
    g. bacteremia
    g. cervicitis
    g. endocarditis
    g. endometritis
    g. epididymitis
    g. gingivitis
    g. hepatitis
    g. infection
    g. meningitis
    g. ophthalmia
    g. orchitis
    g. perihepatitis
    g. peritonitis
    g. pharyngitis
    g. proctitis
    g. prostatitis
    g. salpingitis
    g. salpingo-oophoritis
    g. urethritis
    g. vaginitis
gonococcemia
gonococcus (pl., gonococci)
gonocyte
gonocytoma
gonohemia
gonorrhea
    g. culture
    oropharyngeal g.
    pharyngeal g.
    rectal g.
gonorrheal
    g. heel
    g. ophthalmia
    g. rheumatism
    g. salpingitis

g. tenosynovitis
g. urethritis
Goodell's sign
Goodpasture's stain
Gordius
    G. aquaticus
    G. robustus
Gordon and Sweet stain
Gordon's
    agent
    body
    test
Goriaew's rule
Gorlin's cyst
gorondou
gossypol
GOT — glutamic-oxaloacetic transaminase
Gottron's papule
goundou
gout
    abarticular g.
    articular g.
    calcium g.
    lead g.
    polyarticular g.
    saturnine g.
    tophaceous g.
gouty
    g. arthritis
    g. nephropathy
    g. tophus
    g. urine
Gowers' tract
GP — general paresis
    glucose-6-phosphate
    glycoprotein
    gutta-percha
gp 24 antibody
gp 120/160 antibody
G6P — glucose-6-phosphate
GP-A — glycophorin-A
GPAIS — guinea pig anti-insulin serum
GPC — gastric parietal cell
GP-C — glycophorin-C (glycoconnectin)
GPD or GPDH — glucose phosphate dehydrogenase
G-3-PD — glyceraldehyde-3-phosphate-dehydrogenase

G6PD or
    G6PDH — glucose-6-phosphate dehydrogenase
G6PDA — glucose-6-phosphate dehydrogenase coenzyme variant A
G₀ phase
G_0 phase
G_2 phase
GPI — glucosephosphate isomerase
GPIMH — guinea pig intestinal mucosal homogenate
GPIPID — guinea pig intraperitoneal infectious dose
GPK — guinea pig kidney (antigen)
GPKA — guinea pig kidney absorption (test)
G protein
GPS — guinea pig serum
GPT — glutamic-pyruvic transaminase
GPUT — galactose phosphate uridyl transferase
GR — gastric reaction
    glutathione reductase
gr — grain
GRA — gonadotropin-releasing agent
graafian follicle
gracilis muscle
grade
    ACS g.
    analytical reagent g.
    AR (analytical reagent) g.
    Gleason's tumor g.
    reagent g.
gradient
    average g.
    mitral g.
    ventricular g.
grading
    histologic g.
    tumor g.
graduate
graduated
    g. cylinder
    g. pipet
graft
    allogenic g.
    autogenic g.
    autologous g.
    bone g.
    coronary artery bypass g.
    heterologous g.
    isogenic g.

jejunal g.
material g.
g. rejection
serum chemistry g.
skin g.
split-thickness skin g.
g. versus host
g.-versus-host disease
g.-versus-host reaction
grafting
Graham-Cole test
Graham's
    cells
    law
grain
    g. count halving time
    g. itch
    g. itch mite
    pollen g's
graininess
gram
    g.-calorie
    g.-centimeter
    g.-meter
    g.-molecular weight
    g.-negative
    g.-positive
gramicidin
gram-negative
    g.-n. bacilli
    g.-n. bacteremia
    g.-n. bacteria
    g.-n. bacterium
    g.-n. cocci
    g.-n. intracellular diplococci
    g.-n. rods
gram-positive
    g.-p. bacilli
    g.-p. bacteria
    g.-p. bacterium
    g.-p. cocci
    g.-p. shock
Gram's
    iodine
    method
    solution
    stain
Gram-Weigert stain
granddaughter cyst
grand mal epilepsy
Granger method
granular
    g. atrophy

g. cast
g. cell ameloblastoma
g. cell myoblastoma
g. cell tumor
g. conjunctivitis
g. degeneration
g. dystrophy
g. endoplasmic reticulum
g. kidney
g. layer
g. leukoblast
g. leukocyte
g. megakaryocyte
g. pharyngitis
g. pneumocyte
g. urethritis
g. urinary cast
granulation
    arachnoid g.
    Bayle's g's
    exuberant g.
    pacchionian g.
    Reilly g's
    g. tissue
    toxic g.
granule
    acidophil g.
    acrosomal g.
    albuminous g's
    alpha g's
    Altmann's g.
    amphophil g.
    argentaffin g's
    azurophil g.
    azurophilic g.
    Babés-Ernst g's
    basal g.
    basophil g.
    basophilic g.
    beta g.
    Birbeck's g.
    Bollinger g's
    "bull's-eye" g.
    chromatin g's
    chromatophilic g's
    chromophil g.
    chromophobe g's
    cytoplasmic g's
    delta g.
    dense g.
    g's of developing neutrophils
    Ehrlich-Heinz g's

elementary g.
eosinophil g.
eosinophilic g.
Fordyce's g's
fuchsinophil g.
gamma g's
Grawitz's g's
iodophil g.
juxtaglomerular g's
kappa g.
keratohyalin g.
Kölliker's interstitial g.
Langerhans' g's
lipofuscin g's
lysosome g.
metachromatic g.
neurosecretory g's
Neusser's g.'s
neutrophil g.
oxyphil g.
perichromatin g's
pigment g.'s
primary g.
sand g's
Schüffner's g's
secondary g.
secretory g.
siderocytic g.
siderotic g.
specific g.
sulfur g's
tertiary g.
toxic g.
vermiform g's
Zimmermann's g.
zymogen g's
granuloblast
granuloblastosis
granulocytapheresis
granulocyte
        band-form g.
        basophilic g.
        g. colony–macrophage
            colony–stimulating factor
        g. colony–stimulating factor
        g. concentrate
        eosinophilic g.
        g.-erythroid ratio
        immature g.
        myeloproliferative g.
        neutrophilic g.

segmented g.
        g. transfusion
granulocytic
        g. aplasia
        g. blood cell
        g. cells
        g. hyperplasia
        g. hypoplasia
        g. leukemia
        g. sarcoma
        g. series
granulocytopathy
granulocytopenia
granulocytopoiesis
granulocytopoietic
granulocytosis
        eosinophilic g.
granulogenesis
granuloma
        amebic g.
        g. annulare
        apical g.
        beryllium g.
        bilharzial g.
        calcified g.
        candidal g.
        caseating g.
        coccidioidal g.
        dental g.
        Dürck's g.
        g. endemicum
        eosinophilic g.
        exuberant g.
        g. faciale
        foreign body g.
        g. gangrenescens
        giant cell g.
        giant cell reparative g.
        g. gravidarum
        histiocytic g.
        Hodgkin's g.
        infectious g.
        g. inguinale
        g. inguinale tropicum
        laryngeal g.
        lethal midline g.
        lipoid g.
        lipophagic g.
        Majocchi's g.
        malarial g.
        malignant g.
        midline lethal g.

Mignon's eosinophilic g.
mineral oil g.
multifocal eosinophilic g.
g. multiforme
non-necrotizing g.
oily g.
parasitic g.
periapical g.
peripheral giant cell g.
plasma cell g.
prostatic g.
pseudopyogenic g.
g. pudendi
pyogenic g.
g. pyogenicum
reparative g.
reparative giant cell g.
reticulohistiocytic g.
sarcoid g.
sarcoidal g.
schistosome g.
sea urchin g.
sperm g.
spermatogenic g.
suture g.
swimming pool g.
talc g.
g. telangiectaticum
trichophytic g.
g. trichophyticum
tuberculoid g.
unifocal eosinophilic g.
g. venereum
xanthomatous g.
zirconium g.
granulomatosis
allergic g.
angiitic g.
beryllium g.
g. disciformis chronica et progressiva
g. infantiseptica
Langerhans' cell g.
lipophagic intestinal g.
lymphomatoid g.
Miescher's g.
g. orchitis
g. siderotica
Wegener's g.
granulomatous
g. colitis
g. disease
g. enteritis
g. follicullitis
g. gastritis
g. inflammation
g. mastitis
g. orchitis
g. polyp
g. prostatitis
g. rosacea
g. thymoma
g. thyroiditis
g. uveitis
g. vasculitis
granulomere
granulopenia
granulophthisis
granuloplasm
granuloplastic
granulopoiesis
granulopoietic
granulopoietin
granulosa
g. cell
g. cell carcinoma
g. cell tumor
g.-lutein cells
g. theca cell tumor
granulosis rubra nasi
granulosity
granulovacuolar degeneration
grape mole
graph
Davenport g.
power function g.
graphic
g. analysis
g. terminal
Graphium
grating
replica g.
Gratiolet radiation
grav I — pregnancy one
primigravida
gravel
grave wax
gravid
gravida
gravimetric
Gravindex test
gravitation abscess
gravity
g.-settling culture
specific g.

Gravlee jet wash
Grawitz's
    basophilia
    granules
    tumor
gray
    g. commissures
    g. hepatization
    g. induration
    g. infiltration
    g. patch
    g.-patch ringworm
    g. platelet syndrome
    g. ramus
    g. scale
gray matter
    cerebral g.m.
    cervical spinal cord g.m.
    frontal lobe g.m.
    insula g.m.
    lumbosacral spinal cord g.m.
    occipital lobe g.m.
    paramamillary g.m.
    parietal lobe g.m.
    periventricular g.m.
    spinal cord g.m.
    temporal lobe g.m.
    thoracic spinal cord g.m.
great arteries transposition
green
    g. cancer
    g. hemoglobin
    methylene g.
    g. pus
    g. sickness
    g. sputum
    g. urine
greenstick
    g. compound fracture
    g. fracture
grenz rays
GRF — gonadotropin-releasing factor
    growth hormone–releasing
        factor
GRH — growth hormone–releasing
        hormone
GRID — gay-related immuno-
        deficiency disease
grid
    aligned g.
    Bucky g.
    crossed g.

    focused g.
    g. index
    g. lines
    parallel g.
    Potter-Bucky g.
    g. ratio
Gridley's stain for fungi
griffin claw
Grimelius's argyrophil method
grinders' asthma
grip
    devil's g.
grippe
    Balkan g.
griseofulvin
Grocott-Gomori
    methenamine-silver method
    methenamine-silver stain
groin ulcer
groove
    Harrison's g.
    hippocampal pressure g.
    meningioma of the olfactory g.
    nuclear g.
    g. pressure
    g. sign
Groshong catheter
gross
    g. hematuria
    g. lesion
    g. specimen
Gross virus antigen
ground
    g. glass
    g.-glass appearance
    g.-glass cytoplasm
    g.-glass hepatocyte
    g. itch anemia
    g. state
    g. substance
grounded
groundnut oil
group
    ABO blood g's
    acyloxy g.
    g. agglutinin
    g. A hapten
    alkyl g.
    aryl g.
    g. A streptococci
    g. atrophy
    azo g.

blood g.
Bombay blood g.
g. B streptococci
coli-aerogenes g.
control g.
coryneform g.
dorsal respiratory g.
g. D streptococci
functional g.
guanidinium g.
hydroxyl g.
Kell blood g.
Kell-Cellano blood g.
keto g.
Kidd blood g.
Lewis blood g.
Lutheran blood g.
MNS blood g.
g. N streptococci
P blood g.
peptide g.
plasma blood g.
platinum g.
PLT (psittacosis–lympho-
   granuloma venereum–
   trachoma) g.
prenyl g's
prosthetic g.
proteus g.
Rh blood g.
Runyon's g.
salmonella g.
sulfhydryl g.
symmetry g.
thiocarbonyl g.
g. transfer
ventral respiratory g.
grouping
   antigenic structural g.
   blood g.
   haptenic g.
   Lancefield g.
   reverse g.
   Steinthal's g's
Group I-IV mycobacteria
growing point
growth
   g. acceleration
   g. alteration
   appositional g.
   g. arrest
   g. disorder

exophytic g.
exponential g.
g. factor
g. fraction
gompertzian g.
histiotypic g.
g. hormone
g. hormone deficiency
g. hormone–producing adenoma
g. hormone release–inhibiting
   hormone
g. hormone–releasing factor
g. hormone–releasing hormone
g.-inhibiting factor
interstitial g.
multiplicative g.
new g.
g. rate
g. retardation
GRP — gastrin-releasing peptide
Gruber-Widal reaction
Gruentzig balloon catheter
Gruft's medium
grumous; grumose
gryochrome
G/S — glucose and saline
GSA — Gross virus antigen
   guanidinosuccinic acid
GSC — gas-solid chromatography
   gravity-settling culture
GSD — genetically significant dose
   glycogen storage disease
GSE — gluten-sensitive enteropathy
GSH — reduced glutathione
GSH-Px — glutathione peroxidase
GSR — galvanic skin response
   generalized Shwartzman
   reaction
GSS — Gerstmann-Straussler-
   Schenker syndrome
GSSG — oxidized glutathione
GSSG-R — glutathione reductase
GSSR — generalized Sanarelli-
   Shwartzman reaction
G (hypertelorism-hypospadias) syn-
   drome
GT — generation time
   glucose tolerance
   glutamyl transpeptidase
GTD — gestational trophoblastic
   disease
GTH — gonadotropic hormone
GTN — glyceryl trinitrate

GTP — glutamyl transpeptidase
    guanosine triphosphate
GTT — glucose tolerance test
GU — gastric ulcer
    genitourinary
    gonococcal urethritis
guaiac test
guaiacin
guaiacol
Guama virus
guanase
guanazole
guanethidine
    g. monosulfate
    g. sulfate
guanidinemia
guanidine phosphate
guanidinium group
guanidinoacetate
    g. kinase
    g. methyl-transferase
guanidino-aminovaleric acid
guanido
guanine
    g. cytosine
    g. deaminase
    g. nucleotide
guanosine
    cyclic g. monophosphate
    g. cyclic phosphate
    g. 3′,5′-cyclic phosphate
    g. diphosphate
    g. hydrolase
    g. monophosphate
    g. 5′ phosphate
    g. triphosphate
guanylate cyclase
guanylic acid
guanyl-nucleotide–binding protein
guanylyl
Guarnieri's bodies
Guaroa virus
gubernaculum (pl., gubernacula)
    chorda g.
    g. testis
Gubler's tumor
Gudmand-Hoyer lactose tolerance test
Guilford-Zimmerman personality test
guinea
    g. green B
    g. worm infection
guinea pig
    g.p. anti-insulin serum

g.p. intestinal mucosal homogenate
g.p. intraperitoneal infectious dose
g.p. kidney (antigen)
g.p. kidney absorption (test)
g.p. serum
L-gulonate dehydrogenase
gum
    g. arabic
    g. karaya
gumma (pl., gummas, gummata)
    syphilitic g.
    tuberculous g.
gummatous
    g. abscess
    g. syphilid
    g. ulcer
gummosa
    periarteritis g.
gummy
Gumprecht's shadows
Gun Hill hemoglobin
gunshot wound
Günzberg's
    reagent
    test
GUS — genitourinary system
Gussenbauer's artifical larynx
gustatory
    g. glands
    g. pathway
gustin
GUSTO — Global Utilization of Streptokinase and Tissue Plasminogen Activator for Occluded Coronary Arteries
gut-associated lymphoid tissue
Guthrie's
    bacterial inhibition assay
    test
Gutman unit
guttural gland
Gutzeit's test
GV — gentian violet
GVH — graft versus host
GVH disease
GVHR — graft-versus-host reaction
GVH reaction
GXT — graded exercise test

Gymnoascus
gymnobacterium
gymnocyte
Gymnodinium
gymnoplast
GYN — gynecology
gynandrism
gynandroblastoma
gynandromorphism
gynecogen
gynecography
gynecoid
gynecologic
Gynecological Oncology Group
gynecologist
gynecology
gynecomastia; gynecomasty
gynogenesis
gyrate
gyrus (pl., gyri)
    angular g.
    g. breves insulae
    callosal g.
    callosomarginal g.
    cingulate g.
    dentate g.
    fasciolar g.
    g. fornicatus

    fusiform g.
    hippocampal g.
    inferior frontal g.
    inferior occipital g.
    inferior temporal g.
    intralimbic g.
    lateral occipital g.
    lateral olfactory g.
    lingual g.
    g. longus
    marginal g.
    medial olfactory g.
    middle frontal g.
    middle temporal g.
    occipitotemporal g.
    orbital g.
    parietal g.
    postcentral g.
    posterior parietal g.
    precentral g.
    g. rectus
    subcallosal g.
    superior frontal g.
    superior occipital g.
    superior temporal g.
    supracallosal g.
    supramarginal g.
GZ — Guilford-Zimmerman personality test

H — henry
    Holzknecht unit
    horizontal
    hormone
    Hounsfield unit
    hydrogen
    hypermetropia
H — Hauch (motile microorganism)
H. — *Haemophilus*
^{1}H — protium
^{2}H — deuterium
^{3}H — tritium
H$^+$ — hydrogen ion
h — hour(s)
    Planck's constant
H-2^b mouse cells

HA — headache
    height age
    hemadsorbent
    hemagglutinating antibody
    hemagglutination
    hemolytic anemia
    hyaluronic acid
    hydroxyapatite
Ha — hahnium
HAA — hepatitis-associated antigen
Haagensen and Stout criteria
Haagensen test
HABA — hydroxybenzeneazobenzoic acid
habenula (pl., habenulae)
habenular commissure

habenulopeduncular tract nucleus
Haber-Weiss reaction
habitual abortion
habituation
habitus
          asthenic h.
          hypersthenic h.
          hyposthenic h.
          sthenic h.
Habronema
HAD — hemadsorption
Haemadipsa
Haemagogus
Haemaphysalis
          H. concinna
          H. leporispalustris
          H. spinigera
Haemate P
Haematopinus
haemin
Haemogregarina
Haemonchus
          H. contortus
          H. placei
Haemonetics V50 apheresis machine
Haemophilus
          H. aegyptius
          H. aphrophilus
          H. bovis
          H. bronchisepticus
          H. conjunctivitidis
          H. ducreyi
          H. duplex
          H. gallinarum
          H. haemoglobinophilus
          H. haemolyticus
          H. influenzae
          H. parahaemolyticus
          H. parainfluenzae
          H. parapertussis
          H. paraphrohaemolyticus
          H. paraphrophilus
          H. pertussis
          H. suis
          H. vaginalis
haemophilus
          h. of Koch-Weeks
          h. of Morax-Axenfeld
Haemophilus pertussis vaccine
Haemosporina
Hafnia alvei
hafnium

Hageman factor
H agglutination
H agglutinin
Hahn's oxine reagent
HAHTG — horse antihuman thymus
          globulin
HAI — hemagglutination inhibition
          hemagglutinin inhibition
hair
          h. ball
          beaded h.
          h. bundle
          h. cell
          h. follicle nevus
          h. follicle receptors
          ingrown h.
          lanugo h.
          Schridde's cancer h's
          telogen h.
hairy
          h. cell leukemia
          h. cells
          h. heart
          h. leukoplakia
          h. mole
          h. nevus
hal. — halothane
halazone
Haldane effect
Haldol
Hale's colloidal iron stain
half-bandwidth
half-cell
half-life
          antibody h.-1.
          biologic h.-1.
          drug h.-1.
          effective h.-1.
          physical h.-1.
          terminal h.-1.
half-maximum
half-reaction
half-time
          gastric emptying h.-t.
          plasma iron clearance h.-t.
half-value layer
half-wave
          h.-w. potential
          h.-w. rectifier
halide
halisteresis
halisteretic

Hall's method
hallucination
hallucinatory
hallucinogen
hallux (pl., halluces)
    h. valgus
    h. varus
halo
    anemic h.
    h. melanoma
    h. nevus
halogen
halogenated hydrocarbon assays
halogenation
halometer
haloperidol assay
halophile
haloprogin
halosteresis
halothane
    h. assay
    h. hepatitis
Halsted's mastectomy
hamartia
hamartoblastoma
hamartochondromatosis
hamartoma
    chondromatous h.
    cutaneous h.
    epididymal h.
    fibromyomatous h.
    fibrous h. of infancy
    leiomyomatous h.
    melanotic h.
    pulmonary h.
    sclerosing epithelial h.
hamartomatous
    h. adiposity
    h. polyp
    h. thymoma
hamate
hamatospectroscopy
hamatum
Hamburger's
    interchange
    law
    phenomenon
Hamilton Rating Scale
Hamilton's pseudophlegmon
Hammarsten's reagent
Hammerschlag's method
Hammersmith's hemoglobin

hammer toe
hamster
hamstring
Ham test
hamular
hamulus (pl., hamuli)
H and D curve
H and E — hematoxylin and eosin
H and E staining
hand
    crab h.
    ghoul h.
    h.-foot-and-mouth disease
    h.-foot syndrome
    opera-glass h.
    skeleton h.
    spade h.
    trident h.
handling
    toxic chemical h.
Hand-Schüller-Christian type histiocyte
H and V — hemigastrectomy and vagotomy
Hanes equation
Hangar-Rose skin test antigen
Hanger's test
hanging-block culture
hanging-drop culture
hanging groin
hangnail
Hanker-Yates reagent
Hank's solution
Hanot's cirrhosis
Hansel's secretion stain
Hansemann macrophage
Hansen's bacillus
Hansenula
Hantaan virus
H antigen
HAP — heredopathia atactica polyneuritiformis
    histamine phosphate acid
HAPA — hemagglutinating antipenicillin antibody
hapalonychia
haplodistinct
haploid
    h. genome
    h. number
haploidentical
haploidy

haplophase
Haplorchis
haplosomic
haplotype association studies
hapten
    group A h.
haptenic grouping
haptocorrin
haptoglobin (Hp)
    Hp 1 and Hp 2 assay
haptophore
hard
    h. chancre
    h. papilloma
    h. sore
    h. tissue
    h. tubercle
    h. ulcer
hardened pelvis
harderoporphyrin
Harding-Passey melanoma
hardness
Hardy-Weinberg
    equation
    law
harelip
Hargraves' cell
Harleco synthetic resin
harlequin
    h. color change
    h. fetus
harmaline
harmine
harmonic mean
Harris'
    alum hematoxylin
    hematoxylin
Harris and Ray test
Harrison's
    groove
    spot test
Hartmannella hyalina
Harvard criteria of irreversible coma
harvester's lung
harvest mite
Häser's formula
Hasharon hemoglobin
HASHD — hypertensive arteriosclerotic heart disease
Hashimoto's
    struma
    thyroiditis

hashish
hashitoxicosis
Hassall's corpuscle
Hasselbalch's equation
HAT — heparin-associated thrombocytopenia
    hypoxanthine-aminopterin-thymidine
Hauch (motile microorganism)
haupt-agglutinin
haustrum (pl., haustra)
HAV — hepatitis A virus
Haverhill fever
Haverhillia
    H. moniliformis
    H. multiformis
haversian
    h. canal
    h. glands
    h. lamella
    h. system
Hawaii agent
hawkinsin
hawkinsinuria
Haworth formula
Hayem's
    corpuscle
    hematoblast
    solution
Hayem-Widal anemia
hay fever
Hayflick's limit
Haygarth's nodes
hazard
    h. identification
    radiation h.
    h. symbol
hazardous
    h. concentration
    h. materials
    h. materials labeling
    h. substances
HB — heart block
    hepatitis B
Hb — hemoglobin
HBABA — hydroxybenzeneazobenzoic acid
H band
HBB — hydroxybenzyl benzimidazole
Hb Barts — Bart's hemoglobin
HB_cAg — hepatitis B core antigen
Hb Co — carboxyhemoglobin

HBD or HBDH — hydroxybutyrate
     dehydrogenase
HB_eAg — hepatitis B E antigen
HBF — hepatic blood flow
HbF — fetal hemoglobin
HBI — high serum-bound iron
HBO — hyperbaric oxygen
HbO_2 — oxyhemoglobin
HBP — high blood pressure
HBr — hydrobromic acid
HB_sAg — hepatitis B surface
    antigen
HBV — hepatitis B virus
HBW — high birth weight
HC — hair cell
  head compression
  hepatic catalase
  Huntington's chorea
  hyaline casts
  hydroxycorticoid
HCC — hydroxycholecalciferol
H cell
hCG or HCG — human chorionic
     gonadotropin
  h. α subunit
  h. β subunit
HCH — hexachlorocyclohexane
H chain (heavy chain)
HCHO — formaldehyde
HCL — hairy-cell leukemia
HCl — hydrochloric acid
HCN — hydrocyanic acid
HCO_3 — bicarbonate
H colony
HCP — hepatocatalase peroxidase
  hereditary coproporphyria
hCS or hCSM — human chorionic
     somatomammo-
     tropin
HCT — hematocrit
  homocytotrophic
  hydrochlorothiazide
HCU — homocystinuria
HCVD — hypertensive cardiovascu-
  lar disease
HD — heart disease
  high dosage
  Hodgkin's disease
  hydatid disease
HDAg — hepatitis D antigen
HDC — histidine decarboxylase

HDH — heart disease history
HDL or HDLP — high-density lipo-
    protein
HDN — hemolytic disease of the
    newborn
HDP — hydroxydimethylpyrimidine
HDS — herniated disk syndrome
H & E — hematoxylin and eosin
HE — hereditary elliptocytosis
  human enteric
He — helium
head
  angular h.
  articular h.
  bulldog h.
  coronoid h.
  humeral h.
  infraorbital h.
  lateral h.
  h. louse
  mandibular h.
  medial h.
  Medusa h.
  oblique h.
  plantar h.
  quadrate h.
  radial h.
  scapular h.
  h. space analysis
  transverse h.
  ulnar h.
  zygomatic h.
headache
Heaf test
Health Maintenance Organizations
heart
  abdominal h.
  h. antigen
  armored h.
  h. block
  bony h.
  cervical h.
  h. disease
  disordered action of h.
  drop h.
  extracorporeal h.
  h. failure
  h. failure cells
  fatty h.
  frosted h.
  hairy h.
  h.-hand syndrome

hydroplastic h.
icing h.
h. infusion agar
intracorporeal h.
h.-lung machine
h.-lung preparation
luxus h.
moveable h.
myxedema h.
parchment h.
pendulous h.
h. sound
tiger h.
trilocular h.
h. tumors
valvular disease of h.
heartbeat
heartburn
heartworm
dog h.
HEAT — human erythrocyte agglutination test
heat
h. capacity
h. coagulation test
h. of combustion
h. edema
h. exhaustion
h. of formation
h. of fusion
h. instability test
h. intolerance
h.-killed *Listeria monocytogenes*
h. labile
h. labile test
latent h.
molar h. capacity
h. precipitation test
h. prostration
h. of reaction
h.-resistant glass
h.-shock protein
h. sink
h. of solution
specific h.
specific h. capacity
h. stroke
h. of sublimation
h. unit
h. of vaporization
heat-stable
h.-s. alkaline phosphatase
h.-s. lactic dehydrogenase

heavy
h. chain
h.-chain disease
h. metal poisoning
h. metals
h. metal screen
h. particle therapy
heavy-chain disease
α-heavy-chain disease
β-heavy-chain disease
μ-heavy-chain disease
hebephrenic schizophrenia
Heberden's node
HEC — hydroxyergocalciferol
Hecht's pneumonia
hectogram
hectometer
HED — Haut-Einheits-Dosis (unit of roentgen ray dosage)
heel
cracked h's
gonorrheal h.
Hegar's sign
Hegglin's anomaly
Heidenhain's
azan stain
cell
iron hematoxylin
iron hematoxylin stain
Susa fixative
height
peak h.
Heinz
bodies
body hemolytic anemia
body stain
body test
Heinz-Ehrlich bodies
Heister's valve
HEK — human embryo kidney
human embryonic kidney
Hektoen
agar
enteric agar
HEL — human embryo lung
HeLa cells
Held's
end bulb
space
Heleidae
helenine
helianthine

helical
helicis
Helicobacter pylori
    H.p. serology
    H.p. urease test and culture
helicotrema
heliotrope rash
helium
    h. equilibration time
    h. isotope
helix
    α-h.
    double h.
    right-handed α-h.
    Watson-Crick h.
hellebore
helle Zellen
HELLP — hemolysis, elevated liver
        enzymes, low platelets
HELLP syndrome
Helly's
    fixative
    fluid
helmet cell
helminth identification procedures
helminthiasis
helminthic
    h. appendicitis
    h. disease
    h. infection
helminthism
helminthology
helminthoma
Helminthosporium
Heloderma
Helophilus
helper
    h. cell
    h.-suppressor cell ratio
    h. T cells
    h. T lymphocyte
Helvella esculenta
hemachromatosis
hemachrome
hemachrosis
hemacytometer
hemacytometry
hemadsorption
    mixed h.
    h. test
    h. virus, types 1, 2
hemafacient

hemagglutinating
    h. antibody
    h. anti-penicillin antibody
    h. cold autoantibody
    h. unit
hemagglutination
    h. assay
    indirect h.
    h. inhibition antibody
    h. inhibition test
    passive h.
    reverse passive h.
    h. test
    h. titer
    viral h.
hemagglutinin
    autologous h.
    cold h.
    heterologous h.
    homologous h.
    h. inhibition
    warm h.
Hem-Aliquanter dilutor
hemal lymph glands
Hemalog counter
hemalum
hemanalysis
hemangiectatic hypertrophy
hemangioblast
hemangioblastoma
    cerebral h.
    retinal h.
    spinal h.
hemangioblastomatosis
hemangioendothelial sarcoma
hemangioendothelioblastoma
hemangioendothelioma
    epithelioid h.
    infantile h.
    h. tuberosum multiplex
    vertebral h.
hemangioendotheliosarcoma
hemangiofibroma
hemangiolipoma
hemangioma
    ameloblastic h.
    arterial h.
    arteriovenous h.
    capillary h.
    cavernous h.
    cerebral h.
    h. congenitale

hepatic h.
infantile h.
intramuscular h.
juvenile h.
laryngeal h.
mucosal h.
nuchal h.
h. planum extensum
racemose h.
sclerosing h.
senile h.
h. simplex
strawberry h.
h.-thrombocytopenia syndrome
hemangiomatosis
hemangiopericytic
hemangiopericytoma
hemangiosarcoma
hemapheic
hemaphein
hemapheism
hemapheresis
hemarthritis
hemarthrosis
hemastrontium
hematal
hematapostema
hematein
    Baker's acid h.
    h. test
hematemesis
hematencephalon
Hematest
hematherapy
hemathidrosis
hemathorax
hematic
hematid
hematidrosis
hematimeter
hematin
    acid h.
    acid formaldehyde h.
    h. albumin
    h. crystals
    h. pigmentation
    reduced h.
hematinemia
hematinic principle
hematobilia
hematoblast
    Hayem's h.

hematocele
    parametric h.
    pudendal h.
    retrouterine h.
    scrotal h.
    vaginal h.
hematocelia
hematochezia
hematochlorin
hematochyluria
hematoclasis
hematoclastic
hematocrit
    large vessel h.
    mean circulatory h.
    total body h.
    venous h.
    whole-blood h.
    Wintrobe h.
hematocrystallin
hematocyst
hematocystis
hematocyte
hematocytoblast
hematocytolysis
hematocytometer
hematocytometry
hematocytopenia
hematocyturia
hematodyscrasia
hematodystrophy
hematoencephalic barrier
hematofluorometry
hematogen
hematogenesis
hematogenic
hematogenous
    h. tuberculosis
hematoglobin
hematogone
hematohistioblast
hematohyaloid
hematoid cancer
hematoidin
    h. crystals
    h. pigmentation
hematologic
hematological
hematologist
hematology
hematolymphangioma
hematolysis

hematolytic
hematoma
    chronic subdural h.
    corpus luteum h.
    dissecting h.
    epidural h.
    intramural h.
    organized h.
    subdural h.
hematometra
hematometry
hematonic
hematopathology
hematopathy
hematopenia
hematophilia
hematoplastic
hematopneic index
hematopoiesis
    embryonic h.
    extramedullary h.
    fetal h.
    megaloblastic h.
    myeloid h.
    postnatal h.
hematopoietic
    h. aplasia
    h. cell cytoplasmic alteration
    h. glands
    h. growth factors
    h. hyperplasia
    h. hypoplasia
    h. maturation
    h. maturation alteration
    h. maturation arrest
    h. stem cell
    h. system
    h. tissue
hematopoietin
    panspecific (interleukin-3) h.
hematoporphyrin
hematoporphyrinemia
hematoporphyrinuria
hematosalpinx
hematosepsis
hematoside
hematosis
hematospectroscope
hematospectroscopy
hematospermatocele
hematospermia
hematostasis

hematostatic
hematotoxic
hematotoxicosis
hematotoxin
hematotropic
hematoxin
hematoxylin
    h. body
    Boehmer's h.
    Carazzi's h.
    Clara's h.
    Cole's h.
    Delafield's h.
    h.-eosin stain
    h.-eosin staining
    Harris' alum h.
    Harris' h.
    Heidenhain's iron h. stain
    iron h.
    Lillie's h.
    h.-malachite green-basic
        fuchsin stain
    Mayer's h.
    h.-phloxine B stain
    phosphotungstic acid h.
    Weigert's iron h. stain
hematoxyphil bodies
hematozemia
Hematrak counter
hematuresis
hematuria
    essential h.
    false h.
    gross h.
    initial h.
    microscopic h.
    renal h.
    terminal h.
    total h.
    urethral h.
    vesical h.
hematuric bilious fever
heme
    h. oxygenase
    h. synthesis
    h. synthetase
hemendothelioma
hemerythrins
hemiacardius
hemiacetal
hemianalgesia
hemianesthesia

hemianopia
hemianopsia
    binasal h.
    bitemporal h.
    homonymous h.
hemiaplasia
hemiatrophy
    facial h.
hemiazygos vein
hemiballismus
hemiblock
hemic
    h. calculus
    h. parasite
hemichrome
hemicolectomy
hemidesmosome
hemidiaphoresis
hemidrosis
hemidysplasia
    congenital h.
hemiepiglottis
hemifacial
hemigastrectomy
hemiglobin cyanide
hemiglossal
hemiglossectomy
hemihepatectomy
hemihidrosis
hemihyperhidrosis
hemihypertrophy
hemilaryngectomy
hemilesion
hemimandibulectomy
hemimandibulotomy
hemimaxillectomy
hemimelia
hemin
heminephrectomy
heminephroureterectomy
hemiparesis
hemiplegia
Hemiptera
hemipyonephrosis
hemispheral
    h. lobule
    h. sublobule
hemisphere
    cerebral h.
hemispheric
Hemispora stellata
hemisyndrome

hemizygosity
hemizygous genes
hemoagglutination
hemobartonellosis
hemobilia
hemoblast
    lymphoid h. of Pappenheim
    Pappenheim's lymphoid h.
hemoblastic leukemia
hemoblastosis
hemocatharsis
hemocatheresis
hemocatheretic
Hemoccult test
hemocholecyst
hemocholecystitis
hemochromatoic
hemochromatosis
    exogenous h.
hemochromogen
hemochromometry
hemoclasis; hemoclasia
hemoclastic
    h. reaction
    h. shock
hemocoagulin
hemocoelom
hemoconcentration
hemoconia
hemoconiosis
hemocryoscopy
hemocyanin
    keyhole-limpet h.
hemocystinuria
hemocyt. — hemocytometer
hemocyte
hemocytoblast
hemocytoblastic leukemia
hemocytoblastoma
hemocytocatheresis
hemocytolysis
hemocytoma
hemocytometer
hemocytometry
hemocytophagia
hemocytotripsis
hemodiagnosis
hemodialysis
    peritoneal h.
hemodialyzer
    ultrafiltration h.
hemodiapedesis

hemodilution
hemodynamic
    h. fat embolism
    h. gas embolism
    h. hemorrhage
    h. hyperemia
    h. infarction
    h. pulmonary embolism
    h. shock
    h. system embolism
    h. thrombogenesis
    h. thrombosis
hemodyscrasia
hemodystrophy
hemofiltration
hemoflagellate
hemofuscin pigmentation
hemogenesis
hemogenic
hemoglobin
    h. A_{1a}
    h. A_{1b}
    h. A_{1c}
    h. A_2
    aberrant h.
    acetylated h.
    adult h.
    h. assay
    Bart's h.
    bile pigment h.
    h. Bristol
    h. C
    h. carbamate
    carbon monoxide h.
    carbonyl h.
    h. cast
    h. C-beta thalassemia
    h. C Georgetown
    h. C Harlem
    h. Chesapeake
    h. Constant Spring
    h. C trait
    h. C–type thalassemia
    h. D
    h. demonstration in tissue
    denatured h.
    deoxygenated h.
    h. D Punjab
    h. E
    h. electrophoresis
    embryonic h.
    encapsulated h.

h. E–type thalassemia
h. F
"fast" h's
fetal h.
glycosylated h.
h. Gower-1
h. Gower-2
green h.
Gun Hill h.
h. H
h. Hammersmith
h. Hasharon
hereditary persistence of fe-
    tal h.
h. I
h. identification
h. Indianapolis
intracellular h.
h. J Capetown
h. Kansas
Kenya h.
Köln h.
h. Lepore
h. M
mean cell h.
mean corpuscular h.
muscle h.
mutant h.
nitric oxide h.
oxidized h.
oxygenated h.
oxygen half-saturation pressure
    of h.
h. pigmentation
h. Portland
h. Rainier
reduced h.
h. S
h. SC-alpha thalassemia
h. Seattle
sickle-cell h.
"slow" h's
h. SO Arab sickle disease
stroma-free h.
h. test
h. thalassemia
total circulating h.
un-ionized h.
unstable h.
variant h.
h. Yakima
h. Zurich

hemoglobinated
hemoglobinemia
hemoglobinocholia
hemoglobinolysis
hemoglobinometer
hemoglobinometry
hemoglobinopathy
    heterozygous h.
    homozygous h.
    mixed h.
hemoglobinopepsia
hemoglobinorrhea
hemoglobinous
hemoglobinuria
    bacillary h.
    cold h.
    epidemic h.
    malarial h.
    march h.
    nocturnal h.
    paroxysmal cold h.
    paroxysmal nocturnal h.
    toxic h.
hemoglobinuric
    h. nephropathy
    h. nephrosis
hemogram
hemohistioblast
hemokinesis
hemokinetic
hemolamella
hemoleukocyte
hemolith
hemology
hemolymph
    h. glands
    h. heteroagglutinin
    h. node
hemolymphangioma
hemolysate
hemolysin
    alpha h.
    bacterial h.
    beta h.
    D-L h.
    heterophilic h.
    hot-cold h.
    immune h.
    h. test
    h. unit
hemolysinogen

hemolysis
    alpha h.
    beta h.
    colloid osmotic h.
    compensated h.
    drug-induced h.
    extravascular h.
    extrinsic h.
    gamma h.
    hepatic h.
    hyperbaric h.
    hypotonic h.
    immune-mediated h.
    h. interference
    intramedullary h.
    intravascular h.
    isoimmune h.
    neonatal h.
    nonimmune h.
    osmotic h.
    oxidant h.
    passive h.
    traumatic h.
hemolytic
    h. amboceptor
    h. anemia
    h. anemia of newborn
    h. crisis
    h. disease of newborn
    h. gas
    h. index
    h. jaundice
    h. malaria
    h. reaction
    h. splenomegaly
    β-h. streptococcus
    h. substance
    h. transfusion reaction
    h. unit
    h. uremia
    h. uremic syndrome
hemolyzable
hemolyzation
hemolyze
hemolyzed erythrocyte
hemometry
hemonephrosis
hemopathology
hemopathy
hemoperfusion
hemopericardium
hemoperitoneum

hemopexin
hemophagocyte
hemophagocytic
    h. reticulosis
    h. syndrome
hemophagocytosis
hemophil
hemophilia
    h. A (classic)
    h. B (Christmas disease)
    h. B Leyden
    h. Bm
    h. C
    classic h.
    h. neonatorum
    vascular h.
hemophiliac
hemophilic
    h. arthritis
    h. factor A
hemophilioid
Hemophilus (see *Haemophilus*)
hemophoresis
hemophthalmia
hemophthisis
hemoplastic
hemoplasty
hemopneumopericardium
hemopneumothorax
hemopoiesic diuretic
hemopoiesis
hemopoietic
hemopoietin
hemoprecipitin
hemoprotein
hemopsonin
hemoptysis
    cardiac h.
    endemic h.
    oriental h.
    parasitic h.
    vicarious h.
hemopyelectasis; hemopyelectasia
Hemo-Quant test
hemorepellant
hemorrhage
    antepartum h.
    aortic h.
    cerebral h.
    Duret h.
    extradural h.
    fibrinolytic h.
    gastrointestinal h.

    gingival h.
    hemodynamic h.
    intracerebral h.
    intracranial h.
    intraperitoneal h.
    intraventricular h.
    petechial h.
    postpartum h.
    pulmonary h.
    recurring h.
    renal h.
    retinal h.
    subarachnoid h.
    subdural h.
    transplacental h.
hemorrhagic
    acute h. bronchopneumonia
    acute h. cholecystitis
    acute h. cystitis
    acute h. glomerulonephritis
    acute h. inflammation
    acute h. ulcer
    acute h. ulceration
    h. anemia
    h. ascites
    h. bronchopneumonia
    h. colitis
    h. cyst
    h. cystitis
    h. dengue
    h. diathesis
    h. disease of newborn
    h. diverticulitis
    h. effusion
    h. endovasculitis
    h. fever
    h. fever epidemic
    h. gangrene
    h. gastritis
    h. gastroenteropathy
    h. glomerulonephritis
    h. infarct
    h. infarction
    h. (red) infarction
    h. inflammation
    h. internal pachymeningitis
    h. leukoencephalitis
    h. lobar pneumonia
    h. malaria
    h. necrosis
    h. nephritis
    h. nodule

h. pancreatitis
h. pericarditis
h. plague
h. pleurisy
h. pleuritis
h. pneumonia
h. pneumonitis
h. rickets
h. shock
h. smallpox
h. thrombocythemia
h. ulcer
h. varicella syndrome
hemorrhagicum
    cystic corpus h.
hemorrhagins
hemorrhoid
    cutaneous h's
    external h's
    internal h's
    thrombosed h's
hemorrhoidal
    h. artery
    h. nerve
    h. vein
    h. zone
hemosiderin
    h. deposition
    h.-laden macrophage
    h. pigment
    h. stain
    h. staining
hemosiderinuria test
hemosiderosis
    endogenous h.
    exogenous h.
    hepatic h.
    idiopathic pulmonary h.
    local h.
    pulmonary h.
    secondary pulmonary h.
    systemic h.
    transfusion h.
hemosiderotic
hemospermia
    h. spuria
    h. vera
hemosporian; hemosporidian
hemostasia; hemostasis
hemostat
hemostatic plug
hemotherapy; hemotherapeutics

hemothorax
hemotoxic anemia
hemotoxin
hemotropic
hemotympanum
hemozoin
hempa
HEMPAS — hereditary erythrocytic
                  multinuclearity with
                  positive acidified
                  serum
HEMPAS test
hemuresis
Henderson-Hasselbalch equation
Henle's
    loop
    reaction
Henoch-Schönlein purpura
Henoch's purpura
henpuye
henry
Henry fructose test
Henry's law
Hensen's node
HEPA — high-efficiency particulate
             air (filter)
Hepadenaviridae
hepar (gen., hepatis)
    h. adiposum
    h. lobatum
heparan-N-sulfatase
heparan sulfate
heparin
    h. cofactor
    h. sodium
    h. unit
heparinase
heparinate
heparinemia
heparinic acid
heparinize
heparin-precipitable fraction
heparitin sulfate lyase
heparitin sulphate lyase
hepatatrophia; hepatatrophy
hepatectomy
hepatic
    h. abscess
    h. angiosarcoma
    h. artery
    h. blood flow
    h. branch, vagus nerve

h. capsule
h. capsulitis
h. clearance
h. coma
h. congestion
h. cords
h. cysts
h. docimasia
h. duct
h. encephalopathy/coma
h. failure
h. fibrosis
h. fistula
h. flexure
h. glands
h. glycogen
h. hemangioma
h. hemolysis
h. hemorrhage
h. infarction
h. leukemia
h. lipase
h. lobes
h. lobule
h. lymph nodes
h. ophthalmia
h. osteomalacia
h. parenchyma
h. porphyria
h. portal venous gas
h. prolylhydroxylase
h. sinusoid
h. steatosis
h. triads
h. triglyceride lipase
h. vein
h. veno-occlusive disease
hepatica
    adiposis h.
hepaticojejunostomy
hepatis
hepatitic
hepatitis (pl., hepatitides)
    h. A
    h. A antibody
    acute focal h.
    acute parenchymatous h.
    acute viral h.
    alcoholic h.
    amebic h.
    anicteric h.
    h. antibody

h. antigen
h.-associated antigen
autoimmune h.
A virus h.
h. A virus
h. B
h. B antibody
h. B core antibody
h. B core antigen
h. B E antigen
h. B immune globulin
h. B surface antibody
h. B surface antigen
h. B surface antigen tests
B virus h.
h. B virus
h. C
cholangiolitic h.
cholestatic h.
chronic h.
chronic active h.
chronic interstitial h.
chronic persistent h.
coxsackievirus h.
h. C serology
h. C virus
cytomegalovirus h.
delta h.
drug-induced h.
h. D serology
h. E
epidemic h.
h. externa
fulminant h.
giant cell h.
gonococcal h.
halothane h.
homologous serum h.
icteric h.
infectious h.
ischemic h.
long incubation h.
lupoid h.
lupus h.
neonatal h.
non-A h., non-B h.
h. non-A—non-B virus
peliosis h.
persistent chronic h.
plasma cell h.
post-transfusion h.
serum h.

short incubation h.
Simbu h.
subacute h.
suppurative h.
syphilitic h.
transfusion h.
unresolved h.
viral h.
viral h., type A
viral h., type B
h. virus
hepatization
    gray h.
    red h.
    yellow h.
hepatoadrenal
hepatobiliary
hepatoblastoma
hepatocarcinogenesis models
hepatocarcinoma
hepatocatalase peroxidase
hepatocele
hepatocellular
    h. adenoma
    h. bile carcinoma
    h. carcinoma
    h. cholestasis
    h. injury
    h. jaundice
hepatocholangitis
hepatocuprein
hepatocyte
hepatoduodenal ligament
hepatoerythropoietic porphyria
hepatogenic; hepatogenous
hepatogram
hepatohemia
hepatoid
hepatojugular reflux
hepatolenticular
    h. degeneration
    h. disease
hepatolienography
hepatolienomegaly
hepatolith
hepatolithiasis
hepatoma
    fibrolamellar h.
    malignant h.
hepatomalacia
hepatomegaly; hepatomegalia
hepatomelanosis

hepatonecrosis
hepatonephromegaly
hepatopancreatic
hepatoperitonitis
hepatophlebography
hepatophosphorylase deficiency
hepatophosphorylase deficiency glyco-
    genosis
hepatophyma
hepatopleural fistula
hepatopoietin
hepatoptosis
hepatorenal
    h. glycogenosis
    h. ligament
    h. syndrome
hepatorrhexis
hepatoscan
hepatosplenic candidiasis
hepatosplenitis
hepatosplenography
hepatosplenomegaly
hepatosplenometry
hepatosplenopathy
hepatotomy
hepatotoxemia
hepatotoxicity
heptabarbital
heptachlor epoxide
heptachlorocamphene
heptachlorocyclopentadiene
heptaene
heptane
heptanoate
heptanoic acid
Heptavax B
heptoglobin
heptoglobinemia
herald patch
herbicide
    chlorophenoxy h.
herd immunity
hereditary
    h. adynamia
    h. amyloidosis
    h. angioedema
    h. angioneurotic edema
    h. ataxia telangiectasia
    h. benign intraepithelial dysker-
        atosis
    h. coproporphyria
    h. deforming chondrodysplasia

h. deforming chondrodystrophy
h. elliptocytosis
h. enzymatic-type methemoglobinemia
h. eosinophilia
h. erythroblastic multinuclearity
h. fructose intolerance
h. hemolytic anemia
h. hemorrhagic telangiectasia
h. hemorrhagic thrombasthenia
h. hydrocytosis
h. hyperbilirubinemia
h. hypersegmentation of neutrophils
h. hypocholinesterasemia
h. interstitial nephritis
h. iron-loading anemia
h. lymphedema
h. methemoglobinemia
h. methemoglobinemic cyanosis
h. multiple exostoses
h. multiple trichoepithelioma
h. nephritis
h. nonhemolytic bilirubinemia
b. nonspherocytic hemolytic anemia
h. osteo-onchodysplasia
h. persistence of fetal hemoglobin
h. plasmathromboplastin component
h. plasmathromboplastin component deficiency
h. porphyria
h. progressive arthroophthalmopathy
h. renal-retinal dysplasia
h. sensory motor neuropathy
h. sideroblastic anemia
h. spherocytosis
h. stomatocytosis
heredity
autosomal h.
sex-linked h.
X-linked h.
heredofamilial
heredopathia atactica polyneuritiformis
Herellea vaginicola

Hering-Breuer reflex
Hering's
canal
nerve
heritable
Hermann's fixative
hermaphrodism
hermaphroditism
Hermetia illucens
hermetic seal
HER-2/*neu* oncogene
hernia
diaphragmatic h.
epigastric h.
esophageal h.
femoral h.
hiatal h.
incarcerated h.
inguinal h.
irreducible h.
Morgagni's h.
mucous h.
paraesophageal hiatal h.
peritoneal h.
retrocolic h.
retrosternal h.
Richter's h.
rolling h.
sliding h.
strangulated h.
umbilical h.
hernial aneurysm
herniated
h. disk syndrome
h. nucleus pulposus
herniation
cerebral h.
subfalcine h.
tonsillar cerebellar h.
transtentorial h.
hernioplasty
herniorrhaphy
heroin
herpangina virus
herpes
anorectal h.
h. corneae
h. cytology
h. encephalitis
h. febrilis
h. genitalis
h. gestationis

h. gingivostomatitis
h. iris
h. keratoconjunctivitis
h. labialis
h.-like virus
pharyngeal h.
h. simplex
h. simplex antibody
h. simplex pneumonia
h. simplex virus (1 and 2)
h. simplex virus culture
h. simplex virus isolation
h.-type virus
h. zoster
h. zoster ophthalmicus
h. zoster-varicella infection
h. zoster virus
Herpesviridae
Herpesvirus
    H. hominis
    H. simiae
herpesvirus
    h. antigen
    h. blister
    human h.-6
herpetic
    h. blister
    h. conjunctivitis
    h. esophagitis
    h. gingivostomatitis
    h. keratitis
    h. paronychia
    h. proctitis
    h. stomatitis
    h. viral disease
    h. whitlow
herpetiformis
    dermatitis h.
Herpetomonas
    H. donovani
    H. furunculosa
    H. tropica
Herrick's anemia
Herring bodies
herringbone
herring-worm disease
hertz
Herxheimer's
    reaction
    spiral
Heryng's sign
HES — hydroxyethyl starch
HET — helium equilibration time

hetastarch
HETE — hydroxyeicosatetraenoic
    acid
heterauxesis
heterecious
heteroagglutination
heteroagglutinin
    hemolymph h.
heteroallele
heteroantibody
heteroantigen
heteroatom
Heterobilharzia
heteroblastic
heterobrachial inversion
heterocellular
heterochromatic
heterochromatin
    constitutive h.
    facultative h.
heterochromatinization
heterochromia
heterochromic iridocyclitis
heterochromous
heterochthonous
heterocliticity
heterocrine glands
heterocycle
heterocyclic compound
heterocytotropic antibody
Heterodera
    H. marioni
    H. radicicola
heterodimer
heteroduplex
heterodyne
heterofermentation
heterogamete
heterogametic sex
heterogamy
heterogeneic
heterogeneity
    genetic h.
    intratumor h.
heterogeneous
    h. nuclear RNA
    h. nucleation
    h. radiation
heterogenetic
    h. antibody
    h. antigen
heterogenic

heterogenote
heterogenous nuclear RNA
heteroglobulose
heterogony
heterograft
heterohemagglutination
heterohemagglutinin
heterohemolysin
heteroimmune
heteroimmunity
heterokaryon
heterokaryosis
heterokaryotic twins
heterolactic
heterologous
    h. antigen
    h. chimera
    h. graft
    h. hemagglutinin
    h. serum
    h. tumor
heterology
heterolysis
heterolysosome
heterolytic cleavage
heterometaplasia
heteromorphic
    h. bivalent
    h. chromosomes
heterophagic vacuole
heterophagocytosis
heterophagosome
heterophagy
heterophil; heterophile
    h. agglutinins
    h. antibody test
    h. (Paul-Bunnell) antibody
    h. antigen reaction
    h.-negative mononucleosis
heterophilic
    h. hemolysin
    h. leukocyte
Heterophyes
    H. heterophyes
    H. katsuradai
Heterophyes/Metagonimus
heterophyiasis
heteropinocytosis
heteroplasia
heteroplastic
heteroploid
heteroploidy

heteropolymer
heteropolysaccharide
heteropyknosis
heteropyknotic chromatin
heteroscedasticity
heterosexual
heterosis
heterosomal aberration
heterosome
heterotaxia
    cardiac h.
heterotaxic
heterotaxis; heterotaxy
heterothallism
heterotopia
    adrenal h.
heterotopic
    h. bone
    h. oral gastrointestinal cyst
    h. transplantation
heterotopous
heterotrimer
heterotroph
heterotrophic bacterium
heterotypic mitosis
heterovaccine
heterozygote
    manifesting h.
heterozygosis
heterozygous
    h. gene
    h. hemoglobinopathy
    h. thalassemia
    h. type of hemoglobin disorder
HETP — hexaethyltetraphosphate
Heublein method
Heubner's recurrent artery
heuristic method
hexachloride
    benzene h.
hexachloroacetone
hexachlorobenzene
hexachlorocyclohexane
hexachloroethane
hexachlorophene assay
hexadecanoic acid
hexadecimal
hexaethyl tetraphosphate
hexafluorenium bromide
hexafluorosilicate
    sodium h.
hexamer
hexamethonium bromide

hexamethylenetetramine
hexamethylmelamine
hexamethylpararosanilin
hexamethylphosphoramide
hexamethyl violet
Hexamita
hexane
hexanoate
hexanoic acid
hexaphosphate
    inositol h.
hexapradol
hexavalent
hexazonium salts
hexestrol
hexetidine
hexobarbital
hexocyclium
hexokinase
    h. isoenzyme
    h. method
hexosamine
hexosaminidase
    h. A deficiency
    h. isoenzyme A
hexose
    h. diphosphate
    h. monophosphate
    h. monophosphate pathway
    h. monophosphate shunt
    h.-I-phosphate uridylyl-
        transferase
hexosediphosphatase
hexosephosphate
    h. aminotransferase
    h. dehydrogenase
    h. isomerase
hexosephosphoric esters
hexoside
    ceramide h.
hexosyltransferase
hexulase
hexulose
hexuronate
hexuronic acid
hexylcaine
hexylresorcinol
Heymann's
    glomerulonephritis
    nephritis
HF — Hageman's factor
    hay fever

heart failure
hemorrhagic fever
high flow
high frequency
Hf — hafnium
HFI — hereditary fructose intolerance
HFP — hexafluoropropylene
hFPA — human fibrinopeptide A
Hfr — high-frequency recombination
Hfr mutant
Hg — mercury (L. *hydrargyrum*)
Hg or Hgb — hemoglobin
HGA — homogentisic acid
Hgb — hemoglobin
H (histocompatibility) gene
HGF — hyperglycemic-glycogenolytic
        factor
hGG — human gammaglobulin
hGH — human growth hormone
HGPRT — hypoxanthine guanine
        phosphoribosyl trans-
        ferase
HH — hydroxyhexamide
HHA — hereditary hemolytic anemia
HHb — un-ionized hemoglobin
HHD — hypertensive heart disease
H and Hm — compound hypermetro-
        pic astigmatism
HHT — hereditary hemorrhagic telan-
        giectasia
HI — hemagglutination inhibition
        hydroxyindole
HIA — hemagglutination-inhibition
        antibody
5-HIAA — 5-hydroxyindole-acetic
        acid
hiatal hernia
hiatus
    h. aorticus
    diaphragmatic h.
    h. esophageus
hibernoma
Hickman catheter
Hicks-Pitney thromboplastin genera-
    tion test
hidebound disease
hidradenitis
    h. axillaris of Verneuil
    h. suppurativa
    suppurative h.
hidradenocarcinoma
    clear cell h.

hidradenoma
 clear cell h.
 nodular h.
 papillary h.; h. papilliferum
 solid cystic h.
hidroacanthoma simplex
hidroadenoma
hidrocystoma
 apocrine h.
 eccrine h.
hidrosadenitis
hidrotic ectodermal dysplasia
high
 h.-altitude reaction
 h. birth weight
 h.-density lipoprotein
 h. dosage
 h.-efficiency particulate air
 h.-energy bond
 h.-energy phosphate
 h. eyepoint eyepiece
 h. flow
 h. frequency
 h.-frequency deafness
 h.-frequency recombination
 h.-frequency recombination
  mutant
 h.-grade lymphoma
 h.-grade surface osteosarcoma
 h. level
 h. molecular weight
 h. molecular weight kininogen
 h.-order
 h.-pass filter
 h.-performance liquid chromatography
 h.-peroxidase cells
 h.-power field
 h. pressure
 h.-pressure liquid chromatography
 h. protein
 h.-resolution banding
 h. serum-bound iron
 h.-threshold mechanoreceptor
 h. vacuum
 h. voltage
 h.-voltage electrophoresis
 h.-voltage roentgen therapy
 h.-voltage transformer
 h.-zone tolerance
higher bacteria

Highman's
 Congo red technique
 method for amyloid
Higoumenakia sign
hilar
 h. cell
 h. cell tumor
 h. cell tumor of ovary
 h. cholangiopancreatography
 h. lymph node
 h. node
hilitis
Hill equation
hilum (pl., hila)
hilus (pl., hili)
 h. cells
 h. hepatis
 h. renalis
HIM — hemopoietic inductive micro-
  environment
hindgut
hindrance
 steric h.
Hine-Duley phantom
hinge region
Hinton test
HIOMT — hydroxyindole-O-methyl
  transferase
hip
 h. point
 h. pointer
 snapping h.
Hipeutis
Hippelates
Hippobosca
hippocampal
 h. commissure
 h. fimbria
 h. fissure
 h. gyrus
 h. pressure groove
hippocampus
hippocratic
 h. face
 h. facies
 h. fingers
hippurate
 h. broth
 h. clearance
 h. crystals
 h. hydrolysis test
 h. substrate
hippuria

hippuric
    h. acid
    h. acid excretion test
    h. acid test
Hirano bodies
Hirsch-Pfeiffer stain
hirsutism
    amenorrhea and h.
hirsutoid papilloma
hirud
hirudin
Hirudinea
hirudiniasis
Hirudo (pl., hirudines)
    H. *aegyptiaca*
    H. *medicinalis*
His
    bundle
    space
Hiss's stain
histadyl
Histalog test
histaminase
histamine
    h. acid phosphate
    h. release test
    h.-releasing factor
    h. shock
histaminemia
histaminuria
histidase
histidinase
histidine
    h. alpha-deaminase
    L-h. ammonia-lyase
    analog of h.
    h. decarboxylase
    distal h.
    proximal h.
histidinemia
histidinol dehydrogenase
histidinuria
histidyl
histioblast
histiocyte
    cardiac h.
    Gaucher's-type h.
    Hand-Schüller-Christian-
        type h.
    Niemann-Pick-type h.
    sea-blue h.

histiocytic
    h. granuloma
    h. leukemia
    h. lymphoma
    h. medullary reticulosis
histiocytoma
    cordal h.
    h. cutis
    fibrous h.
    generalized eruptive h.
    malignant fibrous h.
    myxoid malignant fibrous h.
    paratesticular h.
    storiform-pleomorphic malig-
        nant fibrous h.
histiocytosis
    kerasin h.
    kerasin-type h.
    Langerhans' cell h.
    lipid h.
    localized h.
    malignant h.
    nodular non-X h.
    nonlipid h.
    phosphatid h.
    phosphatid-type h.
    regressing atypical h.
    sinus h.
    sinus h. with massive lymph-
        adenopathy
    systemic h.
    h. X
    h. Y
histioid; histoid
histioma
histiotypic growth
histoblast
histochemical stain
histochemistry
histochromatosis
Histoclad
histocompatibility
    h. antigen
    h. complex
    h. gene
    h. locus
    h. testing
histocyte
histocytosis
histodiagnosis
histodifferentiation
histofluorescence

histogenesis
histogram mode
histoid
    h. leprosy
    h. neoplasm
    h. tumor
histoincompatibility
histologic
    h. grading
    h. lesion
    h. staining
histologist
histology
    pathologic h.
histolysis
histolytic
histoma
histometaplastic
Histomonas
histone nucleinate
histonuria
histopathogenesis
histopathology
    synovial h.
Histoplasma
    H. antibody assay
    H. capsulatum
    H. duboisii
    H. farciminosus
histoplasmin-latex test
histoplasmoma
histoplasmosis
    African h.
    disseminated h.
    ocular h.
    progressive disseminated h.
    pulmonary h.
    sclerosing h.
    h. serology
historadiography
history
    pathophysiologic h.
histotechnologist
histotechnology
histotope
histotoxic
    h. anoxia
    h. hypoxia
histotropic
HIT — hemagglutination-inhibition test

hypertrophic infiltrative tendinitis
HIV — human immunodeficiency virus
HIVAGEN test
HIV antigen
hives
    giant h.
HIV I serology
HJ — Howell-Jolly (bodies)
HK — heat-killed
    hexokinase
H^+,K^+-ATPase
HKLM — heat-killed *Listeria monocytogenes*
HL — hearing level
    hearing loss
    histiocytic lymphoma
    histocompatibility locus
    hypermetropia, latent
H & L — heart and lungs
HLA — human leukocyte antigen
    human lymphocyte antigen
HLA
    antigens (loci: -A, -B, -C, -DO, -DP, -DQ, -DZ; subloci: -MB, -MT, $-T_E$)
    B27
    complex
    typing
HLDH — heat-stable lactic dehydrogenase
hLH — human luteinizing hormone
hLT — human lymphocyte transformation
HLV — herpes-like virus
HM — hydatidiform mole
Hm — manifest hyperopia
hm — hectometer
HMD — hyaline membrane disease
HMF — hydroxymethylfurfural
HMG — human menopausal gonadotropin
    hydroxymethylglutaryl
HML — human milk lysozyme
HMM — hexamethylolmelamine
HMO — Health Maintenance Organization
$H-2^b$ mouse cells
HMP — hexose monophosphate
    hexose monophosphate pathway

HMPG — (4-hydroxy-3-methoxy-
phenyl)ethylene glycol
HMPS — hexose monophosphate
shunt
HMSAS — hypertrophic muscular subaortic stenosis
HMW — high molecular weight
HN — hereditary nephritis
hilar node
HN_2 — nitrogen mustard, mechlorethamine
HNP — herniated nucleus pulposus
hnRNA — heterogeneous nuclear
RNA
HNSHA — hereditary nonspherocytic hemolytic
anemia
HO — high oxygen
hyperbaric oxygen
H_2O — water
Ho — holmium
HOA — hypertrophic
osteoarthroscopy
hoarseness
hobnail
h. cell
h. liver
Hoboken's
gemmules
nodules
HOC — hydroxycorticoid
HOCM — hypertrophic obstructive
cardiomyopathy
Hodgkin cycle
Hodgkin's
cell
granuloma
lymphoma
paragranuloma
sarcoma
Hoesch test
hof
Hofbauer cells
Hoffmann's reflex
Hofmann's bacillus
Hogben test
hog cholera serum
holandric
h. genes
h. inheritance
holarthritic
holarthritis

Hollander test
Hollenhorst plaques
Hollerith code
hollow cathode lamp
Holman-Miller sign
Holmes's
alkaline buffer
method
stain
holmium
holoacardius
h. acephalus
h. acormus
h. amorphus
holoantigen
Holobasidiomycetes
Holobasidiomycetidae
holocrine
holoenzyme
hologynic genes
hologynic inheritance
holomorph
Holophyra coli
holoprosencephaly
holosystolic murmur
holotype
Holzer's method
Holzknecht unit
Homalomyia
Homans' sign
homatropine
h. hydrobromide
h. methylbromide
homeopathic symbol for decimal scale
of potencies
homeostasis
electrolyte balance and h.
fluid balance and h.
immunologic h.
homeostatic
homeotypic mitosis
Homer-Wright
pseudorosette
rosette
homing receptor
homme rouge
homoallele
homobiotin
homobrachial inversion
homocarnosine
homochronous inheritance
homocinchonine

homocitrulline
homocyclic
homocysteine desulfhydrase
homocystine
homocystinemia
homocystinuria test
homocytotrophic antibody
homodesmotic
homodimer
homofermentation
homogametic sex
homogenate
homogeneity
homogeneous
    h. immersion
    h. immunoassay
    h. radiation
homogeneously staining region
homogenize
homogenote
homogenous immersion
homogentisate
    h. dioxygenase
    h. 1,2-dioxygenase
    h. oxidase
    h. oxygenase
homogentisic
    h. acid
    h. acid oxidase
homogentisuria
homograft rejection
homolactic
homologous
    h. analog
    h. antigen
    h. artificial insemination
    h. chimera
    h. chromosomes
    h. graft
    h. hemagglutinin
    h. series
    h. serum
    h. serum hepatitis
    h. structures
    h. tumor
homologue
homology unit
homolytic cleavage
homomorphic bivalent
homonymous hemianopsia
homophilic
homopolymer

homorphic
homoscedasticity
homoserine
    h. dehydratase
    h. dehydrogenase
    h. kinase
homosexual
homosexuality
homosomal aberration
homothallism
homotopic transplantation
homotransplantation
homovanillic acid test
homozygosity
homozygote
homozygous
    h. achondroplasia
    h. hemoglobinopathy
    h. thalassemia
    h.-type hemoglobin disorder
    h. typing method
homunculus
hone
    automatic h.
honeycomb
    h. lung
    h. macula
honeymoon cystitis
honey urine
Hong Kong toe
honing
HOOD — hereditary osteo-onycho-
        dysplasia
hood
    fume h.
    laboratory h.
Hooker-Forbes test
Hooke's law
hookworm
    American h.
    h. anemia
    h. disease
    dog h.
    European h.
    New World h.
    Old World h.
HOP — high oxygen pressure
hordeolum
horizontal
Hormodendrum
    H. algeriensis
    H. carrionii

H. *compactum*
H. *dermatitidis*
H. *japonicum*
H. *pedrosoi*
H. *rossicum*
hormonal
  h. evaluation
  h. hyperplasia
  h. therapy
hormone
  adaptive h.
  adenohypophyseal h.
  adipokinetic h.
  adrenocortical h.
  adrenocorticotropic h.
  adrenomedullary h.
  androgenic h.
  anterior pituitary h.
  antidiuretic h.
  antimüllerian h.
  Aschheim-Zondek h.
  bovine growth h.
  chondrotropic h.
  chromaffin h.
  chromatophorotropic h.
  corpus luteum h.
  cortical h.
  corticotropin-releasing h.
  diabetogenic h.
  ectopic h.
  erythropoietic h.
  estrogenic h.
  eutopic h.
  fat-mobilizing h.
  female h's
  follicle h.
  follicle-stimulating h.
  follicle-stimulating hormone-releasing h.
  galactopoietic h.
  gastrointestinal h.
  glycoprotein h's
  gonadotropic h.
  gonadotropin hormone-releasing h.
  gonadotropin-releasing h.
  growth h.
  growth hormone release-inhibiting h.
  growth hormone-releasing h.
  human growth h.
  human luteinizing h.

human pituitary follicle-stimulating h.
hypophysiotropic h.
immunoreactive human growth h.
inappropriate h.
inappropriate antidiuretic h.
inhibiting h's
inhibitory h.
interstitial cell-stimulating h.
juvenile h.
ketogenic h.
lactogenic h.
langerhansian h.
lipolytic h.
luteal h.
luteinizing h.
luteinizing hormone-releasing h.
luteotropic h.
lymphocyte-stimulating h.
male h's
mammotropic h.
melanocyte-inhibiting h.
α-melanocyte-stimulating h.
melanocyte-stimulating hormone release-inhibiting h.
melanocyte-stimulating hormone-releasing h.
melanophore-stimulating h.
neurohypophyseal h.
orchidic h.
ovarian h.
ovine lactogenic h.
oxytocin h.
parathyroid h.
peptide h.
pituitary h.
pituitary growth h.
placental h.
polypeptide h.
posterior pituitary h.
progestational h.
prolactin release-inhibiting h.
prolactin-releasing h.
proparathyroid h.
protein h.
prothoracicotropic h.
h. receptor
releasing h's
h.-secreting tumor
sex h.

somatotropic h.
somatrotropin-releasing h.
steroid h.
testicular h.
thymic h.
thyroid-stimulating h.
thyrotropic h.
thyrotropin-releasing h.
TSH-releasing h.

horn
Ammon's h.
anterior h.
cicatricial h.
cutaneous h.
h. cysts
iliac h.
lateral h.
nail h.
penile h.
posterior h.
sebaceous h.
ventral h.
warty h.

Horner's muscle
hornification
horny
horror autotoxicus
horse
h. antihuman thymus globulin
h. red blood cells
h. serum

horsefly
horseradish peroxidase
horseshoe
h. fistula
h. kidney

Horsley-Clarke apparatus
Hortega's neuroglia stain
HOS — human osteogenic sarcoma
hose
drench h.

hospital
evacuation h.
teaching h.

host
accidental h.
alternate h.
h. defense
definitive h.
graft-versus-h. disease
immunocompromised h.
intermediate h.

h.-parasite relationship
paratenic h.
h. of predilection
h.-range mutation
reservoir h.
h. response
transfer h.

hostility
hot
h. abscess
h. antigen suicide
h. gangrene
h. lesion
h. nodule

Hotchkiss-McManus PAS technique
Hottentot apron
Hounsfield unit
hourglass
h. deformity
h. gallbladder
h. stomach

Houssay
animal
phenomenon

Howard test
Howell-Jolly bodies
Howell's
bodies
method
test
unit

Howship's lacuna
H and P — history and physical
HP — high protein
human pituitary
hp — haptoglobin
HPA — hypothalamic-pituitary-
adrenal
HPAA — hydroxyphenylacetic acid
HPD — hematoporphyrin derivative
HPF — heparin-precipitable fraction
hpf — high-power field
HPFH — hereditary persistence of
fetal hemoglobin
hPFSH — human pituitary follicle–
stimulating hormone
hPG — human pituitary gonadotropin
hPL — human placental lactogen
HPLA — hydroxyphenyllactic acid
HPLC — high-pressure liquid chromatography

HPO — high-pressure oxygen
hypertrophic pulmonary
osteoarthropathy
HPP — hydroxypyrazolopyrimidine
HPPA — hydroxyphenylpyruvic acid
HPPH — hydroxyphenyl-
phenylhydantoin
HPRT — hypoxanthinephosphoribo-
syl transferase
HPS — hematoxylin-phloxine-saffron
hypertrophic pyloric stenosis
HPT — hyperparathyroidism
HPV — *Haemophilus pertussis* vaccine
human papillomavirus
HPVD — hypertensive pulmonary vas-
cular disease
HPVG — hepatic portal venous gas
H.P. Wright method
HR — heart rate
H & R — hysterectomy and radiation
Hr — blood type factor
HRBC — horse red blood cell
H reflex
HRF — histamine-releasing factor
HRIG — human rabies immune
globulin
HRS — Hamilton Rating Scale
HRT — heart rate
Hryniuk's dose-intensity hypothesis
HS — heat-stable
heme synthetase
hereditary spherocytosis
herpes simplex
horse serum
Hurler's syndrome
HSA — human serum albumin
HSF — hydrazine sensitive factor
HSG — hysterosalpingogram
H spike
HSR — homogeneously staining radio-
graphs
H substance
HSV — herpes simplex virus
HSV I — herpes simplex virus I
HSV II — herpes simplex virus II
HSV culture
HSV isolation
HT — hemagglutination titer
hydroxytryptamine
hypermetropia, total
hypertension
hypodermic table

5-HT — 5-hydroxytryptamine
Ht — total hyperopia
ht — heart
height
HTA — hydroxytryptamine
HTC — homozygous typing cell
HTCA — human tumor clonogenic
assay
HTCFA — human tumor
colony–forming assay
HTHD — hypertensive heart
disease
HTLA — human thymus lymphocyte
antigen
HTLV — human T cell leukemia/
lymphoma virus
human T cell lymphotropic
virus
HTLV provirus
HTLV-III/LAV — lymphadenopathy-
associated virus
HTLV-MA — HTLV membrane
antigen
HTP — hydroxytryptophan
HTV — herpes-type virus
HU — heat unit
hemagglutinating unit
hydroxyurea
hyperemia unit
Hucker-Conn
crystal violet solution
stain
Huebener-Thomsen-Friedenreich phenomenon
Hufner's equation
Huhner test
HuIFN — human interferon
Huldshinsky's radiation
hum
venous h.
human
h. antihemophilic factor
h. chorionic gonadotropin infection test
h. chorionic somatomammo-
tropin
h. embryo kidney
h. embryo lung
h. embryonic kidney
h. engineering
h. enteric (virus)
h. erythrocyte agglutination

h. flea
h. gammaglobulin
h. growth hormone
h. herpesvirus-6
h. immunodeficiency virus
h. immunodeficiency virus (HIV) culture
h. leukocyte antigen
h. luteinizing hormone
h. lymphocyte antigen
h. lymphocyte transformation
h. lymphoproliferative disease
h. menopausal gonadotropin
h. milk lysozyme
h. papillomavirus
h. papillomavirus probe test
h. pituitary follicle–stimulating hormone
h. pituitary gonadotropin
h. placental lactogen
h. rabies immune globulin
h. serum
h. serum albumin
h. T-cell leukemia-lymphoma virus
h. T-cell lymphotropic virus
h. thymus antiserum
h. tubercle bacillus
h. tumor clonogenic assay
humectant
humeral
humeroradial joint
humeroscapular joint
humerus (pl., humeri)
humidifier lung
humor (pl., humors, humores)
aqueous h.
plasmoid h.
vitreous h.
humoral
h. immune response
h. immunity
h. pathology
h. thymic factor
Hunner's
cystitis
stricture
ulcer
Hunter's
canal
glossitis
Hunter-Schreger lines

Huntington's chorea
Hunt-Lawrence pouch
Hurler-Scheie compound
hurloid facies
Hurst's dilator
Hürthle
cell
cell adenocarcinoma
cell adenoma
cell carcinoma
cell metaplasia
cell nodule
cell tumor
HUS — hemolytic-uremic syndrome
hyaluronidase unit for semen
Hutchinson's
freckle
melanotic freckle
teeth
triad
-type neuroblastoma
HUTHAS — human thymus anti-serum
huygenian eyepiece
HV — hepatic vein
herpesvirus
HVA — homovanillic acid
HVA test
HVD — hypertensive vascular disease
HVE — high-voltage electrophoresis
HVH — *Herpesvirus hominis*
H-V interval
HVL — half-value layer
HVSD — hydrogen-detected ventricular septal defect
H wave
HX bodies
Hy. — hypermetropia
hyalin
alcoholic h.
hematogenous h.
hyaline
h. arteriolosclerosis
h. body
h. cartilage
h. cast
h. degeneration
h. droplets
h. globule
h. leukocyte
h. membrane

h. membrane disease
h. membrane disease of
newborn
h. necrosis
h. nephrosclerosis
h. perisplenitis
h. thickening
h. thrombus
h. tubercle
h. urinary cast
hyalinization
hyalinized plaque
hyalinizing trabecular adenoma
hyalinosis
systemic h.
hyalinuria
hyalohyphomycosis
hyaloid
h. artery
h. canal
hyalomere
Hyalomma aegyptium
hyaloplasm
hyaloplasmic
hyaloserositis
hyalosome
hyaluronate
hyaluronic acid
hyaluronidase
h. digestion
h. unit for semen
hyaluronoglucosaminidase
hyaluronoglucuronidase
H-Y antigen
hybrid
h. cell
h. orbital
hybridization
cellular h.
competition h.
cross h.
DNA-DNA h.
DNA-RNA h.
filter h.
in-situ h.
liquid (solution) h.
RNA-driven h.
RNA-RNA h.
saturation h.
solution h.
hybridoma
T-lymphocyte h.

hydantoin
hydatid
alveolar h. disease
h. cyst
h. degeneration
h. disease
h. mole
h. of Morgagni
osseous h.
h. polyp
h. rash
sessile h.
unilocular h.
Virchow's h.
hydatidiform mole
hydatidocele
hydatidoma
hydatidosis
hydatiduria
Hydatigera infantis
hydradenitis
hydradenoma
hydralazine
h. hydrochloride
h. lupus
hydramnios
hydranencephaly
hydrargyromania
hydrarthrosis
hydrastine
hydratase
aconitate h.
fumarate h.
hydrate
chloral h.
hydrated
h. alumina
h. erythrocyte
hydration
hydrazide
isonicotinic acid h.
hydrazine
h.-sensitive factor
h. sulfate
h. yellow
hydrazone
Hydrea
hydremia
hydrencephalocele
hydrencephalomeningocele
hydride
hydriodic acid

hydroa
    h. aestivale
    h. vesiculosum
hydroappendix
hydrobromic acid
hydrobromide
    hyoscyamine h.
hydrocalycosis
hydrocarbon
    alicyclic h.
    aliphatic h.
    aliphatic saturated h.
    aliphatic unsaturated h.
    aromatic h.
    carcinogenic h.
    chlorinated h.
    cyclic h.
    polycyclic h.
    saturated h.
    unsaturated h.
hydrocele
    funicular/encysted h.
    paratesticular h.
    h. sac
hydrocephalus
    communicating h.
    noncommunicating h.
    post-traumatic h.
hydrochloric acid
hydrochloride
    acridine h.
    adiphenine h.
    arginine h.
    bacampicillin h.
    captamine h.
    chloroguanide h.
    clonidine h.
    colestipol h.
    cyproheptadine h.
    diphenhydramine h.
    hydromorphone h.
    isoproterenol h.
    loperamide h.
    loxapine h.
    lucanthone h.
    meperidine h.
    minocycline h.
    morphine h.
    phenazopyridine h.
    prazosin h.
    procaine h.
    quinine h.

    semicarbazide h.
    zinterol h.
hydrochlorothiazide
hydrocholecystis
hydrocholeresis
hydrocholeretic
hydrocirsocele
hydrocortamate
hydrocortisone
hydrocyanic acid
hydrocyst
hydrocystoma
hydrocytosis
    hereditary h.
hydroflumethiazide
hydrofluoric acid
hydrogen
    h. acceptor
    h. bacterium
    h. bond
    h. broth test
    h. chloride
    h. cyanide
    h.-detected ventricular septal
      defect
    h. electrode
    h. exponent
    h. fluoride
    h. ion
    h. ion concentration
    h. peroxide
    h. sulfide
    h. sulfide acetyl-transferase
hydrogenase
hydrogenate
hydrogenation
hydrogenlyase
hydrogenolysis
hydrohepatosis
hydrolase
    acetoacetylglutathione h.
    acetyl-CoA h.
    acid h.
    aminoacyl-tRNA h.
    aryl-ester h.
    carboxylic ester h.
    formyl-CoA h.
    guanosine h.
    hydroxyacylglutathione h.
    3-hydroxyisobutyryl-CoA h.
    hydroxyisobutyryl-CoA h.
    hydroxymethylglutaryl-CoA h.

palmitoyl-CoA h.
phosphoric monoester h.
succinyl-CoA h.
hydro-lyase
hydrolysate
    casein h.
    lactalbumin h.
    protein h.
hydrolysis
hydrolytic enzyme
hydrolyze
hydroma
hydromeningocele
hydrometer scale
hydromorphone hydrochloride
hydromphalus
hydromyelia
hydromyoma
hydronephrosis
    congenital h.
hydronephrotic
hydronium
hydronium ion
hydropericardium
hydroperitoneum; hydroperitonia
hydroperoxidase
hydroperoxide
hydroperoxyeicosatetraenoic
    acid
hydrophilic gel
hydrophobia
hydrophobic
    h. chromatography
    h. gel
hydrophthalmos
hydropic
    h. change
    h. degeneration
hydropneumatosis
hydropneumopericardium
hydropneumoperitoneum
hydropneumothorax
hydrops
    h. abdominis
    h. amnii
    h. articuli
    cochlear h.
    endolymphatic h.
    h. fetalis
    h. folliculi
    gallbladder h.
    immune fetal h.

labyrinthine h.
nonimmune fetal h.
h. tubae profluens
hydropyonephrosis
hydroquinone
hydrorchis
hydrosalpinx
hydrosarca
hydrosarcocele
hydrostatic pressure
Hydrotaea
hydrothionemia
hydrothionuria
hydrothorax
    chylous h.
hydrotympanum
hydroureter
hydroxide
    aluminum h.
    h. ion
    potassium h.
    sodium h.
hydroxocobalamin
hydroxy acid
D-2-hydroxyacid dehydrogenase
D-3-hydroxyacyl CoA
L-hydroxyacyl CoA
3-hydroxyacyl–CoA dehydro-
    genase
hydroxyacylglutathione hydrolase
hydroxyamphetamine hydrobromide
11-hydroxyandrosterone
hydroxyanthranilic acid
hydroxyapatite
    h. arthropathy
    calcium h.
    h. crystal
hydroxybenzene
p-hydroxybenzoate esters
hydroxybenzoic acid
p-hydroxybenzoic acid
3-hydroxybutyrate dehydrogenase
hydroxybutyric acid
    3-h.a.
    4-h.a.
    α-h.a.
    β-h.a.
3-hydroxybutyryl-CoA epimerase
2-hydroxy-2,2-*bis*-(4-chlorophenyl)
    ethyl acetate
hydroxychloroquine sulfate

alpha-hydroxycholanate dehydrogenase
25-hydroxycholecalciferol
hydroxycholesterol
hydroxycorticoid
17-hydroxycorticosteroid
    17-h. assay
    17-h. test
17-hydroxycorticosterone
18-hydroxycorticosterone
hydroxycortisol
hydroxydione
β-hydroxydopamine
hydroxyeicosatetraenoic acid
2-hydroxyethanesulfonate
2-hydroxyethanesulfonic acid
hydroxyethyl starch
11-hydroxyetiocholanolone
2-hydroxyglutaratedehydrogenase
hydroxyheptadecatrienoic acid
hydroxyhexamide
5-hydroxyindoleacetic acid
    5-h. a. assay
    5-h. a. test
3-hydroxyisobutyrate dehydrogenase
3-hydroxyisobutyryl–CoA hydrolase
hydroxyketone dye
hydroxykynurenine
hydroxyl
    h. concentration
    h. group
hydroxylamine
hydroxylase
    11-β-h.
    11β-h. deficiency
    11β-h. inhibition
    17-h.
    17-h. deficiency
    18-h.
    21-h.
    21-h. deficiency
    24-h.
    nicotinate 6-h.
    phenylalanine h.
    proline h.
    pyroglutamate h.
hydroxylation
hydroxy-mercurichlorophenol
hydroxy-mercuricresol
hydroxy-mercurinitrophenol

hydroxymethyl
tris(-hydroxymethyl) aminomethane
3-hydroxy-3-methylglutaryl
hydroxymethylglutaryl–CoA
    h–CoA hydrolase
    h.–CoA lyase
    h.–CoA reductase
    h.–CoA synthase
hydroxymethyltetrahydrofolate dehydrogenase
hydroxyperoxycyclophosphamide
hydroxyphenamate
hydroxyphenylacetic acid
o-hydroxyphenylacetic acid
p-hydroxyphenyllactic acid
hydroxyphenyl mercurichloride
p-hydroxyphenylpyruvate
    h. dioxygenase
    h. dydroxylase
    h. oxidase
p-hydroxyphenylpyruvic acid
hydroxyphenyluria
17-hydroxypregnenolone
17-hydroxyprogesterone
17α-hydroxyprogesterone
hydroxyproline
    h. assay
    h. index
    h. oxidase
hydroxyprolinemia
hydroxyprolinuria
hydroxypyruvate
8-hydroxyquinolate
8-hydroxyquinoline
17-hydroxysteroid
3α-hydroxysteroid dehydrogenase
3β-hydroxysteroid dehydrogenase
18-hydroxysteroid dehydrogenase
hydroxysteroid oxidoreductase
3β-hydroxysteroid sulfotransferase
hydroxystilbamidine isethionate
5-hydroxytryptamine
hydroxytryptophan decarboxylase
hydroxyurea
hydroxyvaline
25-hydroxyvitamin D
25-hydroxyvitamin D_3
hydroxyzine
hygienic laboratory coefficient
hygroma (pl., hygromas, hygromata)
    h. axillare
    cervical h.

h. colli cysticum
cystic h.
subdural h.
hygrometer
hygrophilous
hygroscopic
Hylemyia
hylic tumor
hyloma
 mesenchymal h.
 mesothelial h.
hymen
hymenal tag
hymenolepiasis
Hymenolepididae
Hymenolepis
 H. *diminuta*
 H. *fraterna*
 H. *murina*
 H. *nana*
Hymenomycetes
Hymenoptera
Hymorphan
hyoid
 h. arch
 h. bone
hyoscine
hyoscyamine hydrobromide
HYP — hydroxyproline
hypalbuminemia
hypalgesia
Hypaque
hypazoturia
hyperacanthosis
hyperacidity
hyperactive
hyperactivity
 motor h.
hyperacute
 h. rejection
 h. transplantation
hyperadenosis
hyderadiposis; hyperadiposity
hyperadrenalism
hyperadrenocorticism
hyper-β-alaninemia
hyperalbuminemia
hyperalbuminosa polyemia
hyperaldosteronemia
hyperaldosteronism
 congenital h.
 glucocorticoid-suppressible h.

idiopathic h.
primary h.
pseudoprimary h.
secondary h.
hyperalgesia
hyperalimentation
 intravenous h.
hyperallantoinuria
hyperalphaglobulinemia
hyperalphalipoproteinemia
 familial h.
hyperaminoacidemia
hyperaminoaciduria
hyperammonemia
 h. I
 h. II
hyperamylasemia
hyperamylasuria
hyperbaric
 h. chamber
 h. hemolysis
 h. oxygenation
hyperbetaglobulinemia
hyperbetalipoproteinemia
 familial h.
hyperbilirubinemia
 congenital h.
 conjugated h., type III
 constitutional h.
 hereditary h.
 h. I
 h. II
hyperbilirubinuria
 obstructive h.
hyperbola
hyperbradykinism
hypercalcemia
 familial hypocalciuric h.
 idiopathic h.
 idiopathic infantile h.
hypercalcemic
 h. sarcoidosis
 h. uremia
hypercalcinuria
hypercalcitoninemia
hypercalcitoninism
hypercalciuria
 idiopathic h.
hypercapnia
hypercapnic
 h. acidosis
 h. encephalopathy

hypercarbia
hypercardia
hypercarotenemia
hypercellular
hypercellularity
hyperchloremia
hyperchloremic acidosis
hyperchlorhydria
hyperchloruria
hypercholesteremia
hypercholesterinemia
hypercholesterolemia
    essential h.
    familial h.
hypercholesterolia
hypercholia
hyperchromasia
hyperchromatic
    h. anemia
    h. karyokinesis
    h. macrocythemia
hyperchromatism
hyperchromemia
hyperchromia
    macrocytic h.
hyperchromic
    h. anemia
    h. erythrocyte
    h. shift
hyperchylomicronemia
hypercoagulability
hypercoagulable
    h. state
    h. state coagulation screen
hypercorticalism
hypercorticism
hypercortisolism
hypercreatinemia
hypercupremia
hypercupriuria
hypercyanotic
hypercythemia
hypercytochromia
hypercytosis
hyperdiploid chromosome number
hyperdiploidy
hyperdistention
hyperdiuresis
hyperechoic
hyperelastosis cutis
hyperemesis gravidarum

hyperemia
    conjunctival h.
    exercise h.
    hemodynamic h.
    peristaltic h.
    reactive h.
hyperemic
hypereosinophilia
hypereosinophilic syndrome
hypererythrocythemia
hyperesthesia
hyperesthetic zone
hyperestrogenism
hyperferremia
hyperfibrinogenemia
hyperfibrinolysis
    systemic h.
hyperflexion
hyperfunctional adenoma
hypergammaglobulinemia
    monoclonal h.
    polyclonal h.
hypergammaglobulinemic purpura
hypergastrinemia
hypergenesis
hypergenetic
hypergenitalism
hyperglobulia; hyperglobulism
hyperglobulinemia
    polyclonal h.
hyperglobulinemic purpura
hyperglucagonemia
    familial h.
hyperglycemia
    nonketotic h.
hyperglycemic
    h. coma
    h. glycogenolytic factor
hyperglyceridemia
    endogenous h.
    exogenous h.
hyperglycinemia
    ketotic h.
    nonketotic h.
hyperglycinuria
hyperglycosemia
hyperglycosuria
hyperglyoxylemia
hypergonadism
hypergonadotropic hypogonadism
hypergranular promyelocytic leukemia
hypergranulosis

hyperguanidinemia
hyperhemoglobinemia
hyperheparinemia
hyperhydropexy; hyperhydropexis
hypericin
hyperimmune
    h. globulin
    h. serum
hyperimmunity
hyperimmunization
hyperimmunoglobulin
    h. E syndrome
    h. M syndrome
hyperimmunoglobulinemia
    monoclonal h.
    polyclonal h.
hyperindicanemia
hyperinosemia
hyperinosis
hyperinsulinemia
hyperinsulinism
hyperirritability
hyperisotonic
hyperkalemia
hyperkaliemia
hyperkaluresis
hyperkaluria
hyperkeratinization
hyperkeratosis
    h. congenita
    h. eccentrica
    epidermolytic h.
    h. figurata centrifuga atrophica
    h. filiform
    follicular h.
    h. follicularis et parafollicularis
    h. lenticularis perstans
    h. penetrans
hyperkeratotic
    h. dysplasia
    h. papilloma
hyperketonemia
hyperketonuria
hyperkinesis
hyperleukocytosis
hyperlipemia
    endogenous h.
    essential h.
    exogenous h.
hyperlipidemia
    carbohydrate-induced h.
    combined h.

    endogenous h.
    fat-induced h.
    remnant h.
hyperlipidemic
hyperlipoidemia
hyperlipoproteinemia
    familial h.
hyperliposis
hyperlithuria
hyperlucency of bone
hyperlucent lung
hyperlymphocytosis
hyperlysinemia
    h. type I
    h. type II
hyperlysinuria
hypermagnesemia
hypermature
hypermelanosis
hypermenorrhea
hypermethioninemia
hypermetropia
    latent h.
hypermobility
hypermyotrophy
hypernatremia
hyperneocytosis
hypernephroid
hypernephroma
hyperoncotic
hyperonychia
hyperopia
    manifest h.
hyperorchidism
hyperornithinemia
hyperorthocytosis
hyperosmolality
hyperosmolar diabetic coma
hyperosmolarity
hyperosmosis
    nonketotic h.
hyperostosis
    ankylosing h.
    h. corticalis deformans
    h. corticalis deformans juvenilis
    h. corticalis generalisata
    diffuse idiopathic skeletal h.
    flowing h.
    h. frontalis interna
    generalized cortical h.

infantile cortical h.
streak h.
hyperoxaluria
hyperparakeratosis
hyperparathyroidism
    primary h.
    secondary h.
    tertiary h.
hyperperistalsis
    ureteral h.
hyperphenylalaninemia
hyperphosphatasemia
hyperphosphatasia
hyperphosphatemia
hyperphosphaturia
hyperpigmentation
hyperpigmented skin
hyperpipecolatemia
hyperpituitarism
    postpubertal h.
    prepubertal h.
hyperpituitary gigantism
hyperplasia
    adenomatous h.
    adrenal cortical h.
    adrenal medullary h.
    angiofollicular mediastinal
      lymph node h.
    angiolymphoid h.
    atypical h.
    atypical melanocytic h.
    basal cell h.
    basophilic h.
    benign mediastinal lymph
      node h.
    benign prostatic h.
    Castleman's giant lymph
      node h.
    C cell h.
    clear cell intraductal h.
    compensatory h.
    congenital adrenal h.
    congenital lipoid h.
    congenital renal h.
    congenital sebaceous h.
    congenital virilizing adrenal h.
    cortical stromal h.
    cutaneous lymphoid h.
    cystic h.
    cystic h. of breast
    cystic endometrial h.
    diffuse h.

ductal h.
endocervical h.
endometrial h.
eosinophilic h.
epithelial h.
erythroid h.
fibroelastic h.
fibromuscular h.
focal h.
focal nodular h.
follicular h.
giant follicular h.
glandular h.
granulocytic h.
hematopoietic h.
hormonal h.
intracystic h.
intraductal h.
intravascular papillary endothe-
    lial h.
juxtaglomerular cell h.
lentiginous h.
Leydig cell h.
lipoid h.
lipomelanotic reticuloendothe-
    lial cell h.
lobular h.
lymphoid h.
mast cell h.
megakaryocytic h.
mesangial h.
mesenteric h.
microglandular endocervical h.
myeloid h.
neoplastic h.
neutrophilic h.
nodular adrenal h.
nodular adrenocortical h.
nodular lymphoid h.
nodular mesothelial h.
nodular h. of prostate
nodular regenerative h.
papillary h.
papillomatous h.
paracortical lymphoid h.
parathyroid h.
pathologic h.
physiologic h.
plasma cell h.
polypoid h.
primary h.
prostatic h.

pseudocarcinomatous h.
pseudoepitheliomatous h.
reserve cell h.
reticuloendothelial cell h.
reticulum cell h.
sebaceous h.
secondary h.
senile sebaceous h.
squamous h.
stromal h.
Swiss cheese h.
urothelial h.
verrucous h.
vulvar h.
wasserhelle h.
water-clear cell h.
hyperplasmia
hyperplastic
    h. acinus
    h. arteriolitis
    h. arteriosclerosis
    h. bone marrow
    h. cells
    h. cholecystosis
    h. dystrophy
    h. goiter
    h. inflammation
    h. nephrosclerosis
    h. nodular goiter
    h. osteoarthritis
    h. polyp
hyperploid
hyperploidy
hyperpnea
hyperpneic
hyperpolarization
hyperpotassemia
hyperprebetalipoproteinemia
hyperproinsulinemia
hyperprolactinemia
hyperprolinemia
hyperproteinemia
hyperpyrexia
hyperreflexia
hyperreninemia
hypersalemia
hypersarcosinemia
hypersecretion
hypersecretory
    h. gastritis
    h. gastropathy

hypersegmentation
    hereditary h. of neutrophils
    leukocytic h.
hypersegmented neutrophil
hypersensitive
hypersensitivity
    h. angiitis
    delayed h.
    immediate h.
    h. pneumonitis
    h. pneumonitis serology
    h. reaction
    h. vasculitis
hyperserotonemia
hyperskeocytosis
hypersomia
hypersomnia
hypersplenic thrombocytopenia
hypersplenism
hypersplenosis
hypersthenuria
hypertelorism
    ocular h.
hypertension
    arterial h.
    benign intracranial h.
    diastolic h.
    essential h.
    Goldblatt's h.
    idiopathic h.
    malignant h.
    mineralocorticoid h.
    orthostatic h.
    paroxysmal h.
    portal h.
    pulmonary h.
    pulmonary artery h.
    renal h.
    renovascular h.
    secondary h.
    systolic h.
hypertensive
    h. arteriopathy
    h. arteriosclerosis
    h. arteriosclerotic heart disease
    h. cardiovascular disease
    h. crisis
    h. encephalopathy
    h. heart disease
    h. pulmonary vascular disease
    h. retinopathy
    h. vascular disease

hyperthecosis
    testoid h.
hyperthelia
hyperthermia
    malignant h.
hyperthrombinemia
hyperthymic
hyperthymism
hyperthymization
hyperthyroidism
    autoimmune h.
    factitious h.
    iatrogenic h.
    iodine-induced h.
    primary h.
    radiation-related h.
    secondary h.
hyperthyroiditis
hyperthyroxinemia
    dysalbuminemic h.
hypertonia polycythemica
hypertonic
hypertonicity
hypertonus
hypertrichosis
    h. lanuginosa acquisita
    nevoid h.
hypertriglyceridemia
    familial h.
hypertrophia
hypertrophic
    h. amphophil cell
    h. angioma
    h. arthritis
    h. cardiomyopathy
    h. chronic vulvitis
    h. fibrous pachymeningitis
    h. gastritis
    h. gingivitis
    h. hypersecretory gastropathy
    h. infiltrative tendinitis
    h. interstitial neuropathy
    h. lichen planus
    h. lupus erythematosus
    h. muscular subaortic stenosis
    h. obstructive cardiomyopathy
    h. osteoarthropathy
    h. polyneuritic-type muscular
      atrophy
    h. pulmonary osteoarthropathy
    h. pyloric stenosis

    h. scar
    h. subaortic stenosis
hypertrophy
    adaptive h.
    adenomatous h.
    asymmetrical septal h.
    asymmetric septal h.
    benign prostatic h.
    cellular h.
    combined ventricular h.
    compensatory h.
    compensatory h. of heart
    complementary h.
    concentric h.
    diffuse h.
    eccentric h.
    endemic h.
    false h.
    fibrocongestive h.
    focal h.
    functional h.
    giant h. of gastric mucosa
    giant rugal h.
    gingival h.
    hemangiectatic h.
    idiopathic myocardial h.
    left atrial h.
    left ventricular h.
    lipomatous h.
    numerical h.
    physiologic h.
    prostatic h.
    quantitative h.
    right atrial h.
    right ventricular h.
    simple h.
    simulated h.
    true h.
    ventricular h.
    vicarious h.
hypertyrosinemia
    Oregon-type h.
hyperuremia
hyperuresis
hyperuricemia
hyperuricemic
hyperuricosuria
hyperuricuria
hyperurobilinogenemia
hypervalinemia
hypervariable
hypervascular

hyperventilation
hyperviscosity syndrome
hypervitaminosis
hypervolemia
hypesthesia
    tactile h.
    thermal h.
hypha (pl., hyphae)
    racquet h.
hyphal
hyphema; hyphemia
Hyphomyces destruens
Hyphomycetales
hyphomycetoma
hypnagogic hypersynchrony
hypnotic
hypo
hypoacidity
hypoadrenalism
hypoadrenocorticism
    primary h.
    secondary h.
hypoalbuminemia
hypoaldosteronism
hypoaldosteronuria
hypoalphaglobulinemia
hypoazoturia
hypobaric
hypobetaglobulinemia
hypobetalipoproteinemia
    familial h.
hypocalcemia
hypocalcemic
hypocalcification
hypocalciuria
hypocapnia
hypocapnic
hypocarbia
hypocellular
hypocellularity
hypoceruloplasminemia
hypochloremia
hypochloremic azotemia
hypochlorhydria
hypochlorite
hypochlorous acid
hypochloruria
hypocholesteremia
hypocholesterinemia
hypocholesterolemia
hypocholinesterasemia
    hereditary h.

hypochondriac
hypochondriasis
hypochondrium (pl., hypochondria)
hypochondroplasia
hypochromasia
hypochromatic karyokinesis
hypochromatism
hypochromemia
    idiopathic h.
hypochromia
hypochromic
    h. anemia
    h. erythrocyte
    h. microcytic anemia
    h. shift
hypochrosis
hypocitraturia
hypocomplementemia
hypocomplementemic glomerulone-
    phritis
hypocorticoidism
hypocortisolism
hypocupremia
hypocythemia
    progressive h.
hypocytosis
Hypoderma bovis
hypodermic
    h. implantation
    h. needle
hypodermolithiasis
hypodiploid
hypoechoic
hypoeosinophilia
hypoferremia
hypoferric anemia
hypofibrinogenemia
hypogammaglobinemia
hypogammaglobulinemia
    acquired h.
    common variable h.
    physiologic h.
    primary h.
    Swiss-type h.
    transient h.
    transient h. of infancy
    X-linked h.
    X-linked infantile h.
hypoganglionosis
hypogastric
    h. artery
    h. lymph node

h. plexus
h. reflex
h. region
h. vein
hypogastrium
hypogenesis
hypoglobulia
hypoglobulinemia
hypoglossal
    h. muscle
    h. nerve
hypoglycemia
    alimentary h.
    factitious h.
    functional h.
    insulin-induced h.
    leucine h.
    neonatal h.
    postprandial h.
    reactive h.
hypoglycemic
    h. coma
    h. encephalopathy
    h. shock
hypoglycin; hypoglycine
hypogonadism
    hypergonadotropic h.
    hypogonadotrophic h.
    postpubertal h.
hypogonadotropic hypogonadism
hypogranulocytosis
hypohidrotic ectodermal dysplasia
hypohydremia
hypohydrochloria
hypohyloma
hypoinsulinism
hypokalemia
hypokalemic
    h. alkalosis
    h. nephropathy
    h. nephrosis
hypokaluria
hypolepidoma
hypoleukemia
hypoleydigism
hypolipoproteinemia
hypoliposis
hypolymphemia
hypomagnesemia
hypomania
hypomanic
    h. personality

h.-type manic-depressive psy-
    chosis
hypomelanosis of Ito
hypomenorrhea
hypomethioninemia
hyponatremia
hyponatruria
hyponeocytosis
hyponychium
hypo-oncotic
hypo-orthocytosis
hypoparathyroidism
hypopharyngeal
    h. diverticulum
    h. stenosis
hypopharynx
hypophosphatasemia
hypophosphatasia
    congenital h.
hypophosphatemia
    familial h.
    X-linked familial h.
hypophosphaturia
hypophyseal; hypophysial
    h. syndrome
hypophysioprivic
    h. cachexia
hypophysio-sphenoidal syndrome
hypophysiotropic hormone
hypophysis
    h. cerebri
    pharyngeal h.
    h. sicca
    h. staining procedure
hypophysitis
    autoimmune h.
hypopigmentation
hypopituitarism
hypoplasia
    adrenal h.
    cartilage-hair h.
    congenital renal h.
    cytomegalic adrenal h.
    erythroid h.
    focal dermal h.
    germ cell h.
    granulocytic h.
    hematopoietic h.
    Leydig cell h.
    lymphoid h.
    megakaryocytic h.
    myeloid h.

pulmonary h.
renal h.
right ventricular h.
thymic h.
hypoplastic
    h. anemia
    h. bone marrow
    h. heart
hypoploid
hypoploidy
hypopotassemia
hypoproaccelerinemia
hypoproconvertinemia
hypoproteinemia
    prehepatic h.
hypoprothrombinemia
hypopyon
hyporeflexia
hyporeninemia
hyporeninemic
hypersalemia
hyposarca
hyposecretion
hyposegmentation
    leukocytic nuclear h.
hyposensitivity
hyposensitization
hyposialadenitis
hyposkeocytosis
hyposmolality
hyposmotic
hypospadias
    pseudovaginal perineoscrotal h.
hypospermatogenesis
hyposplenism
hypostasis
    postmortem h.
    pulmonary h.
hypostatic
    h. abscess
    h. congestion
    h. ectasia
    h. pneumonia
hyposthenuria
hyposthenuric urine
hyposulfite salt
hypotension
    orthostatic h.
hypotensive shock
hypothalamic
    h. astrocytoma

h. corticotropin-releasing
    factor
h. diabetes insipidis
h. nucleus
h.-pituitary axis
h. sulcus
hypothalamicohypophyseal
hypothalamicothalamic
hypothalamohypophyseal
hypothalamopituitary
hypothalamus
    caudal area of h.
    dorsal nucleus of h.
    dorsomedial nucleus of h.
    infundibulum of h.
    medial nucleus of h.
    nucleus intercalatus of h.
    periventricular gray matter
        of h.
    supraoptic region of h.
    tuberal nucleus of h.
    ventromedial nucleus of h.
hypothenar
hypothermia
hypothermic
hypothesis
    alternative h.
    autocrine h.
    Benditt h.
    biogenic amine h.
    cardionector h.
    chemiosmotic h.
    Goldie-Coldman h.
    Hryniuk's dose-intensity h.
    Lyon's h.
    Norton-Simon h.
    omnibus h.
    one gene–one enzyme h.
    one gene–one polypeptide
        chain h.
    proton-motive h.
    Starling's h.
    h. testing
    unitarian h.
    wobble h.
hypotheticodeductive model
hypothrombinemia
hypothromboplastinemia
hypothyroid cardiomyopathy
hypothyroidism
    drug-associated h.
    radiation-related h.

secondary h.
trophoprivic h.
hypothyroxinemia
hypotonia
vasomotor h.
hypotonic hemolysis
hypotonicity
hypotonus
hypotransferrinemia
hypotriploid
hypouricemia
hypouricuria
hypoventilation
hypovitaminosis
hypovolemia
hypovolemic shock
hypoxanthine
h. guanine phosphoribosyltransferase
h. phosphoribosyltransferase
hypoxemia
arterial h.
hypoxia
anemic h.
cellular h.
histotoxic h.
hypoxic h.

ischemic h.
oxygen affinity h.
stagnant h.
hypoxic
h. anoxia
h. encephalopathy
h. hypoxia
h. nephrosis
hypsarrhythmia
hypsochrome
hypsochromic shift
Hyrtl's canal
hysteratresia
hysterectomy
hysteresis loop
hysteria
conversion h.
hysterocarcinoma
hysterolith
hysteromyoma
hysteromyomectomy
hysterosalpingectomy
hysterosalpingography
hysterosalpingo-oophorectomy
hysterotonin
Hz — hertz
HZV — herpes zoster virus

I

I — intensity of magnetism
iodine
permanent incisor
^{131}I, ^{132}I — radioactive isotopes of iodine
i — deciduous incisor
optically inactive
IA — impedance angle
internal auditory
intra-aortic
intra-arterial
Ia antigen — immune-associated antigen
IABP — intra-aortic balloon pump
IAC — internal auditory canal
IADH — inappropriate antidiuretic hormone

IADHS — inappropriate antidiuretic hormone syndrome
IAEA — International Atomic Energy Agency
IAGP — International Association of Geographic Pathology
IAHA — immune adherence hemaglutination assay
IAM — internal auditory meatus
I and i antibody
I and i antigen
IAP — International Academy of Pathology
IARC — International Agency for Research on Cancer
IAS — interatrial septum
intra-amniotic saline (infusion)

IASD — interatrial septal defect
IAT — invasive activity test
 iodine-azide test
iatrogenic
 i. agent
 i. anemia
 i. hyperthyroidism
 i. infection
iatrotherapy
IB — inclusion body
I band — isotropic band
IBB — intestinal brush border
IBC — iron-binding capacity
IBD — inflammatory bowel disease
IBF — immunoglobulin-binding factor
ibotenic acid
IBR — infectious bovine rhinotracheitis
IBU — international benzoate unit
ibuprofen
IBW — ideal body weight
IC — immune complex
 inspiratory capacity
 integrated circuit
 intercostal
 intermittent claudication
 intracavitary
 intracellular
 intracerebral
 intracranial
 intracutaneous
 irritable colon
 isovolumic contraction
ICA — internal carotid artery
 intracranial aneurysm
ICAO — internal carotid artery occlusion
ICC — immunocompetent cells
 Indian childhood cirrhosis
ICD — International Classification of Diseases
 intrauterine contraceptive device
 isocitric dehydrogenase
ice
 dry i.
 i. point
I cell
I-cell disease
ICF — intracellular fluid
ICG — indocyanine green

ICG excretion test
ICH — intracranial hemorrhage
ichoroid
ichorous pus
ichorrhea
ichthammol
ichthyoacanthotoxism
ichthyohemotoxism
ichthyosarcotoxism
ichthyosis
 acquired i.
 i. congenita
 i. congenita neonatorum
 i. fetalis
 i. hystrix
 i. intrauterina
 lamellar i.
 i. linguae
 nacreous i.
 i. palmaris et plantaris
 i. sauroderma
 i. scutulata
 i. sebacea
 i. sebacea corneae
 i. simplex
 i. spinosa
 i. uteri
 i. vulgaris
 X-linked i.
ichthyotic
ichthyotoxin
icing
 i. heart
 i. liver
ICM — intercostal margin
ICNND — Interdepartmental Committee on Nutrition in National Defense
icosahedral symmetry
ICS — intercostal space
ICSH — International Committee for Standardization in Hematology
 interstitial cell–stimulating hormone
ICSP — International Council of Societies of Pathology
ICT — indirect Coombs' test
 inflammation of connective tissue
 insulin coma therapy
 isovolumic contraction time

ictal
icteric
    i. index
    i. serum
    i. serum hepatitis
icteroanemia
icterogenic spirochetosis
icterohematuria
icterohematuric
icterohemoglobinuria
icterohemolytic anemia
Icterohemorrhagiae leptospirosis
icterohepatitis
icteroid
icterus
    acquired hemolytic i.
    benign familial i.
    chronic familial i.
    congenital familial i.
    congenital hemolytic i.
    cythemolytic i.
    i. gravis
    i. gravis neonatorum
    i. index
    i. index test
    i. interference
    i. melas
    i. neonatorum
    i. precox
ict. ind. — icterus index
ictotest reagent tablet
ictus (pl., ictus)
ICU — intensive care unit
ICW — intracellular water
ID — identification
    immunodiffusion
    infective dose
    inside diameter
    intradermal
I & D — incision and drainage
ID_{50} — median infectious dose
id
IDA — image display and analysis
    iron deficiency anemia
IDDM — insulin-dependent diabetes
    mellitus
ideal body weight
identical twins
identification
    antibody i.
    hazard i.
    hemoglobin i.

identified
identifier
identity pattern
Ide test
IDI — induction-delivery interval
idiochromidia
idiocy
    amaurotic familial i.
    juvenile amaurotic familial i.
    late infantile amaurotic familial i.
    mongolian i.
idiogram
idioheteroagglutinin
idiopathic
    i. Bamberger-Marie disease
    i. cardiomyopathy
    i. etiology
    i. fibrous mediastinitis
    i. fibrous retroperitonitis
    i. generalized glycogenosis
    i. glomerulonephritis
    i. hemosiderosis
    i. hyperaldosteronism
    i. hypercalcemia
    i. hypercalcemia of infants
    i. hypercalcemic sclerosis of infants
    i. hypercalciuria
    i. hypertension
    i. hypertrophic osteoarthropathy
    i. hypertrophic subaortic stenosis
    i. hypochromemia
    i. hypochromic anemia
    i. infantile hypercalcemia
    i. megacolon
    i. myelofibrosis anemia
    i. myocardial hypertrophy
    i. myxedema
    i. nephrotic syndrome
    i. neuralgia
    i. pancreatitis
    i. parkinsonism
    i. paroxysmal rhabdomyolysis
    i. pentosuria
    i. pericarditis
    i. proctitis
    i. pulmonary fibrosis
    i. pulmonary hemosiderosis
    i. respiratory distress syndrome

i. retroperitoneal fibrosis
i. thrombocytopenic purpura
idiopathy
toxic i.
idioretinal light
idiosyncrasy
idiosyncratic
idiot
i. savant
idiotope
idiotoxin
idiotype antibody
idiotypic
idioventricular rhythm
iditol
i. dehydrogenase
i. dehydrogenase assay
IDL — intermediate-density lipoprotein
IDMS — isotope dilution-mass spectrometry
idoxuridine
IDP — inosine diphosphate
IDR — intradermal reaction
id reaction
IDS — immunity deficiency state
IDU — idoxuridine
iododeoxyuridine
iduronate
iduronic
i. acid
i. sulfatase
iduronidase
L-iduronidase
IDVC — indwelling venous catheter
IE — *immunitäts Einheit* (immunizing unit)
immunoelectrophoresis
I/E — inspiratory-expiratory ratio
IEMA — immunoenzymometric assay
IEMG — integrated electromyogram
IEOP — immunoelectroosmophoresis
IEP — immunoelectrophoresis
IF — immunofluorescence
interstitial fluid
intrinsic factor
IFA — immunofluorescence assay
indirect fluorescent antibody
I factor
IFC — intrinsic factor concentrate

IFCC — International Federation of Clinical Chemistry
IFN — interferon
IFR — inspiratory flow rate
IFRA — indirect fluorescent rabies antibody (test)
IFRT — involved field radiotherapy
IFV — intracellular fluid volume
IG — immune globulin
intragastric
Ig — immunoglobulin
Ig gene arrangement
Ig gene assembly
IgA — immunoglobulin A
IgA glomerulonephritis
IgA immunodeficiency
IgA nephropathy
IgA secretory component
IgD — immunoglobulin D
IgE — immunoglobulin E
IGF — insulin-like growth factor
IgG — immunoglobulin G
IgG index
IgG ratios
IgM — immunoglobulin M
IgM antibody
IgM nephropathy
IgM response
ignitability
ignition
i. point
i. source control
i. temperature
IGT — impaired glucose tolerance
IGV — intrathoracic gas volume
IgY — immunoglobulin Y
IH — infectious hepatitis
IHA — indirect hemagglutination
IHBTD — incompatible hemolytic blood transfusion disease
IHC — idiopathic hypercalciuria
IHD — ischemic heart disease
IHO — idiopathic hypertrophic osteoarthropathy
IHR — intrinsic heart rate
IHSA — iodinated human serum albumin
IHSS — idiopathic hypertrophic subaortic stenosis
IIF — indirect immunofluorescence
IJP — internal jugular pressure

Il — illinium
IL-2 — interleukin-2
ILA — insulin-like activity
ILD — ischemic leg disease
 ischemic limb disease
Ile — isoleucine
ileal
  i. artery
  i. intussusception
  i. juice
  i. loop conduit
  i. lumen
  i. mesentery
  i. mucous membrane
  i. submucosa
ileitis
  backwash i.
  distal i.
  regional i.
  terminal i.
ileocecal
  i. intussusception
  i. lymphoma
ileocecum
ileocolic
  i. artery
  i. intussusception
  i. lymph node
ileocolitis ulcerosa chronica
ileocolostomy
ileocystoplasty
ileocystostomy
ileojejunitis
ileorectal
ileosigmoid
ileosigmoidostomy
ileostomy
ileotransversostomy
ileum
  duplex i.
  intestinum i.
ileus
  adynamic i.
  dynamic i.
  gallstone i.
  mechanical i.
  meconium i.
  paralytic i.
  spastic i.
  i. subparta
  ureteral i.
Ilheus virus

iliac
  i. artery
  i. bursa
  i. horn
  i. lymph node
  i. roll
  i. vein
iliocostalis muscle
iliohypogastric
ilioinguinal
iliolumbar ligament
iliolumbocostoabdominal
iliopectineal bursitis
iliopelvic
iliopsoas muscle
ilium (pl., ilia)
ill-defined syndrome
illness
  compressed-air i.
  radiation i.
illuminance
illumination
  critical i.
  diffuse i.
  Köhler i.
illusion
Ilosvay reagent
IM — infectious mononucleosis
 intramedullary
 intramuscular
im- — (indicates presence of) NH
  group
IMA — internal mammary artery
IMAA — iodinated macroaggregated
  albumin
image
  i. display and analysis
  i. intensification
  latent i.
  i. processing
  "ship's wheel" i.
imaging
  electrostatic i.
  magnetic resonance i.
  tomographic i.
IMB — intermenstrual bleeding
imbalance
  autonomic i.
  electrolyte i.
  immunologic i.
  sympathetic i.
  vasomotor i.

IMBC — indirect maximum breathing capacity
imbed
imbibition
imbrication
IMH — idiopathic myocardial hypertrophy
IMHP — 1-iodomercuri-2-hydroxypropane
IMI — intramuscular injection
imidazole carboxamide
imidazolepyruvic acid
imidazolylethylamine
imide
imidecyl iodine
imidodipeptidase
imidodipeptide
imidodipeptiduria
imine
imino acid
iminoacidopathies
iminodipeptidase
iminodipeptide
iminoglycinuria
imipramine
    i. and desipramine assay
    i. hydrochloride
immature
    i. granulocyte
    i. neutrophil
    i. teratoma
immediate
    i. hypersensitivity
    i. principle
immersion
    i. blast injury
    i. foot
    homogeneous i.
    i. objective
    oil i.
    i.-submersion
    i. syndrome
    water i.
imminent abortion
immiscible
immobility
immobilization
immobilized enzyme
immotile cilia syndrome
immotility

immune
    i. adherence
    i. agglutinin
    i. assay
    i. associated antigen
    i. bodies
    i. clearance
    i. complex
    i. complex assay
    i. complex disease
    i. complex glomerulonephritis
    i. complex glomerulopathy
    i. complex nephritis
    i. complex nephropathy
    i. conglutin
    i. cytolysis
    i. deficiency
    i. deficiency state
    i. electron microscopy
    i. elimination
    i. fetal hydrops
    i. globulin
    i. globulin vaccinia
    i. hemolysis
    i. hemolytic anemia
    i. interferon
    i. lactoglobulin
    i.-mediated hemolysin
    i. neutropenia
    i. protein
    i. response
    i. response genes
    i. serum
    i. serum globulin
    i. suppression
    i. surveillance
    i. system
    i. thrombocytopenia
    i. thrombocytopenic purpura
immunity
    antiviral i.
    athreptic i.
    cell-mediated i.
    cellular i.
    genetic i.
    herd i.
    humoral i.
    local i.
    passive i.
    i. substance
    T-cell–mediated i.
    tumor i.

immunization
  passive i.
  prophylactic i.
  Rh i.
immunize
immunizing unit
immunoadjuvant
immunoadsorbent
immunoadsorption
immunoassay
  automated i.
  channelling i.
  cloned enzyme donor i.
  enzyme i's
  enzyme modulator–
    mediated i.
  enzyme-multiplied i.
  fluorescence correlation i.
  fluorescence excitation trans-
    fer i.
  fluorescence polarization i.
  fluorescence protection i.
  fluorescent i.
  homogeneous i.
  light-scattering i's
  nephelometric i.
  nonradioisotopic i.
  particle concentration fluores-
    cence i.
  particle-enhanced turbidimetric
    inhibition i.
  prosthetic group–labeled i.
  radioisotopic i.
  sandwich i.
  solid phase i.
  substrate-labeled fluorescence i.
  thin-layer i.
  turbidimetric i's
immunobiology
immunoblast
immunoblastic
  i. genes
  i. lymphadenopathy
  i. lymphoma
  i. sarcoma
immunoblot
  i. technique
  i. test
immunoblotting
immunocatalysis
immunochemical
  i. analysis
  i. assay

immunochemistry
immunochemotherapy
immunocompetence assessment
immunocompetency
immunocompetent cells
immunocomplex
immunocompromised host
immunoconcentration assay
immunoconglutination
immunoconglutinin
immunocyte
immunocytoadherence
immunocytochemical
immunocytochemistry
immunodeficiency
  cellular i.
  combined i.
  common variable i.
  i. diseases
  human i.
  primary i.
  secondary i.
  severe combined i.
  i. syndrome
  X-linked hyper-IgM i.
immunodeficient
immunodepression
immunodiagnosis
immunodiffusion
  Ouchterlony i.
  Oudin i.
  radial i.
immunodominance
immunodominant
immunoelectro-osmophoresis
immunoelectrophoresis
  counter i.
  countercurrent i.
  crossed i.
  factor VIII–crossed i.
  radio-i.
  reverse i.
  rocket i.
  two-dimensional i.
immunoenzymometric assay
immunoferritin
immunofiltration
  analytical i.
  preparative i.
immunofixation electrophoresis
immunofluorescence
  adenovirus i.

i. assay
i. method
i. microscopy
mixed i.
i. techniques
i. test
immunofluorescent
    i. assay
    i. stain
immunogen
immunogenetics
immunogenic
    i. determinant
    i. determination
immunogenicity
immunoglobulin
    i. A deficiency
    i. A nephropathy
    B-cell i.
    i.-binding factor
    i.-coated erythrocyte
    cytoplasmic i.
    i. D
    i. domains
    i. E
    gamma A i. (IgA)
    gamma D i. (IgD)
    gamma E i. (IgE)
    gamma G i. (IgG)
    gamma M i. (IgM)
    i. G deficiency
    i. G index
    i. M
    monoclonal i.
    platelet-associated i's
    polyclonal i.
    secretory i.
    i. subclass
    thyroid-stimulating i.
    TSH-binding inhibitory i.
immunoglobulinopathy
immunohematology
immunohemolytic anemia
immunohistochemical
    i. staining
    i. techniques
immunohistochemistry
immunohistofluorescence
immunohistologic
immunoincompetent
immunologic
    i. competence

i. enhancement
i. homeostasis
i. imbalance
i. marker
i. memory
i. paralysis
i. pregnancy test
i. self-tolerance
i. surveillance
i. thrombocytopenic purpura
i. tolerance
i. unresponsiveness
immunologically
    i. activated cell
    i. competent cell
immunological surveillance
immunologist
immunology
immunometric assay
immunomodulary
immunomodulating
immunomodulation
immunomodulator
immunomodulatory
immunonephelometry
immunoparalysis
immunoparasitology
immunopathogenesis
immunopathology
immunoperoxidase
    i. staining method
    i. technique
immunophenotype
immunophysiology
immunopotency
immunopotentiation
immunoprecipitation
    automated i.
immunoprecipitin reaction
immunoprobe
immunoproliferative
    i. disorders
    i. small intestinal disease
immunoprophylaxis
immunoradioassay
immunoradiometric assay
immunoradiometry
immunoreactant
immunoreaction
immunoreactive
    i. glucagon
    i. human growth hormone

i. insulin
i. peptide
i. trypsin
immunoreactivity
immunoreagent
immunoregulation
immunoregulatory
immunoselection
immunosenescence
immunosorbent
immunostaining
immunostimulant
immunostimulation
immunosuppressant
immunosuppressed
immunosuppression
immunosuppressive therapy
immunosurveillance
immunotherapy
immunotoxicology
immunotoxin
immunotransfusion
immunovar
Imodium
IMP — inosine-5'-monophosphate
impacted
    i. feces
    i. fracture
    i. tooth
impaction
    fecal i.
    i. lesion
impaired clot retraction
impairment
    functional aerobic i.
impalpable
impatent
impedance
    aortic i.
    electrode i.
    output i.
    i. plethysmography
imperfect yeast
imperforate
    i. anus
    i. hymen
imperforation
impermeable
impetigenization
impetigo
    bullous i.

i. contagiosa
i. neonatorum
implant
    carcinomatous i's
    radium i.
    radon i.
    Silastic i.
implantation
    i. bleeding
    circumferential i.
    i. cyst
    i. dermoid
    hypodermic i.
    interstitial i.
    iodine-125 i.
    iridium-192 i.
    periosteal i.
    radioactive iodine i.
    radioactive iridium i.
    i. site
    superficial i.
    i. test
impotence
    sexual i.
imprecision
impregnation
impression preparation
imprint
    bone marrow i.
impulse sealing
impurity
IMR — infant mortality rate
IMViC tests — indole, methyl red,
                Voges-Proskauer,
                and citrate tests
IN — intranasal
In — indium
inactivated
    i. leukocytolytic serum
    i. poliovaccine
inactivation
    complement i.
inactivator
    anaphylatoxin i.
inactive tuberculosis
INAD — infantile neuroaxonal dys-
             trophy
INAH — isonicotinic acid hydrazide
inanition
inapparent infection
inappropriate
    i. antidiuretic hormone

i. antidiuretic hormone syndrome
i. hormone
inborn error of metabolism
inbred strain
inbreeding coefficient
incarcerated hernia
inch
    pounds per square i.
incidence
    angle of i.
    i. rate
incident light
"incidentalomas"
    adrenal i's
incineration
incised wound
incipient
incision
    paravaginal i.
    Warren's i.
    Weber-Ferguson i.
incisional biopsy
incisor
    deciduous i.
    mandibular i.
    maxillary i.
incl. — including
inclusion
    blenorrhea i.
    i. body
    i. body disease
    i. casts
    cell i's
    i. cell disease
    i. conjunctivitis
    i. conjunctivitis virus
    i. cyst
    cytoplasmic i.
    i. dermoid
    i. disease
    Döhle's i. bodies
    i. encephalitis
    epidermal i. cyst
    epidermoid i. cyst
    epithelial i. cyst
    germinal i. cyst
    germinal epithelial i. cyst
    leukocyte i's
    nuclear i's
    viral i.
incoagulability

incoherent
incompatibility
    ABO i.
    blood group i.
    chemical i.
    physiologic i.
    Rh i.
    Rh antigen i.
incompatible
    i. blood transfusion reaction
    i. chemicals
    i. hemolytic blood transfusion disease
    i. transfusion
incompetence
    aortic i.
    mitral i.
    pulmonary i.
    tricuspid i.
    urinary i.
    valvular i.
incompetency of the cardiac valves
incompetent
    i. aortic valve
    i. cervix
    i. foramen ovale valve
    i. mitral valve
    i. pulmonic valve
    i. tricuspid valve
incomplete
    i. abortion
    i. amnion
    i. amputation
    i. antibody
    i. compound fracture
    i. conjoined twins
    i. differentiation
    i. dislocation
    i. dominance
    i. fistula
    i. fracture
    i. hernia
    i. neurofibromatosis
    i. penetrance
    i. regeneration
    i. right bundle-branch block
    i. transposition
incontinence
    fecal i.
    i. of pigment
    urinary i.

i. aspermatogenesis
i. glomerulonephritis
i. phagocytosis
i. thyroiditis
i. uveitis
inducer T cell
inducible enzyme
inductance
induction
    i. chemotherapy
    enzyme i.
    magnetic i.
inductive
    i. phase
    i. reactance
inductor
indulation
    jugular i.
indulin
indulinophil; indulinophile
indurated
induration
    brown i. of lung
    cyanotic i.
    Froriep's i.
    gray i.
    pigment i. of lung
    plastic i.
    red i.
indurative myocarditis
indusium griseum
industrial
    i. carcinogens
    i. poison
    i. toxicology
indwelling vascular catheterization
INE — infantile necrotizing encephalomyelopathy
ineffective erythropoiesis
inelastic scattering
Inermicapsifer
    I. madagascariensis
inert electrode
inertia
    colonic i.
    uterine i.
inevitable abortion
in extremis
inf. — inferior
    infusion
infancy

infant
    i. death
    "floppy" i.
    low birth weight i.
    i. mortality rate
    postterm i.
    premature i.
    preterm i.
infantile
    i. amaurotic familial idiocy
    i. cortical hyperostosis
    i. digital fibromatosis
    i. fibrosarcoma
    i. glaucoma
    i. hemangioendothelioma
    i. hemangioma
    i. muscular atrophy
    i. myxedema
    i. necrotizing encephalomyelopathy
    i. neuroaxonal dystrophy
    i. obstructive cholangiopathy
    i. paralysis
    i. polycystic disease
    i. progressive spinal muscular dystrophy
    i. respiratory distress syndrome
    i. spasm
    i. syphilis
    i.-type coarctation
    i. uterus
infantilism
    tubal i.
infarct
    acute i.
    anemic i.
    anterior lateral myocardial i.
    anteroseptal myocardial i.
    bile i.
    bland i.
    bone i.
    Brewer's i's
    cerebral i.
    embolic i.
    focal i.
    hemorrhagic i.
    microscopic i.
    myocardial i.
    old i.
    pale i.
    posterior wall i.
    pulmonary i.

recent i.
red i.
ruptured myocardial i.
septic i.
subendocardial i.
thrombotic i.
uric acid i.
watershed i.
white i.
Zahn's i.

infarction
acute myocardial i.
anemic i.
anterior wall i.
anterior wall myocardial i.
atrial i.
bland i.
cerebral i.
hemodynamic i.
hemorrhagic i.
hepatic i.
inferior wall myocardial i.
intestinal i.
mesenteric i.
myocardial i.
nontransmural myocardial i.
old myocardial i.
pulmonary i.
red (hemorrhagic) i.
renal i.
right ventricular i.
septic i.
silent myocardial i.
"stuttering" i.
subendocardial myocardial i.
through-and-through myocardial i.
transmural myocardial i.
venous i.
watershed i.
white (anemic) i.

infect

infected abortion

infection
abortive i.
actinomycetic i.
aerobic-anaerobic i.
airborne i.
anaerobic i.
bacterial i.
chlamydial i.
clostridial i.
colonization i.
contagious i.
cryptogenic i.
cryptosporidial i.
cutaneous i.
disseminated gonococcal i.
dragon worm i.
ectothrix i.
endogenous i.
enteric i.
enterococcal i.
exogenous i.
fever caused by i.
filarial i.
focal i.
fungal i.
gonococcal i.
guinea worm i.
helminthic i.
herpes zoster–varicella i.
iatrogenic i.
inapparent i.
intrauterine i.
medina i.
meningococcal i.
metazoan i.
mycobacterial i.
mycoplasmal i.
nosocomial i.
opportunistic i.
parasitic i.
perinatal i.
persistent tolerant i.
pneumococcal i.
protozoal i.
protozoan i.
pyogenic i.
recurrent upper respiratory tract i.
reoviral i.
rickettsial i.
serpent i.
spirochetal i.
staphylococcal i.
streptococcal i.
treponemal i.
upper respiratory i.
upper respiratory tract i.
urinary tract i.
varicella-zoster i.
viral i.
viral respiratory i.

whipworm i.
zoonotic i.
infectious
i. agent
i. anemia
i. arteritis
i. bovine rhinotracheitis
i. disease
i. endocarditis
i. esophagitis
i. granuloma
i. hemolytic anemia
i. hepatitis
i. lymphocytosis
i. mononucleosis
i. mononucleosis screening test
i. myositis
i. myxoma
i. parotitis
i. warts
i. wastes
Infectious Diseases Society of America
infective
i. dose
i. embolism
i. endocarditis
i. thrombus
infectivity
inferior
i. alveolar nerve
i. aperture
i. brachium
i. cardiac branch
i. cardiac nerve
i. cerebellar peduncle
i. cerebral vein
i. cervical ganglion
i. colliculus
i. complete closed dislocation
i. complete compound dislocation
i. dislocation
i. displacement
i. division, oculomotor nerve
i. epigastric artery
i. esophageal sphincter
i. frontal gyrus
i. frontomarginal sulcus
i. fronto-occipital fasciculus
i. ganglion
i. genicular artery
i. gluteal nerve

i. hemorrhoidal artery
i. hemorrhoidal vein
i. horn, lateral ventricle
i. left pulmonary vein
i. lingular bronchus
i. lipodystrophy
i. longitudinal fasciculus
i. medullary velum
i. mesentery
i. nasal turbinate
i. nucleus, pulvinar
i. oblique muscle
i. occipital gyrus
i. olivary nucleus
i. pancreaticoduodenal artery
i. parietal lobule
i. peduncular interstitial nucleus
i. petrosal sinus
i. phrenic artery
i. phrenic vein
i. preoptic nucleus
i. rectal artery
i. rectal vein
i. rectus muscle
i. right pulmonary vein
i. sagittal sinus
i. segment
i. striate vein
i. temporal gyrus
i. temporal sulcus
i. thyroid artery
i. vena cava
i. wall myocardial infarction
inferolateral
inferomedian
inferoposterior
inferosuperior
inferotemporal
infertility
male i.
primary i.
i. screen
secondary i.
infestation
liver fluke i.
louse i.
mite i.
nematode worm i.
parasitic i.
trematode worm i.

infiltrate
    acute inflammatory i.
    Assmann's tuberculous i.
    eosinophil leukocytic i.
    inflammatory i.
    infraclavicular i.
    leukocytic i.
    lymphocytic inflammatory i.
    monocytic inflammatory i.
    neutrophilic i.
    plasma cell i.
    polymorphonuclear leukocytic i.

infiltrating
    i. comedocarcinoma
    i. duct adenocarcinoma
    i. duct carcinoma
    i. lipoma
    i. lobular carcinoma

infiltration
    adipose i.
    calcareous i.
    cellular i.
    epituberculous i.
    fatty i.
    gelatinous i.
    glycogen i.
    gray i.
    lipomatous i.
    lymphocytic i. of skin
    mesenteric i.
    parenchymal i.
    sanguineous i.
    serous i.
    tuberculous i.

infiltrative
    i. fasciitis
    i. ophthalmopathy

infinite
infinitely miscible
infinitesimal
infinity
infirm
infirmity
inflamed ulcer
inflammable
inflammation
    active chronic i.
    acute i.
    acute and chronic i.
    adhesive i.
    alterative i.
    atrophic i.
    blenorrhagic i.
    bullous i.
    bullous granulomatous i.
    calcified granulomatous i.
    caseating i.
    caseating granulomatous i.
    caseous i.
    catarrhal i.
    cavitating i.
    chronic i.
    circumscribed i.
    confluent i.
    connective tissue i.
    croupous i.
    cystic i.
    cystic acute i.
    cystic chronic i.
    cystic granulomatous i.
    cytopathic i.
    degenerative i.
    diffuse i.
    disseminated i.
    erosive i.
    exanthematous i.
    exudative i.
    exudative granulomatous i.
    fibrinoid necrotizing i.
    fibrinopurulent i.
    fibrinous i.
    fibrocaseous i.
    fibroid i.
    fibrotic i.
    focal granulomatous i.
    follicular i.
    gangrenous i.
    gangrenous granulomatous i.
    gelatinous i.
    granulomatous i.
    gummatous i.
    hemorrhagic i.
    hyperplastic i.
    interstitial i.
    localized i.
    membranous i.
    membranous acute i.
    miliary granulomatous i.
    mononuclear i.
    multifocal i.
    necrotic i.
    necrotizing i.
    necrotizing granulomatous i.

non-necrotizing granulomatous i.
nonspecific chronic i.
obliterative i.
organizing i.
ossifying i.
productive i.
proliferative i.
pseudomembranous i.
pseudomembranous acute i.
purulent i.
pustular i.
recurrent i.
round cell i.
sclerosing i.
serofibrinous i.
serous i.
serous acute i.
subacute i.
subsiding i.
suppurative i.
suppurative acute i.
suppurative chronic i.
suppurative granulomatous i.
transudative i.
ulcerative i.
uremic i.
vesicular i.
vesicular acute i.
vesicular granulomatous i.
inflammatory
   i. adenocarcinoma
   i. bowel disease
   i. breast cancer
   i. carcinoma
   i. cavity
   i. corpuscle
   i. cyst
   i. cystitis
   i. edema
   i. exudate
   i. fistula
   i. infiltrate
   i. lymph
   lymphocytic i. infiltrate
   i. membrane
   monocytic i. infiltrate
   i. necrosis
   i. pelvic disease
   i. perforation
   i. polyp
   i. pseudomembrane

   i. pseudotumor
   i. reaction
   i. rheumatism
   i. rupture
   i. sinus
   i. sinus tract
   i. transudate
inflation
inflection
   point of i.
inflow tract
influenza
   i. A and B titer
   i. virus
   i. virus culture
   i. virus types A, B, C
information
   i. retrieval
   i. theory
informed consent
infra-axillary
infraclavicular infiltrate
infracostal
infradian rhythm
infrahyoid
inframammary
infraorbital
infraorbitomeatal line
infrapatellar
infrared
   i. analyzer
   i. CO_2 analyzer
   i. light
   i. microscope
   i. radiation
   i. ray
   i. spectrometry
   i. spectrophotometry
   i. spectroscopy
   i. tympanic thermography
infrascapular
infraspinatus muscle
infraspinous
infratemporal fossae
infratentorial
infratrochlear
infundibular stenosis
infundibuloneurohypophysitis
   lymphocytic i.
infundibulum (pl., infundibula)
infusion
   brain-heart i.
   total-dose i.

Infusoria
ingestion
ingrown
    i. hair
    i. toenail
inguinal
    i. artery
    i. canal
    i. hernia
    i. ligament
    i. lymph node
    i. region
    i. ring
inguinoabdominal
inguinoscrotal
INH — isoniazid
    isonicotinic acid hydrazide
inhalant
inhalation
    i. burn
    isoproterenol sulfate i.
    i. pneumonia
inherent filter
inheritance
    alternative i.
    amphigonous i.
    autosomal dominant i.
    autosomal recessive i.
    biparental i.
    codominant i.
    complemental i.
    cytoplasmic i.
    dominant i.
    extrachromosomal i.
    holandric i.
    hologynic i.
    homochronous i.
    intermediate i.
    maternal i.
    mendelian i.
    multifactorial i.
    polygenic i.
    quantitative i.
    quasicontinuous i.
    quasidominant i.
    recessive i.
    sex-linked i.
    supplemental i.
    unit i.
    X-linked dominant i.
    X-linked recessive i.
inherited albumin variants

inhibin
inhibit
inhibiting
    i. antibody
    i. hormones
inhibition
    allogenic i.
    allosteric i.
    11-beta-hydroxylase i.
    competitive i.
    contact i.
    enzyme i.
    fertility i.
    hemagglutination i.
    hemagglutinin i.
    i. test
    tetrazolium reduction i.
inhibitor
    activated protein C i.
    $alpha_1$-proteinase i.
    carbonic anhydrase i.
    cell-cycle i.
    C_1 esterase i.
    cholinesterase i's
    C1 i.
    coagulation factor i's
    electron transport i's
    enzyme i.
    factor VIII i.
    factor Xa i.
    fibrolytic i.
    inter-alpha-trypsin i.
    lupus erythematosus i.
    $alpha_2$-macroglobulin i.
    monoamine oxidase i's
    oxidative phosphorylation i's
    $alpha_2$-plasmin i.
    protease i.
    serum i.
    soybean trypsin i.
    i's of translation
    trypsin i.
inhibitory
    i. enzyme
    i. hormone
    i. mold agar
    i. postsynaptic potential
inhomogeneity
inhomogeneous
iniasis
iniencephaly
inion

initial
- i. hematuria
- i. prognostic score
- i. segment
- i. syphilitic lesion

initialization

initiating agent

initiation
- i. codon
- i. factor

initis

injection mass

injury
- birth i.
- blast i.
- cardiac i.
- cellular i.
- cold i.
- compression i.
- crush i.
- decompensation i.
- decompression i.
- hepatocellular i.
- immersion blast i.
- radiation i.
- second-degree radiation i.
- third-degree radiation i.
- torsion i.

innate

innatus
- calor i.

inner
- i. cerebellar funiculus
- i. mesothelial cell
- i. nuclear layer
- i. nuclear membrane alteration
- i. plexiform layer

innervation
- double i.
- law of reciprocal i.
- reciprocal i.

innidiation

innocent tumor

innocuous

innominate
- i. artery
- i. bone
- i. canaliculus
- i. lymph node
- i. vein

innoxious

inoblast

inochondritis

inoculate

inoculation
- protective i.
- smallpox i.

inoculum (pl., inocula)

inocyte

inopectic

inoperable

inorganic
- i. acid
- i. chemistry
- i. phosphate
- i. pyrophosphatase
- i. pyrophosphate

inoscopy

inosemia

inosinase

inosine
- i. cyclohydrolase
- i. dehydrogenase
- i. diphosphate
- i. monophosphate
- i.-5′-phosphate
- i. phosphorylase
- i. phosphorylase deficiency
- i. pranobex
- i. pyrophosphorylase
- i. triphosphate

inosinic acid

inosita
- melituria i.

inositide

inositol
- i. dehydrogenase
- i. hexanitrate
- i. hexaphosphate
- myo-i.
- i. niacinate
- i. 1,4,5-triphosphate

inosituria

inosuria

inotropic state

input/output

INPV — intermittent negative pressure–assisted ventilation

INS — idiopathic nephrotic syndrome

insect bite

insecticide
- organochlorine i.

organophosphate i.
i. poisoning
insemination
homologous artificial i.
insensitivity
androgen i.
insertion
parasol i.
i. sequence
velamentous i.
insertional
i. activity
i. mutation
i. translocation
insheathed
insidious
insipidus
nephrogenic diabetes i.
in situ hybridization
insoluble
insomnia
insonation
insorption
inspiration
inspiratory
i. reserve capacity
i. reserve volume
inspissate
inspissated
inspissation
inspissator
instability
instant thin-layer chromatography
instillation
instrument
instrumentation
insudate
insufficiency
adrenal i.
adrenocortical i.
aortic i.
circulatory i.
coronary i.
metabolic i.
mitral i.
primary adrenal i.
pulmonary i.
renal i.
respiratory i.
tricuspid i.
uteroplacental i.

velopharyngeal i.
venous i.
insufflation
cranial i.
endotracheal i.
perirenal i.
presacral i.
retroperitoneal gas i.
insula (pl., insulae)
insular carcinoma
insulated gate field effect transistor
insulator
insulin
i. antagonist
i. antibody
atypical i.
i. clearance
i. clearance test
i. coma therapy
crystalline i.
i.-dependent diabetes
mellitus
globin i.
i. hypoglycemia test
immunoreactive i.
i.-induced hypoglycemia
i.-like activity
i.-like growth factor
i. lipoatrophy
i. lipodystrophy
protamine i.
protamine zinc i.
i. receptors
i. sensitivity test
i. shock
i. shock therapy
soluble i.
i.-to-glucose ratio
i. tolerance test
i. unit
insulinase
insulinemia
insulinoma
insulinopenic
insulitis
intake and output
integral
i. dose
i. proteins
integrate
integrated circuit
integrating microscope

integration
  large-scale i.
  medium-scale i.
  very large scale i.
integrator
  B1 i.
  B2 i.
  B3 i.
integrin family
integument
in tela (in tissue)
intensification
  i. factor
  image i.
intensifying screen
intensimeter
intensionometer
intensity
  luminous i.
intensive care unit
intention
interaction
  cognate i.
  drug i.
  sample i.
  tumor-host i.
interactive processing
inter-alpha-globulin
inter-alpha-trypsin inhibitor
interatrial
  i. septal defect
  i. septum
interband
intercalary
  i. deletion
  i. neuron
intercalate
intercalated
  i. disk
  i. duct
intercalation
intercapillary
  i. desmosome
  i. glomerulosclerosis
  i. nephrosclerosis
intercapital
intercarpal joint
intercellular
  i. bridge
  i. canaliculus
  i. cement
  i. desmosome

i. junction
i. lymph
i. zonula occludens
γ-intercept
interchange
  Hamburger's i.
interchondral joint
interchromosomal aberration
intercoronary anastomosis
intercostal neuralgia
intercostobrachial nerve
intercranial metastasis
intercristal space
intercurrent
Interdepartmental Committee on Nutrition in National Defense
interdigital space
interelectrode distance
interface
  dineric i.
  EIA (enzyme immunoassay) i.
interfacial canal
interference
  anion i.
  background i.
  cation i.
  centromere i.
  chemical i.
  chromatid i.
  constructive i.
  destructive i.
  drug i.
  i. filter
  hemolysis i.
  icterus i.
  ionization i.
  matrix i.
  i. method
  i. microscope
  negative i.
  i. pattern
  spectral i.
  i. test
interferon
  acid-labile i.
  i.-alpha
  i.-beta
  epithelial i.
  fibroblast i.
  fibroepithelial i.
  i.-gamma

immune i.
leukocyte i.
interfollicular cell
intergene
inter-α-globulin
interhemispheric
interkinesis
interleukin
    i.-1 (IL-1)
    i.-2 (IL-2)
    i.-3 (IL-3)
    i.-4 (IL-4)
    i.-5 (IL-5)
    i.-6 (IL-6)
    i.-7 (IL-7)
    i.-8 (IL-8)
    i.-9 (IL-9)
    i.-10 (IL-10)
    i.-11 (IL-11)
interlobar fissure
interlobitis
interlobular
    i. bile duct
    i. duct
    i. mammary connective tissue
    i. pleurisy
intermaxillary
intermediary metabolism
intermediate
    i. carcinoma
    i. coliform bacteria
    i.-density lipoprotein
    i. filaments
    i. host
    i. inheritance
    i. lobe–inhibiting factor
    i. lymphoma
    malignant teratoma i.
    i. neutron
    i. normoblast
    i. olfactory striae
    reaction i.
intermedin
intermittent
    i. albuminuria
    i. claudication
    i. malaria
    i. malarial fever
    i. parasite
    i. positive pressure breathing
    i. proteinuria
intermuscular lipoma

internal
    i. adhesive pericarditis
    i. arcuate fibers
    i. auditory artery
    i. auditory canal
    i. auditory meatus
    i. auditory vein
    i. capsule
    i. carotid
    i. carotid artery occlusion
    i. cerebral vein
    i. conversion
    i. ear
    i. elastic lamellae
    i. endometriosis
    i. fistula
    i. hemorrhoids
    i. hydrocephalus
    i. hypogastric artery
    i. iliac artery
    i. iliac vein
    i. inguinal ring
    i. jugular vein
    i. limiting membrane
    i. mamillary nucleus
    i. mammary artery
    i. mammary lymphatics
    i. medicine
    i. medullary lamina
    i. nasal branch, nasociliary
      nerve
    i. os
    i. pathology
    i. pudendal artery
    i. pudendal vein
    i. reduction
    i. resistance
    i. rotation
    i. standard
    i. storage
    i. terminal filament
    i. thoracic artery
    i. thoracic vein
    i. urethral orifice
International Academy of Pathology
International Agency for Research on
    Cancer
International Association of Geo-
    graphic Pathology
International Atomic Energy Agency
international benzoate unit
International Classification of Diseases

International Committee for Standard-
ization in Hematology
International Council of Societies of
Pathology
International Federation of Clinical
Chemistry
International Federation of Gynecol-
ogy and Obstetrics
International Normalized Ratio
International Research Information
Service
International Sensitivity Index
International Society for Clinical Lab-
oratory Technology
International Society of Comparative
Pathology
International Society of Hematology
International Society of Microbiolo-
gists
International Society of Pediatric On-
cology
International Standards Organization
International System of Units
International Union Against Cancer
International Union of Biochemistry
Enzyme Commission
International Union of Pure and Applied Chemistry
international unit
interneuron
     inhibitory i.
internodal
    i. segment
    i. tracts
internode
interoanterodorsal nucleus
interoanteromedial nucleus
interoanteroventral nucleus
interocclusal clearance
interoceptor
interocular distance
interorbital
interosseous
interpalpebral zone
interpapillary ridges
interphalangeal joint
interphase
interphyletic
interpolation
interposition
interpreter
interproximal

interpubic
interpupillary
    i. distance
    i. line
interrupt
interrupted respiration
interscapular
intersegmental fibers
intersexuality
interspersed repeats
interspinal
interspinalis muscle
interstice
interstitial
    i. cell
    i. cell of Leydig
    i. cell-stimulating hormone
    i. cell tumor
    i. cell tumor of testis
    i. collagen
    i. conduit
    i. cystitis
    i. deletion
    i. disease
    i. emphysema
    i. fibrosis
    i. fluid
    i. fluke
    i. gastritis
    i. giant cell pneumonia
    i. growth
    i. implantation
    i. inflammation
    i. irradiation
    i. keratitis
    i. mastitis
    i. myositis
    i. nephritis
    i. nephropathy
    i. plasma cell pneumonia
    i. pneumonia
    i. pneumonitis
    i. pulmonary disease
    i. radiation
    i. radiotherapy
    i. tissue
    i. water
interstitium
    renal i.
    testicular t.
intertransversalis muscle
intertrigo

intertropical anemia
inter-α-trypsin inhibitor
intertubercular
interval
    confidence i.
    i. estimate
    reference i.
    rupture-delivery i.
    i. scale
    systolic time i.
    time i.
    tolerance i.
intervening sequence
interventional radiology
interventricular
    i. foramen
    i. septal defect
    i. septum
intervertebral
    i. disc
    i. fibrocartilage
    i. foramen
    i. joint
intervillous
intestinal
    i. adhesion
    i. amebae
    i. atresia
    i. branch, vagus nerve
    i. bypass
    i. ciliates
    i. colic
    i. conduit
    i. emphysema
    i. fistula
    i. flagellates
    i. flora
    i. flow disorder
    i. fluke
    i. infarction
    i. juice
    i. lipodystrophy
    i. lumen
    i. lymphangiectasis
    i. malrotation
    i. metaplasia
    i. mucous membrane
    i. myiasis
    i. nematodes
    i. obstruction
    i. peptide
    i. protozoa

    i. roundworm
    i. sand
    i. sepsis
    i. tract
    i. vein
    i. villi
    i. vomitus
intestine
    large i.
    small i.
intestinum
intima
    aortic tunica i.
intimal
    i. cell
    i. collagen
    i. cushion
intimitis
    proliferative i.
intolerance
    cold i.
    fructose i.
    hereditary fructose i.
    lysine i.
    sucrose i.
intoxication
    acid i.
    alkaline i.
    citrate i.
    roentgen i.
    septic i.
    serum i.
    vitamin D i.
    water i.
intra-adrenal paraganglioma
intra-arterial
intra-articular ligament
intrabiventral fissure
intrabronchial
intracanalicular
    i. fibroadenoma
    i. papilloma
intracapsular ankylosis
intracavitary radiotherapy
intracellular
    i. accumulation
    i. fibroma
    i. fluid
    i. fluid volume
    i. hemoglobin
    i. parasite
    i. water

intracerebral hemorrhage
intrachange
intrachromosomal aberration
intracorporeal heart
intracortical osteosarcoma
intracranial
    i. aneurysm
    i. arachnoid
    i. cholesteatoma
    i. hemorrhage
    i. pressure
    i. subdural space
intracristal space
intraculminate fissure
intracystic
    i. breast cancer
    i. hyperplasia
    i. papilloma
intracytoplasmic inclusion cells
intradermal
    i. nevus
    i. reaction
    i. test
intraductal
    i. carcinoma
    i. hyperplasia
    i. papilloma
    i. papillomatosis
intradural
intraepidermal
    i. basal cell epithelioma
    i. carcinoma
    i. nevus
    i. squamous cell carcinoma
intraepithelial
    i. carcinoma
    i. dyskeratosis
    i. epithelioma
    i. gland
    i. neoplasia
intraerythrocytic
intragastric
intrahepatic
    i. bile duct
    i. cholestasis
intralaminar nucleus
intralaryngeal carcinoma
intraligamentous leiomyoma
intralimbic gyrus
intralobular
    i. bile ductule

    i. duct
    i. mammary connective tissue
intraluminal
intramedullary
    i. hemolysis
    i. lipoma
intramembranous
    i. ossification
    i. space
intramucosal
intramural
    i. hemangioma
    i. hematoma
    i. leiomyoma
    i. leiomyomatosis
    i. lipoma
intramuscular
intranuclear cytoplasmic invagination
intraocular
    i. foreign body
    i. melanoma
    i. pressure
    i. retinoblastoma
intraoperative cell salvage
intraoral
intraorbital
intraosseous
    i. low-grade osteosarcoma
    i. therapy
intraosteal
intraparietal
intrapartum
intraperitoneal
    i. gas
    i. hemorrhage
    i. therapy
intrapleural pressure
intrapulmonary
intrapyramidal fissure
intrascrotal
intraspinal lipoma
intrastitial
intrathecal therapy
intrathenar
intrathoracic
    i. gas volume
    i. goiter
intratracheal carcinoma
intratubal
intratubular
intratumoral
intraurothelial carcinoma

intrauterine
  i. death
  i. device
  i. fetally malnourished
  i. foreign body
  i. growth rate
  i. infection
  i. torsion
  i. transfusion
intravagal paraganglioma
intravaginal
intravasation
intravascular
  i. agglutination
  i. angiomatosis
  i. coagulation screen
  i. consumption coagulopathy
  i. fasciitis
  i. hemolysis
  i. lymph
  i. mass
  i. papillary endothelial hyper-
    plasia
intravenous
  i. glucose tolerance test
  i. hyperalimentation
  i. immune globulin
  i. pyelogram
  i. tolbutamide tolerance test
intravenously
intraventricular
  i. conduction defect
  i. hemorrhage
  i. pressure
intravesical therapy
intravital stain
intrinsic
  i. affinity
  i. association constant
  i. asthma
  i. factor
  i. factor antibody
  i. factor concentrate
  i. laryngeal muscle
  i. light
  i. lingual muscle
  i. pathway
  i. semiconductor
  i. tongue muscle branch
introitus
intron
introsusception

introversion
intubate
intubation
  endotracheal i.
  esophageal i.
  gastrointestinal i.
  rapid duodenal i.
intumesce
intumescence
intumescent cataract
intumescentia
intussusception
  colic i.
  double i.
  ileal i.
  ileocecal i.
  ileocolic i.
  jejunogastric i.
  retrograde i.
intussusceptive
intussusceptum
intussuscipiens
inulase
inulin clearance
in utero
in vacuo
invagination
  intranuclear cytoplasmic i.
invalid
invariant
  i. chain
  I i.
invasin
invasion
invasive
  i. activity test
  i. aspergillosis
  i. carcinoma
  i. fibrous thyroiditis
  i. mole
invasiveness
inverse-square law
inversion
  carbohydrate i.
  chromosomal i.
  heterobrachial i.
  homobrachial i.
  i. of nipple
  overlapping i.
  i. of uterus
  visceral i.
invertase

inverted
    i. ductal papilloma
    i. follicular keratosis
    i. keratosis
    i. papilloma
    i. testis
inverter
invertin
inverting enzyme
invertose
invert sugar
investigation
in vitro
in vivo
involucre
involucrum (pl., involucra)
involuntary
involution
    i. cyst
    i. form
    menstrual i.
    postlactation i.
    senile i.
involutional
    i. melancholia
    i. psychosis
involved field radiotherapy
IO — internal os
    intestinal obstruction
    intraocular
I/O — input/output
    intake and output
Io — ionium
iocarmate meglumine
iocetamic acid
iodamide meglumine
Iodamoeba
    I. bütschlii
    I. williamsi
iodate reaction of epinephrine
iodemia
I/O device
iodic acid
iodide
    i.-associated thyroiditis
    mercuric i.
    i. peroxidase
    saturated solution of potas-
      sium i.
    i. transport defect
iodimetry
iodinase

iodinated
    i. human serum albumin
    i. I-125 serum albumin
    i. I-131 serum albumin
    i. macroaggregated albumin
    i. serum albumin
iodine
    i.-123
    i.-125
    i.-azide test
    butanol-extractable i.
    i. cysts
    i. deficiency
    i. escape peak
    Gram's i.
    imidecyl i.
    i.-induced hyperthyroidism
    i.-125 implant
    i.-131-iodomethyl-19-
      norcholesterol
    i.-131-6 β-iodomethyl-19-
      norcholesterol
    i. mumps
    i. number
    plasma inorganic i.
    protein-bound i.
    radioactive i.
    i. reaction of epinephrine
    serum precipitable i.
    serum protein—bound i.
    i. solution
    i. stain
    i. staining
    i.-131 therapy
    tincture of i.
    i.-131 uptake test
    i. value
iodinophil; iodinophile
iodinophilous
iodipamide
    i. meglumine
    i. sodium
iodized oil
iodoalphionic acid
iodobismuthate
iodochlorhydroxyquin
iodocholesterol I-131
iododeoxyuridine
5-iododeoxyuridine
iodoform
iodohippurate sodium
iodolography

iodometric
iodometry
iodophil granula
iodophilia
iodophor
iodophthalein sodium
iodoplatinate
iodoprotein
iodopsin
iodopyracet
iodoquin
iodothyronine
iodotyrosine
        i. dehalogenase
        i. deiodinase defect
ioduria
IOFB — intraocular foreign body
iometer
ion
        alkoxide i.
        carbonium i.
        carboxylate i.
        i. counter
        dipolar i.
        i. disorder
        i.-exchange chromatography
        i.-exchange membrane
        i.-exchange resin
        gram i.
        hydrogen i.
        hydronium i.
        hydroxide i.
        oxonium i.
        i. pair
        i. product
        i.-selective electrode
ionic
        i. bond
        i. charge
        i. concentration
        i. strength
ionization
        avalanche i.
        i. chamber
        i. constant
        i. interference
        specific i.
ionize
ionized calcium assays
ionizing radiation
ionogen
ionogram

ionometry
ionopherogram
ionophore
iontophoresis
IOP — intraocular pressure
iopamidol
iopanoic acid
iophendylate
iophenoxic acid
IORT — intraoperative electron
        beam radiation therapy
iota
iothalamate
        i. meglumine
        i. sodium
iothiouracil
IP — incisoproximal
        incubation period
        inosine phosphorylase
        instantaneous pressure
        interphalangeal
        intraperitoneally
        isoelectric point
I-para — primipara
IPC — isopropyl chlorophenyl
IPCD — infantile polycystic disease
IPD — inflammatory pelvic disease
ipecac
IPG — impedance plethysmography
IPH — idiopathic pulmonary hemo-
        siderosis
IPL — intrapleural
ipodate
        i. calcium
        i. sodium
ipomea
Ipomoea
IPP — intermittent positive pressure
IPPB — intermittent positive-pressure
        breathing
IPPO — intermittent positive-
        pressure inflation with
        oxygen
IPPR — intermittent positive-pressure
        respiration
IPPV — intermittent positive-
        pressure ventilation
iproniazid
ipronidazole
IPS — initial prognostic score
IPSID — immunoproliferative small
        intestinal disease

ipsilateral
IPSP — inhibitory postsynaptic potential
IPV — inactivated poliovaccine
IR — immunoreactive
    index of response
    infrared
    internal resistance
Ir — immune response
    iridium
IRBBB — incomplete right bundle branch block
IRC — inspiratory reserve capacity
IR drop
IRDS — idiopathic respiratory distress syndrome
    infant respiratory distress syndrome
IRG — immunoreactive glucagon
Ir genes
IRhGH — immunoreactive human growth hormone
IRI — immunoreactive insulin
iridescent
iridium-192 implant
iridocapsulitis
iridochoroiditis
iridocorneal angle
iridocyclectomy
iridocyclitis
    heterochromic i.
    i. septica
iridokeratitis
iridoncus
IRI/G ratio
IRIS — International Research Information Service
iris (pl., irides)
    i. bombé
    Florentine i.
    tremulous i.
    umbrella i.
iritis
IRMA — immunoradiometric assay
iron
    i. absorption
    i. ammonium citrate
    i.-binding capacity test
    bound serum i.
    i. carbohydrate complex
    i. chelation therapy
    i. clearance

i. deficiency
i. deficiency anemia
i. deposition
i. dextran
i. enzymes
ferric i.
ferrous i.
i. hematoxylin
high serum-bound i.
i. index
i. isotope
low serum-bound i.
i. lung
i. metabolism
i. overload
i. oxide
i. pigment
i. pigmentation
i. plasma clearance
i. poisoning
i.-positive pigment demonstration
i. salt–sulfuric acid reagent
i. saturation
serum i.
i. stain
i. storage
i. storage disease
i.-sulfide protein
i. sulfur protein
irovirus
irr. — irradiation
irradiation
    i. change
    i. damage
    interstitial i.
    lymphoid i.
    ultraviolet blood i.
    whole-body i.
irreducible hernia
irregular pulse
irreversible
    i. coma
    i. reaction
    i. shock
irreversibly sickled cell
irrigation
irrigoradioscopy
irritability
irritable
    i. bowel syndrome
    i. colon

irritant
    chemical i.
irritation
    i. cell
    i. fibroma
irritative lesion
irruption
irruptive
IRS — infrared spectrophotometry
IRV — inspiratory reserve volume
IS — intercostal space
    interspace
Isamine blue
isatin
ISC — irreversibly sickled cell
ischemia
    cerebral i.
    mesenteric i.
    myocardial i.
    i. retinae
    testicular i.
    transient cerebral i.
ischemic
    i. bowel disease
    i. cardiomyopathy
    i. colitis
    i. contracture
    i. encephalopathy
    i. heart disease
    i. hepatitis
    i. hypoxia
    i. leg disease
    i. limb disease
    i. maculopathy
    i. muscular atrophy
    i. necrosis
ischial
    i. bursa of gluteus maximus
        muscle
    i. bursa of obturator internus
        muscle
    i. tuberosity
ischiocavernosus muscle
ischiofemoral ligament
ischiogluteal bursitis
ischiopagus
ischiorectal abscess
ischium (pl., ischia)
ISCLT — International Society for
       Clinical Laboratory
       Technology

ISCP — International Society of
       Comparative Pathology
ISD or ISDN — isosorbide dinitrate
ISE — ion-selective electrode
isethionate
    hydroxystilbamidine i.
ISF — interstitial fluid
ISG — immune serum globulin
Is (immune suppressor) genes
ISH — icteric serum hepatitis
    International Society of
       Hematology
island
    blood i.
    erythroblastic i.
islet
    i. alpha cell
    i. beta cell
    i. cell adenoma
    i. cell carcinoma
    i. cell hyperinsulinism
    i. cell hyperplasia
    i. cells
    delta cell i.
    i. delta cell
    i. hormones
    i's of Langerhans
    pancreatic i's
    Walthard's i's
ISM — International Society of
       Microbiologists
ISO — International Standards Orga-
       nization
iso — isoproterenol
isoagglutination
isoagglutinin
isoallele
isoallelism
isoallotypic determinant
isoalloxazine
isoamyl
    i. acetate
    i. nitrate
    i. salicylate
isoamylase
isoanaphylaxis
isoantibody
    platelet i.
isoantigen
    Rh i.
isobar
isobaric

isobestic point
isobornyl thiocyanoacetate
isobuteine
isobutyl alcohol
isobutyric acid
isocarboxazid
isocellular
isochromatic
isochromatid
        i. break
        i. gap
isochromatophil; isochromatophile
isochromic anemia
isochromosome
isochronal rhythm
isochronous
isochroous
isocitrate
        i. dehydrogenase
        i. dehydrogenase assay
        i. lyase
isocitric
        i. acid
        i. dehydrogenase
isocoproporphyrin
isocyanate
isocytosis
isodactylism
isodesmosine
isodose
Isodrin
isoelectric
        i. electrophoresis
        i. focusing
        i. level
        i. point
isoenzyme
        creatine kinase i's
        i. electrophoresis
        lactate dehydrogenase i's
        Regan i.
isoerythrolysis
        neonatal i.
isoetharine
isoflupredone acetate
isoflurane
isoflurophate
isoform
        actin i.
isogamy
isogeneic antigen
isogenic graft

isograft
isohemagglutination
isohemagglutinin
isohydric shift
isohydruria
isohypercytosis
isohypocytosis
isoimmune
        i. hemolytic anemia
        i. thrombocytopenia
isoimmunization
        Rh i. syndrome
isoiodeikon test
isolate
isolated
        i. dextrocardia
        i. dyskeratosis follicularis
        i. levocardia
        i.-organ tuberculosis
        i. parietal endocarditis
        i. proteinuria
        i. sinistrocardia
isolation
        herpes simplex virus i.
isolator system
isoleucine
isoleucyl
isoleucyl-RNA synthetase
isoleukoagglutinin
isologous chimera
isomaltase
isomer
        optical i.
isomerase
        glucosephosphate i.
        hexosephosphate i.
        isopentenylpyrophosphate i.
        5-P-ribose i.
        triosephosphate i.
        uroporphyrin i.
isomeric transition
isomerism
        chain i.
        dynamic i.
        functional group i.
        geometric i.
        nuclear i.
        optical i.
        position i.
        spatial i.
        stereochemical i.
        structural i.

isomerization
isometheptene hydrochloride
isometric period
isomicrogamete
isomorphic gliosis
isomorphous
isomuscarine
isomylamine hydrochloride
isoniazid
    i. assay
    i. phenotype test
isonicotinic acid hydrazide
isonormocytosis
iso-osmotic; isoosmotic
Isopaque
Isoparorchis
    I. hypselobagri
    I. trisimilitubis
isopathy
isopentenyl diphosphate
isopentenylpyrophosphate isomerase
isoperistaltic conduit
isophil antibody
isopleth
isoprene
isoprenoid
isoprinosine
isopropamide iodide
isopropanol
    i. precipitation test
isopropyl
    i. acetone
    i. alcohol poisoning
    i. benzene
    i. cresol
    i. meprobamate
    i. myristate
bis-(isopropylamido) fluorophosphate
isopropyl-*N*-(3-chlorophenyl) carbamate
isopropylmethylprimidyl diethyl thiophosphate
isopropyl-*N*-phenylcarbamate
isoproterenol
    i. hydrochloride
    i. sulfate
isopyknic
isopyknotic
isosbestic point
isoschizomer
isosexual
isosmotic

isosorbide dinitrate
Isospora
    I. belli
    I. hominis
isosporiasis
isosthenuria
isosthenuric urine
isosulfan blue
isothermal
isothromboagglutinin
Isoton diluent
isotone
isotonic
    i. coefficient
    i. sodium chloride solution
isotope
    carbon i.
    i. dilution–mass spectrometry
    nitrogen i.
    radioactive i.
    stable i.
    uranium i.
    zinc i.
isotropic
isotype switch
isotypic exclusion
isovaleric acid
isovalericacidemia
isovaleryl-CoA dehydrogenase
isovolume pressure flow curve
isovolumetric
    i. contraction
    i. relaxation
isovolumic
    i. contraction
    i. relaxation
isoxsuprine hydrochloride
isozyme
ISP — interspace
Israel's
    familial jaundice
    shunt
IST — insulin sensitivity test
    insulin shock therapy
isthmus (pl., isthmi)
    i. of aorta
    i. of fallopian tube
    i. of fauces
    oropharyngeal i.
    pharyngeal i.
    i. of thyroid gland
    i. of uterus

ISW — interstitial water
IT — implantation test
    inhalation test
    inhalation therapy
    intradermal test
    intrathecal
    intratracheal
    intratracheal tube
    intratumoral
    isomeric transition
Itaqui virus
ITC — imidazolyl-thioguanine chemo-
        therapy
itch
    barber's i.
    grain i.
    jock i.
    i. mite
    swimmer's i.
    winter i.
itching
    scrotal i.
iter of Sylvius
iteration
iterative process
ITLC — instant thin-layer chroma-
        tography
Ito's nevus
ITP — idiopathic thrombocytopenic
        purpura
    immune thrombocytopenia
    inosine triphosphate
ITT — insulin tolerance test
IU — immunizing unit
    international unit
    intrauterine
IUCD — intrauterine contraceptive
        device
IUD — intrauterine death
    intrauterine device
IUDR — iododeoxyuridine
IUFB — intrauterine foreign body
IUGR — intrauterine growth rate
IUM — intrauterine fetally malnour-
        ished
IUPAC — International Union of
        Pure and Applied
        Chemistry
[131]I (radioactive iodine) uptake test
IUT — intrauterine transfusion
IV — interventricular
    intervertebral
    intravascular

    intravenous
    intraventricular
    invasive
IVAP — in vivo adhesive platelet
IVC — inferior vena cava
    intravenous cholangiogram
IVCC — intravascular consumption
        coagulopathy
IVCD — intraventricular conduction
        defect
IVCP — inferior vena cava pressure
IVCV — inferior venacavography
IVD — intervertebral disk
IVF — intravascular fluid
IVGG — intravenous gammaglobulin
IVGTT — intravenous glucose toler-
        ance test
IVH — intravenous hyperalimenta-
        tion
    intraventricular hemorrhage
IVIgG — intravenous immune
        globulin G
IVM — intravascular mass
ivory
    i. exostosis
    i. osteoma
IVP — intravenous pyelogram
IVPF — isovolume pressure flow
        (curve)
IVRT — isovolumic relaxation time
IVS — interventricular septum
IVSD — interventricular septal
        defect
IVT — intravenous transfusion
IVTTT — intravenous tolbutamide
        tolerance test
IVU — intravenous urography
Ivy
    bleeding time
    method of bleeding time
    template bleeding time
IWL — insensible water loss
IWMI — inferior wall myocardial in-
        farction
Ixodes
    I. bicornis
    I. cavipalpus
    I. dammini
    I. frequens
    I. holocyclus
    I. pacificus
    I. persulcatus

I. *rasus*
I. *ricinus*
I. *scapularis*
ixodiasis

ixodic
ixodid
Ixodoidea
Izar's reagent

J — Joule's equivalent
JA — juvenile arthritis
Ja$_a$ antigen
J antigen
J$_a$ antigen
Jaccoud's
    arthritis
    arthropathy
jacksonian
    j. epilepsy
    j. march
    j. motor seizure
Jacobson's
    nerve
    organ
Jacquemin's test
Jadassohn's sebaceous nevus
Jadassohn-Tieche nevus
Jaffé's
    assay
    reaction
    test
Jakob-Creutzfeldt pseudosclerosis
Jakobson's malignancy grading
   system
Jaksch's anemia
jalap
Jamaican vomiting sickness
Janeway's
    gastrostomy
    lesion
janiceps
Jansky's classification
janus green B
Japanese B encephalitis virus
jar
    anaerobic j.
    Coplin j.
Jarisch-Herxheimer reaction
Jatropha
jaundice
    acholuric j.

    acute febrile j.
    black j.
    cholestatic j.
    chronic acholuric j.
    chronic familial j.
    chronic idiopathic j.
    congenital familial nonhemo-
      lytic j.
    congenital hemolytic j.
    familial nonhemolytic j.
    hematogenous j.
    hemolytic j.
    hepatocellular j.
    hepatogenous j.
    Israel's familial j.
    leptospiral j.
    malignant j.
    mechanical j.
    nonhemolytic j.
    nonobstructive j.
    obstructive j.
    pathophysiologic j.
    physiologic j.
    regurgitation j.
    retention j.
    spherocytic j.
    spirochetal j.
    toxemic j.
jaw
    lumpy j.
    osteosarcoma of j.
JBE — Japanese B encephalitis
JCAH — Joint Commission on Ac-
    creditation of Hospitals
JCAHO — Joint Commission on Ac-
    creditation of Health-
    care Organizations
J chain
JCML — juvenile chronic myelog-
    enous leukemia
JC virus or JCV

JDM — juvenile diabetes mellitus
Jeanselme's nodules
jejunal
    j. artery
    j. graft
    j. juice
    j. loop
    j. lumen
    j. mesentery
    j. mucous membrane
    j. submucosa
jejunectomy
jejunitis
jejunocecostomy
jejunocolostomy
jejunoesophageal bypass
jejunogastric intussusception
jejunoileal bypass
jejunoileitis
jejunoileostomy
jejunostomy
jejunum
Jendrassik-Grof method
Jenner-Giemsa stain
Jenner-Kay unit
Jenner's stain
Jensen's
    classification
    sarcoma
Jerne
    plaque assay
    plaque technique
jervine
jet lesion
Jewett-Strong staging system
JG — juxtaglomerular
JGC — juxtaglomerular cell
JGI — juxtaglomerular granulation
        index
JH virus
jigger
Jk antigens/antibodies
Jo-1 antibodies
jock itch
jodbasedow phenomenon
Johne's bacillus
joint
    acromioclavicular j.
    astragaloid j.
    j. calculus
    carpometacarpal j.
    cartilaginous j.

cervical vertebral j.
Charcot's j.
Clutton's j.
costotransverse j.
costovertebral j.
fibrous j.
j. fluid
humeroradial j.
humeroscapular j.
intercarpal j.
interchondral j.
interphalangeal j.
intervertebral j.
lumbar vertebral j.
lumbosacral j.
metacarpal j.
metacarpophalangeal j.
metatarsal j.
metatarsophalangeal j.
j. mice
midcarpal j.
midtarsal j.
radiocarpal j.
radioulnar j.
j. receptor
sacrococcygeal j.
sacroiliac j.
sternoclavicular j.
sternocostal j.
synovial j.
talocalcaneonavicular j.
talocrural j.
tarsal j.
tarsometatarsal j.
temporomandibular j.
thoracic vertebral j.
tibiofibular j.
vertebral j.
Joint Commission on Accreditation of
    Healthcare Organizations
Joint Commission on Accreditation of
    Hospitals
Jolles' test
Jolly bodies
Jones'
    criteria
    method
Jones and Campbell staging system
Jones-Cantarow test
Jones-Mote reaction
joule

Joule's
      equivalent
      law
JRA — juvenile rheumatoid
          arthritis
J receptor
J region
jt. — joint
jugular
      j. bodies
      j. foramen
      j. ganglion
      j. glossopharyngeal nerve
      j. indulation
      j. lymph node
      j. tenth cranial nerve
      j. undulation
      j. vagus nerve
      j. vein
      j. venous pulse
jugulodigastric node
jugulotympanic paraganglioma
juice
      cancer j.
      duodenal j.
      gastric j.
      ileal j.
      intestinal j.
      jejunal j.
      pancreatic j.
jump
      conditional j.
      unconditional j.
jumping gene
junction
      j. capacitor
      cardioesophageal j.
      cell j.
      j. field effect transistor
      gap j.
      gastroesophageal j.
      intercellular j.
      j. nevus
      j. potential
      Sertoli cell j.
      tight j.
      j. transistor
      ureteropelvic j.
junctional
      j. automaticity
      j. complex
      j. cyst

      j. escape
      j. nevus
      j. rhythm
      j. tachycardia
Junin virus
juvenile
      j. amaurotic familial idiocy
      j. angiofibroma
      j. carcinoma
      j. cell
      j. chronic myelogenous leu-
          kemia
      j. cirrhosis
      j. diabetes mellitus
      j. elastoma
      j. fibroadenoma
      j. hemangiofibroma
      j. hemangioma
      j. hormone
      j. hyalin fibromatosis
      j. kyphosis
      j. melanoma
      j. nephronophthisis
      j. neutrophil
      j.-onset diabetes
      j. osteoporosis
      j. Paget's disease
      j. palmo-plantar fibromatosis
      j. papillomatosis
      j. pernicious anemia
      j. pilocytic astrocytoma
      j. polyp
      j. polyposis syndrome
      j. rheumatoid arthritis
      j. xanthogranuloma
      j. xanthoma
juxta-articular
      j. nodule
      j. osteoporosis
juxtacortical
      j. chondroma
      j. chondrosarcoma
      j. osteogenic sarcoma
      j. osteosarcoma
juxtaglomerular
      j. apparatus
      j. cell hyperplasia
      j. cell tumor
      j. granulation index
      j. granules
      j. tumor
juxtamedullary nephron

juxtanuclear
juxtaposition
juxtapulmonary-capillary receptor
juxtapyloric
juxtarestiform body

juxtaspinal
juxtavesical
JV — jugular vein
            jugular venous
JVP — jugular venous pulse

K — absolute zero
        electrostatic capacity
        Kell blood system
        kelvin
        potassium
k — constant
KA — kathode (cathode)
        ketoacidosis
        King-Armstrong (units)
kabure
KAF — conglutinogen-activating
            factor
Kahn's test
kainic acid
Kaiserling's fixative
kala-azar
kalemia
kaliopenia
kaliopenic
kalium
kaliuresis
kaliuretic
kallidin
kallikrein
        k.-inhibiting unit
        plasma k.
        k. system
kallikreinogen
kaluresis
kaluretic
Kanagawa phenomenon
kanamycin
kang cancer
kangri
        k. burn carcinoma
        k. cancer
Kansas hemoglobin
K antigen
kaolinosis
kaolin partial thromboplastin time

Kaplan-Meier
        method
        survival curve
Kaposi's
        sarcoma
        varicelliform eruption
kappa
        k. chain
        k. deleting element
        k. factor
        k. granule
        k. rhythm
Kaproski's antigen
Karapandzic flap
Karmen unit
Karnofsky scale
Karwinskia humboldtiana
karyochrome cells
karyoclasis
karyocyte
karyogamic
karyogamy
karyogenesis
karyogenic
karyokinesis
        asymmetrical k.
        hyperchromatic k.
        hypochromatic k.
karyokinetic
karyoklasis
karyoklastic
karyolymph
karyolysis
karyolytic
karyomastigont
karyomegaly
karyomere
karyometry
karyomicrosome
karyomitosis

karyomitotic
karyomorphism
karyon
karyophage
karyoplasm
karyoplasmolysis
karyoplast
karoplastin
karyopyknosis
karyopyknotic index
karyoreticulum
karyorrhectic
karyorrhexis
karyosome
karyostasis
karyotype
    k. aberration
    X k.
    XO k.
    XX k.
    XXX k.
    XXY k.
    XY k.
    XYY k.
karyotypic
karyotyping
karyozoic
Kasten's
    fluorescent Feulgen stain
    fluorescent PAS stain
    fluorescent Schiff reagent
katacalan
katal (kat) unit
Katayama
Katayama's
    fever
    test
katharometer
katolysis
Kato thick smear technique
katzenjammer
KAU — King-Armstrong unit
Kauffman-White
    classification
    scheme
Kay-Bodansky method
Kayser-Fleischer rings
KB — ketone body
kb — kilobase
K-B cell
kbp — kilobase pair
KBr — potassium bromide

KC — kathodal (cathodal) closing
kc — kilocycle
kcal — kilocalorie
K capture
KCC — kathodal (cathodal)-closing
        contraction
K cells
KCG — kinetocardiogram
kCi — kilocurie
KCl — potassium chloride
KCN — (potassium cyanide) broth
        base
kcps — kilocycles per second
KCT — kathodal (cathodal)-closing
        tetanus
KD — kathodal (cathodal) duration
KDT — kathodal (cathodal)-duration
        tetanus
KE — kinetic energy
kedani mite
Keflex
Kefzol
Keith, Wagener, Barker classification
Keith-Wagener classification
kelectome
kelis
Kell
    antigen
    blood group
    blood group system
Kell-Cellano blood group
keloid
    Addison's k.
keloidosis
kelosomia
kelp
Kelthane
Kelvin
    temperature scale
    thermometer
kelvin
Kempson's grading system
Kendall's tau
Kenya hemoglobin
kerasin histiocytosis
keratan sulfate
keratiasis
keratic
keratin
    k. filaments
    k. pearls
    k. staining

keratinase
keratinization
    metaplastic k.
keratinize
keratinocyte
keratinous cyst
keratitic precipitates
keratitis
    acanthamebic k.
    acne rosacea k.
    k. bullosa
    dendritic k.
    disciform k.
    k. disciformis
    herpetic k.
    interstitial k.
    mycotic k.
    parenchymatous k.
    reticular k.
    sclerosing k.
    serpiginous k.
    suppurative k.
    vascular k.
    vesicular k.
    zonular k.
keratoacanthoma
    eruptive k.
    giant k.
    multiple k.
    solitary k
keratoangioma
kerotoatrophoderma
keratocentesis
keratoconjunctivitis
    epidemic k.
    herpes k.
    phlyctenular k.
    k. sicca
    superior limbic k.
keratoconus
keratocyst
    odontogenic k.
keratocyte
keratoderma
    k. acquisitum
    k. blennorrhagicum
    k. climactericum
    k. eccentrica
    lymphedematous k.
    mutilating k.
    k. palmaris et plantaris
    palmoplantar k.

    k. plantare sulcatum
    punctate k.
    senile k.
    k. symmetrica
keratodermatitis
keratoglobus
keratohyalin
    k. granule
    k. granule of epidermis
keratoid
keratolysis exfoliativa
keratolytic
keratoma
    k. disseminatum
    k. hereditaria mutilans
    k. plantare sulcatum
    senile k.
keratomalacia
keratonosis
keratopathy
    band k.
keratose
keratosis (pl., keratoses)
    actinic k.
    arsenic k.
    arsenical k.
    k. blennorrhagica
    k. diffusa fetalis
    follicular k., inverted
    follicularis k.
    inverted k.
    lichenoid k.
    k. nigricans
    k. obturans
    k. palmaris et plantaris
    k. pilaris
    k. punctata
    roentgen k.
    k. rubra figurata
    seborrheic k.
    k. seborrheica
    senile k.
    k. senilis
    solar k.
    tar k.
    k. vegetans
keratotic
    k. balanitis
    k. papilloma
    k. precipitate
Kerckring's valves
kerion celsi

kernicterus
Kernig's sign
Kern's
    isotypic determinant
    plasma relation theory
keroid
kerosene, kerosine
Kerry reducing substance test
ketal
ketamine hydrochloride
ketene
ketimine
keto
    k. acid
    k. group
keto acid
    branched-chain k.a.
    3-k coenzyme A-transferase
ketoacidosis
    diabetic k.
ketoaciduria
    branched-chain k.
ketoacyl
3-ketoacyl-coenzyme A
    thiolase
α-ketoadipate
α-ketoadipic acid
α-ketoadipicaciduria
11-ketoandrosterone
ketoconazole
11-ketoetiocholanolone
ketogenesis
ketogenic
    k. amino acid
    k.-antiketogenic ratio
    k. corticoids test
    k. hormone
    k. steroid
    17-k. steroid assay test
ketogluconokinase
α-ketoglutarate dehydrogenase
ketoglutaric acid
ketohexokinase
ketohexose
ketolaurate testosterone
ketone
    k. body
    k. body test
    k. body formation
    k. body utilization
    dimethyl k.
    methyl butyl k.

    methyl ethyl k.
    methyl isobutyl k.
ketonemia
ketonimine dye
ketonuria
    branched chain k.
ketopentose
ketoprofen
β-ketoreductase
ketose
ketosis
ketosteroid
    17-k. assay test
    17-k. fractionation
Ketostix
ketotetrosealdolase
ketothiolase
ketotic hyperglycinemia
ketotransferase
ketotriose
Kety-Schmidt method
keV — kilo electron volt
keyhole-limpet hemocyanin
Key-Retzius lateral aperture
KFAB — kidney-fixing antibody
kg — kilogram
kg-cal — kilogram-calorie
KGS — ketogenic steroid
khellin
kHz — kilohertz
KI — karyopyknotic index
KIA — Kliger iron agar
Kidd
    antibody
    antigen
    blood group
    blood group system
kidney
    abdominal k.
    k. abscess
    amyloid k.
    Armanni-Ebstein k.
    arteriolosclerotic k.
    arteriosclerotic k.
    artificial k.
    Ask-Upmark k.
    atrophic k.
    autosomal dominant
      polycystic k.
    autosomal recessive
      polycystic k.
    cake k.

k. carbuncle
cicatricial k.
contracted k.
cow k.
crush k.
cystic k.
disk k.
duplex k.
ectopic k.
embryonic k.
end-stage k.
fatty k.
k.-fixing antibody
flea-bitten k.
Formad's k.
fused k.
Goldblatt's k.
granular k.
hemangiopericytoma of k.
horseshoe k.
human embryo k.
human embryonic k.
lump k.
maximal tubular excretory capacity of k's
k. medulla
medullary sponge k.
metanephric k.
mortar k.
multilocular cystic k.
mural k.
pancake k.
pelvic k.
polycystic k.
primary African green monkey k.
k. profile
putty k.
pyelonephritic k.
rabbit k.
rhesus monkey k.
Rose-Bradford k.
scarred/shrunken k.
sclerotic k.
sigmoid k.
k. stones
structural k.
supernumerary k.
thoracic k.
k. transplantation
waxy k.
Kiel classification

Kienböck's
    atrophy
    unit
kieselguhr
Killan's triangle
killed
    heat k.
    k. measles virus vaccine
    k. vaccine
killer
    k. cells
    k. lymphocyte
kilobase pair
kilocalorie
kilocycle
    k's per second
kilodalton
kilo electron volt
kilogram
    k.-calorie
kilohertz
kilohm
kilojoule
kilometer
kilopascal
kilovolt
    k.-ampere
    k. peak
kilovoltage
    peak k.
kilowatt-hour
Kimmelstiel-Wilson lesion
kinase
    adenyl k.
    adenylate k.
    aspartate k.
    creatine k.
    deoxythymidine k.
    macro-creatine k.
    phosphoglycerate k.
    phosphorylase k.
    protein k.
    pyruvate k.
    serum creatine k.
    tyrosinase k.
kindred
kinematic viscosity
kinesin
kinesis
kinesthetic memory
kinetic
    k. analyzer

cellular k's
k. energy
k. measurement
Michaelis-Menten k's
tumor cell k's
kinetochore
kinetocyte
kinetoplasm
kinetoplast
kinetosome
Kinevac
King-Armstrong
 method
 unit
kingdom
Kingella
 K. denitrificans
 K. kingae
King unit
kininase
kininogen
kinin system
kinky hair syndrome
kinocilium (pl., kinocilia)
kinosphere
kinship
Kinyoun carbol fuchsin stain
Kirby-Bauer test
Kirchoff's law
kitasamycin
Kittrich's stain
KIU — kallikrein-inhibiting unit
kj — kilojoule
Kjeldahl's
 method
 technique
Klatskin's tumor
Klebsiella
 K. friedländeri
 K. oxytoca
 K. ozaenae
 K. pneumoniae
 K. rhinoscleromatis
Klebsielleae
Klebs-Löffler bacillus
Kleihauer-Betke test
Kleihauer's
 stain
 test
Klein-Gumprecht shadow nuclei
Klein's
 bacillus
 reaction

Klenow's fragment
KLH — keyhole-limpet hemocyanin
Kliger iron agar
Klinger-Ludwig acid-thionin stain
Klippel-Feil deformity
Klüver-Barrera Luxol fast blue stain
Kluyvera
KM — kanamycin
km — kilometer
Km (kappa marker) allotype
Km allotypic determinant
Km antigen
KMnO — potassium permanganate
KMV — killed measles virus vaccine
knee
 Brodie's k.
 k. cap
 septic k.
knee joint
 lateral meniscus of k.j.
 medial meniscus of k.j.
Knemidokoptes
knife
 k. blade atrophy
 microtome k.
 k.-rest crystal
knizocyte
knob
 malarial k's
 olfactory k.
Knops antigen
Knott's technique
Kobelt's cyst
Kober
 reagent
 test
Kobert's test
KOC
 kathodal (cathodal)-opening
  contraction
Koch's
 bacillus
 ileostomy reservoir
 postulates
Koch-Weeks
 bacillus
 haemophilus
Koebner phenomenon
Koenen's tumor
Koga treatment
Kogoj's abscess
KOH — potassium hydroxide
Köhler illumination

Kohn's
  one-step staining technique
  pores
koilocyte
koilocytosis
koilocytotic
koilonychia
kokoi venom
Kölliker's interstitial granule
Kolmer's test with Reiter protein
Köln hemoglobin
Koplik's spots
Korányi's treatment
Korsakoff's psychosis
Koserella trabulsii
Kossa stain
Kostmann's infantile genetic agranulo-
  cytosis
Kovács' reagent
Kovat's index
KP — keratitic precipitates
kPa — kilopascal
KPTT — kaolin partial thromboplastin time
Kr — krypton
Krabbe's leukodystrophy
kraurosis vulvae
Krause's end bulb
KRB — Krebs-Ringer bicarbonate
  buffer
krebiozen
Krebs'
  cycle
  leukocyte index
Krebs-Henseleit cycle
Krebs-Ringer
  bicarbonate buffer
  phosphate
  solution
"kringles"
Krompecher's
  carcinoma
  tumor
Kronecker's stain
KRP — Kolmer's test with Reiter
  protein
  Krebs-Ringer phosphate
Krukenberg's
  spindle
  tumor
krypton
  k.-85

KS — Kaposi's sarcoma
  ketosteroid
  Klinefelter's syndrome
  Kveim-Siltzbach (test)
KU — Karmen units
KUB — kidney, ureter and bladder
Kühne's methylene blue
Kulchitsky
  cell carcinoma
  cells
Külz's cylinder
Kumba virus
Kunkel's test
Kupffer's
  cells
  cell sarcoma
kurtosis
kuru
Kurzrok-Ratner test
Kussmaul's
  breathing
  respiration
  sign
Küstner's sign
KV — killed vaccine
kV — kilovolt
kVa — kilovolt-ampere
Kveim
  antigen
  reaction
  test
Kveim-Siltzbach
  antigen
  test
kVp — kilovolt peak
KW — Keith-Wagener (classification)
kW — kilowatt
kwashiorkor
KWB — Keith, Wagener, Barker
  (classification)
kW-hr — kilowatt-hour
Kyasanur Forest disease virus
kyestein
kynurenine
  k. aminotransferase
  k. 3-hydroxylase
kyphos
kyphoscoliosis
kyphoscoliotic pelvis
kyphosis
  juvenile k.
  Scheuermann's juvenile k.
kyphotic pelvis

L — coefficient of induction
    left
    length
    lethal
    ligament
    liter
    lumbar
L. — *Lactobacillus*
L — sterically related to
    L-glyceraldehyde
l — levorotatory
    liter
LA — lactic acid
    latex agglutination
    left atrium
    leucine aminopeptidase
    linguoaxial
LAA — leukocyte ascorbic acid
lab — laboratory
Labbé's anastomosing vein
label
    affinity l.
    radioactive l.
    l. variable
labeling
    cohort l.
    hazardous materials l.
    l. index
labia
labia majora
    anterior commissure of l.m.
    posterior commissure of l.m.
labile
    l. cells
    l. factor
    heat l.
labioglossolaryngeal
labioglossopharyngeal
labiomycosis
labioscrotal fold
labium (pl., labia)
labor
    abnormal l.
    postmature l.
    premature l.
laboratorian
laboratory
    clinical l.
    controlled-access l.
    l. diagnosis

    l. hood
    l. reference value
    restricted-access l.
labrocyte
labyrinth
    acoustic l.
    cortical l.
    ethmoidal l.
    membranous l.
    olfactory l.
    perilymphatic l.
    statokinetic l.
    l. vestibule
labyrinthine
    l. defect
    l. hydrops
    l. reflex
labyrinthitis
lac (pl., lacta)
    l. femininum
    l. sulfuris
    l. vaccinum
lacerated wound
laceration
Lachesis
lacis
lac operon
lacrimal
    l. apparatus
    l. artery
    l. calculus
    l. caliculus
    l. canaliculus
    l. duct
    l. fossae
    l. gland
    l. nerve
    l. papilla
    l. sac
    l. secretion
    l. suture
lacrimation
La Crosse virus
lactacidemia
lactacidosis
lactalbumin
    α-l.
    l. hydrolysate
β-lactamase
Lactarius torminosus

lactase
    l. deficiency
    l. test strip
lactate
    calcium l.
    l. dehydrogenase
    l. dehydrogenase assay
    l. dehydrogenase isoenzyme
    l. dehydrogenase isoenzyme de-
       termination
    ferrous l.
    l. oxidase
    l.-pyruvate ratio
    l. racemase
lactated Ringer's solution
lactating
    l. adenoma
    l. breast
lactation
lactational mastitis
lacteal
    l. cyst
    l. fistula
lactescence
lactescent serum
lactic
    l. acid bacteria
    l. acidosis
    l. acid test
    l. dehydrogenase
    l. dehydrogenase test
    l. dehydrogenase virus
lacticacidemia
lacticemia
lactiferous
    l. duct
    l. sinus
Lactobacillaceae
Lactobacilleae
Lactobacillus
    L. acidophilus
    L. arabinosus
    L. bifidus
    L. brevis
    L. bulgaricus
    L. bulgaris
    L. casei
    L. catenaforme
    L. catenaformis
    L. cellobiosus
    L. fermentans
    L. fermenti

    L. fermentum
    L. jensenii
    L. leichmannii
    L. plantarum
lactobacillus of Boas-Oppler
Lactobacillus bulgaricus factor
Lactobacteriaceae
lactocele
lactoferrin
lactogen
    human placental l.
lactogenic hormone
lactoglobulin
    β-l.
    immune l.
lactone dye
lactoperoxidase radioiodination
lactophenol
    l. aniline
    l. cotton blue
lactose
    l. operon
    l. tests
    l. tolerance test
lactoside
    ceramide l.
lactosidosis
    ceramide l.
lactosuria
lactosyl ceramide
lactotroph adenoma
lactoyl
lactoylglutathione lyase
lactulose/mannitol test
lacuna (pl., lacunae, lacunas)
    absorption l.
    cartilage l.
    cerebral l.
    Howship's l.
    osseous l.
    parasinusoidal l's
    trophoblastic l.
lacunar
    l. abscess
    l. cell
    l. resorption
LAD — left anterior descending
      (artery)
    left axis deviation
    leukocyte adhesion defi-
      ciency
Ladd's band
Ladendorff's test

LAE — left atrial enlargement
Laelaps
Laënnec's
     cirrhosis
     pearls
LAF — laminar air flow
          lymphocyte-activating factor
Lafora's bodies
LAG — labiogingival
          lymphangiogram
lag
     nitrogen l.
     l. phase
     l. time
Lagochilascaris minor
lagophthalmos
LAH — lactalbumin hydrolysate
          left atrial hypertophy
LAI — labioincisal
LAIT — latex agglutination-
               inhibition test
LAK — lymphokine-activated killer
          (cells)
lake
     bile l.
laked blood agar
Laki-Lorand factor
Lallemand's bodies
LAMB (lentigines, atrial myxoma, mu-
     cocutaneous myxomas, and blue
     nevi) syndrome
lambda
     l. bacteriophage
     l. chain
     l. wave
lambdoid suture
lambert
Lambert's
     canal
     law
lamblia
lambliasis
Lambl's excrescences
LAMB syndrome
lamella (pl., lamellae)
     annulate l.
     cornoid l.
lamellar
     l. bone
     l. ichthyosis
     l. necrosis

lamina (pl., laminae)
     basal l.
     Bowman's l.
     l. choriocapillaris
     l. cribrosa, sclera
     dental l.
     Descemet's posterior l.
     l. dura
     fibrous nuclear l.
     glomerular basal l.
     medullary l.
     l. papyracea
     l. propria
     l. suprachoroidea
     l. terminalis
     l. vasculosa
laminagram
laminagraph
laminagraphy
laminar
     l. flow burner
     l. necrosis
laminarinase
laminated thrombus
laminectomy
laminin
laminitis
lamp
     Finsen's l.
     hollow cathode l.
     mercury-vapor l.
     spirit l.
     tungsten l.
     tungsten-halogen l.
     Wood's l.
lanatoside C
Lancefield
     classification
     grouping
lanceolate
lancet fluke
lancinating
Landouzy-Déjérine progressive muscu-
     lar dystrophy
Landry's paralysis
Landschutz tumor
land scurvy
Landsteiner-Donath test
Landsteiner's blood group system
Landsteiner-Wiener antigen
Langerhans'
     cell

cell granulomatosis
cell histiocytosis
giant cell
granules
islets
layer
langerhansian
l. adenoma
l. hormone
Lange's
colloidal gold test
solution
test
Langhans'
cells
giant cell
layer
Langmuir expression
language
high-level l.
low-level l.
machine l.
source l.
Lansing virus
lanthanide
lanthanoid
lanthanum nitrate
lanugo hair
LAO — left anterior oblique
LAP — left atrial pressure
leucine aminopeptidase
leukocyte adhesion protein
leukocyte alkaline phosphatase
lyophilized anterior pituitary
laparocolostomy
laparoenterostomy
laparoenterotomy
laparogastroscopy
laparogastrostomy
laparogastrotomy
laparohepatotomy
laparohysterectomy
laparohystero-oophorectomy
laparohysterosalpingo-oophorectomy
laparohysterotomy
laparoileotomy
laparomyomectomy
laparomyositis
laparonephrectomy
laparorrhaphy
laparosalpingectomy

laparosalpingo-oophorectomy
laparosalpingotomy
laparoscope
laparoscopy
laparosplenectomy
laparotome
laparotomy
lapinization
Laplace's law
Laquer's stain for alcoholic hyalin
L-arabinose dehydrogenase
L-arabitol dehydrogenase
lardaceous
l. liver
l. spleen
large
l.-bore needle biopsy
l. calorie
l. cell carcinoma
l. cell immunoblastic lymphoma
l. cleaved cell lymphoma
l. granular lymphocyte
l. intestine
l. noncleaved cell lymphoma
l.-scale integration
l. vessel hematocrit
Laron dwarfism
Larrey's cleft
larva (pl., larvae)
filariform l.
fly l.
lepidopterid l.
l. migrans
rhabditiform l.
larva migrans
spiruroid l.m.
visceral l.m.
laryngeal
l. aperture
l. branch
l. cartilage
l. cavity
l. chondromalacia
l. fibrosarcoma
l. gland
l. granuloma
l. hemangioma
l. leukemia
l. ligament
l. lupus
l. mucus

l. muscle
l. nerve
l. nodule
l. papilloma
l. papillomatosis
l. polyp
l. prominence
l. tuberculosis
l. web
laryngectomy
laryngismus stridulus
laryngitis
laryngocele
laryngoesophageal fistula
laryngofissure
laryngoflex
laryngogram
laryngography
laryngohypopharynx
laryngomalacia
laryngometry
laryngopharyngeal
laryngopharyngectomy
laryngopharyngeus
laryngopharyngitis
laryngopharyngoesophagectomy
laryngopharynx
laryngoplasty
laryngorhinology
laryngorrhagia
laryngorrhaphy
laryngoscleroma
laryngoscope
     Jackson l.
     Rusch l.
laryngoscopic
laryngoscopy
laryngospasm
laryngostat
laryngostenosis
laryngostomy
laryngostroboscopy
laryngotome
laryngotomy
laryngotracheal diphtheria
laryngotracheitis
laryngotracheobronchitis
laryngotracheobronchoscopy
laryngotracheoscopy
laryngotracheotomy
laryngovestibulitis
laryngoxerosis

larynx (pl., larynges)
    fibroelastic membrane of l.
    Gussenbauer's artificial l.
    ligament of l.
    lymphatics of l.
    mucous membrane of l.
    submucosa of l.
    ventricular fold of l.
larynxtrachea
LAS — linear alkylate sulfonate
        lymphadenopathy syndrome
LASER — light amplification by
        stimulated emission of
        radiation
laser
    l. angioplasty
    argon l.
    l. microprobe
    l. microscope
    l. therapy
    l. thermal angioplasty
Lash's casein hydrolysate–serum
  medium
Lasiodiplodia theobromae
Lasiohelea
Lassa
    fever
    virus
lassitude
lat. — lateral
late
    l. infantile amaurotic familial
      idiocy
    l. neonatal death
    l. positive component
    l.-replicating X chromosome
    l. systolic murmur
latency
    l. of activation
    distal l.
    l. period
    REM (rapid eye movement) l.
    sleep l.
    terminal l.
latent
    l. allotype
    l. carcinoma
    l. coccidioidomycosis
    l. empyema
    l. heat
    l. hypermetropia
    l. image

l. iron-binding capacity
l. porphyria
l. virus
lateral
    l. aberrant thyroid carcinoma
    l. aperture
    l. basal branch
    l. basal segment
    l. cerebral fissure
    l. circumflex femoral artery
    l. collateral ligament
    l. column
    l. corticospinal tract
    l. costal branches
    l. displacement
    l. femoral cutaneous nerve
    l. femoral cutaneous vein
    l. fornix
    l. funiculus
    l. geniculate body
    l. gray column
    l. horn
    l. lemniscus
    l. lemniscus nucleus
    l. ligament
    l. lobe, prostate
    l. mammillary nucleus
    l. margin
    l. medullary lamina
    l. meniscus
    l. nasal cartilage
    l. nucleus
    l. occipital gyrus
    l. occipital sulcus
    l. olfactory gyrus
    l. olfactory striae
    l. plantar artery
    l. proper fasciculus
    l. pterygoid nerve
    l. recess
    l. rectus muscle
    l. rectus nerve
    l. sacral artery
    l. sacral vein
    l. segment
    l. spinorubral tract
    l. spinothalamic tract
    l. striate perforating branches
    l. sural cutaneous nerve
    l. thoracic artery
    l. thoracic vein
    l. thyroid

    l. tuberal nucleus
    l. vaginal wall smear
    l. ventricle
    l. ventricular vein
    l. wall, hypopharynx
    l. wall, oropharynx
lateroabdominal
lateromedial
lateroversion
latex
    l. agglutination
    l. agglutination-inhibition test
    l. agglutination test
    l. agglutinin
    l. fixation test
    l. flocculation test
    l. screen
    l. slide agglutination test
lathyrism
Lathyrus
latissimus dorsi muscle
Latrodectus
    L. bishopi
    L. geometricus
    L. mactans
LATS — long-acting thyroid stimu-
        lator
lattice
    dystrophy
    theory
laudanum
laurate
Laurell
    electroimmunoassay
    technique
Lauren classification
lauric acid
lauryl
    l. isoquinolinium bromide
    l. thiocyanate
Lauth's violet
LAV — lymphadenopathy-associated
        virus
lavage
    bladder l.
    bronchial l.
    bronchoalveolar l.
    bronchopulmonary l.
    gastric l.
    peritoneal l.
Laverania

law
> Ambard's l's
> Ångström's l.
> Beer's l.
> Bell-Magendie l.
> Bouguer's l.
> Boyle's l.
> Charles' l.
> Coulomb's l.
> Courvoisier's l.
> Dalton's l.
> Einthoven's l.
> Faraday's l. of electrolysis
> Fick's l.
> Gay-Lussac's l.
> Gibbs-Donnan l.
> Graham's l.
> Hamburger's l.
> Hardy-Weinberg l.
> Henry's l.
> Hooke's l.
> ideal gas l.
> inverse-square l.
> Joule's l.
> Kirchoff's l.
> Lambert's l.
> Laplace's l.
> l. of mass action
> Mendel's l.
> Newton's l. of cooling
> Ohm's l.
> Planck's radiation l.
> Poiseuille's l.
> Raoults' l.
> l. of reciprocal innervation
> right-to-know l.
> Snell's l.
> Starling's l.
> Stefan-Boltzmann l.
> Stokes' l.
> Virchow's l.

Lawless' stain

lawn
> bacterial l.
> l. plate

lawrencium

layer
> cambium l.
> l's of cerebral cortex
> depletion l.
> germ l.
> glomerular l.
> granular l. of cerebral cortex
> granular l. of olfactory bulb
> gray l. of rostral colliculus
> half-value l.
> Langerhans' l.
> Langhans' l.
> mitral cell l.
> molecular l. of olfactory bulb
> nerve fiber l.
> Nitabuch's l.
> nuclear l.
> olfactory nerve fiber l.
> optic l. of rostral colliculus
> palisade l.
> plasma l.
> plexiform l.
> pyramidal l. of cerebral cortex, internal
> somatic l.
> still l.
> subendocardial l.
> visceral l.
> white l. of rostral colliculus

lazarine leprosy

lazy leukocyte syndrome

LBB — left bundle branch

LBBB — left bundle branch block

LBCD — left border of cardiac dullness

LBF — *Lactobacillus bulgaricus* factor

LBI — low serum-bound iron

LBM — lean body mass

LBNP — lower-body negative pressure

LBW — low birth weight

LBWI — low birth weight infant

LC — lethal concentration
lipid cytosomes

LCA — left coronary artery

LCAT — lecithin-cholesterol acyl-transferase

LCAT deficiency

LCD — liquor carbonis detergens

L cells

LCFA — long-chain fatty acid

L (light) chain
> L-c. disease
> L-c. myeloma

LCIS — lobular carcinoma in situ

LCL — Levinthal-Coles-Lillie (bodies)

lymphocytic leukemia
lymphocytic lymphosarcoma
LCM — left costal margin
    lymphatic choriomeningitis
    lymphocytic choriomenin-
        gitis
LCM virus
LCT — long-chain triglyceride
LD — labyrinthine defect
    lactate dehydrogenase
    lactic dehydrogenase
    left deltoid
    legionnaires' disease
    lethal dose
    linguodistal
    living donor
    lymphocyte-defined
L-D — Leishman-Donovan (bodies)
LD_{50} — median lethal dose
LDA — left dorsoanterior
    linear displacement analysis
LDD — light-dark discrimination
LDH — lactate dehydrogenase
LDL; LDLP — low-density lipo-
        protein
L-dopa — levodopa
LDP — left dorsoposterior
LDV — lactic dehydrogenase virus
LE; L.E. — leukoerythrogenetic
    lupus erythematosus
Le^a; Le^b — Lewis antibodies
leaching
lead
    l. acetate
    l. anemia
    l. apron
    l. arsenate
    l. arsenite
    black l.
    l. chromate
    l. demonstration in tissue
    l. dioxide
    l. encephalopathy
    l. fixatives
    l. gout
    l. hydroxide stain
    l. level
    l. neuropathy
    l. oxide
    l. pigmentation
    l. poisoning
    l. stomatitis

    l. tetraethyl
    l. tetramethyl
leading strand
lead-pipe
    l.-p. colon
    l.-p. rigidity
leakage
lean body mass
least
    l. significant bit
    l. significant digit
    l. squares regression
leather-bottle stomach
Leber's
    cells
    optic atrophy
LE (lupus erythematosus) cell test
lecithin
    l.-cholesterol acyltransferase
    l.-cholesterol acyltransferase de-
        ficiency
    l.-sphingomyelin
    l.-sphingomyelin ratio
lecithinase
    l. A
    l. B
    l. C
lecithinemia
lectin
    Ulex europaeus l.
lectotype
LED — lupus erythematosus dissemi-
        natus
Lederer's anemia
leech
Lee-White
    clotting test
    clotting time method
    method
LE factor
left
    l. anterior oblique
    l. atrial enlargement
    l. atrial hypertrophy
    l. axis deviation
    l. bundle branch block
    l. costal margin
    l. posterior oblique
    l. to right ratio
    l. ventricular ejection time
    l. ventricular enlargement

l. ventricular failure
l. ventricular hypertrophy
leg
Barbados l.
elephant l.
milk l.
white l.
Legal nitroprusside reaction
Legal's test
Legionella
L. *bozemanii*
L. *dumoffii*
L. *feeleii*
L. *gormanii*
L. *jordanis*
L. *longbeachae*
L. *micdadei*
L. *pittsburghensis*
L. *pneumophila*
L. *wadsworthii*
Legionella pneumophila
culture
pneumonia
legionellosis
legionnaires' disease
l.d. antibodies
Leibovitz medium (no. 15)
leiodermia
leiomyoblastoma
leiomyofibroma
leiomyoma
bizarre l.
l. cutis
cystic l.
epithelioid l.
intraligamentous l.
intramural l.
parasitic l.
pedunculated l.
submucosal l.
subserosal l.
uterine l.
vascular l.
leiomyomatosis
intramural l.
l. peritonealis disseminata
leiomyomatous hamartoma
leiomyosarcoma
cordal l.
epithelioid l.
paratesticular l.
renal l.

Leipzig yellow
Leishman-Donovan bodies
Leishmania
L. *aethiopica*
L. *braziliensis*
L *caninum*
L. *donovani*
L. *infantum*
L. *major*
L. *mexicana* group
L. *nilotica*
L. *peruviana*
L. *tropica*
L. *tropica mexicana*
leishmaniasis
American l.
l. americana
cutaneous l.
lupoid l.
mucocutaneous l.
naso-oral l.
nasopharyngeal l.
l. recidivans
l. serological test
visceral l.
leishmanicidal
Leishman's
chrome cells
stain
lemmocyte
lemniscus (pl., lemnisci)
lateral l.
medial l.
optic l.
spinal l.
trigeminal l.
Lendrum's
inclusion body stain
phloxine-tartrazine stain
length
focal l.
greatest l.
l.-tension relation
Lennert's
classification
lesion
lymphoma
lens
achromatic l.
aplanatic l.
capsule of l.
cortex of l.

crystalline l.
electron l.
l. ligament
oil immersion l.
l. plate
suspensory ligament of l.
l. vesicle
lenticula
lenticular
    l. fasciculus
    l. follicles
    l. glands
    l. nucleus
    l. opacities
    l. progressive degeneration
    l. proteins
lenticulopapular
lenticulostriate arteries
lentiginosis
    periorificial l.
lentiginous hyperplasia
lentigo (pl., lentigines)
    l. maligna melanoma
    malignant l.
    nevoid l.
lentigomelanosis
Lentivirinae
leonine facies
leontiasis ossea
Leon virus
LEOPARD (lentigines, electrocardiographic abnormalities, ocular hypertelorism, pulmonary stenosis, abnormalities of genitalia, retardation of growth, and deafness) syndrome
leopard
    skin
    spotting
Lepehne-Pickworth stain
leper
lepidic
lepidoma
Lepidoptera
lepidopterid larva
lepidosis
Lepiota morgani
lepocyte
Lepore
    hemoglobin
    thalassemia

lepori pox virus
lepra
    l. cell
    l. manchada
leprechaun facies
leprologist
leprology
leproma
lepromatous leprosy
lepromin
    l. reaction
    l. skin test
    l. test
leprose
leprosy
    l. bacillus
    borderline l.
    cutaneous l.
    dimorphous l.
    dry l.
    histoid l.
    indeterminate l.
    lazarine l.
    lepromatous l.
    Lucio's l.
    macular l.
    Malabar l.
    murine l.
    nodular l.
    smooth l.
    trophoneurotic l.
    tuberculoid l.
leprotic
leprous
Leptoconops
leptocyte
leptocytosis
leptokurtic
leptomeningeal
    l. carcinoma
    l. carcinomatosis
leptomeninges
leptomeningioma
leptomeningitis
Leptomitus
    L. epidermidis
    L. urophilus
    L. vaginae
leptomonad
Leptomonas
leptonema
Leptopsylla segnis

leptoscope
Leptosphaeria senegalensis
Leptospira
  L. australis
  L. autumnalis
  L. biflexa
  L. canicola
  L. culture
  L. grippotyphosa
  L. hebdomidis
  L. hyos
  L. icterohaemorrhagiae
  L. interrogans
  L. pomona
  L. serodiagnosis
leptospiral jaundice
leptospirosis icterohemorrhagica
leptospiruria
leptotene
Leptothrix
Leptotrichia
  L. buccalis
  L. placoides
Leptotrombidium deliense
Leptus
  L. akamushi
  L. irritans
Leri's pleonosteosis
Leser-Trélat sign
lesion
  angiocentric immunoprolifera-
    tive l.
  Antopol-Goldman l.
  Baehr-Lohlein l.
  benign lymphoepithelial l.
  bird's nest l.
  Bracht-Wächter l.
  cavitary pulmonary l.
  central l.
  coin l.
  cold l.
  collar button l.
  Councilman's l.
  Ghon's primary l.
  gross l.
  histologic l.
  hot l.
  impaction l.
  indiscriminate l.
  initial syphilitic l.
  irritative l.
  Janeway's l.

jet l.
Kimmelstiel-Wilson l.
Lennert's l.
Lohlein-Baehr l.
lymphoepithelial l.
Mallory-Weiss l.
molecular l.
multifocal l.
onion scale l.
onion skin l.
organic l.
peripheral l.
precancerous l.
precursor l.
primary l.
radial sclerosing l.
ring-wall l.
skip l.
"soap bubble" l.
space-occupying l.
spontaneous l.
structural l.
systemic l.
target l.
trophic l.
wire-loop l.
lesser
  l. alar cartilage
  l. curvature, stomach
  l. Galen's vein
  l. omentum
  l. pancreas
  l. peritoneal sac
  l. saphenous vein
  l. splanchnic nerve
  l. superficial petrosal nerve
LET — linear energy transfer
lethal
  l. coefficient
  l. concentration
  l. dose
  l. dwarfism
  l. equivalent
  l. midline granuloma
  l. mutation
  l. titer test
Lethane
lethargic encephalitis
lethargy
leucine
  l. aminomutase
  l. aminopeptidase

l. aminopeptidase test
l. aminotransferase
l. hypoglycemia
l. zipper
leucinosis
leucinuria
leucofuchsin
leucomethylene blue
leuco patent blue
leucotomy
leucovorin calcium
leucyl
leucyl-RNA synthetase
leukanemia
leukapheresis
leukasmus
leukemia
  acute granulocytic l.
  acute lymphoblastic l.
  acute lymphoblastic l., B-cell
    type
  acute lymphoblastic l.,
    Burkitt-like
  acute lymphoblastic l., com-
    mon type
  acute lymphoblastic l., null
    cell type
  acute lymphoblastic l., pre–B-
    cell type
  acute lymphoblastic l., T-cell
    type
  acute lymphocytic l.
  acute megakaryoblastic l.
  acute megakaryocytic l.
  acute monoblastic l.
  acute monocytic l.
  acute monomyelocytic l.
  acute myeloblastic l.
  acute myelocytic l.
  acute myelogenous l.
  acute myeloid l.
  acute myelomonocytic l.
  acute nonlymphoblastic l.
  acute nonlymphocytic l.
  acute prelymphocytic l.
  acute progranulocytic l.
  acute promyelocytic l.
  acute undifferentiated l.
  adult T-cell l./lymphoma
  aleukemic l.
  aleukemic granulocytic l.
  aleukemic lymphocytic l.

  aleukemic monocytic l.
  basophilic l.
  basophilocytic l.
  B-cell l.
  bilineage l.
  biphenotypic l.
  blast l.
  blast cell l.
  Burkitt's acute lympho-
    blastic l.
  chronic l.
  chronic basophilic l.
  chronic cell l.
  chronic eosinophilic l.
  chronic granulocytic l.
  chronic lymphatic l.
  chronic lymphocytic l.
  chronic lymphosarcomatous l.
  chronic monoblastic l.
  chronic monocytic l.
  chronic myelocytic l.
  chronic myelogenous l.
  chronic myeloid l.
  chronic myelomonocytic l.
  common acute lympho-
    blastic l.
  compound l.
  congenital l.
  l. cutis
  embryonal l.
  eosinophilic l.
  eosinophilocytic l.
  erythromyeloblastic l.
  extramedullary l.
  gastric l.
  genitourinary l.
  gonadal l.
  granulocytic l.
  hairy cell l.
  hemoblastic l.
  hemocytoblastic l.
  hepatic l.
  histiocytic l.
  hypergranular promyelo-
    cytic l.
  juvenile chronic
    myelogenous l.
  laryngeal l.
  leukopenic l.
  lymphatic l.
  lymphoblastic l.
  lymphocytic l.

LEUKEMIA CLASSIFICATION

	PREFERRED NAME	PREFERRED ABBREVIATION	ALTERNATE NAMES
ACUTE	Acute myelogenous leukemia	AML	Acute myeloblastic leukemia; acute granulocytic leukemia; acute nonlymphocytic leukemia; acute myelocytic leukemia; acute myeloid leukemia
	Acute myeloblastic leukemia	AML-M1	
		AML-M2	
	Acute promyelocytic leukemia	AML-M3	Acute progranulocytic leukemia; APL
	Acute myelomonocytic leukemia	AML-M4	Acute monomyelocytic leukemia; Naegeli-type acute leukemia; AMML
	Acute monoblastic leukemia	AML-M5	Acute monocytic leukemia; pure monoblastic leukemia; Schilling-type acute leukemia; AMoL
	Acute erythroleukemia	AML-M6	Di Guglielmo syndrome
	Acute megakaryoblastic leukemia	AML-M7	AMKL
	Acute lymphoblastic leukemia	ALL	Acute lymphocytic leukemia
	Pre-B cell acute lymphoblastic leukemia	Pre-B ALL	B-lineage ALL
	Common acute lymphoblastic leukemia	cALL	Childhood ALL
	Cytoplasmic immunoglobulin (+) ALL	cIg + ALL	Pre-B ALL
	Philadelphia chromosome (+) ALL	Ph + ALL	

T cell	T-ALL	
B cell	B-ALL	Burkitt's leukemia (L3); "lymphosarcoma cell" leukemia
Acute unclassifiable leukemia	AUL	Stem cell leukemia; acute undifferentiated leukemia
CHRONIC		
Chronic myelocytic leukemia	CML	Chronic granulocytic leukemia; chronic myelogenous leukemia
Chronic phase of CML	CML	
Metamorphosis of CML		
Accelerated ± myelofibrosis	CML-BC	Blastic crisis
Lymphoblastic transformation	CML-BC lymphoblastic	
Myeloblastic transformation	CML-BC myeloblastic	
Megakaryoblastic transformation	CML-BC megakaryoblastic	
Juvenile chronic granulocytic leukemia	Juv.-CML	
Chronic eosinophilic leukemia	CEL	
Chronic basophilic leukemia	CBL	
Chronic lymphocytic leukemia	CLL	Chronic lymphoid leukemia
B cell	B-CLL	
T cell	T-CLL	
Hairy cell leukemia	HCL	Leukemic reticuloendotheliosis
Prolymphocytic leukemia	PLL	
Plasma cell leukemia	PCL	Leukemic phase of multiple myeloma
Sézary syndrome	SS	Leukemic phase of mycosis fungoides
Adult T-cell leukemia/lymphoma	ATL	

From Henderson, E. S., and Lister, T. A.: Leukemia, 5th ed. Philadelphia, W. B. Saunders, 1990, p. 14.

lymphogenous l.
lymphoid l.
lymphosarcoma cell l.
mast cell l.
mature cell l.
megakaryoblastic l.
megakaryocytic l.
meningeal l.
micromyeloblastic l.
mixed l.
mixed cell l.
mixed-lineage l.
monoblastic l.
monocytic l.
monomyelocytic l.
musculoskeletal l.
myeloblastic l.
myelocytic l.
myelogenic l.
myelogenous l.
myeloid l.
myeloid granulocytic l.
myelomonocytic l.
Naegeli-type monocytic l.
neonatal l.
neutrophilic l.
ocular l.
pancreatic l.
pituitary l.
plasma cell l.
plasmacytic l.
polylymphocytic l.
polymorphocytic l.
pre–B-cell l.
progranulocytic l.
prolymphocytic l.
promyelocytic l.
prostatic l.
pulmonary l.
refractory l.
relapsed l.
Rieder cell l.
Schilling's l.
Schilling-type monocytic l.
smoldering l.
splenic l.
splenomedullary l.
stem cell l.
subacute myelomonocytic l.
subleukemic l.
subleukemic granulocytic l.
subleukemic lymphocytic l.
subleukemic monocytic l.
T-cell l.
testicular l.
thrombocytic l.
thymic l.
thyroid l.
undifferentiated l.
l. virus
leukemic
l. cells
l. erythrocytosis
l. myelosis
l. reticuloendotheliosis
l. reticulosis
l. retinopathy
leukemid
leukemogen
leukemogenesis
leukemogenic
leukemoid
leukemoid reaction
lymphocytic l.r.
monocytic l.r.
myelocytic l.r.
plasmacytic l.r.
leukencephalitis
Leukeran
leukexosis
leukin
leukoagglutinating antibody
leukoagglutinin
leukobilin
leukoblast
granular l.
leukoblastosis
leukochloroma
leukocidin
Panton-Valentine l.
leukocrit
leukocytal
leukocyte
acidophilic l.
l. acid phosphatase stain
l. adherence assay test
l. adhesion deficiency
l. adhesion protein
l. agglutinin
agranular l.
l. alkaline phosphatase
l. alkaline phosphatase
methods
l. alloantibodies

l. antigens
l. ascorbic acid
l. bactericidal assay test
basophilic l.
broken l.
l. common antigen
contracted l.
l. cream
cryopreserved l.
cystinotic l.
l. cytochemistry
l. differential count
endothelial l.
eosinophilic l.
l. esterase
filament polymorphonuclear l.
l. function-associated anticoagulation
l. function-related anticoagulation
globular l.
granular l.
heterophilic l.
l. histamine release test
hyaline l.
l. inclusions
l. inhibitory factor
interferon l.
lymphoid l.
mast l.
mononuclear l.
motile l.
multinuclear l.
neutrophilic l.
nonfilament polymorphonuclear l.
nongranular l.
nonmotile l.
oxyphilic l.
passenger l's
polymorphonuclear l.
polynuclear l.
l.-poor erythrocyte
l.-poor red blood cells
segmented l.
l. transfusion
transitional l.
Türk's l.
Türk's irritation l.
leukocythemia
cryopreserved l.

leukocytic
l. crystals
eosinophilic l. infiltrate
l. hypersegmentation
l. infiltrate
l. margination
l. marrow
l. maturation
l. maturation alteration
l. nuclear hypersegmentation
l. nuclear hyposegmentation
polymorphonuclear l. infiltrate
l. sarcoma
leukocytoblast
leukocytoclasis
leukocytoclastic
l. angiitis
l. vasculitis
leukocytogenesis
leukocytoid lymphocyte
leukocytolysis
venom l.
leukocytolytic
leukocytoma
leukocytometer
leukocytopenia
leukocytophagy
leukocytoplania
leukocytopoiesis
leukocytosis
absolute l.
agonal l.
basophilic l.
digestive l.
distribution l.
eosinophilic l.
lymphocytic l.
monocytic l.
neutrophilic l.
l. of newborn
pathologic l.
physiologic l.
l.-promoting factor
reactive l.
relative l.
terminal l.
toxic l.
leukocytotactic
leukocytotaxis
leukocytotherapy
leukocytotoxicity
leukocytotropic

leukocyturia
leukoderma
    acquired l.
    l. acquisitum centrifugum
leukodystrophy
    adrenal l.
    globoid cell l.
    Krabbe's l.
    metachromatic l.
    metachromatic-type l.
    spongy degenerative-type l.
    sudanophilic l.
leukoedema
leukoencephalitis
    acute hemorrhagic l.
    necrotizing hemorrhagic l.
leukoencephalopathy; leukoencephaly
    multifocal progressive l.
    necrotizing l.
    progressive multifocal l.
leukoerythroblastic anemia
leukoerythroblastosis
leukoerythrogenetic
leukogram
leukokeratosis
leukokinesis
leukokinetics
leukokinin
leukokoria
leukokraurosis
leukolymphosarcoma
leukoma
leukomaine
leukomainemia
leukomalacia
    periventricular l.
leukomatous
leukomonocyte
leukomyelitis
leukomyelopathy
leukon
leukonecrosis
leukonychia
leukoparakeratosis
leukopathia; leukopathy
    acquired l.
leukopedesis
leukopenia
    autoimmune l.
    basophilic l.
    congenital l.
    eosinophilic l.

    lymphocytic l.
    monocytic l.
    neutrophilic l.
    pernicious l.
leukopenic
    l. factor
    l. index
    l. leukemia
    l. myelosis
leukophlegmasia dolens
leukophoresis
leukoplakia
    l. buccalis
    dysplastic l.
    glottic l.
    hairy l.
    l. lingualis
    oral hairy l.
    speckled l.
    urothelial l.
    l. vulvae
leukoplakic vulvitis
leukopoiesis
leukopoietic
leukopoietin
leukoprecipitin
leukorrhea
leukosarcoma
leukosarcomatosis
leukosis
    lymphoid l.
    myeloblastic l.
    myelocytic l.
Leukosporidium
leukostasis
leukostatic hemorrhage
leukotactic assay
leukotaxine
leukotaxis
leukothrombin
leukotic
leukotomy
leukotoxicity
leukotoxin
leukotriene
    l. A
    l. B
    bioactive l's
    l. C
    l. D
leukovirus
leukovorin

Leu-Ml antigen
leuprolide
Levaditi's
    method
    stain
levallorphan tartrate
levamisole
levamphetamine
levan
levarterenol bitartrate
levator
    l. ani muscle
    l. glandulae thyroideae muscle
    l. muscle of scapula
    l. muscle of thyroid gland
    l. palpebrae branch, oculomotor nerve
    l. palpebrae superioris muscle
    l. scapulae muscle
level
    antibiotic l.
    barbiturate l.
    Clark's l.
    complement l.
    confidence l.
    ethanol l.
    high l.
    isoelectric l.
    lead l.
    low l.
    minimal bactericidal l.
    pH l.
    salicylate l.
    serum urate l.
    signal l.
    significance l.
Levey-Jennings control chart
Levinson test
Levin's tube
Levinthal-Coles-Lillie bodies
levoatrio-cardinal vein
levocardia
    isolated l.
levodopa
Levo-Dromoran
levonordefrin
levopropoxyphene
levorotatory
levorphanol
levothyroxine sodium
levulosemia
levulose tolerance test

levulosuria
Lewis
    acid
    antibodies, Le^a, Le^b
    antigens
    base
    blood group
    gene
    procedure
    substance
lewisite
Lewy body
Leyden's
    crystals
    β-hemophilia
Leydig cell
    adenoma
    hyperplasia
    hypoplasia
    nodule
    tumor
Leydig-Sertoli cell tumor
Leydig's interstitial cells
LF — laryngofissure
    limit flocculation
LFA — left femoral artery
    left frontoanterior
    leukocyte function–associated
        anticoagulation
LFN — lactoferrin
L-form
LFP — left frontoposterior
LFT — latex flocculation test
    left frontotransverse
    liver function test
LG — left gluteal
    linguogingival
LGB — Landry-Guillain-Barré (syndrome)
LGN — lateral geniculate nucleus
LGV — lymphogranuloma venereum
LH — luteinizing hormone
Lhermitte's sign
LHL — left hepatic lobe
LH-RF — luteinizing hormone–releasing factor
LH-RH — luteinizing hormone–releasing hormone
LI — linguoincisal
LIA — leukemia-associated inhibitory activity

LIAFI — late infantile amaurotic
familial idiocy
LIBC — latent iron-binding capacity
libido
Libman-Sacks endocarditis
library
cDNA l.
gene l.
LIC — limiting isorrheic concentration
lichen
l. amyloidosis
l. annularis
atrophic l. planus
bullous l. planus
hypertrophic l. planus
l. myxedematosus
l. nitidus
l. pilaris
l. planopilaris
l. planus
l. planus, atrophic
l. planus, bullous
l. planus, hypertrophic
l. sclerosus et atrophicus
l. scrofulosorum
l. simplex chronicus
l. striatus
lichenase
lichenification
lichenization
lichenoid
l. dermatitis
l. eczema
l. keratosis
pigmented purpuric l. dermatitis
Lichtheimia corymbifera
lid
granular l.
l. lag
lidocaine
l. assay
l. hydrochloride
Lieberkühn's crypts
Liebermann-Burchard
reaction
test
lienomedullary
lienomyelogenous
Liesegang rings

LIF — left liac fossa
leukocyte inhibitory factor
life
average l.
mean l.
mean effective l.
l. table
technologic l.
useful l.
lig. — ligament
ligament
acromioclavicular joint l.
alar l.
ankle joint l.
annular l.
arcuate l.
broad l.
capsular l.
carpometacarpal joint l.
clitoral l.
coccygeal l.
conoid l.
Cooper's suspensory l's
coronary l.
cruciate l.
deltoid l.
dentate l.
denticulate l.
diaphragmatic l.
distal tibiofibular joint l.
elbow joint l.
epididymal l.
falciform l.
flaval l.
gastrocolic l.
gastrohepatic l.
gastrophrenic l.
gastrosplenic l.
hepatoduodenal l.
hepatorenal l.
hip joint l.
iliolumbar l.
inguinal l.
interphalangeal joint l.
intra-articular l.
ischiofemoral l.
knee joint l.
laryngeal l.
lateral collateral l.
lens l.
liver l.
Lockwood's l.

lower extremity l.
lumbosacral joint l.
lung l.
metacarpophalangeal joint l.
metatarsophalangeal joint l.
midcarpal joint l.
midtarsal joint l.
neck l.
nuchal l.
omental l.
ossicular l.
ovarian l.
patellar l.
pectinate l.
l. of penis
l. of perineum
phrenicocolic l.
proximal tibiofibular joint l.
quadrangular l.
l. of pubic symphysis
pulmonary l.
radiocarpal joint l.
round l.
sacrococcygeal joint l.
sacroiliac joint l.
shoulder l.
sternoclavicular joint l.
superior radioulnar joint l.
suspensory l.
talocalcaneonavicular joint l.
talocrural joint l.
tarsometatarsal joint l.
tracheal l.
trapezoid l.
triangular l.
trunk l.
umbilical l.
upper extremity l.
uterine l.
uterosacral l.
Whitnall's l.
ligamentum (pl., ligamenta)
l. arteriosum
l. denticulatum
l. flavum
l. nuchae
l. teres
l. venosum
ligand
ligandin
ligase
DNA l.
polynucleotide l.

ligate
ligation
ligature needle
light
actinic l.
l. chain
l.-chain disease
l.-chain nephropathy
coherent l.
cold l.
Finsen's l.
idioretinal l.
incident l.
infrared l.
intrinsic l.
l. microscope
l. microscopy
monochromatic l.
l. pen
l. pipe
polarized l.
l. reaction
l. reflex
refracted l.
l.-scattering analyzer
l.-scattering immunoassay
stray l.
strobe l.
transmitted l.
ultraviolet l.
visible l.
Wood's l.
ligneous
l. struma
l. thyroiditis
lignocerate
lignoceric acid
ligroin
ligula intestinalis
Liley test
Lillie's
allochrome connective tissue
stain
allochrome method
azure-eosin stain
ferrous iron stain
hematoxylin
sulfuric acid Nile blue stain
limb
anacrotic l.
l. bud
catacrotic l.

flail l.
l.-girdle muscular dystrophy
phantom l.
Roux-en-Y l.
thoracic l.
limbic system
limbus (pl., limbi)
limen insulae
limit
assimilation l.
l. check
l. dextrin
l. dextrinosis
explosive l's
l. flocculation
gas storage l's
Hayflick's l.
permissible exposure l's
quantum l.
l. of resolution
saturation l.
storage l's
within normal l's
limitations
container size l.
limiting
l. isorrheic concentration
l. reactant
Limnatis
L. granulosa
L. mysomelas
L. nilotica
limonene
limulus lysate test
Limulus polyphemus
limulus test
lincomycin
lindane
Lindau's tumor
line
absorption l.
Beau's l's
canthomeatal l.
cell l.
cement l.
cervical l.
D l.
delay l.
l. of demarcation
diploid cell l's
Eberth's l's
emission l.

equipotential l.
l. filter
l. focus
Gennari's l.
Hunter-Schreger l's
M l.
Muercke's l.
l. number
Ohngren's l.
regression l.
Reid's base l.
resonance l.
l. spectrum
l.-spread function
l. test
Ullmann's l.
Wegner's l.
Z l.
Zahn's l's
linea (pl., lineae)
lineae albicantes
lineae atrophicae
linear
l. accelerator
l. attenuation coefficient
l. discriminant analysis
l. energy transfer
l. equation
l. focus
l. fracture
l. IgA bullous disease in children
l. regression
l. sebaceous nevus syndrome
linearity
l. check
photometric l.
Lineweaver-Burk equation
linguae
anthracosis l.
lingual
l. artery
l. branch
l. goiter
l. gyrus
l. muscle
l. nerve
l. papillae
l. thyroid
l. tonsil
Linguatula serrata
linguatuliasis

linguatulid
Linguatulidae
lingula (pl., lingulae)
lingular
    l. branch
    l. bronchus
linitis plastica
linkage
    chromosomal l.
    l. disequilibrium
    l. group
    l. map
    peptide l's
linoleate
linoleic acid
linolenate
linolenic acid
linseed
Linstowiidae
liomyoma
liothyronine
liotrix
LIP — lymphocytic interstitial pneu-
    monitis
lip
    cleft l.
    rhombic l.
liparocele
lipase
    l. assay
    clearing factor l.
    gastric l.
    hepatic l.
    hepatic triglyceride l.
    lipoprotein l.
    pancreatic l.
    serum l.
    l. test
    triacylglycerol l.
lipedema
lipemia
    absorptive l.
    alimentary l.
    diabetic l.
    postprandial l.
    l. retinalis
lipemic
lipid
    accumulation of complex l's
    l. assay
    l. bilayer
    l. cell tumor

Ciaccio-positive l's
    l. cytosomes
    l. degeneration
    l. depletion
    l. disorder
    l. embolism
extracellular aggregate alter-
    ation l.
glycerol l.
l. histiocytosis
l.-laden macrophage
l. nephrosis
nuclear aggregate l.
    l. peroxidation
    l. pigments
    l. pneumonia
    l. profile
    l. proteinosis
    l.-rich adenoma
    l. stains
    l. storage disease
    l. test
    l. transport
    l. transport disorder
    l. tubular adenoma
lipidase
lipidemia
lipidosis
    cerebroside l.
    glycolipid l.
    sphingomyelin l.
    sulfatide l.
Lipid Research Clinics Program
lipiduria
lipiodol
lipoadenoma
lipoamide dehydrogenase
lipoarthritis
lipoate acetyltransferase
lipoatrophia
    l. annularis
    l. circumscripta
lipoatrophic diabetes
lipoatrophy
    insulin l.
    partial l.
lipoblast
lipoblastic lipoma
lipoblastoma
lipoblastomatosis
lipocele
lipochondrodystrophy

lipochondroma
lipochromemia
lipochrome pigmentation
lipocrit
lipocyte
lipodystrophia
     l. intestinalis
     l. progessiva
lipodystrophy
     congenital l.
     congenital total l.
     inferior l.
     insulin l.
     intestinal l.
     partial l.
     progressive l.
lipoedema
lipofibroma
lipofuscin
     l. granules
     l. pigment
lipofuscinosis
lipogenesis
lipogenic
lipogranuloma
     sclerosing l.
lipogranulomatosis
     disseminated l.
     Farber's l.
lipohemia
lipoic acid
lipoid
     l. degeneration
     l. dermatoarthritis
     l. dystrophy
     l. granuloma
     l. hyperplasia
     l. nephrosis
     l. pneumonia
     l. proteinosis
lipoidemia
lipoidosis
lipolipoidosis
lipolysis regulation
lipolytic
     l. enzyme
     l. hormone
lipoma
     l. annulare colli
     l. arborescens
     atypical l.
     l. capsulare

     l. cavernosum
     cordal l.
     fetal l.
     fetal fat cell l.
     l. fibrosum
     infiltrating l.
     intermuscular l.
     intramedullary l.
     intramuscular l.
     intraspinal l.
     lipoblastic l.
     l. myxomatodes
     l. ossificans
     paratesticular l.
     l. petrificans
     pharyngeal l.
     pleomorphic l.
     l. sarcomatodes
     l. sarcomatosum
     spindle cell l.
     telangiectatic l.
lipomatoid
lipomatosis
     encephalocraniocutaneous l.
     multiple symmetric l.
     l. neurotica
     pelvic l.
lipomatous
     l. hypertrophy
     l. infiltration
     l. myxoma
     l. polyp
lipomelanic reticulosis
lipomelanotic reticuloendothelial cell
     hyperplasia
lipomicron
lipomucopolysaccharidosis
lipomyohemangioma
lipomyoma
lipomyxoma
liponisus (see Lyponyssus)
lipopenia
lipopenic
lipophage
lipophagia granulomatosis
lipophagic
     l. granuloma
     l. intestinal granulomatosis
lipophagy
lipophilic
lipopolysaccharide

lipoprotein
    l. assay
    α-l.
    β-l.
    l. chylomicron
    l. electrophoresis
    "floating β"-l.
    high-density l.
    intermediate-density l.
    l. lipase
    l. lipase deficiency
    low-density l.
    pre-β l.
    serum l.
    sinking pre-β l.
    very-high-density l.
    very-low-density l.
    l.-X
lipoproteinemia
lipoproteinosis
liposarcoma
    cordal l.
    dedifferentiated l.
    myxoid l.
    paratesticular l.
    pleomorphic l.
    retroperitoneal l.
    round cell l.
    well-differentiated l.
liposis
liposome
lipotrophic
lipotropic
lipotropin
β-lipotropin
lipotropy
lipoxin
lipoxygenase pathway
lipping
Lipschütz's
    cell
    ulcer
lipuria
lipuric
LIQ — lower inner quadrant
liquefacient
liquefaction
    l. degeneration
    l. necrosis
liquefactive
    l. degeneration
    l. necrosis

liquid
    l. chromatography
    combustible l.
    l. crystal
    l.-in-glass thermometer
    l. ion-exchange membrane
    l. junction potential
    l.-liquid chromatography
    l. scintillation counter
    l. scintillator
    l. (solution) hybridization
Lisch nodules
Lison-Dunn
    method
    stain
lissamine rhodamine B 200
Lissauer's tract
lissencephaly
list
    l. mode
    l. structure
Listerella
Listeria monocytogenes
listeriosis; listerosis
liter
    l's per minute
    millimoles per l.
literal
lithiasis
    l. conjunctivae
    pancreatic l.
lithic acid
lithium
    l.-associated thyroiditis
    l. carbonate
    l. carmine
    l. citrate
    l.-drifted detector
    l. poisoning
    l. tungstate
lithocholate
lithocholic acid
lithogenesis
lithogenic
lithogenous
lithogeny
lithoid
lithonephritis
lithopedion
lithotomy
lithotroph
lithuresis

lithureteria
lithuria
litmus whey
littoral cell
Littre's gland
littritis
livedo
        lupus l.
        l. racemosa
        l. reticularis
        l. reticularis idiopathica
        l. reticularis symptomatica
        l. telangiectatica
        l. vasculitis
livedoid
liver
        l. battery
        caudate lobe of l.
        l. cell adenoma
        l. cell carcinoma
        central veins of l.
        cirrhotic l.
        fatty l.
        l. fibrosis
        l. flocculation test
        l. fluke
        l. fluke infestation
        frosted l.
        l. function test
        l. grooves
        hobnail l.
        icing l.
        lardaceous l.
        left lobe of l.
        ligament of l.
        lymphatics of l.
        l. membrane protein
        nutmeg l.
        l. palm
        polycystic l.
        l. profile
        quadrate lobe of l.
        right lobe of l.
        septal fibrosis of l.
        l.-specific protein
        sugar-icing l.
        "Swiss cheese" l.
        wandering l.
        waxy l.
lividity
        postmortem l.
living donor

livor mortis
lixiviation
lizard skin
LJM — Löwenstein-Jensen medium
LK — left kidney
LL — left leg
        left lung
        lower lobe
        lysolecithin
LLF — Laki-Lorand factor
LLL — left lower lobe
LLM — localized leukocyte mobili-
        zation
Lloyd's reagent
LLQ — left lower quadrant
LLV — lymphoid leukosis virus
LM — light microscopy
        linguomesial
LMA — left mentoanterior
LMF — lymphocyte mitogenic factor
LMM — lentigo maligna melanoma
LMP — left mentoposterior
LMT — left mentotransverse
LMW — low molecular weight
LMWD — low molecular weight
        dextran
LN — lipoid nephrosis
        lupus nephritis
        lymph node
LNPF — lymph node permeability
        factor
LO — linguo-occlusal
LOA — left occipitoanterior
load factor
loading
        l. dose
        salt l.
loaiasis
Loa loa
lobar
        l. cerebral atrophy
        l. pneumonia
        l. pulmonary atrophy
        l. sclerosis
lobation
lobe
        azygos l.
        cerebellar l.
        cruciate l.
        cuneiform l.
        digastric l.
        ear l.

flocculonodular l.
frontal l.
hepatic l's
lateral l.
occipital l.
parietal l.
Riedel's l.
temporal l.
thyroid l.
lobectomy
lobeline
lobitis
Loboa loboi
lobomycosis
lobster claw deformity
lobular
    l. adenocarcinoma
    l. breast cancer
    l. carcinoma
    l. carcinoma in situ
    l. duct
    l. glomerulonephritis
    l. hyperplasia
    infiltrating l. carcinoma
    l. neoplasia
    l. pneumonia
lobulation
    fetal l.
lobule
    hemispheral l.
    hepatic l.
    parietal l.
    peripheral l.
lobulus (pl., lobuli)
    l. biventer
    l. simplex
lobus (pl., lobi)
local
    l. anaphylaxis
    l. anemia
    l. anesthesia
    l. death
    l. exhaust ventilation
    l. glomerulonephritis
    l. hemosiderosis
    l. immunity
localization
    eye tumor l.
localized
    l. fibrous mesothelioma
    l. histiocytosis
    l. inflammation

    l. leukocyte mobilization
    l. myeloma
    l. nodular tenosynovitis
    l. osteitis fibrosa
    l. peritonitis
    l. plaque formation
    l. scleroderma
locant
location
    storage l.
lochia
Locke-Ringer solution
Locke's solution
lockjaw
Lockwood's ligament
locomotor ataxia
locoregional
loculated empyema
loculation
loculus (pl., loculi)
locus (pl., loci)
    l. coeruleus
    histocompatibility l.
    major histocompatibility l.
    minor histocompatibility l.
LOD (logarithm of the odds) score
Loeb's deciduoma
Loevit's cells
Löffler's; Loeffler's
    agar
    blood culture medium
    blood serum
    caustic stain
    coagulated serum medium
    endocarditis
    eosinophilia
    fibroplastic endocarditis
    methylene blue
    myocarditis
    pneumonia
    stain
Logan's procedure
logarithm
    common l.
    napierian l.
logarithmic
    l. amplifier
    l. curve
    l. phase
    l. response
logic
    CMOS (complementary metal
      oxide semiconductor) l.

emitter-coupled l.
transistor-transistor l.
tristate l.
logical record
logit transformation
lognormal distribution
Lohlein-Baehr lesion
loiasis
Lomidine
Lomotil
lomustine
long-acting thyroid stimulator
long arcuate fibers
long association fibers
long-chain
   l.-c. fatty acid
   l.-c. triglyceride
long-incubation hepatitis
longiradiate
longissimus muscle
longitudinal
   l. caudate vein
   l. cerebral fissure
   l. duct of epoophoron
   l. fasciculi of pons
Long's
   coefficient
   formula
long-term potentiation
longus
   l. capitis muscle
   l. colli muscle
loop
   capillary l's
   l. diuretic
   feedback l.
   Henle's l.
   hysteresis l.
   J. l.
   R-l.
   ventricular l.
looping
Looser's transformation zones
loose skin
LOP — left occipitoposterior
loperamide hydrochloride
Lophophora
lophotrichous
LOQ — lower outer quadrant
lorazepam
lordoscoliosis
lordosis

lordotic
   l. albuminuria
   l. pelvis
loss
   blood l.
   estimated blood l.
   transepidermal water l.
LOT — left occipitotransverse
Lotrimin
Louisiana pneumonia
louping ill virus
louse (pl., lice)
   l. bite
   l.-borne typhus
   chicken l.
   crab l.
   dog l.
   head l.
   l. infestation
   pubic l.
   sucking l.
lousiness
low
   l.-actinic glass
   l. birth weight
   l. birth weight infant
   l.-compliance bladder
   l.-density lipoprotein
   l.-density lipoprotein cholesterol
   l.-grade lymphoma
   l. ionic strength salt solution
   l. level
   l. molecular weight
   l. molecular weight dextran
   l. order
   l.-level language
   l.-power field
   l. protein
   l. serum-bound iron
   l.-voltage foci
   l.-zone tolerance
Löwenstein-Jensen-Gruft medium
Löwenstein-Jensen medium
lower
   l. extremity
   l. nephron nephrosis
   l. respiratory fluids
   l. respiratory spaces
   l. respiratory tract
   l. respiratory tract smear

l. trunk
l. uterine segment
Lowry assay
loxapine
l. hydrochloride
l. succinate
Loxosceles
L. laeta
L. reclusa
LP — latency period
leukocyte-poor
light perception
linguopulpal
lipoprotein
low protein
lumbar puncture
lymphoid plasma
L/P — lactate-pyruvate ratio
LPA — left pulmonary artery
LPC — late positive component
lysophosphatidylcholine
LPE — lipoprotein electrophoresis
lysophosphatidylethanolamine
LPF — leukocytosis-promoting factor
localized plaque formation
low-power field
lymphocytosis-promoting
factor
LPH — lipotropin
L-phase variant
LPL — lipoprotein lipase
Lpm; lpm — liters per minute
LPO — left posterior oblique
LPS — lipopolysaccharide
LPT — lateral position test
LPV — left pulmonary veins
Lp-X — lipoprotein-X
LR — laboratory reference
lactated Ringer's (solution)
light reaction
Lr — lawrencium
L/R — left to right ratio
L & R — left and right
L → R — left to right
LRF — luteinizing hormone–releasing
factor
LRH — luteinizing hormone–
releasing hormone
LRQ — lower right quadrant
LRS — lactated Ringer's solution
LRT — lower respiratory tract

LS — lumbosacral
lymphosarcoma
L/S (amniotic fluid lecithin to
sphingomyelin) ratio
LSA — left sacroanterior
lymphosarcoma
LSA/RCS — lymphosarcoma–
reticulum cell
sarcoma
LSB — left sternal border
LScA — left scapuloanterior
LScP — left scapuloposterior
LSCS — lower segment cesarean
section
LSD — lysergic acid diethylamide
LSH — lymphocyte-stimulating
hormone
LSM — late systolic murmur
LSP — left sacroposterior
L/S ratio — lecithin-sphingomyelin
ratio
LST — left sacrotransverse
LSV — left subclavian vein
LT — levothyroxine
lymphotoxin
LTB — laryngotracheobronchitis
LTF — lymphocyte-transforming
factor
LTH — lactogenic hormone
luteotropic hormone
lt. lat. — left lateral
LTPP — lipothiamide pyrophosphate
LU — left upper
Lu — lutetium
L & U — lower and upper
Lubarsch's crystals
lucanthone hydrochloride
lucidification
Lucilia
Lucio's
leprosy
phenomenon
Lückenschädel
Lücke's test
Ludwig's angina
Luer connector
lues
luetic
l. aneurysm
l. aortitis
Luft's potassium permanganate fixative

Lugol's
    iodine solution
    solution
Luke antigen
Lukes and Butler classification
Lukes-Collins classification
LUL — left upper lobe
lumbago
lumbar
    l. appendicitis
    l. artery
    l. lymph node
    l. myotome
    l. nerve
    l. plexus
    l. puncture
    l. spinal cord
    l. splanchnic nerve
    l. spondylosis
    l. sympathetic nervous system
    l. vein
    l. vertebra
    l. vertebral joint
lumbosacral
    l. joint
    l. plexus
    l. spinal cord
lumbricales pedis muscles
lumbrical muscle
lumbricosis
lumbricus (pl., lumbrici)
lumen (pl., lumina, lumens)
    bronchial l.
    colonic l.
    duodenal l.
    epididymal l.
    esophageal l.
    fallopian tube l.
    gastric l.
    ileal l.
    intestinal l.
    jejunal l.
    rectal l.
    seminal vesicle l.
    tracheal l.
    ureteral l.
    urethral l.
    vas deferens l.
luminal
luminescence
luminescent
luminophore

luminous
    l. flux
    l. flux density
    l. intensity
lump kidney
lumpy jaw
Luna-Ishak stain
lunate bone
Lundh meal
lung
    l. abscess
    acinic cell tumor of l.
    bilobed l.
    black l.
    coal-miner's l.
    collier's l.
    cystic disease of l.
    diffusing capacity of l's
    "end-stage" l.
    eosinophilic l.
    eosinophilic granuloma of l.
    farmer's l.
    fibroid l.
    l. fluke
    harvester's l.
    "honeycomb" l.
    human embryo l.
    humidifier l.
    hyperlucent l.
    l. ligament
    mason's l.
    miner's l.
    mushroom picker's l.
    nocardiosis of l.
    rudimentary l.
    l. scan
    shock l.
    silo-filler's l.
    thresher's l.
    l. tumors
    uremic l.
    welder's l.
    wet l.
Lunyo virus
lupiform
lupinine
lupoid
    l. hepatitis
    l. leishmaniasis
    l. rosacea
    l. ulcer
lupous

lupus
    l. anticoagulant
    chilblain l.
    chronic discoid l. erythema-
       tosus
    l. cystitis
    discoid l. erythematosus
    disseminated l. erythematosus
    l. erythematodes
    l. erythematosus
    l. erythematosus cell
    l. erythematosus cell test
    l. erythematosus, cutaneous
    l. erythematosus, discoid
    l. erythematosus disseminatus
    l. erythematosus, hypertrophic
    l. erythematosus inhibitor
    l. erythematosus profundus
    l. erythematosus tumidus
    l. hepatitis
    hydralazine l.
    l. hypertrophicus
    laryngeal l.
    l.-like anticoagulant
    l. livedo
    l. lymphaticus
    l. mutilans
    neonatal l.
    l. nephritis
    l. panniculitis
    l. papillomatosus
    l. pernio
    l. profundus
    l. psoriasis
    l. sclerosis
    l. sclerosus
    l. sebaceus
    l. serpiginosus
    l. superficialis
    systemic l. erythematosus
    l. tuberculosus
    l. tumidus
    l. verrucosus
    l. vulgaris
    l. vulgaris erythematoides
LUQ — left upper quadrant
Luschka's
    bursa
    crypts
    ducts
    foramen
Luse bodies

luteal
    l. cyst
    l. function
    l. hormone
lutein
    l. cells
    serum l.
luteinization
luteinized follicular cyst
luteinizing
    l. hormone
    l. hormone assay
    l. hormone–releasing factor
    l. hormone–releasing hormone
    l. principle
luteinoma
luteolysis
luteolytic
luteoma
    pregnancy l.
    stromal l.
luteotropic hormone
luteotropin
lutetium
luteum
    cystic corpus l.
Lutheran
    antibodies
    antigens
    blood group
    blood group system
lututrin
lux
luxation
Luxol fast blue stain
luxus heart
Luys' nucleus
LV — left ventricle
    leukemia virus
    live virus
LVDP — left ventricular diastolic
       pressure
LVE — left ventricular enlargement
LVEDP — left ventricular end-
       diastolic pressure
LVEDV — left ventricular end-
       diastolic volume
LVET — left ventricular ejection
       time
LVF — left ventricular failure
    low-voltage fast
    low-voltage foci

LVH — large vessel hematocrit
    left ventricular hypertrophy
LVP — left ventricular pressure
    lysine vasopressin
LVS — left ventricular strain
LVSP — left ventricular systolic
    pressure
LVSV — left ventricular stroke
    volume
LVSW — left ventricular stroke work
LVW — left ventricular work
LVWI — left ventricular work index
LW — Lee-White method
LW antigen
LX — local irradiation
Ly antigens
lyase
    argininosuccinate l.
    heparan sulfate l.
    isocitrate l.
lycopene
lycopenemia
Lycoperdaceae
Lycoperdon
lye
Lygidakis' procedure
Ly1 B cell
Lymantria
Lyme borreliosis
Lymnaea
lymph
    aplastic l.
    blood l.
    l. cell
    l. corpuscle
    corpuscular l.
    croupous l.
    dental l.
    l. embolism
    euplastic l.
    fibrinous l.
    l. gland
    glycerinated l.
    inflammatory l.
    intercellular l.
    intravascular l.
    l. node
    l. node, inguinal
    l. node, innominate
    l. nodule
    plastic l.
    l. scrotum

    tissue l.
    vaccine l.
    l. varix
lympha
lymphaden
lymphadenectasis
lymphadenectomy
lymphadenitis
    acute nonspecific l.
    chronic nonspecific l.
    dermatopathic l.
    mesenteric l.
    paratuberculous l.
    reactive l.
    tuberculous l.
lymphadenoid goiter
lymphadenoma
lymphadenomatosis
lymphadenopathy
    angioimmunoblastic l.
    dermatopathic l.
    immunoblastic l.
    persistent generalized l.
    l. syndrome
    tuberculous l.
lymphadenosis
    aleukemic l.
    benign l.
    malignant l.
lymphadenotomy
lymphadenovarix
lymphangeitis
lymphangiectasis; lymphangiectasia
    cavernous l.
    cystic l.
    intestinal l.
    simple l.
lymphangiectatic
lymphangiectodes
lymphangiitis
lymphangioadenography
lymphangioendothelial sarcoma
lymphangioendothelioma
lymphangiofibroma
lymphangiography
    bipedal l.
lymphangiology
lymphangioma
    l. capillare varicosum
    capillary l.
    l. cavernosum
    cavernous l.

l. circumscriptum
cystic l.
l. cysticum
fissural l.
peripelvic l.
l. simplex
l. superficium simplex
l. tuberosum multiplex
l. xanthelasmoideum
lymphangiomatosis
lymphangiomatous
lymphangiomycomatosis
lymphangiomyoma
lymphangiophlebitis
lymphangiosarcoma
lymphangitis carcinomatosa
lymphapheresis
lymphatic
l. anchoring filaments
l. angina
l. capillaries
l. choriomeningitis
l. cord
l. corpuscle
l. dissemination theory of
endometriosis
l. duct
l. dyscrasia
l. edema
l. follicle
l. glands
l. leukemia
l. nevus
l. sarcoma
l. sporotrichosis
l. system
l. trunks
l. vessels
lymphatitis
lymphatogenous
lymphatolysis
lymphatolytic
lymphectasia
lymphedema
congenital l.
hereditary l.
obstructive l.
penoscrotal l.
l. praecox
primary l.
lymphedematous keratoderma
lymphemia

lymphenteritis
lymphepithelioma
lymphmonocyte
lymph node
l.n. abscess
l.n. adenocarcinoma
l.n. biopsy
l.n. capsule
Cloquet's l.n.
epitrochlear l.n.
germinal center of l.n.
hepatic l.n's
hilar l.n.
ileocolic l.n.
iliac l.n.
inguinal l.n.
innominate l.n.
lumbral l.n.
mesenteric l.n.
obturator l.n.
perithyroidal l.n's
l.n. permeability factor
retropharyngeal l.n's
Rosenmüller's l.n.
lymphoadenoma
lymphoblast
nonleukemic l.
reticular l.
lymphoblastic
l. leukemia
l. lymphoma
l. lymphosarcoma
lymphoblastoma
giant follicular l.
lymphoblastomid
lymphoblastosis
lymphocele
lymphocerastism
lymphocyst
lymphocytapheresis
lymphocyte
activated l.
l.-activating factor
l. activation
atypical l.
autoreactive l.
B l.
l. blastogenic factor
circulating atypical l.
cytotoxic T l's
l.-detected membrane antigen
Downey-type l.

helper T l.
killer l.
large granular l.
leukocytoid l.
l.-mediated cytotoxicity
l. microcytotoxicity assay
natural killer l.
nodular poorly differentiated l.
null l.
plasmacytoid l.
l. recirculation
reticular l.
Rieder's l.
l.-stimulating hormone
stress l.
l. subset enumeration
suppressor T l.
T l.
T-cell l.
thymus-dependent l's
thymus-independent l's
l. transfer test
l. transformation test
tumor-infiltrating l's
lymphocythemia
lymphocytic
l. blood cells
l. cells
l. choriomeningitis
l. choriomeningitis virus
l. infiltration of skin
l. inflammatory infiltrate
l. infundibuloneurohypophysitis
l. interstitial pneumonitis
l. leukemia
l. leukemoid reaction
l. leukocytosis
l. leukopenia
l. lymphoma
l. lymphosarcoma
l. marrow
l. meningitis
l. series
l. thymoma
l. thyroiditis
l. tissue
l. transformation
lymphocytoblast
lymphocytolysis
lymphocytoma
benign l. cutis

lymphocytopenia
lymphocytopoiesis
lymphocytorrhexis
lymphocytosis
B-cell l.
infectious l.
neutrophilic l.
l.-promoting factor
lymphocytotoxic
l. antibody
l. assay
lymphocytotoxicity
lymphocytotoxin
lymphocytotropic
lymphoderma perniciosa
lymphoepithelial
l. cyst
l. lesion
lymphoepithelioma
nasal l.
nasopharyngeal l.
lymphoepithelium
lymphogenesis
lymphogenic
lymphogenous
l. embolism
l. leukemia
l. metastasis
lymphoglandula
lymphogram
lymphogranuloma
l. benignum
l. inguinale
l. malignum
Schaumann's l.
venereal l.
l. venereum
l. venereum antibody
l. venereum titer
l. venereum virus
lymphogranulomatosis
benign l.
l. cutis
l. inguinalis
l. maligna
lymphography
lymphohematopoiesis
lymphohematopoietic
lymphohistiocytosis
familial erythrophagocytic l.
lymphoid
appendiceal l. nodule

l. cell
colonic solitary l. nodule
l. corpuscle
l. follicle
l. hemoblast of Pappenheim
l. hyperplasia
l. hypoplasia
l. interstitial pneumonitis
l. irradiation
l. leukemia
l. leukocyte
l. leukosis
l. neoplasm
l. nodule
l. plasma
l. polyp
l. reactivity
rectal solitary l. nodule
l. series
l. stem cell
l. tissue
lymphoidocyte
lymphokine-activated killer cells
lymphokinesis
Lympho-Kwik
lympholeukemia
lympholeukocyte
lymphology
lympholysis
cell-mediated l.
lymphoma
adult T-cell leukemia/l.
adult T-cell l.
African l.
allogeneic l.
allogenic l.
autologous l.
B-cell l./
benign l.
benign l. of rectum
Burkitt-like l.
Burkitt's l.
cardiac l.
centroblastic/centrocytic l.
composite l.
convoluted T-cell l.
cutaneous T-cell l.
l. cutis
diffuse histiocytic l.
diffuse, large cell l.
diffuse, mixed small and large
cell l.

diffuse, poorly differentiated l.
diffuse, small cleaved cell l.
extranodal l.
follicular l.
follicular, mixed small cleaved
and large cell l.
follicular, predominantly large
cell l.
follicular, predominantly small
cleaved cell l.
giant follicular l.
high-grade l.
histiocytic l.
Hodgkin's l.
ileocecal l.
immunoblastic l.
intermediate l.
large cell l.
large cell, immunoblastic l.
large cleaved cell l.
large noncleaved cell l.
Lennert's l.
l.-like thyroiditis
low-grade l.
lymphoblastic l.
lymphocytic l.
lymphoplasmacytoid l.
lymphosarcoma-type malig-
nant l.
macrofollicular l.
malignant l.
mantle zone l.
Mediterranean l.
metastatic l.
mixed lymphocytic histiocytic l.
nodular l.
nodular histiocytic l.
non-Burkitt's l.
non-Hodgkin's l.
plasmacytoid lymphocytic l.
pleomorphic l.
poorly differentiated lymphocytic l.
primary l.
secondary l.
Sézary l.
signet ring cell l.
small cell l.
small cleaved cell l.
small lymphocytic l.
small noncleaved cell l.

splenic l.
stem cell l.
T-cell lymphoblastic l.
transfusion-related l.
U-cell l.
undifferentiated l.
well-differentiated lympho-
    cytic l.
lymphomatoid
    l. granulomatosis
    l. papulosis
lymphomatosis
lymphomatous polyposis
lymphomyeloma
lymphomyxoma
lymphopathia venereum
lymphopenia
lymphopenic thymic dysplasia
lymphoplasia
    cutaneous l.
lymphoplasmacytoid lymphoma
lymphoplasmapheresis
lymphopoiesis
lymphopoietic
lymphoproliferative
    l. disorders
    l. syndrome
lymphoreticular
    l. disorders
    l. system
lymphoreticulosis
lymphorrhea
lymphorrhoid
lymphosarcoma
    l. cell leukemia
    fascicular l.
    follicular l.
    lymphoblastic l.
    lymphocytic l.
    reticulum cell l.
    sclerosing l.
    l.-type malignant
        lymphoma
lymphosarcomatosis
lymphosis
lymphostatic verrucosis
lymphotoxicity
lymphotoxin
lymphotrophy
lymphotropic retrovirus

lymphuria
lyonization
Lyon's
    effect
    hypothesis
lyophilization
lyophilize
lyophilized anterior pituitary
Lyponyssus
lys — lysine
lysate
lyse
lysemia
lysergic
    l. acid diethylamide
    l. acid diethylamide assay
lysin
    β-l.
lysine
    l. dehydrogenase
    l. intolerance
    l. iron agar
    l. ketoglutarate reductase
    L-l. : NAD$^+$ oxidoreductase
    l. oxidoreductase
    l.-2-oxoglutaryl reductase
    procollagen l.
    l. racemase
lysinemia
lysing agent
lysinuria
lysis
    l. centrifugation system
    clot l.
    colloid-osmotic l.
    fibrin plate l.
    reactive l.
    red-cell l.
lysochrome
Lysodren
lysogen
lysogenic bacterium
lysogeny
lysokinase
lysolecithin acylmutase
lysophosphatidate
lysophosphatide
lysophosphatidylcholine
lysophosphatidylethanolamine
lysophospholipase

lysophospholipid
lysosomal storage
   disease
lysosome
      l. alteration
      l. granules
      l. α-L-iduronase
      primary l.
      secondary l.
lysostaphin

lysozyme
      l. assay
      egg-white l.
      human milk l.
lysylbradykinin
lysyloxidase-RNA synthetase
Lyt antigen
lytic
Lytta
lzm — lysozyme

M — macerate
    male
    maximal
    maximum
    mega
    minim
    molar
    mucoid
    multipara
    murmur
    muscle
    myopia
    permanent molar
    strength of pole
    thousand (mil-, milli-)
M. — *Micrococcus*
    Microsporum
    Mycobacterium
    Mycoplasma
m — meter
M_1 — mitral first sound
MΩ — megohm
μ — micron
    mu
MA — mandelic acid
      mean arterial (blood pressure)
      Miller-Abbott (tube)
Ma — masurium
mA or ma — milliampere
MAA — macroaggregated albumin
MABP — mean arterial blood
        pressure
MAC — maximum allowable concen-
        tration

    membrane attack complex
    minimum alveolar concen-
        tration
Macaca
macaque
MacCallum's patch
Macchiavello's stain
MacConkey agar
macerated
      m. fetus
      m. stillbirth
maceration
Machado-Guerreiro test
Mache unit
machine
      amino apheresis m.
      Cobe/IBM 2997 m.
      Cobe Spectra m.
      m. error
      Haemonetics V50 apheresis m.
      m. language
Machupo virus
Macleod's capsular rheumatism
maclurin
MacNeal's tetrachrome blood stain
Macracanthorhynchus hirudinaceus
macradenous
macrencephaly
macroadenoma
macroaggregate
macroaggregated albumin
macroaleuriospore
macroamylase
macroamylasemia

macroangiopathic
Macrobdella
macroblast
macrocephaly
macrocheilia; macrochilia
macrochemistry
macrochylomicron
macrocolon
macroconidium (pl., macroconidia)
macrocranium
macro-creatine kinase
macrocryoglobulin
macrocryoglobulinemia
macrocyclic
macrocyst
macrocyte
macrocythemia
　　hyperchromatic m.
macrocytic
　　m. achylic anemia
　　m. anemia
　　m. anemia of pregnancy
　　m. erythrocyte
　　m. hyperchromia
macrocytosis
macrodystrophia lipomatosa
macroerythroblast
macroerythrocyte
macrofollicular
　　m. adenoma
　　m. lymphoma
macrogamete
macrogametocyte
macrogastria
macrogenia
macrogenitosomia
　　m. praecox
　　m. praecox suprarenalis
macroglia
macroglobulin assay
macroglobulinemia
　　Waldenström's m.
macroglossia gigantism
macrogyria
macrohomology
macro-Kjeldahl method
macrolabia
macroleukoblast
macrolide antibiotic
macrolides
macrolymphocyte
macrolymphocytosis

macromastia
macromelanosome
macromethod of Wintrobe
macromolecular
macromolecule
　　m. aggregate alteration, extra-
　　　cellular
　　crystalline m. alteration
　　nuclear m's
Macromonas
　　M. *bipunctata*
　　M. *mobilis*
macromonocyte
macromyeloblast
macronodular cirrhosis
macronormoblast
macronormochromoblast
macronucleus
macroorchidism
macropathology
macropenia
macrophage
　　activated m.
　　m.-activating factor
　　m. agglutination factor
　　alveolar m.
　　anti-tumor m.
　　armed m.
　　m. chemotactic factor
　　m. colony–stimulating factor
　　m.-derived growth factor
　　epithelioid-type m.
　　m. fusion factor
　　m. growth factor
　　Hansemann m.
　　hemosiderin-laden m.
　　m.-inhibiting factor
　　lipid-laden m.
　　m. migration inhibition factor
　　monocyte-m.
　　m. proliferation
　　pulmonary alveolar m.
　　suppressor m.
macrophagocyte
Macrophoma
macropolycyte
macroprolactinoma
macropromyelocyte
macroreticulocyte
macroscopic agglutination
macrosigmoid
macrosis

macrosomia
Macrostoma mesnili
macrostomia
macrothrombocyte
macrothrombocytopathia
macrovesicular steatosis
macula (pl., maculae)
> acoustic m.
> m. adherens
> m. albida (pl., maculae albidae)
> m. atrophica
> m. cerulea (pl., maculae ceruleae)
> m. cribrosa
> m. densa
> m. gonorrhoeica
> honeycomb m.
> m. lactea
> m. lutea
> mongolian m.
> m. occludens
> m. retinae
> Saenger's m.
> m. tendinea
macular
> m. amyloidosis
> m. atrophy
> m. degeneration
> m. dystrophy
> m. eruption
> m. fibers
> m. leprosy
maculatum
> atrophoderma m.
macule
maculoerythematous
maculopapular eruption
maculopathy
> ischemic m.
madder
Madelung's neck
Madura foot
Madurella
> M. *grisea*
> M. *mycetomi*
maduromycetoma
maduromycosis
maduromycotic mycetoma
maedivirus
MAF — macrophage-activating factor

mafenide
MAFH — macroaggregated ferrous hydroxide
magaldrate
Magendie's foramen
magenta
> acid m.
> basic m.
> m. I, II, III
> m. O
MAggF — macrophage agglutination factor
maggot
> Congo floor m.
> rat-tail m.
magnesia
> m. alba
> m. calcinata
> m. carbonatada
> m. usta
magnesium
> m.-activated ATPase
> m. ammonium phosphate
> m. carbonate
> m. chloride
> m. citrate
> m. fluoride
> m. hydrate
> m. hydroxide
> m. isotope
> m. oxide
> m. phosphate crystals
> m. poisoning
> m. salt
> m. sulfate
> m. test
> m. trisilicate
> m. urate
magnet
magnetic
> m. beads
> m. core
> m. core memory
> m. field
> m. field strength
> m. flux
> m. induction
> m. moment
> m. radiation
> m. resonance imaging
> m. resonance spectroscopy

m. susceptibility
m. tape
magnetization
magneton
Bohr m.
nuclear m.
magnification
magnify
magnitude
signed m.
Magon dye
MAHA — microangiopathic hemolytic anemia
main
m. en griffe
m. en lorgnette
maintenance
Mainz's pouch
MAIS — *Mycobacterium avium-intracellulare-scrofulaceum*
Majocchi's granuloma
major
m. basic protein
m. gene
m. histocompatibility antigen
m. histocompatibility complex
m. histocompatibility locus
m. tranquilizer
mal
m. de Cayenne
m. de San Lazaro
Malabar leprosy
malabsorption
glucose-galactose m.
m. syndrome
malachite green
malacia
malacic
malacoplakia; malakoplakia
m. vesicae
malacosis
malacotic
maladie de Roger
maladjustment
malaise
malaria
algid m.
benign tertian m.
bilious remittent m.
bovine m.
double tertian m.
falciparum m.

m. film test
gastric m.
gastric algid m.
hemolytic m.
hemorrhagic m.
intermittent m.
malignant tertian m.
ovale m.
pernicious m.
quartan m.
quotidian m.
remittent m.
m. smear
tertian m.
vivax m.
malariacidal
malarial
m. cachexia
m. deposition pigment
m. dysentery
m. fever
m. granuloma
m. hemoglobinuria
m. knobs
m. parasite
m. pigment
m. pigment deposition
m. pigment stain
m. rosette
Malassezia
M. *furfur*
M. *macfadyani*
M. *ovalis*
M. *pachydermatis*
M. *tropica*
malassimilation
malate
decarboxylating m. dehydrogenase
m. dehydrogenase
m. oxidase
malathion
Malayan
filariasis
pit viper venom
maldigestion
Maldonado–San Jose stain
male
m. breast cancer
m. castration
m. genital fluids
m. genitalia

m. genital spaces
m. hormones
m. infertility
m. phenotype
m. pseudohermaphroditism
m. rudimentary uterus
m. sex chromatin pattern
m. Turner's syndrome
m. urethra
maleic hydrazide
4-maleylacetoacetate isomerase
malformation
    Arnold-Chiari m.
    arteriovenous m.
    bile duct plate m.
    cardiac valvular m.
    cardiovascular m.
    Chiari's m.
    congenital m.
    cutaneous m.
    Dandy-Walker m.
    Ebstein's m.
    m. syndrome
    Taussig-Bing m.
malfunction
Malherbe's calcifying epithelioma
malic
    m. acid
    m. dehydrogenase
    m. enzyme
maligna
    cynanche m.
malignancy
    B-cell m.
malignant
    m. adenoma
    m. ameloblastoma
    m. anemia
    m. astrocytoma
    m. atrophic papulosis
    m. breast tumors
    m. carbuncle
    m. carcinoid syndrome
    m. dyskeratosis
    m. edema
    m. endocarditis
    m. ependymoma
    m. epithelioma
    m. external otitis
    m. fibrous histiocytoma
    m. focal glomerulosclerosis
    m. giant cell tumor of bone

m. giant cell tumor of soft
    parts
m. glioma
m. globulin
m. glomerulonephritis
m. granuloma
m. hepatoma
m. histiocytoma
m. histiocytosis
m. hypertension
m. hyperthermia
m. jaundice
m. lentigo
m. lentigo melanoma
m. lymphadenosis
m. lymphocytoma
m. lymphoma
m. lymphoma, lymphosarcoma
    type
m. malnutrition
m. melanoma
m. melanoma in situ
m. meningioma
m. mesenchymal nephroma
m. mesenchymoma
m. mesothelioma
m. midline reticulosis
m. mixed mesodermal tumor
m. mole
m. neoplasm
m. nephrosclerosis
m. neurilemoma
m. pseudothyroiditis
m. pustule
m. schwannoma
m. small pox
m. synovioma
m. teratoma
m. teratoma intermediate
m. tertian fever
m. tertian malaria
m. trophoblastic teratoma
m. tumor
malignin
mallein test
malleolar
    m. artery
    m. bursa
malleolus (pl., malleoli)
Malleomyces
    M. *mallei*

M. *pseudomallei*
M. whitmori
malleomycosis
mallet finger
malleus
Mallophaga
Mallory's
    aniline blue stain
    bodies
    collagen stain
    iodine stain
    phloxine stain
    phosphotungstic acid hematoxy-
        lin stain
    stain for *Actinomyces*
    stain for hemofuchsin
    trichrome stain
    triple stain
Mallory-Weiss
    lesion
    tear
mallotoxin
Malmejde's test
malnourished
    intrauterine fetally m.
malnutrition
    malignant m.
    protein-calorie m.
    protein-energy m.
malocclusion
malonate
    m. broth
    m. coenzyme A transferase
malonic acid
malonyl coenzyme A
malonyl–coenzyme A decarboxylase
malpighian
    m. body
    m. follicle
malposition
malrotation
    intestinal m.
MALT — mucosa-associated
        lymphoid tissue
Malta fever
malt agar
maltase
Maltese cross appearance
maltose 4-glucosyltransferase
maltoside
maltosuria
maltotriose

malum
    m. articulorum senilis
    m. coxae senile
MAM — methylazoxymethanol
M + Am — myopic astigmatism
mam — milliampere-minute
mamillary
    m. bodies
    m. peduncle
    m. peduncular nucleus
mammal
mammalgia
Mammalia
mammalian
mammary
    m. artery
    m. calculus
    m. connective tissue
    m. duct
    m. duct ectasia
    m. dysplasia
    m. fistula
    m. fluids
    m. gland lymphatics
    m. lobule
    m. lymphatics
    m. neuralgia
    m. Paget's disease
    m. tumor virus
mammillary body
mammillitis
mammitis
mammography
    digital m.
mammosomatotropic adenoma
mammotropic hormone
mammotropin
management
Mancini method
Mandelin's reagent
mandible
mandibular
    m. arch
    m. condyle
    m. cyst
    m. gingiva
    m. incisor
    m. joint neuralgia
    m. lymph node
    m. molar
    m. nerve

m. ramus
m. torus
mandibulectomy
mandibuloacral dysostosis
mandibulofacial
m. dysostosis
m. dysotosis syndrome
m. dysplasia
mandibulo-oculofacial
m.-o. dysmorphia
m.-o. syndrome
mandibulotomy
mandibulopharyngeal
maneuver
Adson's m.
Osler's m.
Valsalva's m.
manganese
m. ethylene bis-dithiocar-
bamate
m. isotope
m. poisoning
m. salt
manganic
manganism
manganous
mange
sarcoptic m.
manic-depression
manifestation
manifest hyperopia
manifesting heterozygote
mannans
mannitol
m. dehydrogenase
m. fermentation
m. hexanitrate
m.-1-phosphate dehydrogenase
mannoheptulose
mannoheptulosuria
mannokinase
mannosamine
mannosazone
mannose-6-phosphate
mannosephosphate isomerase
α-mannosidase
mannosidosis
Mann's methyl blue-eosin stain
Mann-Whitney rank sum statistic
manometer
manometric flame
manometry

MANOVA — multivariate analysis
of variance
Mansonella
M. ozzardi
M. perstans
mansonelliasis
Mansonia
Mansonioides
Manson's
blood fluke
schistosomiasis
M_2 antibodies
M antigen
mantle layer, embryonic
mantle zone lymphoma
Mantoux
conversion
diameter
pit
skin test
test
manubrium (pl., manubria)
manuum
MAO — maximal acid output
monoamine oxidase
MAOI — monamine oxidase inhibitor
MAP — mean aortic pressure
mean arterial pressure
megaloblastic anemia of
pregnancy
methylacetoxyprogesterone
methylaminopurine
muscle-action potential
map
chromosome m.
conjugation m.
cytogenetic m.
genetic m.
linkage m.
restriction m.
transduction m.
m. unit
MAPF — microatomized protein food
maphosphamide
maple
m. bark disease
m. syrup urine
m. syrup urine disease
mapping
genetic m.
maprotiline

Maragiliano body
marantic
    m. atrophy
    m. endocarditis
    m. thrombosis
    m. thrombus
marasmic
    m. thrombosis
    m. thrombus
marasmus
marble
    m. bone disease
    m. bones
marbled state of brain
Marburg
    agent
    fever
    variant of multiple sclerosis
    virus
marcescens
march
    m. albuminuria
    m. hemoglobinuria
    jacksonian m.
Marchand's
    adrenals
    rest
Marchiafava-Micheli anemia
Marchi's
    fixative
    reaction
    stain
marcid
marcy agent
marfanoid hypermobility syndrome
Margaropus
margin
    left costal m.
marginal
    m. excision
    m. granulocyte pool
    m. gyrus
    m. insertion of umbilical cord
    m. layer, embryonic
    m. sulcus
    m. ulcer
    m. venous sinus
margination
    leukocytic m.
marijuana; marihuana
marine protein concentrate
Marituba virus

Marjolin's ulcer
mark
    port-wine m.
    m. sense reader
    strawberry m.
    tape m.
    Unna's m.
marker
    allotypic m.
    B-cell m's
    biological m.
    cell m.
    m. chromosome
    clonal m.
    cytogenetic m.
    cytoplasmic m.
    DNA m.
    fecal m.
    genetic m.
    immunologic m.
    molecular m.
    oncofetal m.
    prognostic m.
    m. rescue
    serological tumor m's
    surface m's
    tumor m.
Marme's reagent
marmoratus
    status m.
Marochetti's blisters
Marquis reagent
marrow
    aplastic bone m.
    basophilic m.
    bone m.
    eosinophilic m.
    erythrocytic m.
    gelatinous m.
    leukocytic m.
    lymphocytic m.
    monocytic m.
    neutrophilic m.
    m. platelets
    reticulocytic m.
    spinal m.
Marshall's method
marsh fever
marsupial
marsupialization
"martial arts thyroiditis"
Martinez's technique

Martin-Lester agar
Martinotti's cell
Martius
  scarlet blue
  yellow
mas or mA-s — milliampere-second
maschaladenitis
maschaloncus
masculinization
  ovarian m.
masculinovoblastoma
maser — microwave amplification
    by stimulated emission
    of radiation
  molecular application by
    stimulated emission of
    radiation
mask
  m. of pregnancy
  tropical m.
  Venturi m.
masked
  m. message
  m. virus
Mason Pfizer monkey virus
mason's lung
mass
  m. action law
  adrenal m.
  atomic m.
  m. attenuation coefficient
  body m.
  carbon gelatin m.
  m. concentration
  critical m.
  erythrocyte m.
  exchangeable m.
  fat-free m.
  filar m.
  flank m.
  m. fragmentography
  injection m.
  intravascular m.
  lean body m.
  molar m.
  molecular m.
  m. number
  red blood cell m.
  m. reflex
  relative molecular m.
  scrotal m.
  m. spectrograph

  m. spectrometer
  m. spectrometry
  m. spectroscopy
  m. storage
massage
  cardiac m.
  m. effect
massa intermedia
masseter
  m. fascia
  m. muscle
masseteric
massive
  m. collapse
  m. embolus
  m. hepatic necrosis
  m. transfusion
  m. vitreous retraction
Masson
  argentaffin stain
  pseudoangiosarcoma
  stain
  trichrome method
  trichrome stain
Masson-Fontana ammoniacal silver
  stain
mast
  m. cell
  m. cell disease
  m. cell hyperplasia
  m. cell leukemia
  m. cell sarcoma
  m. cell staining
  m. cell tumor
  m. leukocyte
mastadenitis
mastadenoma
mastadenovirus
mastalgia
mastatrophy; mastatrophia
mastauxe
mastectomy
  Auchincloss-Madden m.
  Halsted's m.
  Meyer's m.
  palliative m.
  partial m.
  Patey m.
  prophylactic m.
  radical m.
  salvage m.
  Scanlon m.

segmental m.
simple m.
subcutaneous m.
total m.
Master two-step exercise test
mastication
mastic test
Mastigomycotina
Mastigophora
mastigophorous
mastigote
mastitis
    acute m.
    chronic cystic m.
    cystic m.
    fibrocystic m.
    gargantuan m.
    glandular m.
    granulomatous m.
    interstitial m.
    lactational m.
    m. neonatorum
    parenchymatous m.
    periductal m.
    phlegmonous m.
    plasma cell m.
    puerperal m.
    retromammary m.
    submammary m.
    suppurative m.
mastocarcinoma
mastochondroma
mastocyte
mastocytogenesis
mastocytoma
mastocytosis
    diffuse cutaneous m.
    systemic m.
mastodynia
mastography
mastoid
    m. abscess
    m. antrum
    m. canaliculus
    m. cells
mastoidectomy
mastoiditis
mastoncus
mastopathy
    cystic m.
    fibrocystic m.
Mastophora

mastoplasia
mastorrhagia
mastoscirrhus
mastosquamous
mastostomy
Masugi's nephritis
Masugi-type nephrotoxic serum
    nephritis
material
    biuret-reactive m.
    control m's
    cross-reacting m.
    explosive m.
    extracellular m.
    fluorescent m.
    gonadotropin-inhibitory m.
    m. graft
    hazardous m's
    labeling of hazardous m's
    neurosecretory m.
    particulate crystalline m.
    primary reference m's
    reactive m.
    reference m's
    m. safety data sheet
    secondary reference m's
    vasodepressor m.
    vasoexcitor m.
maternal
    m. death
    m. inheritance
    m. mortality rate
mathematical
    m. genetics
    m. logic
mating
    assortative m.
    consanguineous m.
    negative assortative m.
    positive assortative m.
    random m.
matrass
matrilineal
matrix
    m. antigen
    m. calculus
    collagen m.
    cytoplasmic m.
    m. interference
    mitochondrial m.
    myxoid m.

m. production
sarcoplasmic m.
matrix alteration
bone m.a.
cartilage m.a.
extracellular m.a.
fibrocartilage m.a.
matt; matte
matter
maturate
maturation
affinity m.
m. arrest
m. division
m. factor
m. index
sexual m.
sperm m.
testicular m.
maturation alteration
hematopoietic m.a.
leukocytic m.a.
mature
m. abnormal chorion
m. abnormal chorionic villi
m. abnormal placenta
m. cell leukemia
m. neutrophil
m. ovarian follicle
m. teratoma
maturity-onset diabetes
Maurer's
clefts
dots
max. — maximum
maxilla (pl., maxillae)
maxillary
m. antrum
m. artery
m. crest
m. gingiva
m. incisor
m. molar
m. nerve
m. ostia
m. process
m. sinus
maxillectomy
maxillitis
maxilloethmoidectomy
maxillofacial prosthesis
maxillolabial

maxillomandibular
maxillopalatine
maxillopharyngeal
maxillotomy
maximal
m. acid output
m. breathing capacity
m. expiratory flow rate
m. expiratory flow volume
m. growth temperature
m. Histalog test
m. midexpiratory flow rate
m. midflow rate
m. permissible dose
m. tubular excretory capacity
of kidneys
m. tubular reabsorption of
glucose
m. voluntary ventilation
Maximow's
fixative
stain for bone marrow
maximum (pl., maxima)
m. cell
m. impurities reagents
m. inhibiting dilution
m. permissible concentration
m. thermometer
m. urea clearance
m. urinary concentration
maxwell
Mayaro virus
mayer
Mayer's
acid alum hematoxylin stain
hemalum stain
hematoxylin
mucicarmine stain
mucihematein stain
waves
mayfly
May-Grünwald-Giemsa stain
May-Grünwald stain
May-Hegglin
anomaly
body
mazoplasia
Mazzini's test
Mazzotti
reaction
test

MB — mesiobuccal
  methylene blue
  microbiological assay
Mb — myoglobin
m.b. — mix well
MBA — methylbovine albumin
M band
mbar — millibar
MBAS — methylene blue active substance
MBC — maximal breathing capacity
  minimal bactericidal concentration
MbCO — myoglobin combination with carbon monoxide
MBD — methylene blue dye
  minimal brain damage
  minimal brain dysfunction
  Morquio-Brailsford disease
MBF — myocardial blood flow
MBK — methyl butyl ketone
MBL — minimal bactericidal level
MBO — mesiobucco-occlusal
MbO_2 — myoglobin combination with oxygen
MBP — antigen prepared from *Brucella melitensis, B. bovis,* and *B. suis*
  mean blood pressure
  mesiobuccopulpal
  myelin basic protein
MBSA — methylated bovine serum albumin
MC — mast cell
  maximum cell
  maximum concentration
  metacarpal
  mineralocorticoid
  myocarditis
  mytomycin-C
Mc — megacurie
  megacycle
mC — millicoulomb
mc; mCi; MCU — millicurie
MCA — methylcholanthrene
  middle cerebral artery
  multichannel analyzer
MCB — membranous cytoplasmic body
MCBR — minimum concentration of bilirubin

MCC — mean corpuscular hemoglobin concentration
  minimum complete-killing concentration
McCallum's plaque
McCollough effect
MC (mean corpuscular) concentration
MCD — mean cell diameter
  mean of consecutive differences
  mean corpuscular diameter
  medullary cystic disease
M cell
MCF — macrophage chemotactic factor
MCFA — medium-chain fatty acid
mcg; μg — microgram
Mcf isotypic determination
MCH — mean cell hemoglobin
  mean corpuscular hemoglobin
mch — millicurie-hour
MCHC — mean cell hemoglobin concentration
  mean corpuscular hemoglobin concentration
MCHg — mean corpuscular hemoglobin
MCI — mean cardiac index
mCi — millicurie
mCi-hr — millicurie-hour
MCL — midclavicular line
  midcostal line
McLeod
  blood group system
  phenotype
McMaster technique
McNeer classification
M colony
M component
M concentration
MCP — metacarpophalangeal
  mitotic-control protein
McPhail test
Mcps — megacycles per second
MCR — metabolic clearance rate
M-CSF — macrophage colony–stimulating factor
MCT — mean cell threshold
  mean circulation time
  mean corpuscular thickness
  medium-chain triglyceride

medullary carcinoma of thyroid
MCTD — mixed connective-tissue disease
MCV — mean cell volume
mean corpuscular volume
MD — malic dehydrogenase
Mantoux diameter
Marek's disease
movement disorder
muscular dystrophy
myocardial damage
myocardial disease
Md — mendelevium
MDA — mentodextra anterior
methylenedioxyamphetamine
motor discriminative acuity
MDC — minimum detectable concentration
MDF — mean dominant frequency
myocardial depressant factor
MDH — malic dehydrogenase
MDHV — Marek's herpesvirus disease
MDP — mentodextra posterior
methylene diphosphonate
muramyl dipeptide
MDS — myelodysplastic syndrome
MDT — median detection threshold
mentodextra transversa
MDTR — mean diameter-thickness ratio
MDUO — myocardial disease of unknown origin
ME — mercaptoethanol
2-ME — 2-mercaptoethanol
M/E; M : E — myeloid-erythroid ratio
Me — methyl
MEA — mercaptoethylamine
multiple endocrine adenomatosis
meal
Lundh m.
test m.
mean
arithmetical m.
m. arterial pressure
m. cell diameter
m. cell hemoglobin
m. cell hemoglobin concentration
m. cell threshold

m. cell volume
m. circulation time
m. circulatory hematocrit
m. of consecutive differences
m. corpuscular diameter
m. corpuscular hemoglobin
m. corpuscular hemoglobin concentration
m. corpuscular thickness
m. corpuscular volume
m. deviation
m. diameter-thickness ratio
m. dominant frequency
m. dose
m. dose per unit cumulated activity
m. effective life
m. generation time
geometric m.
harmonic m.
m. hemolytic dose
m. life
m. platelet volume
m. square deviation
m. time between failures
trimmed m.
windsorized m.
measles
m. antibody
black m.
German m.
three-day m.
m. virus
measly
measurable
measure
measurement
blood volume m's
end-point m.
kinetic m.
oxygen saturation m's
measuring pipet
meatal stenosis
meat fibers
meatus (pl., meatus, meatuses)
external auditory m.
internal acoustic m.
nasal m.
urethral m.
urinary m.
mebendazole
mebutamate

mecamylamine
MeCbl — methylcobalamin
mechanical
>m. diuretic
>m. fragility
>m. ileus
>m. jaundice
>m. nociceptor
>m. styptic
>m. ventilation

mechanism
>countercurrent m.
>Frank-Starling m.
>oculogyric m.
>ping-pong m.
>somatic m.
>splanchnic m.
>Starling m.

mechanocyte
mechanoreceptor
>high-threshold m.

mechanosensory
mechlorethamine hydrochloride
mecillinam
Mecistocirrhus
Meckel's
>cartilage
>diverticulum
>scan

Mecke's reagent
meclizine hydrochloride
mecobalamine
meconium
>m. aspiration
>m. extravasation
>m. ileus
>m. periorchitis
>m. peritonitis
>m. retention

mecrylate
MED — minimal erythema dose
med. — median
media
>aerotitis m.
>aortic tunica m.
>aqueous mounting m.
>bilateral otitis m.
>culture m.
>otitis m.
>secretory otitis m.
>serous otitis m.
>suppurative chronic otitis m.

medial
>m. arteriosclerosis
>m. calcification
>m. calcific sclerosis
>m. cystic necrosis
>m. degeneration
>m. fasciculus
>m. lemniscus
>Mönckeberg's m. calcification
>m. necrosis
>m. necrosis cystica of aorta
>m. nucleus

median
>m. aperture
>m. bar of Mercier
>m. cubital vein
>m. curative dose
>m. detection threshold
>m. effective dose
>m. eminence
>m. fatal dose
>m. forebrain
>m. infectious dose
>m. lethal dose
>m. lobe branch
>m. nerve
>m. raphe cyst
>m. rhomboid glossitis
>m. tissue culture dose
>m. tissue culture infective dose
>m. unbiased estimate

mediastinal
>m. artery
>m. cyst
>m. emphysema
>m. fibrosis
>m. germinoma
>m. lymph node
>m. neuroblastoma
>m. pericarditis
>m. pleura
>m. shift
>m. teratocarcinoma
>m. vein

mediastinitis
>idiopathic fibrous m.
>sclerosing m.

mediastinogram
mediastinography
mediastinopericarditis
>adhesive m.

mediastinoscope

mediastinoscopic biopsy
mediastinoscopy
mediastinum (pl., mediastina)
    m. spinalis
    m. testis
mediate agglutination
mediators
    chemical m.
medical
    m. genetics
    m. record
Medical Internal Radiation Dose
medicinal scarlet red
medicine
    forensic m.
    preventive m.
medina infection
mediolateral
medionecrosis
    m. aortae idiopathica cystica
    cystic m.
    m. of aorta
Mediterranean
    M. anemia
    familial M. fever
    M. fever
    M.-hemoglobin E disease
    M. lymphoma
    M. stomatocytosis
medium (pl., media)
    Apathy's gum syrup m.
    Balamuth's culture m.
    Boeck-Drbohlav-Locke egg
       serum m.
    Bordet-Gengou m.
    brain-heart infusion broth m.
    chopped meat m.
    clearing m.
    contrast m.
    culture m.
    dermatophyte test m.
    differential m.
    dispersive m.
    Eagle's basal m.
    Eagle's minimum essential m.
    egg-base culture m.
    enrichment m.
    Farrant's m.
    Fletcher's m.
    m. frequency
    glycerol gelatin m.
    Gruft's m.

HAT (hypoxanthine,
    aminopterin, and thymi-
    dine) m.
Lash's casein hydro-
    lysate–serum m.
Leibovitz m. (no. 15)
Löeffler's blood culture m.
Löeffler's coagulated serum m.
Löwenstein-Jensen m.
Löwenstein-Jensen-Gruft m.
Middlebrook's m.
minimum essential m.
Mitchison m.
mounting m.
nitrate m.
Novy, MacNeal, and
    Nicolle's m.
nutrient m.
oxidation-fermentation m.
passive m.
Petragnani m.
Proteose peptone m.
PVA lacto-phenol m.
radiopaque m.
Rees's culture m.
refracting m.
m.-scale integration
selective m.
separating m.
sodium chloride culture m.
support m.
tellurite m.
Thayer-Martin m.
thioglycollate m.
tissue culture m.
Tobie, von Brand, and Mehl-
    man's diphasic m.
transport m.
virus transport m.
Weinman's m.
Wisconsin m.
xylose-lysine-deoxycholate m.
medium-chain
    m.-c. fatty acid
    m.-c. triglycerides
medorrhea
medroxyprogesterone
medulla (pl., medullae)
    adrenal m.
    kidney m.
    m. nodi lymphatici
    m. ossium

m. ossium flava
m. ossium rubra
ovarian m.
renal m.
spinal m.
suprarenal m.
thymic m.

medulla oblongata
arcuate nucleus of m.o.
dorsal lateral sulcus of m.o.
dorsal median sulcus of m.o.
dorsal spinocerebellar tract of m.o.
dorsal spinothalamic tract of m.o.
external arcuate fibers of m.o.
fasciculus cuneatus of m.o.
fasciculus gracilis of m.o.
internal arcuate fibers of m.o.
lateral nucleus of m.o.
medial lemniscus of m.o.
medial longitudinal fasciculus of m.o.
raphe of m.o.
reticular formation of m.o.
tectospinal tract of m.o.
ventral lateral sulcus of m.o.
ventral median fissure of m.o.
ventral spinocerebellar tract of m.o.
ventral spinothalamic tract of m.o.

medullary
m. adenocarcinoma
m. breast cancer
m. carcinoma
m. carcinoma of thyroid
m. chromaffinoma
m. cystic disease
m. ductal ectasia
m. fibroma
m. fibrosarcoma
m. follicular cyst
m. histiocytic reticulosis
m. lamina
m. necrosis
m. paraganglioma
m. rays
m. renal cyst
m. reticulosis
m. sarcoma

m. sponge kidney
m. velum

medullated neuroma
medullectomy
medullization
medulloarthritis
medulloblast
medulloblastoma
medulloepithelioma
adult m.

Medusa head
MEF — maximal expiratory flow
MEFR — maximal expiratory flow rate
MEFV — maximal expiratory flow volume
MEG — megakaryocyte
megabladder
megacaryocyte; megakaryocyte
megacolon
acquired m.
aganglionic m.
chronic idiopathic m.
congenital m.; m. congenitum
idiopathic m.
toxic m.

megacycle
megacystic syndrome
megacystis-microcolon intestinal hypoperistalsis syndrome
megadolichocolon
megaelectron volt
megaesophagus
megahertz
megakaryoblast; megacaryoblast
megakaryoblastic leukemia
megakaryocyte; megacaryocyte
basophilic m.
dwarf m.
granular m.

megakaryocytic
m. aplasia
m. blood cell
m. cells
m. hyperplasia
m. hypoplasia
m. leukemia
m. myelosis

megakaryocytopoiesis
extramedullary m.

megakaryocytosis
megalencephaly

megalgia
megaloblast of Sabin
megaloblastic
    m. anemia
    m. anemia of pregnancy
    m. crisis
    m. erythropoiesis
megaloblastoid
megaloblastosis
megalobulbus
megalocystis
megalocyte
megalocythemia
megalocytic anemia
megalocytosis
megalodactyly
megaloenteron
megalogastria
megaloglossia
megalohepatia
megalokaryocyte
megalopenis
Megalopyge
megalosplenia
megalosyndactyly
megalothymus
megaloureter
megalourethra
megamitochondria
meganucleus
megarectum
Megaselia
megasigmoid
Megasphaera
megathrombocyte
megaureter
megaurethra
megavolt
megavoltage
Meg-CSA — megakaryocyte col-
              ony–stimulating
              activity
megestrol acetate
meglumine
    m. diatrizoate crystals
    iodipamide m.
    m. iodipamide
    iothalamate m.
    m. iothalamate
megohm
megoxycyte
megoxyphil; megoxyphile

meibomian
    m. cyst
    m. gland
    m. stye
meibomitis; meibomianitis
Meinicke turbidity reaction
meiocyte
meiogenic
meiosis
meiotic
    m. chromosome
    m. phase
    m. recombination
Meissner's
    corpuscle
    nerve plexus
MEK — methyl ethyl ketone
melancholia
    involutional m.
melanemia
Melania
melaniferous phagocyte
melanin
    artificial m.
    m. bleaching methods
    factitious m.
    m. pigment
    m. pigmentation
    m. staining methods
    m. test
melanism
melanoacanthoma
melanoameloblastoma
melanoblast
melanoblastoma
melanocarcinoma of anus
melanocortin
melanocyte
    dendritic m.
    m.-inhibiting factor
    m.-inhibiting hormone
    α-m.–stimulating hormone
    β-m.–stimulating hormone
    m.-stimulating hormone–re-
      lease-inhibiting hormone
    m.-stimulating hormone–re-
      leasing factor
    m.-stimulating hormone–re-
      leasing hormone
melanocytic
    m. nevus
    m. proliferation

melanocytoma of optic disk
melanoderma
    m. cachecticorum
    m. chloasma
    senile m.
melanodermatitis
melanodermic
melanogenemia
melanogenesis
melanogen test
melanoglossia
melanoid
Melanoides
melanokeratosis
Melanolestes picipes
melanoleukoderma
melanoma
    acral lentiginous m.
    amelanotic m.
    balloon cell m.
    benign juvenile m.
    chorionic m.
    Cloudman m.
    cutaneous malignant m.
    desmoplastic m.
    epithelioid cell m.
    halo m.
    Harding-Passey m.
    intraocular m.
    juvenile m.
    lentigo maligna m.
    malignant m.
    malignant m. in situ
    malignant lentigo m.
    minimal deviation m.
    mucosal m.
    multiple m.
    nodular m.
    ocular m.
    spindle-cell m.
    subungual m.
    superficial spreading m.
    uveal m.
melanomatosis
melanonychia
melanopathy
melanophage
melanophore-stimulating hormone
melanoplakia
melanosarcoma
melanosis
    m. circumscripta precancerosa

    m. coli
    m. corii degenerative
    m. iridis
    neurocutaneous m.
    oculodermal m.
    precancerous m. of Dubreuilh
    Riehl's m.
    vagabond's m.
melanosome
    giant m.
melanotic
    m. ameloblastoma
    m. cancer
    m. carcinoma
    m. freckle
    m. freckle of Hutchinson
    m. hamartoma
    m. neuroectodermal tumor
    m. pigment
    m. progonoma
    m. whitlow
melanotroph
melanuria
melanuric
melarsonyl potassium
melarsoprol
melasma universale
melatonin
melena vera
Meleney's
    gangrene
    ulcer
melengestrol acetate
melicera
meliceris
melioidosis
melitis
melitose
melituria
    glycosuric m.
    m. inosita
    nondiabetic glycosuric m.
    nonglucose m.
Meloidae
Meloidogyne javanica
melon seed body
Melophagus
melorheostosis
melphalan
melting
    m. point
    m. temperature

MEM — macrophage electrophoretic
          mobility
          minimum essential medium
membranacea
          placenta m.
membrane
          acute inflammatory m.
          acute pyogenic m.
          artificial rupture of m's
          m. antigens
          basement m.
          Bowman's m.
          Bruch's m.
          Bruch's basal m.
          m. capacitance
          cell m.
          cellular m's
          cloacal m.
          m. control protein
          croupous m.
          cytoplasmic m.
          decidual m.
          Descemet's m.
          diphtheritic m.
          epithelial basement m.
          erythrocyte m.
          excitable m.
          exocelomic m.
          false m.
          fetal m's
          m. filter
          m. filter techniques
          glassy m.
          m. glycoprotein P 170
          hyaline m.
          inflammatory m.
          ion-exchange m.
          jejunal mucous m.
          mucous m.
          oropharyngeal m.
          placental m.
          plasma m.
          postsynaptic m.
          m. potential
          premature rupture of fetal m's
          presynaptic m.
          prolonged rupture of fetal m's
          prophylactic m.
          m. protein
          pupillary m.
          pyogenic m.
          Reissner's m.

          rupture of m's
          semipermeable m.
          Shrapnell's m.
          "m. skeleton"
          spiral m.
          synovial m.
          tectorial m.
          m. transport
          tympanic m.
          undulating m.
          unit m.
          urethral m.
membranectomy
membranelle
membranoproliferative glomerulone-
          phritis
membranous
          m. acute inflammation
          m. ampulla
          m. cytoplasmic body
          m. glomerulonephritis
          m. inflammation
          m. labyrinth
          m. nephropathy
          m. pharyngitis
          m.-proliferative glomerulone-
             phritis
          m. uretha
memory
          kinesthetic m.
          magnetic core m.
MEN — multiple endocrine neoplasia
menadiol sodium diphosphate
menadione
          m. reductase
          m. sodium bisulfite
menaquinone
menarche
mendelevium
mendelian
          m. character
          m. genetics
          m. inheritance
Mendel's law
Menghini needle
Mengo virus
meningeal
          m. artery
          m. carcinoma
          m. carcinomatosis
          m. leukemia
          m. sarcoma

m. sarcomatosis
m. spaces
meningematoma
meningeocortical
meninges
meningioma
    anaplastic m.
    angioblastic m.
    angioblastomatous m.
    angiomatous m.
    cerebellopontine angle m.
    clival m.
    convexity m's
    cutaneous m.
    cystic m.
    diffuse m.
    falcine m.
    falx m.
    fibroblastic m.
    fibrous m.
    malignant m.
    meningothelial m.
    meningotheliomatous m.
    m. of olfactory groove
    papillary m.
    parasagittal m.
    posterior fossa m.
    post-radiation m.
    psammomatous m.
    m. of sphenoid ridge
    suprasellar m.
    syncytial m.
    tentorial m.
    transitional m.
    m. of tuberculum sellae
meningiomatosis
meningismus
meningitic neurosyphilis
meningitis (pl., meningitides)
    amebic m.
    aseptic m.
    bacterial m.
    Candida m.
    candidal m.
    cerebrospinal m.
    chemical m.
    chronic m.
    cryptococcal m.
    fungal m.
    gonococcal m.
    lymphocytic m.
    meningococcal m.

mycobacterial m.
mycotic m.
pneumococcal m.
pyogenic m.
subacute m.
syphilitic m.
torular m.
tuberculous m.
viral m.
meningoblastoma
meningocele
    cranial m.
meningocerebritis
meningococcal
    m. bacteremia
    m. infection
    m. meningitis
    m. septicemia
meningococcemia
meningococcin
meningococcus (pl., meningococci)
    m. conjunctivitis
meningocyte
meningoencephalitis
    amebic m.
    cryptococcal m.
    eosinophilic m.
    m. mumps
meningoencephalocele
meningoencephalomyelitis
meningoencephalopathy
    carcinomatous m.
meningomyelitis
meningomyelocele
meningomyeloencephalitis
meningomyeloradiculitis
meningo-osteophlebitis
meningopathy
meningorrhea
meningothelial meningioma
meningotheliomatous meningioma
meningovascular neurosyphilis
meninguria
meniscectomy
meniscitis
meniscocyte
meniscocytosis
meniscus (pl., menisci)
    degenerated m.
    lateral m.
menometrorrhagia

menopausal
    m. endometrium
    m. gonadotropin
    m. syndrome
menopause
   delayed m.
menorrhagia
menostasis
menses
menstrual
    m. colic
    m. cycle
    m. disorder
    m. endometrium
    m. fluid
    m. involution
    m. sclerosis
menstruation
   vicarious m.
MEN (multiple endocrine neoplasia)
   syndrome
mental
    m. deficiency
    m. disturbance
    m. retardation
Mentha
menthol
mentolabial
Menzies's method
mep. — meperidine
meparfynol
mepazine acetate
mepenzolate
meperidine hydrochloride
mephenesin
mephenoxalone
mephentermine
mephenytoin
mephobarbital
mepivacaine hydrochloride
MEPP — miniature end-plate
        potential
meprobamate
   isopropyl m.
meprylcaine hydrochloride
mEq or meq — milliequivalent
MER — mean ejection rate
       methanol-extruded residue
MER-29 — triparanol
meralluride
M : E (myeloid-erythroid) ratio; M/E
   ratio
merbromin

mercaptan
mercapto
mercaptoacetic acid
mercaptoethanol
2-mercaptoethanol
mercaptoethylamine
mercaptoethylguanidine
mercaptomerin sodium
6-mercaptopurine
mercaptopyrazidopyrimidine
3-mercaptopyruvate sulfurtransferase
mercocresols
mercumatilin
mercuriacetate
mercurialism
mercurial thermometer
mercuric
    m. acetate
    m. chloride poisoning
    m. cyanide
    m. cyanoguanidine
    m. dicyanodiamine
    m. fixative
    m. iodide
    m. oxide
    m. phosphate
    m. salt
mercurichloride
   hydroxyphenyl m.
mercurimetric method
mercurous chloride
mercury
   ammoniated m.
    m. bichloride
    m. chloride
    m. isotope
   methyl m.
    m. oxycyanide
    m. phosphate
    m. poisoning
    m.-vapor lamp
    m.-wetted relay
merethoxylline procaine
merge
meristic variation
Merkel-Ranvier cell
Merkel's
   cell
   cell carcinoma
   cell tumor
   corpuscle
   tactile disk

mermithid
Mermithidae
Mermithoidea
merocrine gland
merocyst
Merodicein
merogony
 diploid m.
 parthenogenetic m.
meromelia
meromicrosomia
meromyarial
meromyosin
meronecrosis
merozoite antigens
merozygote
mersalyl
Merthiolate
Merulius lacrimans
mesangial
 m. hyperplasia
 m. lupus glomerulonephritis
 m. nephritis
 m. proliferative glomerulonephritis
mesangiocapillary glomerulonephritis
mesangium
 extraglomerular m.
 glomerular m.
mesaortitis
mesarteritis
mesaxon
mescal
mescaline
mesectic
mesencephalic reticular formation
mesencephalitis
mesencephalon
mesenchyma
mesenchymal
 m. cancer
 m. cells
 m. hyloma
 m. neoplasia
 m. tumor
 m. villous core
mesenchyme
 urogenital m.
mesenchymoma
 benign m.
 malignant m.

mesenteric
 m. adenitis
 m. artery
 m. cyst
 m. hyperplasia
 m. infarction
 m. ischemia
 m. lymphadenitis
 m. lymph node
 m. nodes
 m. panniculitis
 m. plexus
 m. pseudocyst
 m. thrombosis
 m. vascular obstruction
 m. vein
mesenteritis
mesentery
 dorsal m.
 ileal m.
 inferior m.
 m. infiltration
 jejunal m.
 sigmoid colon m.
 small intestinal m.
mesiodistal
mesion
mesoappendix
mesobacterium
mesobilifuscin
mesobilirubin
mesobilirubinogen
mesoblast
 primitive m.
mesoblastema
mesoblastic nephroma
mesocardia
mesocardium
Mesocestoides variabilis
Mesocestoididae
mesocolon
 sigmoid m.
 transverse m.
meso compound
mesocyst
mesocytoma
mesoderm
mesodermal
 m. mixed tumor
 m. tumor
mesogastric
mesogastrium

Mesogastropoda
mesoglioma
mesohyloma
mesolepidoma
mesomelia
mesomelic dwarfism
mesometanephric carcinoma
mesomere
mesometritis
mesometrium
meson
mesonephric
    m. adenocarcinoma
    m. adenoma
    m. carcinoma
    m. cyst
    m. duct
    m. remnant
    m. rest
    m. tubules
mesonephroid tumor
mesonephroma
mesonephros (pl., mesonephroi)
mesophile
mesophilic bacteria
mesophlebitis
mesoridazine besylate
mesosalpinx
mesosigmoiditis
mesosome
mesotendineum
mesotestis
mesothelial
    m. cells
    m. cyst
    m. hyloma
    m. sarcoma
mesothelioma
    benign m. of genital tract
    benign fibrous m.
    cordal m.
    diffuse m.
    fibrous m.
    localized fibrous m
    malignant m.
    nodular m.
    papillary m.
    paratesticular m.
    peritoneal m.
    pleural m.
    m. of testis
    m. of tunica vaginalis

mesothelium
    epithelial type/m.
    pericardial m.
    peritoneal m.
    pleural m.
    sarcomatoid-type m.
mesothorium
mesovarium
message
    masked m.
messenger RNA
mesylate
    deferoxamine m.
    ergoloid m.
Met or M — methionine
meta-analysis
metabiosis
metabisulfite test
metabolic
    m. acidemia
    m. acidosis
    m. alkalosis
    m. antagonism
    m. antagonist
    m. bone disease
    m. burst
    m. clearance rate
    m. coma
    m. craniopathy
    m. detoxification
    m. encephalopathy
    m. indican
    m. inhibition test
    m. insufficiency
    m. mucinosis
    m. myopathy
    m. pathway
    m. pool
metabolism
    aerobic m.
    anaerobic m.
    basal m.
    divalent ion m.
    glucose m.
    glycine m.
    inborn errors of m.
    intermediary m.
    iron m.
    oxygen m.
    propionate m.
metabolite
    catecholamine m.
    terpenal m's

metabolizable
metabutethamine
metabutoxycaine
metacarpal
    m. index
    m. joint
metacarpophalangeal joint
metacarpus (pl., metacarpi)
metacentric chromosome
metacercaria (pl., metacercariae)
metachromasia; metachromia
    alpha m.
    beta m.
    gamma m.
metachromatic
    m. bodies
    m. dye
    m. granule
    m. leukodystrophy
    m. stain
metachromatism
metachromatophil
metachromophil; metachromophile
metachronal rhythm
metachronous
metachrosis
metacresylacetate
metagenesis
metagglutinin
metaglobulin
metagonimiasis
Metagonimus
    M. *ovatus*
    M. *yokogawai*
metal
    alkali m.
    alkaline earth m.
    m. fume fever
    heavy m's
    m. sol
metaldehyde
metallic
    m. bond
    m. foreign body
    m. thermometer
metalloenzyme
metalloflavoprotein
metallophil cells
metallophilia
metalloprotein
metamorphosis
    fatty m.
    viscous m.

metamyeloblast
metamyelocyte
    basophilic m.
    eosinophilic m.
    neutrophilic m.
metanephric kidney
metanephrine assay
metanephros (pl., metanephroi)
metaneutrophil
metaniline yellow
metanil yellow
metaphase
    m. chromosome
    m. plate
metaphosphoric acid
metaphyseal
    m. dysostosis
    m. dysplasia
    m. fibrous defect
metaphysis (pl., metaphyses)
metaphysitis
metaplasia
    agnogenic myeloid m.
    apocrine m.
    autoparenchymatous m.
    Barrett's m.
    cartilaginous m.
    chondroid m.
    decidual m.
    endothelial m.
    epidermoid m.
    glandular m.
    Hürthle cell m.
    intestinal m.
    mucous m.
    myeloid m.
    myelosclerosis with myeloid m.
    nephrogenic m.
    osseous m.
    osteoid m.
    ovarian theca m.
    primary myeloid m.
    pseudopyloric m.
    pseudosarcomatous m.
        secondary myeloid m.
    squamous m.
    squamous m. of amnion
    stromal m.
    symptomatic myeloid m.
    thecal m.
    transitional cell m.
    urethral m.

urothelial m.
vaginal m.
metaplasis
metaplasm
metaplastic
    m. anemia
    m. carcinoma
    m. cartilage
    m. keratinization
    m. ossification
    m. polyp
Metaprel
metaproterenol sulfte
metaraminol
metarubricyte
    pernicious anemia–type m.
metastable state
metastasis (pl., metastases)
    bone m.
    calcareous m.
    contralateral axillary m.
    cutaneous m.
    hematogenous m.
    intracranial m.
    ocular m.
    osteoblastic m.
    pulsating m's
    satellite m.
    visceral m.
metastasize
metastasizing mole
metastatic
    m. abscess
    m. calcification
    m. cancer
    m. carcinoid syndrome
    m. carcinoma
    m. cascade
    m. lymphoma
    m. mumps
    m. neoplasm
    m. ophthalmia
    m. orchitis
    m. panniculitis
    m. pneumonia
    m. prostatic adenocarcinoma
    m. thermometer
    m. tumor
Metastrongylus elongatus
metatarsalgia
metatarsal joint
metatarsectomy

metatarsophalangeal joint
metatarsus
metatropic
metatypical carcinoma
metaxeny
metazoa (sing., metazoon)
metazoan
    m. infection
    m. parasite
Metchnikoff's (Mechnikov's) cellular
    immunity theory
metencephalon
meteorism
meter
    count rate m.
    d'Arsonval m.
    flow m.
    gram-m.
    oxygen saturation m.
    pH m.
    rate m.
    survey m.
meter-kilogram-second
    m.-k.-s. system
    m.-k.-s. unit
methacholine
methacrylate
    butyl m.
    glycol m.
    methyl m.
    polymethyl m.
methacycline
methadone hydrochloride
methallenestril
methamphetamine hydrochloride
methandrostenolone
methane
Methanobacterium
Methanococcus
methanol
    m. assay
    m.-extruded residue
    m. fixative
    m. poisoning
methantheline
methapyrilene
methaqualone assay
metharbital
methazolamide
MetHb or metHb — methemoglobin
methdilazine hydrochloride
methemalbumin assay

methemalbuminemia
methemalbuminuria
metheme
methemoglobin
    m. elution test
    m. reductase
methemoglobinemia
    acquired m.
    congenital m.
    enterogenous m.
    hereditary m.
    hereditary enzymatic-type m.
    primary m.
    secondary m.
    toxic m.
methemoglobinuria
methenamine
    m. hippurate
    m. mandelate
    periodic acid–silver m.
    m. silver
    m. silver stain
methenyltetrahydrofolate cyclohy-
    drolase
methicillin
methimazole
methine dye
methiodal sodium
methionine
    m. adenosyltransferase
    N-formyl m.
    m. malabsorption syndrome
    m. synthase
methionyl
methionyl-RNA synthetase
methisazone
methitural
methixene hydrochloride
methocarbamol
methocycline
method
    Abell m.
    Abell-Kendall m.
    acid anhydride m.
    acid-fast staining m's
    acridine orange m.
    agar diffusion m.
    alkaline phosphatase m.
    antialkaline phosphatase m.
    Ashby's differential agglutina-
      tion m.
    Ashby's m.

Austin and Van Slyke's m.
axon-staining m's
Ayoub-Shklar m.
bacterial agar m.
bacterial antigen detection m.
Baker's Sudan black m.
Barnett-Bourne acetic alcohol–
    silver nitrate m.
Barrnett-Seligman dihydroxydi-
    naphthyl disulfide m.
Barrnett-Seligman indoxyl
    esterase m.
Barroso-Moguel and Costero
    silver m.
Baumgartner m.
Beaver direct smear m.
Bengston's m.
Bennett's sulfhydryl m.
Bennhold's Congo red m.
Bensley's aniline–acid
    fuchsin–methyl green m.
benzo sky blue m.
Berg's chelate removal m.
Bethesda m.
bidiazotized benzidine m.
Bielschowsky's m.
biuret m.
black periodic acid m.
Bodian's m.
Borchgrevink m.
Brecher-Cronkite m.
bromcresol m.
Brown m.
Cajal's gold-sublimate m.
Cajal's uranium silver m.
Caldwell-Moloy m.
Camp-Gianturco m.
carbolfuchsin–methylene blue
    staining m.
cellophane tape m.
cell separation m's
Chang's aniline–acid fuch-
    sin m.
checker-board m.
cherry m.
Chiffelle and Putt m.
chloranilate m.
chloride m's
cholesterol staining m's
chromate m.
chrome alum–hematoxy-
    linphloxine m.

chromolytic (dyed-starch) m.
Ciaccio's m.
Clauss m.
clean-catch collection m.
cobalt nitrite m.
Colcher-Sussman m.
collagen-staining m.
constitutive heterochro-
　matin m.
cooled-knife m.
Cope m. of bronchography
copper sulfate m.
coverglass m.
Craigie's tube m.
Credé's m.
Crippa's lead tetraacetate m.
cysteic acid m.
Dale-Laidlaw's clotting
　time m.
Dane's m.
definitive m.
De Galantha's m. for urates
diazo staining m.
Dieterle's m.
diffusion m.
digitonin m.
Duke's m. of bleeding time
dyed starch m.
enzymatic digestion m's
enzyme demonstration m's
esterase staining m's
Fahey m.
Feulgen m.
fibrin degradation products m.
fibrinogen m.
field m.
Fite's m.
fixed sediment m.
flat substrate m.
fluoroimmunometric m.
Fontana-Masson staining m.
Foot's reticulin m.
formaldehyde-induced fluores-
　cence m.
formalin-ether sedimenta-
　tion m.
m's for sulfates
freeze-cleave m.
freeze-etch m.
freeze-fracture-etch m.
frozen section m.
glass-bead retention m.

glucose oxidase m.
glycerin m.
Gomori's m. for chromaffin
Gram's m
Granger m.
Grimelius's argyrophil m.
Grocott-Gomori methenamine-
　silver m.
Hall's m.
Hammerschlag's m.
Heublein m.
hexokinase m.
Highman's m. for amyloid
Holmes's m.
Holzer's m.
homozygous typing m.
Howell's m.
H.P. Wright m.
immunofluorescence m.
immunoperoxidase staining m.
indophenol m.
interference m.
Ivy's m. of bleeding time
Jendrassik-Grof m.
Jones's m.
Kaplan-Meier m.
Kay-Bodansky m.
Kety-Schmidt m.
King-Armstrong m.
Kjeldahl's m.
Lee-White m.
Lee-White clotting time m.
leukocyte alkaline phospha-
　tase m's
Levaditi's m.
Lillie's allochrome m.
Lison-Dunn m.
macro-Kjeldahl m.
Mancini m.
Marshall's m.
Masson trichrome m.
melanin bleaching m's
melanin staining m's
Menzies' m.
mercurimetric m.
micro-Kjeldahl m.
Monte Carlo m.
Movat's pentachrome m.
myelin-staining m's
myoglobin identification m's
Nichols m.
Nikiforoff's m.

Nimeh's m.
Ouchterlony m.
panning m.
Penfield's m.
peroxidase staining m's
Pfeiffer-Comberg m.
Pisano m.
Pizzolato's peroxide-silver m.
plasma-thrombin clot m.
polyvinyl alcohol fixative m.
protein separation m's
Puchtler's alkaline Congo
    red m.
Puchtler's Sirius red m.
PVA fixative m.
Quick's m.
Rees-Ecker m.
reference m.
Rideal-Walker m.
Sahli's m.
Salzman m.
Schales and Schales m. for
    chloride
Schoenheimer-Sperry m.
Scotch tape m.
Shaffer-Hartman m.
Shihabi-Bishop m.
Somogyi m.
special reference m.
Spin-cool filter m.
spinner m.
Stovall-Black m.
suction m.
Sweet's m.
Thoms m.
Tietz-Fiereck m.
trihydroxyindole m.
two-slide m.
ultropaque m.
Van Slyke and Cullen's m.
von Kossa's m.
wedge m.
Welker's m.
Westergren m.
Westergren sedimentation
    rate m.
Whipple's m.
Wintrobe and Landsberg's m.
Wintrobe's method
Wintrobe's sedimentation
    rate m.
Zeeman's correction m.

zeta sedimentation ratio m.
zinc-sulfate flotation m.
ZSR m.
methodology
methohexital
methotrexate
methotrimeprazine
methoxamine
methoxsalen
methoxy
methoxyamphetamine
p-methoxyamphetamine assay
4-methoxybenzene-diazonium
methoxychlor
methoxyethyl mercuriacetate
methoxyflurane
3-methoxy-4-hydroxymandelic acid
3-methoxy-4-hydroxymandelic acid
    test
3-methoxy-4-hydroxyphenyl glycol
methoxyphenamine
methoxypromazine
methscopolamine
methsuximide
methyclothiazide
methyl
    m. acetate
    m. alcohol
    m. alcohol poisoning
    m. aldehyde
    m. blue
    m. bromide
    m. butyl ketone
    m. chloride
    m. chloroform
    m. chlorophenoxyacetic acid
    m. cyclohexane
    m. demeton
    m. ethyl ketone
    m. formate
    m. green
    m. green–pyronin stain
    m. *p*-hydroxybenzoate
    m. hydroxybutyric acid
    m. iodide
    m. isobutyl ketone
    m. mercuric cyanoguanidine
    m. mercuric dicyanodiamine
    m. mercury
    m. methacrylate
    m. orange indicator
    m. parathion

m. phenol
m. phenylethylhydantoin
m. polysiloxane
m. red broth
m. red indicator
m. red test
m. salicylate
m. testosterone
m. violet
m. yellow
N-methylacetamide
N-methylacetamide green
methylacetic acid
α-methylacetoacetic acid
α-methylacetoacetyl acid
N-methyl-aminoacid oxidase
methylaminoheptane
p-methylaminophenol hydrochloride
p-methylaminophenol sulfate
N-methyl-D-aspartate
methylaspartate mutase
methylated naphthalene
methylation
methylazoxymethanol
methylbenzene
methylbenzethonium
methylcellulose
methylcholanthrene
methylcobalamin
3-methylcrotonyl
methylcrotonoyl–coenzyme A carboxylase
methyldopa
methylene
m. azure
m. blue
m. blue active substance
m. blue dye
m. blue stain
m. blue test
m. chloride
m. dichloride
m. diphosphonate
m. green
m. tetrahydrofolate
m. violet
m. white
methylene blue
Kühne's m.b.
Löffler's m.b.
new m.b.

polychrome m.b.
m.b. test
methylenedioxyamphetamine
3,4-methylenedioxyamphetamine
assay
5,10-methylenetetrahydrofolate
methylenetetrahydrofolate reductase
methylenophil; methylenophile
methylenophilic; methylenophilous
methylergonovine
methylformamide
N-methylformamide
methylglutaconyl–coenzyme A hydratase
methyglyoxal
1-methyl-histidine
3-methyl-histidine
methylmalonate
methylmalonic
m. acid
m. acidemia
m. aciduria
m. acid screening test
methylmalonyl-CoA decarboxylase
methylmalonyl-CoA mutase
S-methylmalonyl-CoA mutase
methylmercaptan
methylmercury
α-methylmetatyrosine
methylmorphine
methylnicotinamide
N'-methylnicotinamide
methylnitrosourea
α-methylnorepinephrine
methylparaben
methylparafynol
methylpentose
methylphenidate assay
methylphenylethylhydantoin
methylprednisolone
5-methylresorcinol
methylrosaniline chloride
methyltestosterone
5-methyltetrahydrofolate
methylthiouracil
methyltransferase
nicotinamide m.
tetrahydropteroylglutamate m.
5-methyluracyl
methylxanthine
methyprylon
methysergide

metMb — metmyoglobin
metmyoglobin
metocurine iodide
Metopirone test
Metopium
metoprolol tartrate
metoxenous
metoxeny; metaxeny
metraterm
metratrophy; metratrophia
metria
metric
    m. data
    m. system
metritis
metrizamide
metrizoate
metrocarcinoma
metrocele
metrocyte
metrofibroma
metrolymphangitis
metromalacia
metromalacoma; metromalacosis
metronidazole assay
metroperitoneal assay
metroperitoneal fistula
metroperitonitis
metrorrhagia
metrosalpingitis
metrotrophic test
metula
metyrapone stimulation test
MeV — megaelectron volt
mev — million electron volts
mevaldate reductase
mevalonate kinase
mevinphos
Mexican
    hat cell
    hat corpuscle
mexiletine
Meyenburg's complex
Meyers-Kouvenaar bodies
Meyer's mastectomy
Meynet's nodes
mezlocillin
MF — medium frequency
    mycosis fungoides
    myelin figure
mF — millifarad
mf — microfilaria

μf; μfd — microfarad
MFB — metallic foreign body
MFH — malignant fibrous histio-
    cytoma
MFP — monofluorophosphate
MFR — mucus flow rate
MG — menopausal gonadotropin
    mesiogingival
    methyl glucoside
    Michaelis-Gutmann (bodies)
    muscle group
    myasthenia gravis
Mg — magnesium
mg — milligram
mg% — milligrams per deciliter
    milligrams per 100 milliliters
Mg agglutinin
MGBG — methylglyoxal
    bisguanylhydrazone
MGC — minimum gelling
    concentration
MGF — macrophage growth factor
MGGH — methylglyoxal
    guanylhydrazone
MGH or mgh — milligram-hour
mgm — milligram
MGN — membranous
    glomerulonephritis
MGP — marginal granulocyte pool
MGR — modified gain ratio
MGUS — monoclonal gammopathy
    of undetermined signifi-
    cance
MH — malignant histiocytosis
    mammotropic hormone
mH — millihenry
MHA — methemalbumin
    microangiopathic hemolytic
    anemia
    mixed hemadsorption
MHA-TP — microhemagglutination–
    Treponema pallidum
MHA-TP test
MHb — methemoglobin
MHC — major histocompatibility
    complex
    major histocompatibility
    (locus)
MHD — mean hemolytic dose
    minimum hemolytic
    dose
MHN — massive hepatic necrosis

MHP — 1-mercuri-2-hydroxpropane
MHPG — methoxyhydroxyphenyl-
glycol
MHR — maximal heart rate
MHz — megahertz
MI — mercaptoimidazole
mitral incompetence
mitral insufficiency
myocardial infarction
Mibelli's
angiokeratoma
porokeratosis
MIC — minimal inhibitory concentration
minimal isorrheic concen-
tration
micaceous balanitis
mice
joint m.
New Zealand m.
pneumonia virus of m.
micelle
ferruginous m.
Michaelis-Gutmann bodies
Michaelis-Menten
equation
kinetics
miconazole
microabscess
Munro's m.
Pautrier's m.
microadenocarcinoma
microadenoma
microadenopathy
microaerophile
microaerophilic streptococcus
microaggregate filter
microalbinuria
microalbuminuria
microaleuriospore
microampere
microanalysis
microaneurysm
retinal m.
microangiopathic hemolytic
anemia
microangiopathy
diabetic m.
thrombotic m.
Microascaceae
Microascales
Microbacterium

microbar
microbe
microbial
m. antagonism
m. variation
microbic dissociation
microbicidal
microbioassay
microbiol. — microbiological
microbiological
m. assay
m. culture
microbiologist
microbiology
m. automation
m. identification system
microbiotic
microblast
microbody
microbroth
microburet
microcalcifications
microcarcinoid
microcarcinoma
papillary m.
microcell
microcephalic
microcephaly
microchemistry
microchromosome
microcirculation
microcirculatory thrombosis
Micrococcaceae
Micrococcus
M. *flavus*
M. *intracellularis*
M. *pyogenes* var. *aureus*
M. *tetragenus*
microcolitis
microcolony
microcomputer
microconidium (pl., microconidia)
microcoulomb
microcrystalline
microcurie
microcurie-hour
microcyst
microcystic disease of renal
medulla
microcyte
microcythemia

microcytic
    m. anemia
    m. erythrocyte
    m. hypochromic anemia
microcytosis
microcytotoxicity assay
microdensitometer
microdiffusion analysis
microdissection
microdochectomy
microdrepanocytic anemia
microdrepanocytosis
microecology
microelectrode
microelectrophoresis
microembolic
microerythrocyte
microfarad
microfibril
microfiche
microfilament
microfilaremia
microfilaria (pl., microfilariae)
    m. bancrofti
    m. streptocerca
microfilariasis
microflora
microfollicular
    m. adenoma
    m. goiter
microgamete
microgametocyte
microglandular
    m. adenosis
    m. endocervical hyperplasia
microglia
microglial
    m. cell
    m. nodule
microgliocyte
microglioma
microgliomatosis
β-microglobulin
    β_2-m.
    β_{12}-m.
microglossia
micrognathia
microgram
micrograph
    electron m.
microgyria
microhemagglutination assay

microhemagglutination–*Treponema pallidum* test
microhematocrit
microhenry
microhistology
microhm
microhomology
microimmunofluorescent test
microincineration
microinfarct
microinvasion
microinvasive
    m. breast cancer
    m. carcinoma
micro-Kjeldahl method
microlactinoma
microlesion
microleukoblast
microliter
microlith
microlithiasis
    pulmonary alveolar m.
microlymphocytotoxicity
    m. assay
    m. test
micromegakaryocyte
micromelia
micromelic dwarfism
micrometastasis
micrometastatic disease
micrometer
    ocular m.
micromethod
    buffy coat m.
micrometry
micromicrocurie
micromicron
micromillimeter
micromole
Micromonospora
    M. faeni
    M. inyoensis
Micromonosporaceae
micromulticystic renal disease
micromyeloblast
micromyeloblastic leukemia
micromyelolymphocyte
micron (pl., microns; micra; abbreviated μ)
microneedle
micronodular cirrhosis
micronucleus (pl., micronuclei)

microorganism
micropapillary carcinoma
micropathology
micropenis
microphage
microphagocyte
microphthalmia; microphthalmos
micropinocytotic vesicles
micropipette
microplania
microplethysmography
micropolygyria
Micropolyspora faeni
microprecipitation test
micropredation
micropredator
microprobe
    electron m.
    laser m.
microprocessor
microprogram
micropromyelocyte
microprotein
micropyle
microradiography
microrefractometer
microroentgen
microscope
    binocular m.
    color-contrast m.
    comparison m.
    compound m.
    darkfield m.
    darkground m.
    electron m.
    fluorescent m.
    infrared m.
    integrating m.
    interference m.
    laser m.
    light m.
    Nomarski m.
    operating m.
    Oto-Microscope
    polarizing m.
    reflecting m.
    simple m.
    slit-lamp m.
    stereoscopic m.
    trinocular m.
    ultraviolet m.
    x-ray m.

microscopic
    m. agglutination
    m. hematuria
    m. infarct
    m. polyarteritis
    m. syphilis
microscopy
    brightfield m.
    electron m.
    fluorescence m.
    immune electron m.
    immunofluorescence m.
    light m.
    phase-contrast m.
    polarized light m.
microsecond
microsomal
    m. antibodies
    m. enzyme
    m. enzyme system
    m. thyroid antibody
microsome
microspectrophotometry
microspectroscope
microsphere
    aggregated m's
microspherocyte
microspherocytosis
microsplanchnic
microsplenia
microspore
Microsporidia
microsporidian
microsporidiosis
Microsporon
microsporosis
Microsporum
    M. audouinii
    M. canis
    M. felineum
    M. ferrugineum
    M. fulvum
    M. furfur
    M. gypseum
    M. lanosum
    M. nanum
microstomia
Microsulfon
microsurgery
microsyringe
microtia

microtome
    cold m.
    freezing m.
    m. knife
    rocker m.
    rotary m.
    sliding m.
microtonometer
microtubule
Microtus
microunit
microvascular
microvasculopathy
microvesicle
microvesicular steatosis
microvillus (pl., microvilli)
microviscosimeter
microvolt
microwatt
microwave
microxycyte
microxyphil
Micrurus
micturition
    m. attack
    m. reflex
MID — maximum inhibiting dilution
    mesioincisodistal
    minimum infective dose
midbody
midbrain
midcarpal joint
midcolic lymph node
mid-diastolic
Middlebrook-Dubos hemagglutination
    test
Middlebrook's
    agar
    broth
    media
midge
midline
    m. lethal granuloma
    m. malignant reticulosis
    m. nucleus
midlobular region
midpalmar space
midsagittal plane
midsternal line
midtarsal joint
midzonal necrosis
Mielke bleeding time

Miescheria
Miescher's
    elastoma
    granulomatosis
MIF — macrophage-inhibiting factor
    melanocyte-stimulating
      hormone–inhibiting factor
    migration-inhibiting factor
    mixed immunofluorescence
MIFR — maximal inspiratory flow
    rate
Mignon's eosinophilic granuloma
migraine
migrainous neuralgia
migrating
    m. abscess
    m. thrombophlebitis
migration inhibition
    m.i. factor
    m.i. test
migratory
    m. arthritis
    m. cells
    m. inhibiting factor
    m. phlebitis
    m. pneumonia
    m. polyarthritis
    m. thrombophlebitis
Mikulicz's
    cells
    clamp
    pack
    pyloroplasty
mild silver protein
milia
miliaria
    apocrine m.
    m. profunda
    m. rubra
miliary
    m. abscess
    m. aneurysm
    m. carcinosis
    m. dissemination
    m. embolism
    m. granulomatous inflam-
      mation
    m. tuberculosis
milieu
milium (pl., milia)
    colloid m.
    m. cyst

milk
>   m. alkali syndrome
>   m. anemia
>   biundulant m. fever
>   m. cyst
>   m. fat globulin
>   m. leg
>   m. spots

milker's nodules
Milkman's fracture
milky
>   m. ascites
>   m. urine

Millar's asthma
Miller-Abbott tube
millers' asthma
milliammeter
milliamperage
milliampere-second
millibar
millicoulomb
millicurie
millicurie-hour
milliequivalent
millifarad
milligram
milligram-hour
milligram
>   m's per deciliter
>   m's per 100 milliliters

millihenry
millilambert
milliliter
millimeter
>   cubic m.
>   m's of mercury
>   m's partial pressure

millimicrocurie
millimicrogram
millimicron
millimolar
millimole
>   m's per liter

millinormal
milliosmol; milliosmole
milliosmolal
Millipore filter
millirad
millirem
milliroentgen
millisecond
milliunit

millivolt
milliwatt
Millon-Nasse test
Millon's reagent
Miltenberger antigen
Mima polymorpha
Mimeae
mimicry
>   molecular m.

min. — minute(s)
mineral
>   m. deficiency
>   m. excess
>   m. foreign body
>   m. nutrients
>   m. oil foreign body
>   m. oil granuloma

mineralization
mineralocorticoid
>   m. hypertension
>   m.-secreting adenoma

miners'
>   m. asthma
>   m. lung

Ming's classification
minicell
minify
minimal
>   m. bactericidal concentration
>   m. bactericidal level
>   m. brain damage
>   m. brain dysfunction
>   m.-change disease
>   m.-change nephrotic syndrome
>   m. deviation melanoma
>   m. erythema dose
>   m. growth temperature
>   m. inhibitory concentration
>   m. isorrheic concentration
>   m. lethal concentration
>   m. lethal dose
>   m. morbidostatic dose

minimum
>   m. complete-killing concentration
>   m. concentration of bilirubin
>   m. detectable concentration
>   m. dose causing death or malformation of 100% of fetuses
>   m. essential medium
>   m. hemolytic dose
>   m. infective dose

m. lethal concentration
m. lethal dose
m. mycoplasmacidal concentration
m. thermometer

minocycline
m.-associated pigment
m. hydrochloride

minor
m. calyx
m. epilepsy
m. histocompatibility antigen
m. histocompatibility complex
m. histocompatibility locus
m. inferior aperture
m. pelvis
m. salivary gland
m. sublingual duct
m. superior aperture
m. tranquilizer
variola m.
m. vestibular gland

Minor's starch-iodine test
Minot-Murphy treatment
minoxidil
Mintezol

minute
counts per m.
cycles per m.
double m's
liters per m.
revolutions per m.
m. volume

minuthesis
mionectic
miosis
MIP — maximum inspiratory pressure
miracidium (pl., miracidia)
schistosomal m.
MIRD — Medical Internal Radiation
Dose
Mirex
mirror-image cell
miscarriage
miscibility
miscible
infinitely m.
partially m.
missed abortion
missense mutation
missile wound
MIT — monoiodotyrosine

Mitchison medium

mite
m. bite
grain itch m.
harvest m.
m. infestation
m. itch
kedani m.
parasitoid m.
predaceous m.
red m.
trombiculid m.

mithramycin
miticidal
miticide

mitochondrial
m. antibody
m. aspartate aminotransferase
m.-rich cell
m. cristae alteration
m. encephalomyopathy
m. enzyme
m. matrix alteration
m. membrane alteration
m. myopathy
m. thymopathy

mitochondrion (pl., mitochondria)
mitocromin

mitogen
B-cell m's
pokeweed m.
T-cell m's

mitogenic
m. factor
m. radiation

minogenicity
mitogillin
mitokinetic
mitomalcin
mitome
mitomycin C
mitoplasm

mitosis (pl., mitoses)
heterotypic m.
homeotypic m.
m.-karyorrhexis index
multicentric m.
pathologic m.
pluripolar m.
three-part m.

mitosome
mitotane

mitotic
    m. arrest
    m.-control protein
    m. cycle
    m. figure
    m. index
    m. poison
mitral
    m. anulus calcification
    m. atresia
    m. gradient
    m. incompetence
    m. incompetence and stenosis
    m. insufficiency
    m. orifice
    m. regurgitation
    m. ring
    m. stenosis
    m. valve calcification
    m. valve prolapse
Mitsuda
    antigen
    reaction
mittelschmerz
Mittendorf's dots
mixed
    m. acid fermentation
    m. agglutination reaction
    m. anhydride
    m. calculus
    m. carcinoma
    m. cell leukemia
    m. chancre
    m. connective tissue disease
    m. cryoglobulin syndrome
    m. culture
    m. glioma
    m. hemadsorption
    m. hemoglobinopathy
    m. hepatocellular carcinoma
    m. immunofluorescence
    m. leukemia
    m. leukocyte culture
    m. lineage lesion
    m. lymphocyte culture
    m. lymphocyte culture test
    m. lymphocyte reaction
    m. lymphocytic-histiocytic
        lymphoma
    m. medullary-follicular car-
        cinoma
    m. mesodermal tumor

    m. papillary follicular car-
        cinoma
    m. squamous cell carcinoma
        and adenocarcinoma
    m. test
    m. thalassemia
    m. thrombus
    m. tumor
    m. tumor of salivary gland
    m. tumor of skin
    m. venous
    m. venous blood
    m. venous PCO_2
    m. venous PO_2
mixoploid
    developmental m.
    proliferative m.
mixoploidy
mixotrophic
mixture
    Brompton's m.
    dextrose solution m.
    dichloropropene-
        dichloropropene m.
    racemic m.
    toxoid-antitoxin m.
Miyagawanella
    M. *illinii*
    M. *louisianae*
    M. *lymphogranulomatosis*
    M. *ornithosis*
    M. *pneumoniae*
    M. *psittaci*
MK — monkey kidney
MKS — meter-kilogram-second
MKV — killed-measles vaccine
ML — mesiolingual
M:L — monocyte-lymphocyte ratio
mL — millilambert
    milliliter
ml — milliliter
μL or μl — microliter
MLA — mento-laeva anterior
    mesiolabial
    monocytic leukemia, acute
MLAI — mesiolabioincisal
MLAP — mean left atrial pressure
MLC — minimum lethal concentra-
        tion
    mixed leukocyte culture
    mixed lymphocyte culture
    multilamellar cytosome

                    myelomonocytic leukemia,
        chronic
MLD — metachromatic leukodystro-
            phy
        minimum lethal dose
MLI — mesiolinguoincisal
M line
MLNS — mucocutaneous lymph
            node syndrome
MLO — mesiolinguo-occlusal
MLP — left mentoposterior (mento-
            laeva posterior)
        mesiolinguopulpal
MLR — mixed lymphocyte reaction
MLS — myelomonocytic leukemia,
            subacute
MLT — left mentotransverse (mento-
            laeva transversa)
MLV — Moloney's leukemogenic
            virus
        mouse leukemia virus
MM — malignant melanoma
        medial malleolus
        mediastinal mass
        mucous membrane
        multiple myeloma
        muscularis mucosa
        myeloid metaplasia
mM — millimolar
        millimole
mm — millimeter
mμ — millimicron
$\mu\mu$ — micromicron
MMA — methylmalonic acid
MMC — minimal medullary concen-
            tration
mμc — millimicrocurie (nanocurie)
$\mu\mu$c — micromicrocurie (picocurie)
MMD — minimal morbidostatic dose
MMEF — maximal midexpiratory
            flow
MMEFR — maximal midexpiratory
            flow rate
MMF — maximal midexpiratory flow
MMFR — maximal midexpiratory
            flow rate
        maximal midflow rate
mμg — millimicrogram (nanogram)
μm — micrometer
μmg — micromilligram
$\mu\mu$g — micromicrogram (picogram)
mm Hg — millimeter(s) of mercury

mM/L or mM/l — millimoles per
                liter
MMM — myeloid metaplasia with
            myelofibrosis
        myelosclerosis with myeloid
            metaplasia
μmm — micromillimeter
M-mode echo
mmol — millimole
mmpp — millimeters partial pressure
MMPR — methylmercaptopurine
            riboside
MMR — mass miniature radiography
        myocardial metabolic rate
MMTV — mouse mammary tumor
            virus
MM virus
MN — multinodular
        myoneural
Mn — manganese
mN — millinormal
MN blood group system
MNCV — motor nerve conduction
            velocity
mnemonic code
MNU — methylnitrosourea
MO — mesio-occlusal
Mo — molybdenum
mo; mos — month(s)
Moberg's arthrodesis
mobile
        m. cecum
        m. genes
        m. phase
mobility
        electrophoretic m.
mobilization
        localized leukocyte m.
        m. test
mobilometer
Mobiluncus
MOD — mesio-occlusodistal
modal
modality
mode
        B-m.
        conversational m.
        decay m.
        histogram m.
        list m.
model
        Cox proportional hazards m.

fluid mosaic m.
hepatocarcinogenesis m.
hypotheticodeductive m.
modem
moderator band
modification
    racemic m.
modified
    m. amino acid
    m. smallpox
modifier
    biologic response m.
modifying gene
modiolus
modular
modulate
modulation
    antigenic m.
    m. transfer function
module
modulus
Moellerella wisconsensis
Mohr pipette
Mohs' technique
moiety
moist
    m. gangrene
    m. papule
    m. wart
mol — mole
molal
molality
molar
    m. absorption coefficient
    m. absorptivity
    m. concentration
    deciduous m.
    m. extinction coefficient
    m. heat capacity
    mandibular m.
    m. mass
    maxillary m.
    m. pregnancy
    m. weight
molarity
mold
mole
    BK m.
    blood m.
    Breus m.
    carneous m.
    cystic m.

false m.
fleshy m.
m. fraction
grape m.
hairy m.
hydatid m.
hydatidiform m.
invasive m.
malignant m.
metastasizing m.
spider m.
vesicular m.
molecular
    m. anemia
    m. biology
    m. cloning
    m. dispersion
    m. distillation
    m. exclusion chromatography
    m. genetics
    m. hybridization probe
    m. layer
    m. lesion
    m. marker
    m. mass
    m. mimicry
    m. pathology
    m. sieve
    m. sieve chromatography
    m. weight
molecule
    adhesion m's
    T-4 m.
molindone hydrochloride
Molisch's test
Mollicutes
mollities
Moll's gland
molluscous
molluscum (pl., mollusca)
    m. body
    m. contagiosum
    m. contagiosum virus
    m. corpuscle
    m. fibrosum
    m. fibrosum gravidarum
    m. sebaceum virus
    m. verrucosum
mollusk
Moloney's
    leukemogenic virus
    sarcoma virus

mol. wt. — molecular weight
molybdate
molybdenum
    m. blue
    m. isotope
molybdic
molybdous
MOMA — methoxyhydroxymandelic
        acid
moment
    dipole m.
    magnetic m.
momentum
monad
Monadina
monamide
monaminergic
monaminuria
monarthritis
    acute m.
    m. deformans
Monas
monaster
monaxonic
Mönckeberg's
    arteriosclerosis
    calcification
    degeneration
    medial calcification
    medial sclerosis
mongol
mongolian
    m. idiocy
    m. idiot
    m. macula
    m. spot
mongolism
mongoloid
monilated
monilethrix
Monilia sitophila
monilial esophagitis
moniliasis
moniliform
Moniliformis moniliformis
moniliid
monitor
    air m.
monitoring
    atmospheric m.
    drug m.
    transcutaneous m.

monkey
    m. B virus
    m. kidney cells
monoacylglycerol
monoallelic
monoamine
    m. oxidase
    m. oxidase inhibitors
monoaminodicarboxylic acid
monoaminomonocarboxylic acid
monoaminuria
monoamniotic placenta twins
monobasic
    m. acid
    m. potassium phosphate
monobenzone
monoblast
monoblastic leukemia
monoblastoma
monobutyl
    m. biphenyl sodium monosul-
        fonate
    m. phenyl phenol sodium
        monosulfonate
monocarboxylic acid
monocentric
monocephalic cranial duplication
monocephalus
    m. tetrapus dibrachius
    m. tripus dibrachius
monochorionic
    m. diamniotic placenta
    m. diamniotic placenta twin
    m. monoamniotic placenta
    m. placenta twins
monochroic
monochromatic
    m. light
    m. radiation
    m. ray
monochromatism
monochromatophil
monochromator
monochromic
monochromophil
monoclonal
    m. antibodies
    m. band
    m. gammopathy
    m. hypergammaglobulinemia
    m. hyperimmunoglobulinemia
    m. immunoglobulin

m. paraproteinemia
m. peak
m. tumor
monocyte
    m. function test
    m.-lymphocyte ratio
    m.-macrophage
monocytic
    m. angina
    m. blood cell
    m. cells
    m. inflammatory infiltrate
    m. leukemia
    m. leukemoid reaction
    m. leukocytosis
    m. leukopenia
    m. marrow
    m. tissue
monocytoid cell
monocytopenia
monocytopoiesis
monocytosis
5-monodeiodinase
monodermal teratoma
monodermoma
monoenergetic radiation
monoenoic fatty acid
monoester
monoethylglycinexylidide
monofluoroacetate salt
monogenic character
monoglutamate
monoglyceride
monohistiocytic series
monohydric alcohol
monohydrochloride
    arginine m.
monohydrolase
    orthophosphoric ester m.
monoiodothyronine
monoiodotyrosine
3-monoiodo-L-tyrosine
monokaryote
monokaryotic
monokine
monolayer
monomer
    fibrin m.
monomeric
monomethyl-*p*-aminophenol sulfate
monomorphic adenoma
monomorphism

monomyelocytic leukemia
monomyositis
Mononchus
mononeuritis multiplex
mononeuropathy
mononuclear
    m. inflammation
    m. leukocyte
    m. phagocyte
    m. phagocyte system
    m. pleocytosis
mononucleate
mononucleosis
    cytomegaloviral m.
    heterophil-negative m.
    infectious m.
    post-transfusion m.
mononucleotide
    flavin m.
monooxygenase
    flavin m.
β-monooxygenase
monopenia
monophasic
    m. anaplasia
    m. wave
monophosphate
    adenosine m.
    adenosine 3′,5′-cyclic m.
    cyclic adenosine m.
    cyclic guanosine m.
    cytidine m.
    deoxyadenosine m.
    deoxycytidine m.
    deoxyguanosine m.
    deoxyuridine m.
    fludarabine m.
    guanosine m.
    hexose m.
    inosine m.
    thymolphthalein m.
    uridine m.
    xanthosine m.
3′,5′-monophosphate
monophosphoglyceromutase
monophyletic theory
monophyletism
monoplast
monoplegia
monoploid
monopolar
monoptychial

monorecidive chancre
monosaccharide
monosodium
     m. glutamate
     m. urate crystals
     uric m.
monosome
monosomic cells
monosomy
monospecific antiserum
Monosporium apiospermum
Monospot test
monostotic fibrous dysplasia
monosynaptic
monotetrazolium
monotreme
Monotricha
monotrichous
monotropic
monounsaturated fatty acids
monovalent antiserum
monoxide
     carbon m.
monozygotic twins
Monro's
     abscess
     foramen
mons (pl., montes)
     m. pubis
     m. ureteris
     m. veneris
monster
     anencephalic m.
Monte Carlo method
Montenegro skin test
Montevideo unit
moon facies
MOPP — nitrogen mustard, On-
     covin, prednisone, pro-
     carbazine
MOPV — monovalent oral poliovirus
     vaccine
Morand's foot
Moranyl
Morax-Axenfeld
     bacillus
     diplococcus
     haemophilus
Moraxella
     M. *bovis*
     M. *(Branhamella)*
      catarrhalis

     M. *kingae*
     M. *lacunata*
     M. *liquefaciens*
     M. *nonliquefaciens*
     M. *osloensis*
     M. *phenylpyruvica*
     M. *urethralis*
morbidity rate
morbility
morbillivirus
morbus
morcellation
mordant
Morgagni's
     column
     crypt
     cyst
     hernia
     hydatid
     nodules
     prolapse
     spheres
morgagnian cataract
morgan
Morganella morganii
Morgan's bacillus
morin
Mörner's test
morococcus
morphallactic regeneration
morphea
     m. acroterica
     m. alba
     m. guttata
     m. herpetiformis
     m. linearis
     m. pigmentosa
morphine hydrochloride
morphodifferentiation
morphogenesis
morpholine
morphologic abnormality
morphology
morphometry
morrhuic acid
mors (gen., mortis) thymica
mortality rate
mortar kidney
Mortierella wolfii
Mortierellaceae
mortification
mortified

Morton's
> neuralgia
> neuroma
> toe

morula
> endometrial m.

morular

morule

mOs — milliosmolal

mosaic
> m. fungus
> m. pattern
> m. wart

mosaicism

Mosenthal's test

Mosler's diabetes

mOsm — milliosmol; milliosmole

mosquito

mosquitocidal

mosquitocide

Moss's classification

mossy foot

mote
> blood m's

mother cyst

motile
> m. colony
> m. leukocyte
> m. serum

motilin

motility
> gastrointestinal m.

motion
> brownian m.
> range of m.

motoneuron
> beta m's

motor
> m. aphasia
> m. cortex
> m. end plate
> m. hyperactivity
> m. neuron
> m. neuron disease
> m. nucleus, trigeminal
>   nerve
> m. pathway
> m. root

Mott
> bodies
> cell

mottled enamel

mottling

Motulsky dye reduction test

moulage

mould

mount

mountain fever

mountant

mounting medium

mouse
> m. cancer
> cancer-free white m.
> m. leukemia virus
> m. mammary tumor virus
> m.-specific lymphocyte antigen
> m. unit
> m. uterine units

mouth
> tapir m.
> trench m.

movable
> m. heart
> m. testis

Movat's pentachrome method

movement
> ameboid m.
> m. artifact
> athetoid m.
> ballistic m's
> brownian m.
> euglenoid m.
> streaming m.

moving
> m. boundary electrophoresis
> m. phase

Mowry's colloidal iron stain

MP — mean pressure
> melting point
> menstrual period
> mercaptopurine
> mesiopulpal
> metacarpophalangeal
> monophosphate
> mucopolysaccharide
> multiparous

6-MP — 6-mercaptopurine

MPA — main pulmonary artery
> medroxyprogesterone acetate
> methylprednisolone acetate

MPAP — mean pulmonary arterial
> pressure

MPC — marine protein concentrate
> maximum permissible con-
> centration

meperidine, promethazine,
chlorpromazine
minimum mycoplasmacidal
concentration
MPD — maximal permissible dose
MPEH — methylphenylethylhy-
dantoin
MPGM — monophosphoglycerate
mutase
MPGN — membranoproliferative glomerulonephritis
M (meiotic) phase
MPJ — metacarpophalangeal joint
MPL — mesiopulpolingual
MPLA — mesiopulpolabial
MPMV — Mason Pfizer monkey virus
MPO — myeloperoxidase
MPP — mercaptopyrazidopyrimidine
M protein
MPS — mononuclear-phagocyte (reticuloendothelial) system
mucopolysaccharide
mucopolysaccharidosis
MPS storage diseases I–VII
MPV — mean platelet volume
MR — metabolic rate
methyl red
mitral reflux
mitral regurgitation
mortality rate
mortality ratio
muscle relaxant
mR — milliroentgen
mrad — millirad
MRAP — mean right atrial pressure
mrem — millirem
MRF — melanocyte-stimulating
hormone–releasing factor
mesencephalic reticular formation
mitral regurgitant flow
MRI — magnetic resonance imaging
mRNA — messenger RNA
MRVP — mean right ventricular
pressure
MS — mass spectrometry
mitral stenosis
morphine sulfate
mucosubstance
multiple sclerosis
musculoskeletal

MSA — multiplication-stimulating
activity
MSB — Martius scarlet blue
most significant bit
MSB trichrome stain
MSD — most significant digit
msec — millisecond
MSER — mean systolic ejection rate
MSG — monosodium glutamate
MSH — melanocyte-stimulating hor-
mone
melanophore-stimulating
hormone
MSH-IF — melanocyte-stimulating
hormone–inhibiting
factor
MSH-RF — melanocyte-stimulating
hormone–releasing
factor
MSK — medullary sponge kidney
MSL — midsternal line
MSLA — mouse-specific lymphocyte
antigen
MSU — monosodium urate
MSUD — maple syrup urine disease
MSV — Moloney's sarcoma virus
murine sarcoma virus
MT — malignant teratoma
membrana tympani
metatarsal
methyltyrosine
MTBF — mean time between failures
MTF — maximum terminal flow
modulation transfer function
MTHF — 5-methyltetrahydrofolate
acid
MTI — malignant teratoma interme-
diate
MTP — metatarsophalangeal
MTR — Meinicke turbidity reaction
MTT — malignant trophoblastic ter-
atoma
methyltetrazolium
monotetrazolium
MTU — methylthiouracil
MTV — mammary tumor virus
MTX — methotrexate
MU — Mache unit
Montevideo unit
mu heavy-chain disease
mU — milliunit
mu — micron
mouse unit

MUC — maximum urinary concentration
mucase
mucicarmine stain
mucicarminophilic
mucigen
mucihematein
    Mayer's m.
mucilloid
    psyllium hydrophilic m.
mucin
    m. clot test
    m. test
mucinase
mucinemia
muninoid degeneration
mucinosa
    alopecia m.
mucinosis
    follicular m.
    localized m.
    metabolic m.
    papular m.
    reticular erythematous m.
    secondary m.
mucinous
    m. adenocarcinoma
    m. adenoma
    m. atrophy
    m. breast cancer
    m. carcinoma
    m. cystadenocarcinoma
    m. cystadenoma
    m. degeneration
    m. tumor
mucinuria
mucitis
mucocele
mucociliary escalator
mucoclasis
mucocutaneous
    m. candidiasis
    m. herpes simplex
    m. leishmaniasis
    m. lymph node syndrome
mucocyst
mucoenteritis
mucoepidermoid
    m. carcinoma
    m. tumor
mucoepithelial dysplasia

mucoglobulin
mucoid
    m. adenocarcinoma
    m. colony
    m. cyst
    m. degeneration
    m. medial degeneration
mucolipidosis
    m. I
    m. II
    m. III
    m. IV
mucolytic
mucomembranous
mucopeptide
muoperiosteal flap
mucopolysaccharidase
mucopolysaccharide
    acid m.
    m. staining
    m. storage disease
    sulfated acid m.
    m. test
mucopolysaccharidosis
    type I m.
    type IS m.
    type II m.
    type III m.
    type IV m.
    type V m.
    type VI m.
    type VII m.
mucopolysacchariduria
    abnormal m.
mucoprotein
    m. assay
    Tamm-Horsfall m.
    m. test
mucopurulent exudate
mucopus
Mucor
    M. circinelloides
    M. corymbifer
    M. indicus
    M. mucedo
    M. pusillus
    M. racemosus
    M. ramosus
    M. rhizopodiformis
Mucoraceae
mucormycosis
    cerebral m.
    rhinocerebral m.

mucosa
    alveolar m.
    buccal m.
    gallbladder m.
    gastric m.
    gastrointestinal m.
    muscularis m.
    olfactory m.
    oral m.
    respiratory m.
    seminal vesicle m.
    strawberry m.
    vas deferens m.
mucosal
    m. hemangioma
    m. melanoma
    m. neuroma
    m. neuroma syndrome
mucosanguineous; mucosanguinolent
mucoserous
mucositis necroticans agranulocytica
mucosocutaneous
mucosubstance
mucosulfatidosis
mucous
    m. cast
    m. colitis
    m. connective tissue
    m. cyst
    m. gland
    m. hernia
    m. membrane
    m. membrane gland
    m. membrane, ileal
    m. membrane, intestinal
    m. metaplasia
    m. neck cell
    m. papule
    m. patch
    m. plug
    m. polyp
    m. threads
mucoviscidosis
Mucuna
mucus
    accessory sinus m.
    bronchial m.
    cervical m.
    colonic m.
    endocervical m.
    epiglottic m.
    esophageal m.

    m. extravasation
    laryngeal m.
    lower respiratory tract m.
    nasal m.
    nasopharyngeal m.
    pharyngeal m.
    rectal m.
    m. retention
    tracheal m.
    upper respiratory tract m.
Mueller-Hinton
    agar
    broth
Mueller's arteries
mulberry calculus
mule-spinner's cancer
muliebria
müllerian
    m. adenosarcoma
    m. duct
    m. inhibitory factor
    m. mixed tumor
    m. rest
    m. tumor
Müller's
    capsule
    duct
    fixative
    muscle
    radial cell
    tubercle
multicellular
multicentric
    m. breast cancer
    m. mitosis
    m. osteosarcoma
    m. reticulohistiocytosis
Multiceps
    M. *glomeratus*
    M. *multiceps*
    M. *serialis*
multichannel analyzer
multicore disease
multicystic ameloblastoma
multidrug radioiron
multifactorial inheritance
multifocal
    m. breast cancer
    m. encephalitis
    m. eosinophilic granuloma
    m. fibrosis
    m. granulomatous folliculitis

m. inflammation
m. lesion
m. osteitis fibrosa
m. progressive leukoencephalopathy
multiformatter
multiform neuron
multigravida
multilamellar body
multilobar
multilobate placenta
multilobular
multilocular; multiloculate
    m. cyst
    m. cystic kidney
    m. hydatid cyst
multimeric analysis
multimeter
multimodal
    m. convergence
    m. neuron
multinodular
    m. adrenal cortex
    m. goiter
multinuclear leukocyte
multinuclearity
    erythroblastic m.
multinucleated
    m. giant cell
    m. rhabdomyoblast
multinucleosis
multip.
    (multipara) — pregnant woman who has borne two or more children
multipara
multipartita
    placenta m.
multiphasic screening
multiplane tomographic scanner
multiple
    m. access
    m. adenoma
    m. adenomatous polyps
    m. allele
    m. colloid goiter
    m. drug radioiron
    m. endocrine adenomatosis
    m. endocrine neoplasia syndromes, types I, II, IIA, IIB, III
    m. endocrinoma

m. endocrinopathy
m. epiphyseal dysplasia
m. event curve
m. exostosis
m. fission
m. fractures
m. hamartoma syndrome
m. hemorrhagic sarcoma
m. idiopathic hemorrhagic sarcoma
m. intestinal polyposis
m. keratoacanthoma
m. lentigines syndrome
m. melanoma
m. meningiomas
m. mucosal neuroma syndrome
m. myeloma
m. myelomatosis
m. myositis
m. neurofibromatosis
m. osteochondromas
m. osteochondromatosis
m.-point electrode
m. polyps
m. polyposis
m. sclerosis
m. self-healing squamous epithelioma
m. serositis
m. spike complex
m. spike foci
m. stage random sample
m. stain
m. symmetric lipomatosis
multiplex
    mononeuritis m.
multiplication
    m.-stimulating activity
    vegetative m.
multiplicative growth
multiplicator
multipolar
    m. neuron
    m. spindle
multipotential
    m. primary sarcoma of bone
    m. stem cells
multi-rule technique
multisensory neuron
Multistix test
multitrichous
multivalent
multivariate analysis of variance

multivesicular body
multiwire proportional chamber
multi-X chromosome disorder
mummification necrosis
mumps
    m. antibody titer
    iodine m.
    meningoencephalitis m.
    metastatic m.
    m. orchitis
    m. serology
    m. virus
    m. virus culture
Munro's
    abscess
    microabscess
mural
    m. aneurysm
    m. endocarditis
    m. kidney
    m. papilloma
    m. thrombosis
    m. thrombus
muralium
muramic acid
muramidase
Murchison-Pel-Ebstein
    fever
Muercke's lines
murein
murexide
muriatic acid
muriform
murine
    m. leprosy
    m. sarcoma virus
    m. T-cell phenotype
    m. typhus
murmur
    aortic m.
    apical m.
    Austin Flint m.
    basal m.
    cardiac m.
    cardiovascular m.
    continuous m.
    diastolic m.
    ejection m.
    holosystolic m.
    late systolic m.
    regurgitant m.
    systolic m.

    venous m.
    ventricular filling m.
    vesicular m.
Murphy-Pattee test
Murray Valley encephalitis virus
Musca
    M. *domestica*
muscae volitantes
muscarine receptor
muscarinic
Muscidae
muscle
    m. action potential
    m. biopsy
    cardiac m.
    constrictor m.
    m. contractile protein
    cremasteric m.
    detrusor m.
    extrafusal fiber of m.
    extraocular m.
    m. fibers, types I and II
    m. filament
    m. hemoglobin
    Horner's m.
    intermediate fiber of stri-
        ated m.
    intrafusal fiber of m.
    lingual m.
    lubrical m.
    masseter m.
    Müller's m.
    mylohyoid m.
    oblique m.
    ocular m.
    omohyoid m.
    m. palsy
    platysma m.
    pterygoid m.
    quadrate m.
    receptor m.
    Riolan's m.
    m. serum
    skeletal m.
    smooth m.
    spinal m.
    m. spindle
    sternocleidomastoid m.
muscular
    m. artery
    m. atrophy
    m. dystrophy

m. fibrillation
m. rheumatism
m. rigidity
m. subaortic steosis
muscular atrophy
    Charcot-Marie-Tooth m.a.
    hypertrophic polyneuritic type
        m.a.
    infantile m.a.
    peroneal m.a.
    progressive m.a.
muscular dystrophy
    Becker's m.d.
    distal-type m.d.
    Duchenne-type m.d.
    facioscapulohumeral-type m.d.
    Landouzy-Dejerine progressive
        m.d.
    limb girdle–type m.d.
    myotonic m.d.
    ophthalmoplegic-type m.d.
muscularis
    m. mucosa
    m. propria
    tunica m.
musculoaponeurotic fibromatosis
musculocutaneous
musculomembranous
musculophrenic
musculoskeletal
    m. leukemia
    m. system
musculotendinous
musculotropic
mushroom
    m. picker's lung
    m. poisoning
mustard
    m. gas
    nitrogen m.
    phosphoramide m.
    uracil m.
mutagen
    chromosomal m.
mutagenesis
mutagenic
mutagenicity test
Mutamycin
mutant
    m. gene
    m. hemoglobin
    hfr m.

high-frequency recombina-
    tion (hfr) m.
mutarotation
mutase
    2,3-diphosphoglycerate m.
    S-methylmalonyl-CoA m.
    6-phosphoglycerate
mutation
    amber m.
    auxotrophic m.
    clear plaque m.
    cold-sensitive m.
    conditional lethal m.
    constitutive m.
    deletion m.
    feedback inhibition m.
    forward m.
    frameshift m.
    genetic m.
    host-range m.
    insertional m.
    lethal m.
    missense m.
    nonsense m.
    ochre m.
    phage-resistant m.
    pleiotropic m.
    point m.
    polyadenylation signal m.
    radiation-induced m.
    rapid-lysis m.
    m. rate
    reverse m.
    semilethal m.
    sex-reversed m.
    silent m.
    somatic m.
    spontaneous m.
    subvital m.
    suppressor m.
    temperature-sensitive m.
    transition m.
    transversion m.
    ultraviolet light–induced m.
mutilating
    m. keratoderma
    m. wound
mutism
    akinetic m.
muton
mutualism
mutualist

MUU — mouse uterine unit
muzzled sperm
MV — megavolt
      minute volume
      mitral valve
      mixed venous
mV — millivolt
μV — microvolt
MVM — microvillose membrane
MVP — mitral valve prolapse
MVR — massive vitreous retraction
MVV — maximal voluntary
           ventilation
MW — molecular weight
mW — milliwatt
mw — microwave
M wave
Mx — maxwell
My — myopia
my — mayer (unit of heat capacity)
myalgia
myasis
myasthenia gravis
myatrophy
Mycelex
Mycelia sterilia
mycelial fungus
mycelium (pl., mycelia)
mycetismus
      m. cerebralis
      m. cerebris
      m. choleriformis
      m. gastrointestinalis
      m. nervosus
      m. sanguinarius
mycetogenic; mycetogenous
mycetoma
      actinomycotic m.
      eumycotic m.
      maduromycotic m.
mycetosis
mycoagglutinin
Mycobacteriaceae
mycobacterial
      m. adjuvant
      m. infection
      m. meningitis
mycobacteriosis
Mycobacterium
      M. *abscessus*
      M. *africanum*
      M. *aquae*

M. *asiaticum*
M. *avium-intracellulare*
M. *balnei*
M. *berolinenis*
M. *borstelense*
M. *bovis*
M. *brunense*
M. *buruli*
M. *butyricum*
M. *chelonae*
M. *flavescens*
M. *fortuitum*
M. *gastri*
M. *giae*
M. *gordonae*
M. *habana*
M. *haemophilum*
M. *intracellulare*
M. *intracellulare-avium*
M. *johnei*
M. *kansasii*
M. *leprae*
M. *lepraemurium*
M. *littorale*
M. *luciflavum*
M. *malmoense*
M. *marianum*
M. *marinum*
M. *microti*
M. *nonchromogenicum*
M. *paraffinicum*
M. *paratuberculosis*
M. *peregrinum*
M. *phlei*
M. *platypoecilus*
M. *ranae*
M. *scrofulaceum*
M. *simiae*
M. *smegmatis*
M. *szulgai*
M. *terrae*
M. *terrae-nonchromogenicum-*
  triviale
M. *triviale*
M. *tuberculosis*
M. *tuberculosis* var. *avium*
M. *tuberculosis* var. *bovis*
M. *tuberculosis* var. *hominis*
M. *tuberculosis* var. *muris*
M. *ulcerans*
M. *xenopi*

mycobacterium (pl., mycobacteria)
  anonymous m.
  atypical m.
  Battey-type m.
  m. culture
  Group I–IV m.
  nonphotochromogenic m.
  nontuberculous m.
  photochromogenic m.
  scotochromogenic m.
mycobactin
mycobiotic agar
Mycocandida
Mycococcus
Mycoderma
  M. *aceti*
  M. *dermatitidis*
  M. *immite*
mycolic acid
mycologist
mycology
mycomyringitis
myc oncogene amplification
Myconostoc gregarium
Mycoplana
  M. *bullata*
  M. *dimorpha*
Mycoplasma
  M. *buccale*
  M. *faucium*
  M. *fermentans*
  M. *genitalium*
  M. *hominis*
  M. *orale*
  M. *pharyngis*
  M. *pneumoniae*
  M. *salivarium*
mycoplasma
  T-strain m.
mycoplasmal
  m. infection
  m. pneumonia
  m. serology
Mycoplasmataceae
Mycoplasmatales
mycopus
mycosel agar
mycoside
mycosis
  m. fungoides
  m. fungoides d'emblée
  Gilchrist's m.

  m. intestinalis
  Posada m.
  splenic m.
mycostasis
Mycostatin
mycotic
  m. abscess
  m. aneurysm
  m. arthritis
  m. keratitis
  m. meningitis
mycotica
  otitis m.
mycotoxicosis
mycotoxin
mydriasis
myelapoplexy
myelemia
myelencephalon
myelin
  m. basic protein
  m. degeneration
  m. figures
  m. protein
  m. sheath
  m. staining methods
myelinated axon
myelination
myelinic degeneration
myelinolysis
  central pontine m.
myelitis
  radiation m.
  transverse m.
myeloablation
myeloablative
myeloblast
myeloblastemia
myeloblastic
  m. granulocytic sarcoma
  m. leukemia
  m. leukosis
myeloblastoma
myeloblastomatosis
myeloblastosis
myelocele
myeloclast
myelocyst
myelocystic
myelocystocele
myelocystomeningocele

myelocyte
    m. A
    m. B
    basophilic m.
    m. C
    eosinophilic m.
    neutrophilic m.
myelocythemia
myelocytic
    m. crisis
    m. leukemia
    m. leukemoid reaction
    m. leukosis
myelocytoma
myelocytomatosis
myelocytosis
myelodysplasia
myelodysplastic syndrome
myeloencephalitis
    eosinophilic m.
    epidemic m.
myelofibrosis
myelogenic
    m. leukemia
    m. osteopathy
    m. sarcoma
myelogenous
    m. callus
    m. leukemia
myelogeny
myelogone
myelogonium
myelogram
myelography
    gas m.
    opaque m.
    radionuclide m.
myeloid
    m. antigen
    m. cell
    m. depression
    m.-erythroid ratio
    m. granulocytic leukemia
    m. hyperplasia
    m. hypoplasia
    m. leukemia
    m. metaplasia
    m. metaplasia, agnogenic
    m. metaplasia with myelofibrosis
    m. metaplasia with polycythemia vera

m. reticulosis
m. sarcoma
m. series
m. stem cells
m. tissue
myeloidosis
myelokathexis
myeloleukemia
myelolipoma
myelolymphocyte
myelolysis
myeloma
    Bence Jones m.
    endothelial m.
    giant cell m.
    indolent m.
    L-chain m.
    localized m.
    multiple m.
    m. nephrosis
    nonsecretory m.
    plasma cell m.
    plasmacytic m.
    m. protein
    sclerosing m.
    solitary m.
myelomalacia
myelomatoid
myelomatosis
    multiple m.
myelomeningitis
myelomeningocele
myelomonoblast
myelomonocyte
myelomonocytic leukemia
myelomyces
myeloneuropathy
myelopathic
    m. anemia
    m. polycythemia
myelopathy
    carcinomatous m.
    paracarcinomatous m.
    transverse m.
    vacuolar m.
myeloperoxidase
    m. deficiency
    m. system
myelophthisic anemia
myelophthisis
myeloplast

myelopoiesis
 ectopic m.
 extramedullary m.
myelopoietic
myeloproliferative
 m. disorder
 m. granulocyte
 m. syndromes
myeloradiculitis
myelorrhagia
myelosarcoma
myelosarcomatosis
myeloschisis
myelosclerosis with myeloid metaplasia
myelosis
 aleukemic m.
 chronic nonleukemic m.
 erythremic m.
 leukemic m.
 leukopenic m.
 megakaryocytic m.
 nonleukemic m.
 subleukemic m.
myelosuppression
myelosyringosis
myelotomy
 commissural m.
myelotoxic
myenteric plexus
myenteron
MyG — myasthenia gravis
myiasis
 cutaneous m.
 facial m.
 gastric m.
 genitourinary m.
 intestinal m.
 nasal m.
 sanguivorous m.
myiosis
myitis
Mylar capacitor
mylohyoid muscle
Mylone
myoatrophy
myobacterial bacteremia
myoblastic myoma
myoblastoma
 granular cell m.
myocardial
 m. anoxia

m. bridge
m. damage
m. depressant factor
m. disease
m. disease of unknown origin
m. dysfunction
m. infarct
m. infarction
m. infarction on H-form
m. ischemia
m. necrosis
myocarditis
 acute isolated m.
 Fiedler's m.
 fragmentation m.
 giant cell m.
 indurative m.
 Löffler's m.
 rheumatic m.
 viral m.
myocardium
myocardosis
myocele
myocelitis
myocellulitis
myocerosis
myoclonic epilepsy
myoclonus
 nocturnal m.
myocutaneous flap
myocyte
 Anichkov's (Anitschkow's) m.
myocytolysis
 coagulative m.
 m. of heart
myocytoma
myodegeneration
myodemia
myodiastasis
myoendocarditis
myoepithelial cell
myoepithelioma
myoepithelium
myofascial syndrome
myofascitis
myofiber
myofibril
myofibroblast
myofibroma
myofibromatosis
myofibrosis cordis
myofibrositis

myofilament
myoglobinemia
myoglobin identification
    methods
myoglobinuria
    acute paroxysmal m.
myoglobinuric
    m. nephropathy
    m. nephrosis
myoglobulin
myoglobulinuria
myohemoglobin
myo-inositol oxygenase
myoischemia
myokerosis
myokinase
myokymia
myolipoma
myolysis
    cardiotoxic m.
myoma (pl., myomas, myomata)
    myoblastic m.
    uterine m.
myomalacia
myomatous polyp
myomectomy
myomelanosis
myometrial gland
myometritis
myometrium
myonecrosis
    clostridial m.
myoneme
myoneural
myoneuroma
myonosus
myopachynsis
myopathic glycogen storage
    disease
myopathy
    alcoholic m.
    carcinomatous m.
    centronuclear m.
    congenital m.
    corticosteroid m.
    distal m.
    endocrine m.
    fiber-type disproportion m.
    metabolic m.
    mitochondrial m.
    myotubular m.
    nemaline m.

    rod body m.
    thyrotoxic m.
myopericarditis
myoperitonitis
myophosphorylase deficiency glycoge-
    nosis
myopia
myorrhexis
myosalpingitis
myosarcoma
myosclerosis
myoseism
myosin filament
myosis
    endolymphatic stromal m.
    stromal m.
myositic
myositis
    acute disseminated m.
    autoimmune m.
    clostridial m.
    m. fibrosa
    infectious m.
    interstitial m.
    multiple m.
    m. ossificans
    m. ossificans circumscripta
    m. ossificans progressiva
    ossifying interstitial m.
    proliferative m.
myospherulosis
myosteoma
myotenositis
myotome
    caudal m.
    cervical m.
    lumbar m.
    occipital m.
    sacral m.
    thoracic m.
myotonia
    m. acquisita
    m. atrophica
    m. congenita
    m. dystrophica
    m. neonatorum
myotonic muscular dystrophy
myotubular myopathy
Myriangiales
myriapod
Myriapoda

myringitis
    bullous m.
myringomycosis
myristate
    isopropyl m.
myristic acid
Myrmecia
myrmecia
myrosulfatase
Myrtophyllum hepatis
Mysoline
myxadenitis
myxadenoma
myxedema
    m. heart
    idiopathic m.
    infantile m.
    pituitary m.
    pretibial m.
myxedematoid
myxedematous coma
myxemia
myxochondrofibrosarcoma
myxochondroma
myxocystoma
myxocyte
myxoenchondroma
myxoendothelioma
myxofibroma
    odontogenic m.
myxofibrosarcoma
myxoglioma
myxoid
    m. chondrosarcoma
    m. cyst

m. degeneration
m. fibroma
m. liposarcoma
m. malignant fibrous histio-
    cytoma
myxolipoma
myxoliposarcoma
myxoma (pl., myxomas, myxomata)
    atrial m.
    cardiac m.
    cystic m.
    m. enchondromatosum
    enchondromatous m.
    erectile m.
    m. fibrosum
    infectious m.
    m. lipomatosum
    lipomatous m.
    odontogenic m.
    m. sarcomatosum
    vascular m.
myxomatosis
    cardiac valve m.
myxomatous degeneration
myxomyoma
myxopapillary ependymoma
myxopapilloma
myxopod
myxosarcoma
myxosarcomatous
Myxosporidia
myxovirus
Myzomyia
Myzorhynchus
MZ — monozygotic

N — newton
    nitrogen
    normal
    unit of neutron dosage
N. — *Neisseria*
    Nocardia
n — index of refraction
    neutron
    normal

NA — neutralizing antibody
    Nomina Anatomica
    noradrenalin
    numerical aperture
Na — sodium
NAA — neutron activation analysis
NAACLS — National Accrediting
    Agency for Clinical
    Laboratory Sciences

nabam
nabilone
nabothian
> n. cyst
> n. follicle

Naboth's glands
NaBr — sodium bromide
NAC — neoadjuvant chemotherapy
NAC-EDTA — N-acetyl-L-cysteine ethylenedi-aminetetra-acetic acid
NaCl — sodium chloride
NaClO — sodium hypochlorite
$NaClO_3$ — sodium chlorate
Na_2CO_3 — sodium carbonate
$Na_2C_2O_4$ — sodium oxalate
nacreous ichthyosis
NAD — nicotinamide adenine dinucleotide
> normal axis deviation

NADH — nicotinamide-adenine dinucleotide (reduced form)
NADH-cytochrome b5 reductase
NADH-dependent methemoglobin reductase
Nadi reaction
nadolol
NADP — nicotinamide adenine dinucleotide phosphate
NADPH — nicotinamide adenine dinucleotide phosphate (reduced form)
Naegeli's
> chromatophore nevus
> leukemia
> microblast

Naegeli-type monocytic leukemia
Naegleria fowleri
naepaine
nafcillin
nafoxidine hydrochloride
Naganol
Nägele's pelvis
Nageotte's cells
Nager's acrofacial dysostosis
Nagler's reaction
NaI — sodium iodide
nail
> n. horn
> n.-patella syndrome

> shell n.
> yellow n.

Naja
Nakanishi's stain
nalbuphine hydrochloride
NALC — N-acetyl-L-cysteine
nalidixic acid
nalorphine hydrochloride
naloxone hydrochloride
NAME — nevi, atrial myxoma, myxoid neurofibroma, and ephelides
NAME syndrome
NANA — N-acetylneuraminic acid
nandrolone
nanism
Nannizzia
> *N. cajetani*
> *N. grubia*
> *N. gypsea*
> *N. incurvata*
> *N. obtusa*

nanocurie
nanofarad
nanogram
nanoliter
nanomelia
nanometer
nanomole
nanosecond
N antigen
NAPA — N-acetyl-p-aminophenol
nape nevus
naphazoline hydrochloride
naphtha
naphthalene
naphthamine
> olfactory n.

naphthol
> n. ASD chloroacetate esterase
> n. poisoning
> n. yellow S

α-naphthol
β-naphthol
naphthyl
> α-N-acetate esterase
> α-N-butyrate esterase

naphthylamidase
β-naphthylamine
naphthylpararosaniline
N-1-naphthyl phthalmic acid
N-1-naphthyl sodium salt

1(1-naphthyl)-2-thiourea
Napier formol-gel test
napierian logarithm
naproxen
narceine
narcolepsy
narcosis
    carbon dioxide n.
    nitrogen n.
narcotic
    n. antagonist
    n. blockade
naris (pl., nares)
NAS — National Academy of
    Sciences
nasal
    n. airway
    n. antrum
    n. cavity
    n. choana
    n. fossa
    n. glands
    n. glioma
    n. lymphoepithelioma
    n. meatus
    n. mucus
    n. myiasis
    n. plasmacytoma
    n. polyp
    n. turbinate
    n. vestibule
nascent
nasion
nasociliary
    n. nerve
    n. neuralgia
nasogastric tube
nasolabial
    n. flap
    n. fold
    n. tube
nasolacrimal
naso-oral leishmaniasis
nasopalatine duct cyst
nasopharyngeal
    n. angiofibroma
    n. carcinoma
    n. cavity
    n. culture
    n. fibroma
    n. gland
    n. leishmaniasis

    n. lymphoepithelioma
    n. mucus
    n. pituitary gland
    n. submucosa
    n. swab
nasopharyngitis
nasopharyngography
nasopharynx
nasoscope
nasosinusitis
nasotracheal
National Academy of Sciences
National Accrediting Agency for Clinical Laboratory Sciences
National Association of Medical Examiners
National Cancer Institute
National Certification Agency for Medical Laboratory Personnel
National Cholesterol Education Program
National Committee for Clinical Laboratory Standards
National Council of Health Laboratory Services
National Diabetes Data Group
National Formulary
National Institute of Allergy and Infectious Diseases
National Institutes of Health
National Registry in Clinical Chemistry
National Registry of Microbiologists
National Society for Histotechnology
native albumin
natremia
natrium
natriuresis
natriuretic factor
natural
    n. death
    n. dyes
    n. killer cells
    n. killer lymphocyte
    n. selection
nausea
Nauta's stain
navicular
    n. arthritis
    n. cells
NB — newborn
    nitrous oxide–barbiturate

Nb — niobium
NBS — normal blood serum
NBT — nitroblue tetrazolium
NBTE — nonbacterial thrombotic
      endocarditis
NBT test
NBW — normal birth weight
nc — nanocurie
NCA — neurocirculatory asthenia
NCAMLP — National Certification
      Agency for Medical
      Laboratory Personnel
NCF — neutrophil chemotactic
      factor
NCHLS — National Council of
      Health Laboratory
      Services
NCI — National Cancer Institute
nCi — nanocurie
NCV — nerve conduction velocity
ND — neonatal death
    Newcastle disease
    nondisabling
Nd — neodymium
n_D — refractive index
NDA — no data available
    no demonstrable antibodies
NDGA — nordihydroguaiaretic acid
NDI — nephrogenic diabetes
      insipidus
NDMA — nitrosodimethylamine
NDP — net dietary protein
NDV — Newcastle disease virus
NE — nerve ending
    neurologic examination
    nonelastic
    norepinephrine
Ne — neon
nearsightedness
nebulizer
    ultrasonic n.
nebulous urine
Necator americanus
necatoriasis
neck
    buffalo n.
    bull n.
    n. ligament
    Madelung's n.
    n. reflexes
    webbed n.
    wry n.

Necrobacterium necrophorum
necrobiosis lipoidica diabeticorum
necrobiotic
    n. ray
    n. xanthogranuloma
necrocytosis
necrocytotoxin
necrogenic wart
necrogenous
necrogranulomatous
necrolysis
    toxic epidermal n.
necrolytic migratory erythema
necropathy
necrophagocytosis
necrophilic
necropsy; necroscopy
necrose
necrosis (pl., necroses)
    acute inflammatory n.
    acute tubular n.
    aseptic n.
    avascular n.
    Balser's fatty n.
    brain n.
    bridging n.
    bridging hepatic n.
    caseation n.
    caseous n.
    cellular n.
    central n.
    central hemorrhagic n.
    centrilobular n.
    cerebral laminar n.
    coagulation n.
    coagulative n.
    colliquative n.
    contraction band n.
    cortical n.
    cystic medial n.
    cytodegenerative n.
    cytotoxic n.
    diffuse n.
    "drop-out" n.
    epiphyseal aseptic n.
    fat n.
    fibrinoid n.
    focal n.
    gangrenous n.
    hemorrhagic n.
    hepatic n.
    hyaline n.

inflammatory n.
ischemic n.
lamellar n.
laminar n.
liquefactive n.
massive hepatic n.
medial n.
medial cystic n.
medullary n.
midzonal n.
mummification n.
myocardial n.
nephrotoxic acute tubular n.
pancreatic n.
papillary n.
peripheral n.
periportal n.
piecemeal n.
postpartum pituitary n.
progressive emphysematous n.
radiation n.
radium n.
renal cortical n.
renal medullary n.
renal papillary n.
sclerosing hyaline n.
scrotal fat n.
septic n.
simple n.
subcutaneous fat n. of newborn
suppurative n.
total n.
toxic acute tubular n.
tubular n.
tumor n.
Zenker's n.
zonal n.
necrospermia
necrosteosis
necrotic
    n. cirrhosis
    n. cyst
    n. inflammation
necrotizing
    n. angiitis
    n. arteriolitis
    n. bronchopneumonia
    n. cellulitis
    n. encephalomyelopathy
    n. enteritis
    n. enterocolitis
    n. factor

n. fasciitis
n. glomerulitis
n. glomerulonephritis
n. granulomatous inflammation
n. granulomatous sinusitis
n. hemorrhagic leukoencepha-
    litis
n. herpetic tracheobronchitis
n. inflammation
n. leukoencephalopathy
n. lobar pneumonia
n. pancreatitis
n. papillitis
n. pneumonia
n. sialometaplasia
n. ulcerative gingivitis
n. ulcerative gingivostomatitis
n. vasculitis
NED — no evidence of disease
needle
    Abrams's n.
    aneurysm n.
    aspirating n.
    n. aspiration cytology
    n. biopsy
    Chiba n.
    Cope's n.
    n. culture
    Hagedorn's n.
    hypodermic n.
    ligature n.
    Menghini's n.
    Reverdin's n.
    Seldinger's n.
    Silverman's n.
    spinal n.
    Vim-Silverman n.
NEFA — nonesterified fatty acid
neg. — negative
negative
    n. afterimage
    n. assortative mating
    n. base excess
    n. catalyst
    n. control enzyme induction
    n. control repression
    n. cytotaxis
    n. eyepiece
    false-n.
    gram-n.
    n. interference
    n. neutrotaxis

n. pressure
n. pressure lavage
Rh n.
Rhesus factor n.
n. stain
n. variation
negatron beta decay
Negri bodies
Neisseria
    N. catarrhalis
    N. caviae
    N. cinerea
    N. flava
    N. flavescens
    N. gonorrhoeae
    N. intracellularis
    N. lactamica
    N. meningitidis
    N. mucosa
    N. ovis
    N. perflava
    N. pharyngis
    N. sicca
    N. subflava
neisseria
    anaerobic n.
Neisseriaceae
Neisser's
    diplococcus
    reaction
    stain
Neivamyia
Nelson's tumor
NEM — *N*-ethylmaleimide
nema
nemaline myopathy
nemathelminth
Nemathelminthes
nematocide
Nematoda
nematode
    intestinal n's
    n. worm infestation
nematodiasis
Nematodirus
Nematomorpha
nematosis
neoadjuvant
    n. chemotherapy
    n. therapy
neoantigen
neocerebellum

neocinchophen
neocyte
neocytosis
neodymium
neoformation
neogenesis
neomembrane
neomycin
neon
neonatal
    n. anemia
    n. bilirubin
    n. cholestasis
    n. death
    n. hemolysis
    n. hepatitis
    n. hypoglycemia
    n. isoerythrolysis
    n. leukemia
    n. lupus
    n. mortality rate
    n. necrotizing enterocolitis
    n. screening
    n. thrombocytopenia
    n. torsion
    n. transfusion
neonate
neonatorum
    atelectasis n.
    blennorrhea n.
    conjunctivitis n.
    ophthalmia n.
    pemphigus n.
neopathy
neoplasia
    cervical intraepithelial n.
    esophageal intraepithelial n.
    gestational trophoblastic n.
    lobular n.
    mesenchymal n.
    multiple endocrine n., type I
    multiple endocrine n., type II
    multiple endocrine n.,
      type IIA
    multiple endocrine n., type IIB
    multiple endocrine n., type III
    neuroendocrine n.
    trophoblastic n.
neoplasm
    adnexal n's
    adrenal n.
    B-cell n.

benign n.
epithelial n.
glandular n.
histoid n.
lymphoid n.
malignant n.
metastatic n.
ovarian granulosa cell n.
renal n.
sclerosing epithelial n.
transitional cell n.
urachal n.
neoplastic
    n. acinus
    n. fibrosis
    n. hyperplasia
    n. papillae
neoprecipitin test
neopterin
neostigmine
    n. bromide
    n. methylsulfate
Neotestudina
Neotran
neotype
neovascularization
nephelometer
nephelometric
    n. immunoassay
    n. immunoprecipitin technique
    n. inhibition assay
nephelometry
nephradenoma
nephrectasis; nephrectasia
nephrectomy
nephredema
nephrelcosis
nephritic
    n. calculus
    n. factor
    n. syndrome
nephritis (pl., nephritides)
    acute n.
    acute interstitial n.
    analgesic n.
    antiglomerular basement membrane n.
    anti-kidney serum n.
    bacterial n.
    chronic n.
    chronic interstitial n.
    circulating immune complex n.

drug-induced n.
Ellis types 1 and 2 n.
focal n.
glomerular n.
n. gravidarum
hemorrhagic n.
hereditary interstitial n.
Heymann's n.
immune complex n.
interstitial n.
lupus n.
Masugi's n.
Masugi-type nephrotoxic
    serum n.
mesangial n.
nephrotoxic n.
nonstreptococcal glomerular n.
radiation n.
scarlatinal n.
serum n.
subacute n.
suppurative n.
syphilitic n.
transfusion n.
tuberculous n.
tubular n.
tubular interstitial n.
tubulointerstitial n.
uranium n.
vascular n.
nephroblastoma
    rhabdomyosarcomatous n.
nephroblastomatosis
nephroblastosis
nephrocalcinosis
nephrocapsectomy
nephrocystanastomosis
nephrogenesis
nephrogenic
    n. adenoma
    n. blastema
    n. diabetes insipidus
    n. metaplasia
    n. zone
nephrogenous
nephrogram
nephrography
nephrohydrosis
nephrolith
nephrolithiasis
nephrology

nephroma
    congenital mesoblastic n.
    cystic n.
    embryonal n.
    malignant mesenchymal n.
    mesoblastic n.
nephromalacia
nephromegaly
    congenital m.
nephron
    cortical n.
    juxtamedullary n.
nephronophthisis–uremic medullary
    cystic disease complex
nephropathy
    acute uric acid n.
    analgesic n.
    Balkan n.
    Danubian endemic familial n.
    diabetic n.
    gouty n.
    hemoglobinuric n.
    hypokalemic n.
    immune complex n.
    immunoglobulin A n.
    immunoglobulin M n.
    interstitial n.
    light-chain n.
    membranous n.
    myoglobinuric n.
    reflux n.
    sickle cell n.
    tubulointerstitial n.
    urate n.
    uric acid n.
nephrophthisis
    juvenile n.
nephropoietin
nephroptosis; nephroptosia
nephropyelitis
nephropyelography
nephropyosis
nephrorrhagia
nephrosclerosis
    arterial n.
    arteriolar n.
    benign n.
    hyaline n.
    hyperplastic n.
    intercapillary n.
    malignant n.
    senile n.

nephrosclerotic
nephrosis (pl., nephroses)
    acute n.
    amyloid n.
    bile n.
    cholemic n.
    familial n.
    glomerular lipoid n.
    hemoglobinuric n.
    hypokalemic n.
    hypoxic n.
    lipid n.
    lipoid n.
    lower nephron n.
    myeloma n.
    myoglobinuric n.
    osmotic n.
    toxic n.
    tubular n.
    vacuolar n.
nephrospasia; nephrospasis
nephrostomy
nephrotic syndrome
nephrotome
nephrotomography
nephrotoxic
    n. acute tubular necrosis
    n. antibody
    n. nephritis
    n. serum nephritis, Masugi
       type
nephrotoxicity
nephrotoxin
nephrotuberculosis
nephroureterectomy
nephrourography
neptunium
Nernst equation
nerve
    Arnold's n.
    n. block
    cochlear n.
    n. conduction velocity
    n. cord
    n. fiber
    n. growth factor
    Hering's n.
    Jacobson's n.
    jugular glossopharyngeal n.
    jugular tenth cranial n.
    jugular vagus n.
    lacrimal n.

lingual n.
lumbar n.
median n.
oculomotor n.
ophthalmic n.
optic n.
n. papilla
petrosal n.
radial n.
n. sheath tumor
splanchnic n.
ulnar n.
vagus n.
Wrisberg's n.
zygomatic n.
nervonate
nervonic acid
nervosa
anorexia n.
nervous system
aminergic n.s.
autonomic n.s.
central n.s.
parasympathetic n.s.
peptidergic n.s.
peripheral n.s.
sympathetic n.s.
nervus (pl., nervi)
nesidioblast
nesidioblastoma
nesidioblastosis
nesslerization
nesslerize
Nessler's reagent
nest
Brunn's n's
Brunn's epithelial n's
cell n's
epithelial n.
solid cell n's
net
achromatic n.
Chiari's n.
chromidial n.
n. dietary protein
n. protein ratio
n. protein utilization
netilmicin sulfate
network
Chiari's n.
chromatin n.
n. theory

Neubauer ruling
neural
n. breast
n. cell
n. crest
n. tube
n. tube defect
neuralgia
cardiac n.
cervicobrachial n.
cervico-occipital n.
cranial n.
geniculate n.
glossopharyngeal n.
idiopathic n.
intercostal n.
mammary n.
mandibular joint n.
migrainous n.
Morton's n.
nasociliary n.
peripheral n.
postherpetic n.
sphenopalatine n.
stump n.
supraorbital n.
trifacial n.
trigeminal n.
vidian n.
visceral n.
neuralgic amyotrophy
neuraminic acid
neuraminidase
neurapraxia
neurasthenia
neuraxis
neurectoderm
neurilemma
neurilemmitis
neurilemoma; neurilemmoma
acoustic n.
ameloblastic n.
malignant n.
neurilemosarcoma
neurinoma
acoustic n.
neuritic
n. atrophy
n. plaque
neuritis
allergic n.
branchial n.

experimental allergic n.
optic n.
paralytic brachial n.
neuroacanthocytosis
neuroamine-neuropeptide
neuroanatomic
neuroarthropathy
neuroastrocytoma
neuroblast
   sympathetic n.
neuroblastic nodule
neuroblastoma
   adrenal n.
   cerebral n.
   Hutchison-type n.
   n. in situ
   mediastinal n.
   olfactory n.
   paratesticular n.
neurochitin
neurochoroiditis
neurocirculatory asthenia
neurocristopathy
neurocutaneous
   n. melanosis
   n. phacomatosis
   n. phacomatosis syndrome
neurocysticercosis
neurocytoma
neurodegenerative disease
neurodermatitis
neuroectodermal tumor
neuroencephalomyelopathy
neuroendocrine
   n. carcinoma
   n. cells
   n. cell tumor
   n. dysplasia
   n. neoplasia
   n. tumor
neuroendocrinology
neuroepithelial
neuroepithelioma
neuroepithelium
   undifferentiated n.
neurofibril
neurofibrillary tangles
neurofibroma
   plexiform n.
   storiform n.
neurofibromatosis
   abortive n.

incomplete n.
multiple n.
von Recklinghausen's n.
neurofibrosarcoma
neurofilament
   cellular n's
   protein n.
neurogenic
   n. arthropathy
   n. bladder
   n. diabetes insipidus
   n. dysplasia
   n. muscular atrophy
   n. sarcoma
   n. shock
neuroglia
neurogliocyte
neurogliocytoma
neuroglioma ganglionare
neurogliosis
neurohypophyseal hormone
neurohypophysis
neuroid nevus
neuroimmunology
neurokeratin
neurolemmoma
neuroleptanalgesia
neuroleptanesthesia
neuroleptic malignant syndrome
neuroleukin
neurologic; neurological
neurologic cretinism
neurology
neuroma
   acoustic n.
   amputation n.
   n. cutis
   false n.
   medullated n.
   Morton's n.
   mucosal n.
   plexiform n.
   traumatic n.
neuromalacia
neuromere
neuromodulator
neuromuscular
neuromyelitis optica
neuromyopathy
   carcinomatous n.
neuromyositis
neuromyotonia

neuron
    afferent n.
    alpha motor n.
    bipolar n.
    central n.
    efferent n.
    fusimotor n's
    Golgi's n.
    intercalary n.
    motor n.
    multiform n.
    multimodal n.
    multipolar n.
    multisensory n.
    piriform n's
    polymorphic n.
    postganglionic n.
    preganglionic n.
    primary sensory n.
    Purkinje's n's
    pyramidal n.
    red n's
    secondary sensory n.
    sensory n.
    n.-specific enolase
    spiny n.
    unipolar n.
neuronal
neuronevus
neuronophagia
neuro-oncology
neuro-ophthalmic
neuro-ophthalmology
neuroparalysis
neuropathic
    n. albuminuria
    n. arthritis
neuropathology
neuropathy
    amblyopia n.
    amyloid n.
    arsenical n.
    arsenic n.
    autonomic n.
    demyelinating n.
    diabetic n.
    entrapment n.
    hereditary sensory motor n.
    hypertrophic interstitial n.
    lead n.
    optic n.
    paraneoplastic n.

    periaxial n.
    peripheral n.
    retrobulbar n.
    sensorimotor n.
    subacute myelo-optical n.
    toxic n.
    vincristine n.
neuropeptide Y
neurophysin
neurophysiologic; neurophysiological
neurophysiology
neuropil
neuroplasm
neuropsychiatric
neuroradiologic; neuroradiological
neuroretinitis
neuroretinopathy
neurosarcoma
neurosclerosis
neurosecretion
neurosecretory
    n. cell
    n. granules
    n. material
neurosis
    anxiety n.
    compensation n.
    obsessive-compulsive n.
    phobic n.
neuroskeletal
Neurospora sitophila
neurosurgery
neurosurgical
neurosyphilis
    meningitic n.
    meningovascular n.
    parenchymatous n.
    paretic n.
neurotendinous organ
neurotensin
neurothekeoma
neurotoxicity
neurotoxin
    enzyme-derived n.
    eosinophilic n.
neurotransducer
neurotransmission
neurotransmitter
neurotrophic atrophy
neurotubule
neurovascular
Neusser's granules

neutral
  n. buffered formalin fixative
  n. lipid storage disease
  n. protamine Hagedorn (insulin)
  n. red indicator
  n. stain
neutralism
neutralization test
neutralizing antibody
neutrino
neutron
  n. activation analysis
  n. beam therapy
  epithermal n.
  intermediate n.
  slow n.
  thermal n.
neutropenia
  autoimmune n.
  cyclic n.
  immune n.
  neonatal n.
  periodic n.
  splenic n.
neutropenic angina
neutrophil; neutrophile
  n. alkaline phosphatase
  n. antibody test
  band n.
  n. chemotactic factor
  filamented n.
  giant n.
  n. granule
  hypersegmented n.
  immature n.
  juvenile n.
  mature n.
  polymorphonuclear n.
  rod n.
  segmented n.
  stab n.
neutrophilia
  giant n.
neutrophilic
  n. granulocyte
  n. hyperplasia
  n. infiltrate
  n. leukemia
  n. leukemoid reaction
  n. leukocyte
  n. leukocytosis

  n. leukopenia
  n. lymphocytosis
  n. marrow
  n. metamyelocyte
  n. myelocyte
  n. promyelocyte
neutrophilopenia
neutrophilous
neutrotaxis
  indifferent n.
  negative n.
nevocarcinoma
nevocellular nevus
nevocyte
nevocytic nevus
nevoid
  n. elephantiasis
  n. hypertrichosis
  n. lentigo
nevolipoma
nevose; nevous
nevoxanthoendothelioma
  scrotal n.
nevus (pl., nevi)
  achromic n.
  acquired n.
  amelanotic n.
  n. anemicus
  n. angiomatodes
  n. arachnoideus
  araneus n.
  balloon cell n.
  basal cell n.
  bathing trunk n.
  Becker's n.
  blue n.
  blue rubber-bleb n.
  capillary n.
  n. cavernosus
  n. cell
  cellular blue n.
  n. comedonicus; comedo n.
  compound n.
  congenital n.
  connective tissue n.
  dermal n.
  dermal-epidermal n.
  dysplastic n.
  n. elasticus of Lewandowsky
  epidermal n.
  epidermic-dermic n.
  epithelioid n.

epithelioid cell n.
faun tail n.
flame n.; n. flammeus
n. follicularis keratosis
giant blue n.
giant pigmented n.
hair follicle n.
halo n.
intradermal n.
intraepidermal n.
Ito's n.
Jadassohn's sebaceous n.
Jadassohn-Tièche n.
junctional n.
junction n.
n. lipomatodes; n. lipomatosus
lymphatic n.
n. lymphaticus
melanocytic n.
nape n.
neuroid n.
nevocellular n.
nevocytic n.
organoid n.
Ota's n.
pigmented n.
pigmented hair epidermal n.
n. pigmentosus
n. pilosus
sebaceous n.; n. sebaceus
spider n.
spindle cell n.
Spitz n.
spongy n.
strawberry n.
Sutton's n.
n. syringocystadenomatosus
    papilliferus
systematized n.
n. unius lateris
Unna's n.
vascular n.
n. venosus
verrucous n.
newborn
    n. crossmatch
    hemolytic disease of n.
    n. hemorrhagic disease
    icterus gravis of n.
    n. respiratory distress syndrome
    n. screen
Newcastle virus disease

Newcastle-Manchester bacillus
Newcomer's fixative
New International Staging System
newton
Newton's law of cooling
New World hookworm
New Zealand mice
nexus (pl., nexus, nexuses)
Nezelof's T-cell deficiency
Nezelof-type thymic alymphoplasia
NF — National Formulary
nF — nanofarad
NFTD — normal full-term delivery
NG — nasogastric
ng — nanogram
NGF — nerve growth factor
NGU — nongonococcal urethritis
NHA — nonspecific hepatocellular
    abnormality
NHANS — National Health and
    Nutrition Survey
NHC — nonhistone chromosomal
    (protein)
NHL — non-Hodgkin's lymphoma
NHS — normal horse serum
    normal human serum
Ni — nickel
NIA — nephelometric inhibition
    assay
niacinamide
niacin test
NIAID — National Institute of
    Allergy and Infectious
    Diseases
nialamide
niche
    ecologic n.
Nichols
    method
    reagent
nickel
    n. carbonyl
    Raney n.
Nickerson-Kveim test reaction
Nicklès' test
Nicollella
Nicolle's stain for capsules
Nicol prism
Nicotiana
nicotinamide
    n. adenine dinucleotide

n. adenine nucleotide
n. methyltransferase
n. mononucleotide adenylyltransferase
n. mononucleotide pyrophosphorylase
n. phosphoribosyltransferase
nicotinate
n. 6-hydroxylase
n. phosphoribosyltransferase
n. ribonucleotide
nicotine
nicotinic
n. acid
n. receptor
nidal
NIDDM — non–insulin-dependent
diabetes mellitus
nidus (pl., nidi)
Niemann-Pick
cell
disease
Niemann-Pick-type histiocyte
nifedipine
nifuroxime
niger seed agar
nightsweats
nigra
nigrities linguae
nigrosin; nigrosine
Nigrospora
nigrostriate fibers
NIH — National Institutes of Health
NIG 3T3 cells
nikethamide
Nikiforoff's method
Nikolsky's sign
nil disease
Nile blue
N.b. A
N.b. fat stain
N.b. sulfate
Nimeh's method
Ninhydrin
N.-Schiff reaction
N.-Schiff stain
ninth cranial nerve
niobium
nipple
n. discharge cytology
inversion of n.
supernumerary n.

Nippostrongylus
niridazole
Nissl
bodies
substance alteration
Nissl's stain
Nitabuch's layer
nitrate
n. agar
n. ester reductase
isoamyl n.
n. media
n. reduction test
uranium n.
n. utilization test
nitric
n. acid
n. oxide
n. oxide hemoglobin
nitrifying bacterium
nitrile
nitrilotriacetic acid
nitrite
butyl n.
nitritoid reaction
nitrituria
nitroaniline poisoning
Nitrobacter
Nitrobacteraceae
p-nitrobenzene diazonium
p-toluene
nitrobenzyl thioinosine
nitroblue tetrazolium
nitrochlorobenzene
Nitrocystis
nitro dye
nitroethane
nitrofurans
nitrofurantoin
nitrofurazone
nitrofurfuryl methylether
nitrogen
alkali-soluble n.
alpha-amino acid n.
amide n.
n. balance
blood urea n.
n. dilution
n. distribution
n. dioxide
n. equivalent
n. fixation

n. isotope
n. lag
n. mustard
n. narcosis
nonprotein n.
n. partition
n. pentoxide
n. phosphorus
n. pressure
serum urea n.
n. tetroxide
n. trioxide
undetermined n.
urea n.
urinary n.
nitroglycerin
nitromersol
nitromethane
O-nitrophenol-β-galactoside
p-nitrophenylic acid
4-nitrophenyl-phosphate
2-nitropropane
nitroprusside
sodium n.
n. test
nitrosamine
N-nitrosodimethylamine
N-nitrosodiphenylamine
nitroso dye
nitrosonaphthol test
nitrosulfathiazole
nitrosourea
nitrosyl chloride
nitrous
n. acid
n. oxide
nits
NIXIE tube
Nizoral
NK — natural killer
NK (natural killer) cells
NKH — nonketotic hyperos-
mosis
Nl — normal
nl; nL — nanoliter
NLA — neuroleptanalgesia
NLP — no light perception
NLT — normal lymphocyte transfer
(test)
NM — neuromuscular
not measurable
nuclear medicine

nm — nanometer
NMA — neurogenic muscular atrophy
nmol — nanomole
NMP — normal menstrual period
NMR — nuclear magnetic resonance
N : N — (indicates presence of) the
azo group
NND — neonatal death
New and Nonofficial Drugs
NNN — Novy, MacNeal, and Ni-
colle's (medium)
NO — nitric oxide
N_2O — dinitrogen monoxide (nitrous
oxide)
No — nobelium
no demonstrable antibodies
no evidence of distant metastases
no evidence of primary tumor
no reflow phenomenon
no significant abnormality
no significant difference
nobelium
Noble's stain
Nocardia
N. asteroides
N. brasiliensis
N. caviae
N. coeliaca
N. farcinica
N. lutea
N. madurae
N. minutissima
N. otitidis-caviarum
N. pelletieri
N. tenuis
Nocardiaceae
nocardial
n. abscess
n. empyema
n. pleuritis
n. pneumonia
nocardioform
n. actinomycetes
nocardiosis
lung n.
Nocard's bacillus
nociception
nociceptive
nociceptor
C-fiber n.
cutaneous n's

mechanical n.
signal n.
Virchow's n.

nocturia

nocturnal
   n. dyspnea
   n. emission
   n. hemoglobinuria
   n. myoclonus

nodal cells

node
   Aschoff-Tawara n.
   atrioventricular n.
   Babès's n's
   Bouchard's n's
   Delphian n.
   Dürck's n's
   Haygarth's n.
   Heberden's n.
   Hensen's n.
   hepatic lymph n's
   hilar n.
   jugular lymph n.
   jugulodigastric n.
   lymph n.
   mesenteric n's
   Meynet's n's
   Osler's n's
   pelvic lymph n.
   potato n.
   pulmonary lymph n.
   Ranvier's n's
   retropharyngeal lymph n's
   Rotter's n.
   Rouvière's n.
   SA (sinoatrial) n.
   sentinel n.
   signal n.
   singer's n.
   sinoatrial n.
   Troisier's n.
   Virchow's n.

nodosa
   epididymitis n.
   periarteritis n.
   trichorrhexis n.

nodose
   n. ganglion
   n. rheumatism

nodositas

nodosity

nodular
   n. adrenal cortex
   n. adrenal hyperplasia
   n. adrenocortical hyperplasia
   n. calcific aortic stenosis
   n. calcific stenosis
   n. colloid goiter
   n. dysplasia
   n. embryo
   n. fasciitis
   n. fibromyositis
   n. fibrosis
   n. glomerulosclerosis
   n. goiter
   n. hidradenoma
   n. hyperplastic goiter
   n. lymphoid hyperplasia
   n. lymphoma
   n. mesothelioma
   n. nonsuppurative panniculitis
   n. periorchitis
   n. renal blastema
   n. sclerosis
   n. sclerosis Hodgkin's disease
   n. sclerotic disease
   n. tenosynovitis
   n. vasculitis

nodulate; nodulated

nodulation

nodule
   adenomatoid n.
   adenomatous n.
   appendiceal lymphoid n.
   apple jelly n's
   Aschoff's n.
   Babès's n.
   Bohn's n.
   Brenner n's
   Caplan's n's
   cold n.
   colonic solitary lymphoid n.
   Dalen-Fuchs n's
   fibrocalcific n.
   fibrosiderotic n.
   fibrous n.
   follicular n.
   Gandy-Gamna n's
   glial n's
   hemorrhagic n.
   Hoboken's n's
   hot n.
   Hürthle cell n.

Jeanselme's n's
juxta-articular n.
laryngeal n.
Leydig cell n.
Lisch n's
lymph n.
lymphoid n.
microglial n.
milker's n's
Morgagni's n's
neuroblastic n.
papillary hyperplastic n.
pigmented n.
rectal solitary n.
rheumatic n.
rheumatoid n.
Schmorl's n.
Sertoli cell n.
siderofibrotic n's
siderotic n's
Sister Joseph's n.
solitary n.
spindle cell n.
stromal n's
subcutaneous n.
thyroid n.
nodulous; nodose
nodulus (pl., noduli)
Noguchia granulosis
noma
Nomarski microscope
nomenclature
binomial n.
chromosome n.
Nomina Anatomica
nominal
n. variable
n. wave length
nomogram
acid-base n.
blood volume n.
cartesian n.
Radford n.
Siggaard-Andersen n.
Siggaard-Andersen alignment n.
nomograph
nonadapting receptor
nonaesthenic
nonagglutinating vibrio
non-A hepatitis
nonalcoholic tropical pancreatitis

nonbacterial
n. gastroenteritis virus
n. thrombotic endocarditis
n. verrucous endocarditis
non-B hepatitis
non-Burkitt lymphoma
nonchromaffin paraganglioma
noncleaved cell
noncommunicating hydrocephalus
noncoronary cusp
nondiabetic glycosuric melituria
nondisabling
nondisjunction
chromosomal n.
nondrying oil
nonelectrolyte
nonencapsulated
n. nerve ending
nonendemic goiter
nonenzymatic glycosylation
nonerythroid cells
nonesterified fatty acid
nonfilament polymorphonuclear leukocyte
nonfunctional
n. adenoma
n. tumor
nonfunctioning tumor
nonglucose melituria
nongonococcal urethritis
nongranular leukocyte
nongranulomatous uveitis
nonhemolytic
n. jaundice
n. streptococci
n. transfusion
nonhistone chromosomal protein
non-Hodgkin's lymphoma
nonimmune
n. fetal hydrops
n. hemolysis
noninfectious vasculitis
noninfiltrating lobular carcinoma
noninflammatory edema
non—insulin-dependent diabetes mellitus
noninvasive
non-ionizing radiation
nonisolated proteinuria
nonkeratinizing carcinoma
nonketotic
n. hyperglycemia

n. hyperglycinemia
n. hyperosmolar coma
n. hyperosmosis
nonleukemic
    n. lymphoblast
    n. myelosis
nonlipid histiocytosis
nonlymphocytic
nonmalignant
nonmotile
    n. leukocyte
    n. organism
nonmyelinated
non-necrotizing
    n.-n. granuloma
    n.-n. granulomatous inflammation
non-neoplastic; nonneoplastic
nonnucleated erythrocyte
nonobstructive jaundice
nonossifying fibroma
nonoxynol-9
nonpalpable
nonparametric
nonpathogenic amebae
nonpermissive culture media
nonphotochromogenic mycobacteria
nonpituitary
nonprotein
    n. nitrogen
    n. nitrogen test
nonradioisotopic immunoassay
nonreactive
nonreaginic asthma
nonrenal
    n. azotemia
    n. death
nonrespiratory alkalosis
nonretractable prepuce
nonrotation
    n. of intestine
    n. of kidney
nonsecreting adenoma
nonsecretor
nonsecretory
    n. adenoma
    n. myeloma
nonseminomatous germ cell tumor
nonsense mutation
nonseptate
nonshivering thermogenesis
nonsister chromatid

non–small cell carcinoma
non–small cell lung carcinoma
nonspecific
    n. acute splenitis
    n. chronic inflammation
    n. epididymitis
    n. hepatocellular abnormality
    n. orchitis
    n. thyroiditis
    n. urethritis
nonspherocytic hemolytic anemia
nonsteroidal anti-inflammatory drugs
nonstreptococcal glomerular nephritis
nonstructural genes
nonsuppressible insulin-like activity
nonsuppurative thyroiditis
nonsymptomatic
nonthrombocytopenic purpura
nontoxic nodular goiter
nontransmural myocardial infarction
nontreponemal spirochete
nontropical
    n. idiopathic splenomegaly
    n. sprue
nontuberculous
nonunion fracture
nonvascular
nonviable
nonviral
nonvisceral
noradrenalin
noradrenergic
norbormide
norbornane
norcodeine
nordefrin hydrochloride
norepinephrine
norethandrolone
norethindrone
norethynodrel
norfloxacin
normal
    n. antithrombin
    n. blood serum
    n. body temperature
    n. cholesteremic xanthomatosis
    n. distribution
    n. flora
    n. horse serum
    n. human plasma
    n. human serum

n. human serum albumin
n. lymphocyte transfer test
n. plasma
n. probability
n. rabbit serum
n. reference serum
n. single dose
n. sinus rhythm
upper limits of n.
n. values
normetanephrine
normoblast
    acidophilic n.
    basophilic n.
    eosinophilic n.
    intermediate n.
    orthochromatic n.
    orthochromatophilic n.
    oxyphilic n.
    polychromatic n.
    polychromatophilic n.
normoblastic
normoblastosis
normocalcemia
normocalcemic
normocapnia
normocapnic
normocholesterolemia
normocholesterolemic
normochromasia
normochromia
normochromic
    n. anemia
    n. erythrocyte
normocrinic
normocyte
normocytic
    n. anemia
    n. erythrocyte
normocytosis
normoerythrocyte
normoglycemia
normoglycemic glycosuria
normokalemia
normolipemic xanthoma planum
normolipidemic
normo-orthocytosis
normoplasia
normorphine
normoskeocytosis
normothermia
normovolemia

nornicotine
norpropoxyphene
Norris's corpuscles
North American
    blastomycosis
    coral snake antivenin
North Asian tick typhus
Northern
    blot analysis
    blot technique
    blotting
Norton endotracheal tube
Norton-Simon hypothesis
nortriptyline
Norwalk
    agent
    virus
Norwegian scabies
NOS — not otherwise specified
noscapine
Nosema
nosocomial
    n. anemia
    n. bacteremia
    n. infection
    n. pneumonia
nosology
nosomycosis
Nosopsyllus fasciatus
notation
    scientific n.
notencephalocele
notencephalus
notochord
Notoedres
novobiocin
Novy, McNeal, and Nicolle's medium
noxious
NP — nasopharyngeal
    nasopharynx
    neuropathology
    neuropsychiatric
    nitrogen-phosphorus
    normal plasma
    nucleoplasmic index
    nucleoprotein
    nucleoside phosphorylase
Np — neptunium
NPB — nodal premature beat
NPC — nasopharyngeal carcinoma
    near point of convergence
NPD — Niemann-Pick disease

NP detector
NPDL — nodular, poorly differenti-
    ated lymphocytes
NPH — neutral protamine Hagedorn
    (insulin)
NPN — nonprotein nitrogen
N-point potentiometer
4-NPP — 4-nitrophenylphosphate
NPR — net protein ratio
NPT — neoprecipitin test
NPU — net protein utilization
NR — nonreactive
    no radiation
    no response
    normal
    not recorded
    not resolved
NRBC — nucleated red blood cell
NRC — National Research Council
    normal retinal correspon-
      dence
    Nuclear Regulatory Com-
      mission
NRCC — National Registry in Clini-
    cal Chemistry
NRD — nonrenal death
NREM — nonrapid eye movement
NREM sleep
NRM — National Registry of Microbi-
    ologists
NRS — normal rabbit serum
    normal reference serum
NS — nephrotic syndrome
    nervous system
    neurologic survey
    nonspecific
    nonsymptomatic
    normal saline
    not significant
    not sufficient
N/S — normal saline
ns, nsec — nanosecond
NSA — no serious abnormality
    no significant abnormality
NSAID — nonsteroidal anti-
    inflammatory drugs
NSC — no significant change
NSCLC — non–small cell lung car-
    cinoma
NSD — nominal single dose
    normal single dose
    normal spontaneous delivery

    no significant defect
    no significant deviation
    no significant difference
    no significant disease
NSE — neuron-specific enolase
NSGCT — nonseminomatous germ
    cell tumor
NSH — National Society for Histo-
    technology
NSILA — nonsuppressible insulin-
    like activity
NSM — neurosecretory material
NSND — nonsymptomatic, nondis-
    abling
NSQ — not sufficient quantity
NSR — normal sinus rhythm
NSS — normal saline solution
    not statistically significant
NSU — nonspecific urethritis
NT — nasotracheal
    neutralization test
    neutralizing
NTAB — nephrotoxic antibody
Ntaya virus
NTG — nontoxic goiter
NTN — nephrotoxic nephritis
NTP — normal temperature and
    pressure
nubecula
nuchal
    n. fascia
    n. hemangioma
    n. ligament
    n. region
    n. rigidity
Nuck's canal
nuclear
    n. aggregate
    n. aggregate lipid
    n. alteration
    n. antibodies
    n. antigens
    n. aplasia
    n. bag fiber
    n. chain fiber
    n. crystalline aggregate
    n. cytoplasmic asynchrony
    n. cytoplasmic ratio alteration
    n. dust
    n. enlargement
    n. envelope
    n. enzyme

n. groove
n. inclusion body
n. isomerism
n. layer
n. lipid aggregate
n. macromolecules
n. magnetic resonance
n. magnetic resonance spec-
    trometer
n. magneton
n. membrane alteration
n. pleomorphism
n. ploidy
n. pore alteration
n. reactor
n. resonance imaging
n. sap alteration
n. shape alteration
n. size alteration
n. stain
n. transplantation
n. vacuolization
Nuclear Regulatory Commission
nuclease
nucleated
    n. erythrocyte
    n. red blood cell
nucleation
    heterogeneous n.
nucleic
    n. acid
    n. acid probe
nucleinate
    histone n.
nucleochylema
nucleocytoplasmic
nucleography
nucleohistone
nucleoid
nucleolar
    n. alteration
    n.-associated chromatin
    n. organizer
    n. satellite
nucleolinus (pl., nucleolini)
nucleolonema
nucleolus (pl., nucleoli)
nucleon
nucleophagocytosis
nucleophile
nucleoplasmic index
nucleoprotein antigen

Nucleopore filter
nucleosidase
nucleoside
    n. analogue
    n. diphosphatase
    n. monophosphate kinase
    n. phosphorylase
    n. triphosphate
nucleosidediphosphate kinase
nucleosidemonophosphate kinase
nucleosis
nucleosome
nucleospindle
nucleotidase
5'-nucleotidase
nucleotide
    adenine n.
    n. cyclase
    cyclic n's
    diphosphopyridine n.
    Duval's n.
    nicotinamide adenine n.
    n. polymerase
    pyridine n.
    n. pyrophosphatase
nucleotidylexotransferase
    DNA n.
nucleotidyl transferase
    DNA n.
    RNA n.
nucleotoxin
Nuclepore filter
nucleus (pl., nuclei)
    accessory n.
    n. ambiguus
    n. amygdalae
    Balbiani's n.
    caudate n.
    cerebriform n.
    Clarke's n.
    cuneate n.
    Darkshevich's n.
    Deiters' n.
    dentate n.
    diploid n.
    Duval's n.
    Edinger-Westphal n.
    n. gracilis
    hypothalamic n.
    intralaminar n.
    Klein-Gumprecht shadow
        nuclei

lateral n.
lenticular n.
n. of Luys
motor n.
oculomotor n.
olivary n.
peduncular n.
pontine n.
preoptic n.
pseudoclear n.
n. pulposus
Roller's n.
sensory n.
shadow n.
stripped n.
n. thoracicus
trophic n.
ventromedial n.
vesicular n.
vestibular n.
wrinkled n.
nuclide
NUG — necrotizing ulcerative gingivitis
null
    n. cell adenoma
    n. lymphocyte
nullipara
number
    acid n.
    atomic n.
    Avogadro's n.
    color index n.
    complex n.
    CT n.
    diploid n.
    haploid n.
    iodine n.
    line n.
    mass n.
    neutron n.
    oxidation n.
    random n.

real n.
Reynold's n.
turnover n.
wave n.
numbering
    stereospecific n.
numbness
numerical
    n. aperture
    n. hypertrophy
nummiform
nummular
    n. eczema
    n. sputum
nummulation
nutmeg liver
nutrient
    n. agar
    n. broth
    n. medium
    mineral n's
nutrition
    parenteral n.
nutritional
    n. cirrhosis
    n. macrocytic anemia
    n. obesity
    n. therapy
nux vomica
NV — negative variation
NVD — Newcastle virus disease
NWTS — National Wilms' Tumor Study
nyad
nyctalopia
Nygmia
nylidrin hydrochloride
nylon wool adherence procedure
nymphitis
nympholabial
nymphoncus
Nyssorhynchus
nystagmus
nystatin

O — oxygen
O — nonmotile organism
OA — occipital artery
    osteoarthritis
    oxalic acid
OAAD — ovarian ascorbic acid
    depletion
OAD — obstructive airway disease
OAF — osteoclast-activating factor
OAG — oleylacylglycerol
O agglutination
O agglutinin
O antigen
O antistreptolysin
OAP — osteoarthropathy
oasthouse
    o. syndrome
    o. urine disease
oat cell
    o.c. breast cancer
    o.c. carcinoma
OAV — oculoauriculovertebral (dys-
    plasia)
O & B — opium and belladonna
Obermayer's test
Obermeier's spirillum
Obermüller's test
obesity
    nutritional o.
obex
object
    o. code
    o. program
objective
    achromatic o.
    aplanatic o.
    apochromatic o.
    flat-field o.
    fluorite o.
    immersion o.
    semiapochromatic o.
obl. — oblique
obligate
    o. aerobe
    o. anaerobe
    o. autotroph
    o. parasite
oblique
    o. fracture
    o. inferior branch, oculomotor
      nerve

    o. interlobar fissure
    o. muscle
obliquus
    o. capitis muscle
    o. externus abdominis muscle
    o. internus abdominis muscle
obliterating
    o. arteritis
    o. endarteritis
obliteration
    fibrous o.
obliterative
    o. bronchiolitis
    o. bronchitis
    o. endarteritis
    o. endocarditis
    o. glomerulosclerosis
    o. inflammation
    o. pericarditis
    o. pleuritis
OBS — organic brain syndrome
obscuration
obstetrical
obstipation
obstructed testis
obstruction
    ball-valve o.
    biliary o.
    bladder neck o.
    bowel o.
    chronic airway o.
    closed-loop o.
    colonic o.
    complete o.
    extrahepatic o.
    intestinal o.
    mesenteric vascular o.
    pancreatic ductal o.
    partial o.
    superior vena cava o.
    ureteropelvic o.
    ureterovesical o.
    urethral o.
    urethral outlet o.
    urinary o.
    venous o.
obstructive
    o. airway disease
    o. appendicitis
    o. atelectasis

o. cholestasis
o. cirrhosis
o. diverticulitis
o. emphysema
o. hyperbilirubinuria
o. hypertrophic cardiomy-
    opathy
o. jaundice
o. lymphedema
o. overinflation
o. pulmonary disease
o. pulmonitis
o. pyelonephritis
o. sialadenitis
o. uropathy
obstruent
obtunded
obturation
obturator
o. artery
o. internus muscle
o. lymph node
o. muscle
o. nerve
prosthetic o.
o. vein
OC — occlusocervical
    oral contraceptive
OC 125 antibody
O$_{2cap}$ — oxygen capacity
occipital
o. artery
o. bone
o. gyrus
o. horn
o. lobe
o. lymph node
o. myotome
o. nerve
o. pole
o. region
o. sinus
o. sulcus
o. vein
occipitalization
occipitoanterior
occipitocervical
occipitofrontal projection
occipitopontine fibers
occipitoposterior
occipitotemporal gyrus
occipitothalamic radiation

occiput
occlusal
occlusion
    internal carotid artery o.
    thrombotic o.
    o. time
occlusive thrombosis
occult
o. bleeding
o. blood
o. blood test
o. breast cancer
o. carcinoma
o. filariasis
occupational lung disease
Occupational Safety and Health Ad-
    ministration
OCG — oral cholecystogram
ochratoxin
ochre mutation
Ochromyia anthropophaga
ochronosis
ochronotic
o. arthritis
o. pigment
O colony
OCR — optical character recognition
OCT — ornithine carbamoyltrans-
    ferase
    oxytocin challenge test
octachlorocyclohexenone
octadecanoic acid
Octadecyl silane
octamethyl pyrophosphoramide
octane
octanoic acid
Octomitus hominis
Octomyces etiennei
octopamine
octopeptide
N-octylbicycloheptene dicarboximide
octyl cresol
N-octyl isosafrole sulfoxide
ocular
o. albinism
o. cytology
o. histoplasmosis
o. hypertelorism
o. leukemia
o. melanoma
o. metastasis
o. micrometer

o.-mucous membrane syndrome
o. muscle
o. muscle dystrophy
o. muscle palsy
o. pemphigus
o. pseudolymphoma
o. syndrome
oculoauriculovertebral dysplasia
oculobuccogenital syndrome
oculocardiac reflex
oculocerebrorenal syndrome
oculocutaneous albinism
oculodentodigital
o. dysplasia
o. syndrome
oculodermal melanosis
oculoglandular
o. syndrome
o. tularemia
oculomandibulodyscephaly
oculomotor
o. nerve
o. nucleus
oculomycosis
oculovertebral
o. dysplasia
o. syndrome
OD — optical density
outside diameter
ODA — occipitodextra anterior
ODD — oculodentodigital dysplasia
Oddi's sphincter
odditis
ODM — ophthalmodynamometry
odontoameloblastoma
odontoblast
odontoblastoma
odontogenic
o. cyst
o. fibroma
o. fibrosarcoma
o. keratocyst
o. myxofibroma
o. myxoma
o. tumor
odontology
odontoma
ameloblastic o.
complex o.
compound o.

embryoplastic o.
fibroameloblastic o.
odoratism
ODP — occipitodextra posterior
ODT — occipitodextra transversa
odynometer
odynophagia
OER — oxygen enhancement ratio
Oesophagostomum
O. *apiostomum*
O. *bifurcum*
O. *stephanostomum*
Oestridae
Oestrus
O. *hominis*
O. *ovis*
OF — osmotic fragility
Ovenstone factor
OFC — occipitofrontal circumference
OFD — oral-facial-digital (syndrome)
OGTT — oral glucose tolerance test
17-OH-corticoids test
17-OHCS — 17-hydroxycortico-
steroid
ohm
ohmmeter
Ohm's law
Ohngren's line
OHP — oxygen under high pressure
17-OHP — 17-hydroxyprogesterone
OI — opportunistic infection
osteogenesis imperfecta
Oidiomycetes
oidiomycosis
OIF — oil immersion field
OIH — orthoiodohippurate
oil
anise o.
bergamot o.
canola o.
cedar o.
chenopodium o.
clove o.
croton o.
o. cyst
distilled o.
o. embolism
essential o.
eucalyptus o.
fatty o.
fixed o.
flaxseed o.

o. immersion
o. immersion field
o. immersion lens
nondrying o.
rapeseed o.
o. red O
safflower o.
sandalwood o.
santal o.
semidrying o.
sesame o.
o. tumor
turpentine o.
volatile o.
o.-water ratio
ointment
    Credé's o.
Okazaki's segments
OKN — optokinetic nystagmus
OKT 4 cells
OKT 8 cells
OLA — occipitolaeva anterior
Old World hookworm
oleaginous
oleandomycin
oleandrin
oleate
olecranarthropathy
olecranon
olefin
oleic acid
    o.a. I-125
    o.a. uptake test
oleogranuloma
oleoma
oleoresin
    aspidum o.
    capsicum o.
oleovitamin A and D
oleoyl
olfactory
    o. bulb
    o. cells
    o. esthesioneuroblastoma
    o. gland
    o. gyrus
    o. knob
    o. labyrinth
    o. mucosa
    o. naphthamine
    o. nerve
    o. neuroblastoma

o. pathway
o. receptor
o. sensory epithelium
o. striae
o. sulcus
o. system
o. tract
o. trigone
OLH — ovine lactogenic hormone
oligemia
oligemic
olighemia
oligoamnios
oligoarthritis
oligoblast
oligocardia
oligochromemia
oligoclonal banding
oligocystic
oligocythemia
oligocytosis
oligodactyly
oligodendroblastoma
oligodendrocyte
oligodendroglia staining
oligodendroglioma
oligodynamic
oligoencephalon
oligogenic
oligo-1,6-glucosidase
oligoglucoside
oligohydramnios sequence
oligohydruria
oligomeganephronia
oligomenorrhea
oligomer
oligomeric plasmid
oligonucleotide
    allele-specific o.
    o. probe
oligopeptide
oligophrenia
    phenylpyruvic o.
oligosaccharide
    asparagine-linked o.
oligospermatism
oligospermia
oligotrophic
oligozoospermatism
oligozoospermia
oliguria
O-linked saccharide

oliva cerebellaris
olivary nucleus
olive
    cerebellar o.
    inferior o.
    spurge o.
    superior o.
olivocerebellar
    o. atrophy
    o. fibers
olivopontocerebellar atrophy
olophonia
OLP — occipitolaeva posterior
OM — otitis media
omagra
OMD — ocular muscle dystrophy
omental
omentectomy
omentitis
omentoportography
omentovolvulus
omentum
    gastrocolic o.
    gastrohepatic o.
    gastrosplenic o.
    pancreaticosplenic o.
    splenogastric o.
O-methyltransferase
OMI — old myocardial infarction
omicron
omitis
Ommaya's reservoir
OMNISTIK (blood gas syringe)
omohyoid muscle
OMPA — octamethylpyrophosphora-
       mide
    otitis media, purulent,
      acute
Omphalalotus olearius
omphalelcosis
omphalitis
omphalocele
omphaloma
omphalomesenteric
    o. artery
    o. duct
    o. vein
    o. vessels
omphalophlebitis
Omsk hemorrhagic fever
Omsk hemorrhagic fever virus
onc gene

Onchocerca
    O. caecutiens
    O. cervicalis
    O. lienalis
    O. volvulus
onchocerciasis-type filariasis
onchocercosis
oncocyte
oncocytic
    o. adenoma
    o. hepatocellular tumor
    o. papillary cystadenoma
oncocytoma
    renal o.
oncocytosis
oncodnavirus
oncofetal
    o. antigen
    o. marker
    o. protein
oncogene
    Abelson's o.
    cellular o's
    erb-A o.
    erb-B o.
    fms o.
    o. gene
    HER-2/neu o.
    myc o.
    ras o.
    retroviral o.
oncogenesis
    viral o.
oncogenic
    o. protein
    o. virus
oncogenicity
oncogenous
    o. osteomalacia
    o. radius
oncoides
oncolipid
oncologist
oncology
oncolysate
oncolysis
oncolytic
oncoma
Oncomelania
oncoprotein
oncornavirus
oncosis

oncosphere
oncotherapy
oncothlipsis
oncotic pressure
oncotomy
oncotropic
Oncovin
Oncovirinae
oncovirus
one-stage prothrombin time
one-tailed test
onion
  o. bodies
  o. scale lesion
  o. skin lesion
onkinocele
ONPG tablets
Onthophagus
ontogeny
onychatrophia
onychia
onychitis
onychoheterotopia
onycholysis
onychoma
onychomycosis
onycho-osteodysplasia
onychopathic
onychopathology
onychophosis
onychorrhexis
onychoschizia
O'nyong-nyong
  fever
  fever virus
onyxis
onyxitis
ooblast
oocyst
oocyte
oocytin
oogenesis
oogonium
oolemma
oophorectomy
oophoritis parotidea
oophorocystosis
oophoroma folliculare
oophoropathy
oophorosalpingitis
oophorus
  cumulus o.

Oospora
ootid
OP — opening pressure
  osmotic pressure
O & P — ova and parasites
opacification
opacities
  corneal o.
  lenticular o.
opalescent
opalgia
opaque
open
  o. angle glaucoma
  o. circuit
  o. loop reflex
  o. spina bifida
  o. tuberculosis
opening snap
operand
operculum
operation
operator gene
operon
  arabinose o.
  lactose o.
  transfer o.
OPG — ocular plethysmography
  oxypolygelatin
ophiasis
ophidism
ophryogene
  ulerythema o.
ophthalmatrophia
ophthalmencephalon
ophthalmia
  actinic ray o.
  Brazilian o.
  catarrhal o.
  flash o.
  gonococcal o.
  gonorrheal o.
  granular o.
  hepatic o.
  metastatic o.
  mucous o.
  o. neonatorum
  neuroparalytic o.
  phlyctenular o.
  scrofulous o.
  strumous o.
  sympathetic o.

ophthalmic
- o. artery
- o. nerve
- o. pathology
- o. vein

ophthalmicus

ophthalmitis
- sympathetic o.

ophthalmoblennorrhea

ophthalmodynamometry

ophthalmologist

ophthalmology

ophthalmomandibulomelic dysplasia

ophthalmomycosis

ophthalmopathy
- external o.
- infiltrative o.
- internal o.

ophthalmoplegia

ophthalmoplegic-type progressive muscular dystrophy

ophthalmoscopy

ophthalmosteresis

ophthalmotrope

ophthalmovascular

opiate
- o. assay
- o. receptor

opioid
- o. agonist
- o. peptide; o. peptid
- o. receptor

opisthorchiasis

opisthorchosis

Opisthorchiidae

Opisthorchioidea

Opisthorchis
- *O. felineus*
- *O. gudyaquilensis*
- *O. noverca*
- *O. viverrimi*

opisthorchosis

opisthotonos

opium

OPK — optokinetic

opponens
- o. digiti minimi muscle
- o. pollicis muscle

opportunistic
- o. infection
- o. dermatophytosis

- o. fungus
- o. pathogen

opsin

opsinogen

opsoclonus

opsomyoclonus

opsonic
- o. action
- o. index
- o. therapy

opsonin
- bacterial o.

opsonization

optic
- o. atrophy
- o. chiasm
- o. cup
- o. disc; o. disk
- o. glioma
- o. nerve
- o. neuritis
- o. neuropathy
- o. papillitis
- o. radiation
- o. recess
- o. stalk
- o. tract
- o. vesicle

optical
- o. activity
- o. character reader
- o. character recognition
- o. density
- o. glass
- o. isomer
- o. isomerism
- o. path
- o. purity
- o. rotary dispersion
- o. rotation
- o. scanner

optics
- geometric o.
- physical o.

optimal growth temperature

optimizing compiler

Optochin
- disk
- susceptibility test

OPV — oral poliovaccine
- oral poliovirus vaccine

OR — orosomucoid

ora (pl., orae)
    o. serrata
oral
    o. antibiotic
    o. cavity
    o. cholecystogram
    o. commissure
    o. contraceptive
    o. epithelium
    o.-facial-digital
    o. gland
    o. glucose tolerance test
    o. hairy leukoplakia
    o. lactose tolerance test
    o. mucosa
    o. mucous membrane
    o. pathology
    o. pharynx
    o. smear
    o. thrust
    o. vestibule
orange
    acridine o.
    ethyl o.
    o. G
    methyl o.
    o. peel change
    victoria o.
orangeophil
orbicularis
    oculi muscle
    o. oris muscle
orbiculus (pl., orbiculi)
orbit
orbita (pl., orbitae)
orbital
    o. abscess
    o. gyrus
    hybrid o.
    o. pneumotomography
    o. rhabdomyosarcoma
    o. septum
    o. sulcus
    o tubercle
    o. varix
orbitography
orbitomeatal
orbitoparietal
orbitotomy
orbivirus
orcein
    acetic o.
    acid o.

orchella
orchiatrophy
orchidic hormone
orchiditis
orchidoblastoma
orchidoepididymectomy
orchidoncus
orchidoptosis
orchiectomy
orchiepididymitis
orchil
orchioblastoma
orchiocele
orchiomyeloma
orchioncus
orchiopathy
orchiopexy
orchioscirrhus
orchitic
orchitis
    autoimmune o.
    congenital syphilitic o.
    gonococcal o.
    granulomatous o.
    metastatic o.
    mumps o.
    nonspecific o.
    spermatogenic granuloma-
      tous o.
    syphilitic o.
    traumatic o.
    o. variolosa
orcin
orcinol test
ORD — optical rotary dispersion
ordinal variable
ordinate
orexigenic
ORF — open reading frame
orf virus (sheep pox virus)
organ
    accessory o.
    Chievitz's o.
    Corti's o.
    floating o.
    Golgi tendon o.
    Jacobson's o.
    neurotendinous o.
    o. percussion
    o. perfusion
    ptotic o.
    spiral o.

supernumerary o.
target o.
tendon o.
o. tolerance dose
o. transplantation
vestibulocochlear o's
vestigial o.
vomeronasal o.
wandering o.
Zuckerkandl's o's
organelle
organic
    o. acid
    o. acidemia
    o. aciduria
    o. brain syndrome
    o. chemistry
    o. contracture
    o. dust
    o. phosphate
organism
    anaerobic o.
    Arizona o.
    indicator o.
    nonmotile o.
    photosynthetic o.
    pleuropneumonia-like o.
    Rickett's o.
    transgenic o.
    Vincent's o.
organized
    o. hematoma
    o. pneumonia
    o. thrombus
organizer
    nucleolar o.
    procentriole o.
organochlorine
    o. insecticide
    o. pesticides
organogenesis
organography
organoid
    o. nevus
    cytoplasmic o's
    o. tumor
organoma
organomegaly
organomercury compound
organometallic compound
organon

organophosphate
    o. compound
    o. insecticide
    o. poisoning
organophosphorous compound
organothiophosphate compound assay
organotroph
organotropic bacterium
organotropism
organum vasculosum of the lamina terminalis
Oriboca virus
oriental
    o. blood fluke
    o. body fluke
    o. hemoptysis
    o. lung fluke
    o. lung fluke disease
    o. rat flea
    o. tropical sore
orienting
    o. reflex
    o. response
orifice
    aortic o.
    atrioventricular o.
    auriculoventricular o.
    duodenal o.
    mitral o.
    pulmonary o.
    ureteral o.
    uterine o.
    vesicourethral o.
origanum oil
origin
    amyloid of immunoglobulin o.
    amyloid of unknown o.
    anomalous o.
    fever of undetermined o.
    fever of unknown o.
    myocardial disease of unknown o.
    polyphyletic o.
    pyrexia of unknown o.
oris
    pachyderma o.
ornithine
    o. aminotransferase
    o. carbamoyltransferase
    o. carbamoyltransferase assay
    o. carbamoyltransferase deficiency

o. decarboxylase
o.-ketoacid aminotransferase
o. oxo-acid aminotransferase
o. transcarbamoylase
o. transcarbamoylase deficiency
ornithinemia
ornithinuria
Ornithobilharzia
Ornithodoros
    O. coriaceus
    O. kellyi
Ornithonyssus
ornithosis virus
orodigitofacial dystosis
orofaciodigital
orogenital
oropharyngeal
    o. dysplasia
    o. gonorrhea
    o. isthmus
    o. membrane
oropharynx
Oropouche virus
orosomucoid
orotate
    o. calcium
    o. phosphoribosyltransferase
orotic
    o. acid
    o. acidosis
    o. aciduria
orotidine 5-phosphate decarboxylase
orotidine 5'-phosphate pyrophosphorylase
orotidylate decarboxylase
orotidylic
    o. acid
    o. decarboxylase
    o. pyrophosphorylase
Oroya fever
orphan
    o. receptor
    o. virus
orphenadrine
Ortalidae
orthochlorobenzene
orthochromatic
    o. erythroblast
    o. erythrocyte
    o. normoblast
orthochromatophilic normoblast
orthochromophil

orthochromophile
orthocytosis
orthodiagraphy
ortho-dianisidine
orthodromic conduction
orthoglycemic
orthoiodohippurate
orthokeratosis
orthomolecular
ortho multichannel hematology analyzer
Ortho-mune
orthomyxovirus
orthophosphoric
    o. acid
    o. ester monohydrolase
orthopnea
Orthopodomyia
orthopoxvirus
Orthoptera
orthoptic transplantation
orthoroentgenography
Orthorrhapha
orthostatic
    o. albuminuria
    o. edema
    o. hypertension
    o. hypotension
    o. proteinuria
orthostereoscope
orthotolidine
orthotopic
orthovoltage
Orth's
    fixative
    fluid
    stain
Os — osmium
os (pl., ossa, *which see*)
    o. acromiale
    o. basilare
    o. calcis
    o. capitatum
    o. carpale
    o. coccygis
    o. coxae
    o. cuboideum
    o. cuneiforme
    o. ethmoidale
    o. frontale
    o. hamatum
    o. ilium

o. interparietale
o. lacrimale
o. lunatum
o. nasale
o. naviculare
o. occipitale
o. penis
o. pubis
o. sacrum
o. unguis
o. zygomaticum
osazone test
oscheitis
oschelephantiasis
oscheocele
oscheohydrocele
oscheoma
oscillation
oscillator
oscillogram
oscillograph
oscillometer
oscillometry
oscillopsia
oscilloscope
OSHA — Occupational Safety and
          Health Administration
Osler's
    erythema
    maneuver
    node
    triad
OSM — oxygen saturation meter
Osm — osmole
osmic acid
osmicate
osmication
osmification
osmiophilic
osmiophobic
osmium tetroxide
osmol clearance
osmolal clearance
osmolality
    calculated serum o.
    delta o.
osmolar
osmolarity
osmole
osmolute
osmometer
    dew point o.

    freezing point depression o.
    vapor pressure depression o.
osmometry
osmosis
    reverse o.
osmotic
    o. coefficient
    o. diuretic
    o. fragility
    o. fragility test
    o. hemolysis
    o. nephrosis
    o. pressure
    o. shock
ossa (*see also* os)
    o. carpi
    o. cranii
    o. digitorum
    o. faciei
    o. membri
    o. metacarpalia
    o. metatarsalia
    o. sesamoidea
    o. suprasternalia
    o. tarsi
osseofibrous
osseous
    o. ankylosis
    o. dysplasia
    o. hydatid
    o. hydatid cyst
    o. labyrinth
    o. metaplasia
    o. polyp
ossicle
    auditory o.
ossicular
    o. ligament
    o. muscle
ossification
    abnormal endochondral o.
    endochrondral o.
    intramembranous o.
    metaplastic o.
ossifying
    o. fibroma
    o. inflammation
    o. interstitial myositis
ostealgia
ostectomy
osteitic

osteitis
- o. albuminosa
- carious o.
- o. carnosa
- caseous o.
- central o.
- condensing o.
- o. condensans
- cortical o.
- o. deformans
- o. fibrosa
- o. fibrosa circumscripta
- o. fibrosa cystica
- o. fibrosa disseminata
- o. fibrosa localisata
- o. fibrosa osteoplastica
- Garré's o.
- o. granulosa
- gummatous o.
- hematogenous o.
- necrotic o.
- rarefying o.
- sarcomatous o.
- sclerosing o.
- o. tuberculosa multiplex cystica

ostemia

ostempyesis

osteoarthritis
- erosive o.
- hyperplastic o.

osteoarthropathy
- familial o.
- hypertrophic o.
- hypertrophic pulmonary o.
- idiopathic hypertrophic o.
- pneumogenic o.
- pulmonary o.
- secondary hypertrophic o.

osteoarthroscopy
- hypertrophic o.

osteoarthrosis

osteoblast

osteoblastic
- o. osteosarcoma
- o. metastasis
- o. tumor

osteoblastoma

osteocalcin

osteocarcinoma

osteocartilaginous exostosis

osteocele

osteochondral

osteochondritis
- calcaneal o.
- o. deformans juvenilis
- o. deformans juvenilis dorsi
- o. dissecans
- o. ischiopubica
- o. necroticans
- syphilitic o.

osteochondrodystrophia deformans

osteochondrodystrophy

osteochondroma

osteochondromatosis
- multiple o.
- synovial o.

osteochondromyxoma

osteochondropathy

osteochondrosarcoma

osteochondrosis

osteoclasia

osteoclasis

osteoclast-activating factor

osteoclastic
- o. giant cells
- o. resorption

osteoclastoma

osteocomma

osteocope

osteocystoma

osteocyte

osteodermatopoikilosis

osteodermatous

osteodermia

osteodysplasty

osteodystrophia

osteodystrophy
- Albright's hereditary o.
- renal o.

osteoectasia
- familial o.

osteofibrochondrosarcoma

osteofibroma

osteofibromatosis
- cystic o.

osteofibrosis

osteogenesis
- o. imperfecta
- o. imperfecta congenita
- o. imperfecta cystica
- o. imperfecta tarda

osteogenic
- o. fibroma
- o. sarcoma

osteogram
osteography
osteohalisteresis
osteohydatidosis
osteohypertrophic nevus flammeus
osteohypertrophy
osteoid
    o. matrix of bone
    o. metaplasia
    o. osteoma
    o. seam
    o. tumor
osteoinduction
osteolathyrism
osteolipochondroma
osteolipoma
osteolysis
osteolytic
osteoma
    o. cutis
    o. durum
    o. eburneum
    fibrous o.
    giant osteoid o.
    ivory o.
    o. medullare
    osteoid o.
    parosteal o.
    o. sarcomatosum
    o. spongiosum
osteomalacia
    hepatic o.
    infantile o.
    juvenile o.
    oncogenous o.
    osteogenic o.
    puerperal o.
    renal tubular o.
    senile o.
osteomalacic pelvis
osteomatoid
osteomere
osteomucoperiosteal flap
osteomyelitis
    diffuse sclerosing o.
    focal sclerosing o.
    Garré's sclerosing o.
    pyogenic o.
    salmonella o.
    sclerosing nonsuppurative o.
    tuberculous o.
    typhoid o.

osteomyelodysplasia
osteomyelofibrotic syndrome
osteomyelography
osteomyelosclerosis
osteomyxochondroma
osteon
osteonecrosis
osteonectin
osteonosus
osteo-odontoma
osteo-onychodysplasia
    hereditary o.
osteopathia
    o. condensans
    o. hemorrhagica infantum
    o. striata
osteopathy
    alimentary o.
    disseminated condensing o.
    myelogenic o.
osteopenia
osteoperiostitis
osteopetrosis acro-osteolytica
osteopetrotic
osteophlebitis
osteophyma
osteophyte
osteopoikilosis
osteoporosis
    o. circumscripta
    o. circumscripta cranii
    juvenile o.
    juxta-articular o.
    postmenopausal o.
    post-traumatic o.
    senile o.
osteoporotic
osteopsathyrosis
osteopulmonary arthropathy
osteoradionecrosis
osteosarcoma
    chondroblastic o.
    classic o.
    extraosseous o.
    extraskeletal o.
    fibroblastic o.
    high-grade surface o.
    intracortical o.
    intraosseous low-grade o.
    o. of jaw
    juxtacortical o.
    multicentric o.

osteoblastic o.
parosteal o.
periosteal o.
primary o.
secondary o.
small cell o.
telangiectatic o.
variant o.
osteosarcomatosis
osteosarcomatous
osteosclerosis
o. congenita
o. fragilis
o. myelofibrosis
osteosclerotic anemia
osteosis
o. cutis
o. eburnisans monomelica
parathyroid o.
osteospongioma
osteosteatoma
osteotelangiectasia
osteothrombosis
osteotomy
Ostertag
streptococcus of O.
Ostertagia
ostitic
ostitis
ostosis
ostraceous
ostium (pl., ostia)
maxillary o.
o. primum
o. secundum
o. uteri
Ostwald viscosimeter
OT — occlusion time
old tuberculin
orotracheal
otalgia
Ota's nevus
OTC — ornithine transcarbamoylase
oxytetracycline
OTD — organ tolerance dose
otic
o. abscess
o. ganglion
o. vesicle
otitic
otitis
o. desquamativa

o. diphtheritica
o. externa
o. labyrinthica
malignant external o.
o. mastoidea
o. media
o. media, purulent, acute
mucosis o.
mucosus o.
o. mycotica
o. sclerotica
staphylococcal o.
viral o.
Otobius
otoconia
Otodectes
otodynia
otolaryngology
otolith
otomandibular
o. dysostosis
o. syndrome
Otomyces
O. *hageni*
O. *purpureus*
otomycosis aspergillina
otopathy
otorhinolaryngology
otorhinology
otorrhagia
otorrhea
otosclerosis
otoscope
ototoxic
ototoxicity
OTR — Ovarian Tumor Registry
Otto's pelvis
ouabain
Ouchterlony
immunodiffusion
method
technique
Oudin's
immunodiffusion
resonator
technique
OURQ — outer upper right quadrant
outbreeding
outer nuclear membrane alteration
outflow
urinary o.

outlet
    urethral o.
outlier
output
    basal acid o.
    o. capacitor
    carbon dioxide o.
    cardiac o.
    CO_2 o.
    energy o.
    o. exposure rate
    o. impedance
    maximal acid o.
    peak acid o.
    stroke o.
    urinary o.
ova
ovalbumin
ovale
    anatomically patent foramen o.
    o. malaria
    prematurely closed foramen o.
oval fat bodies
ovalocyte
ovalocytic anemia
ovalocytosis
ovarialgia
ovarian
    o. artery
    o. ascorbic acid depletion
    o. ascorbic acid depletion test
    o. cycle
    o. cyst
    o. dysgerminoma
    o. dysfunction
    o. follicle
    o. germ cell–stromal sex cord tumor
    o. granulosa cell neoplasm
    o. hormone
    o. ligament
    o. masculinization
    o. medulla
    o. pregnancy
    o. teratoma
    o. theca metaplasia
    o. thyroid
    o. tubular adenoma
    o. tumor
    o. varicocele
    o. vein
Ovarian Tumor Registry

ovariocele
ovarioncus
ovariopathy
ovariosalpingitis
ovaritis
ovarium masculinum
ovary
    adenocystic o.
    oyster o's
    polycystic o.
    streak o.
Ovenstone factor
overflow
    o. aminoaciduria
    o. proteinuria
overinflation
    obstructive o.
overload
    circulatory o.
    iron o.
oviduct
ovine lactogenic hormone
OVLT — organum vasculosum of the lamina terminalis
ovotestis
Ovotran
ovotransferrin
ovulation
ovulational sclerosis
ovulatory
ovum (pl., ova)
    blighted o.
    pathologic o.
    schistosomal o.
O/W — oil in water
    oil-water ratio
oxacillin sodium
oxalacetate transacetase
oxalate
    ammonium o.
    calcium o.
    o. calculus
    o. coenzyme A–transferase
    o. crystals
    potassium o.
    sodium o.
oxalemia
oxalic
    o. acid
    o. acid assay
oxalism
oxaloacetate decarboxylase

oxaloacetic acid
oxalosis
oxalosuccinate
oxaluria
oxamniquine
oxanamide
oxandrolone
oxazepam
oxazine dye
oxazolidinedione compound
oxethazaine
Oxford unit
oxidant hemolysis
oxidase
     aldehyde o.
     D-amino acid o.
     L-amino acid o.
     benzidine o.
     coproporphyrinogen o.
     cytochrome o.
     glucose o.
     homogentisic acid o.
     p-hydroxyphenylpyruvate o.
     hydroxyproline o.
     lysol o.
     monoamine o.
     o.-positive glucose
       fermenter
     proline o.
     protoporphyrinogen o.
     o. reaction
     sulfite o.
     o. test
     urate o.
     xanthine o.
oxidation
     alpha o.
     fatty acid o.
     o.-fermentation test
     periodate o.
     o.-reducing potential
     o. reduction indicator
     o.-reduction reaction
oxidative
     o. phosphorylation
     o. phosphorylation inhibitors
     o. phosphorylation uncouplers
oxide
     aluminum o.
     chloroethylene o.
     chloropropylene o.
     ethylene o.

     iron o.
     mercuric o.
     nitrous o.
     vitamin K_1 o.
     zinc o.
oxidize
oxidized hemoglobin
oxidizer
     glucose o.
oxidizing
     o. agent
     o. gas
oxidoreductase
     L-lysine:NAD+ o.
oxidosis
oximeter
     cuvette o.
     intracaradiac o.
     whole blood o.
oximetry
     pulse o.
oximinotransferase
oxine
oxirane
oxisuran
oxmotaxis
oxo acid
3-oxo-adipate coenzyme
     A-transferase
oxogluconate dehydrogenase
oxoglutarate dehydrogenase
2-oxoglutaric acid
oxohydroxybutyrate aldolase
2-oxoisovalerate dehydrogenase
oxolinic acid
oxonium ion
oxophenarsine hydrochloride
5-oxoprolinase
5-oxoproline
4-oxoproline reductase
5-oxoprolinuria
oxtriphylline
oxybiotin
oxybutyria
oxybutyric acid
3-oxybutyric acid
oxycephaly
oxychromatic
oxychromatin
oxycodone hydrochloride
oxycyanide

oxygen
    o. acceptor
    o. affinity anoxia
    o. affinity hypoxia
    o. analyzer
    o. capacity of blood
    cerebral metabolic
       rate of o.
    o. consumption
    o. content of blood
    o. deprivation
    o. dissociation curve
    o. effect
    o. electrode method
    o. enhancement ratio
    o. equilibrium
    o. excess
    o. half-saturation pressure of
       hemoglobin
    o.-hemoglobin dissociation
       curve
    high-pressure o.
    hyperbaric o.
    o. metabolism
    molecular o.
    o. poisoning
    o. pressure
    o. quotient
    o. saturation
    o. saturation measure-
       ments
    o. saturation meter
    singlet o.
    o. tension
    o. therapy
    o. toxicity
    o. transport
    o. under high pressure
    o. uptake
    o. utilization
oxygenase
    heme o.
oxygenate
oxygenated hemoglobin
oxygenation
    hyperbaric o.
oxygenator
oxyhemoglobin
    o. dissociation curve
    o. method
oxyhemogram
oxyhemograph

oxyhydrocephalus
oxyhyperglycemia
oxymel
oxymetholone
oxymorphone hydrochloride
oxyntic
    o. cell
    o. gland
oxyosis
oxyphenbutazone
oxyphencyclimine hydro-
    chloride
oxyphenisatin
oxyphenonium bromide
oxyphil
    o. adenoma
    o. cell
    o. chromatin
    o. granule
    o. inclusion body
oxyphilic
    o. erythroblast
    o. leukocyte
    o. normoblast
oxypolygelatin
oxyprocaine
oxypurine
oxypurinol
oxyquinoline
Oxyspirura
oxysteroid
oxysulfide
    carbon o.
oxytalan
    o. fiber
    o. fiber stain
oxytalanolysis
oxytetracycline
oxytocin
    o. challenge test
    o. hormone
    o. secretion
Oxytrema
oxytropism
Oxyurata
oxyuriasis
Oxyuridae
Oxyuris
    O. incognita
    O. vermicularis
Oxyuroidea

Oz
    antigen
    isotypic determinant
oz. — ounce
ozena
ozolinone

ozone
ozonide
ozonization
ozonolysis
ozonophore
Ozzard's filaria

P

P — partial pressure
    pharmacopeia
    phosphorus
    plasma
    position
    postpartum
    premolar
    presbyopia
    pressure
    primipara
    probability
    protein
    pulse
    pupil
P. — *Pasteurella*
    Plasmodium
    Proteus
P_1 — parental generation
P_2 — pulmonic second sound
^{32}P — radioactive phosphorus
P_{Na} — plasma sodium
p- — para-
PA — paralysis agitans
    pathology
    pernicious anemia
    posteroanterior
    pregnancy-associated
    primary amenorrhea
    primary anemia
    pulmonary artery
    pulpoaxial
Pa — pascal
    protactinium
PAB; PABA — para-aminobenzoic
               acid
PAC — premature auricular con-
               traction
pacchionian granulation
pacemaker
    p. cell

    p. current
    wandering p.
pachyacria
pachycephalia
pachycephalic; pachycephalous
pachycephaly
pachychromatic
pachydactylia
pachydactylous
pachydactyly
pachyderma
    p. laryngis
    p. lymphangiectatica
    p. oris
    p. verrucosa
    p. vesicae
pachydermatocele
pachydermatosis
pachydermatous
pachydermia
pachydermic
pachydermoperiostitis
pachydermoperiostosis
pachygyria
pachyhymenia
pachyhymenic
pachyleptomeningitis
pachylosis
pachymenia
pachymenic
pachymeningitis
    adhesive chronic p.
    cerebral p.
    chronic adhesive p.
    fibrous hypertropic p.
    hemorrhagic internal p.
    purulent p.
pachymeningopathy
pachymeninx (pl., pachymeninges)

pachynema
pachynsis
pachyntic
pachyonychia congenita
pachyperiostitis
pachyperitonitis
pachypleuritis
pachysalpingitis
pachysalpingo-ovaritis
pachysomia
pachytene
pachyvaginalitis
pachyvaginitis cystica
pacing
    cardiac p.
pacinian corpuscle
paciniform
    p. corpuscles
    p. receptors
pacinitis
pack
    cold p.
    dry p.
    Mikulicz's p.
    periodontal p.
package
    dual-in-line p.
packed
    p. cell volume
    p. erythrocytes
    p. human blood cells
    p. red blood cells
    p. red cells
packet
packing ratio
Padgett's dermatome
Padykula-Herman stain for myosin
    ATPase
Paecilomyces
paecilomycosis
Paederus
PAF — platelet-activating factor
    platelet-aggregating factor
    pulmonary arteriovenous
      fistula
PAFIB — paroxysmal atrial fibril-
    lation
PAGE — polyacrylamide gel electro-
    phoresis
Paget-Eccleston stain
pagetic

pagetoid
    p. cells
    p. dysplasia
    p. reticulosis
Paget's
    carcinoma
    cells
    disease of bone
    disease of breast
    disease of vulva
    test
PAGMK — primary African green
    monkey kidney
PAH — para-aminohippuric acid
    polycyclic aromatic hydro-
      carbon
    pulmonary artery hyper-
      tension
PAHA — para-aminohippuric acid
PAHO — Pan American Health Or-
    ganization
PAIDS — pediatric AIDS
Paigen test
pain
    fulgurant p's
    heterotopic p.
    homotopic p.
    ideogenous p.
    lancinating p.
    phantom limb p.
    p. receptor
    referred p.
    terebrating p.
painless jaundice
P-A interval
pair
    base p.
    conjugate redox p.
    electron p.
    ion p.
    kilobase p.
    p. production
pairing
    base p.
    exchange p.
    p. segment
    somatic p.
PAL — posterior axillary line
PALA — N-phosphonacetyl
    L-asparate
Palaemonetes
palatal flap

palate
    cleft p.
    gothic p.
    premaxillary p.
    soft p.
palatine
    p. arch
    p. bone
    p. gland
    p. mucous membrane
    p. muscle
    p. process
    p. tonsil
palatitis
palatognathous
palatography
palatomaxillary
palatonasal
palatopharyngeal
palatoplasty
pale
    p. infarct
    p. thrombus
    p. urine
paleocerebellum
paleopathology
PALI — Programmed Accelerated
        Laboratory Investigation
        system
palindrome
palindromia
palindromic rheumatism
palisade layer
palisading
palladium chloride
palliation
palliative
    p. mastectomy
    p. treatment
pallidofugal fibers
pallium
pallor
palm
    liver p.
palmar
    p. aponeurosis
    p. artery
    p. crease
    p. erythema
    p. fibromatosis
    p. metacarpal artery
    p. reflex

    p. skin
    p. vein
palmaris
    p. brevis muscle
    p. longus muscle
palmellin
Palmgren's silver impregnation stain
palmitate
palmitic acid
palmitin
palmitoleate
palmitoleic acid
palmitone
palmitoyl-coenzyme A hydrolase
palmoplantar keratoderma
palpation thyroiditis
palpebra (pl., palpebrae)
palpebral
    p. artery
    p. conjunctiva
    p. glands
palpitation
palsy
    Bell's p.
    bulbar p.
    cerebral p.
    Erb's p.
    facial p.
    muscle p.
    ocular muscle p.
    progressive bulbar p.
    progressive supranuclear p.
    pseudobulbar p.
    supranuclear p.
paludal fever
Paludina
paludism
PAM — crystalline penicillin G in
        2% aluminum monoste-
        arate
        phenylalanine mustard
        pralidoxime
        pulmonary alveolar macro-
        phage
        pulmonary alveolar micro-
        lithiasis
        pyridine aldoxime meth-
        iodide
pampiniform plexus
pampinocele
PAN — periodic alternating nys-
        tagmus

peroxyacetyl nitrate
polyarteritis nodosa
panacinar emphysema
panagglutinable
panagglutination
panagglutinin
Pan American Health Organization
panangiitis
panarteritis
panarthritis
panatrophy
pancake kidney
pancarditis
pancervical smear
Pancoast's tumor
pancreas (pl., pancreata)
    aberrant p.
    accessory p.
    annular p.
    Aselli's p.
    Baggenstoss change in p.
    cystic fibrosis of p.
    p. divisum
    dorsal p.
    endocrine p.
    exocrine p.
    lesser p.
    pulmonary p.
    renal cortical p.
    uncinate process of p.
    ventral p.
    Willis' p.
    Winslow's p.
pancreatectomy
pancreatemphraxis
pancreatic
    p. abscess
    p. acinus
    p. amylase
    p. calculus
    p. cancer
    p. carcinoma
    p. cholera
    p. colic
    p. colipase
    p. cyst
    p. duct
    p. ductal obstruction
    p. fluid
    p. interstitial tissue
    p. islet cell antibody test
    p. islets

    p. islet stain
    p. juice
    p. lipase
    p. lithiasis
    p. necrosis
    p. oncofetal antigen
    p. polypeptide cells
    p. pseudocyst
    p. RNase
    p. tumor
pancreaticoduodenal
    p. artery
    p. vein
pancreaticosplenic
    p. glands
    p. omentum
pancreatin
pancreatitis
    acute p.
    acute hemorrhagic p.
    calcifying p.
    chronic p.
    edematous p.
    familial hereditary p.
    hemorrhagic p.
    idiopathic p.
    necrotizing p.
    nonalcoholic tropical p.
    relapsing p.
    tropical p.
pancreatoblastoma
pancreatoduodenectomy
pancreatogram
pancreatography
    endoscopic retrograde p.
pancreatolith
pancreatolithiasis
pancreatomegaly
pancreatopeptidase E
pancreatosplenic lymph node
pancrelipase
pancreolith
pancreoprivic
pancreozymin
    p.-cholecystokinin
    p.-secretin test
pancuronium bromide
pancytopenia
    autoimmune p.
    Fanconi's p.
pandemic

Pandy's
    reaction
    test
panel
panencephalitis
    subacute sclerosing p.
panendoscope
Paneth's cells
Pangonia
panhematolymphoid antigen
panhematopoietic
panhemocytophthisis
panhyperemia
panhypogammaglobulinemia
panhypopituitarism
    autoimmune p.
    postpubertal p.
    prepubertal p.
panleukopenia
    autoimmune p.
    p. virus
panlobular emphysema
panlymphopenia
panmixis
panmyelopathy
panmyelophthisis
panmyelosis
panniculitis
    cytophagic p.
    factitial p.
    febrile nodular p.
    lupus p.
    mesenteric p.
    metastatic p.
    nodular nonsuppurative p.
    relapsing febrile nodular p.
    Weber-Christian p.
panniculus
    p. adiposus
    p. carnosus
"panning method"
pannus
panography
panophthalmitis
panoptic stain
PANS — puromycin amino-
        nucleoside
pansclerosis
panspecific (interleukin-3) hematopoietin
Panstrongylus
pantachromatic

pantalgia
pantaloon embolism
pantatrophia; pantatrophy
pantetheine kinase
pantetheinephosphate adenylyltransferase
P antibodies
P antigen
p24 antigen
pantomography
Panton-Valentine leukocidin
pantothenate calcium
pantothenic
    p. acid assay
    p. acid unit
pantothenoylcysteine decarboxylase
pantoyl-β-alanine
panuveitis
panzerherz
panzootic
PAO — peak acid output
P_AO_2 — alveolar oxygen pressure
PAOD — peripheral arterial occlu-
        sive disease
        peripheral arteriosclerotic
        occlusive disease
PAP — peroxidase-antiperoxidase
        positive airway pressure
        primary atypical pneumonia
        prostatic acid phosphatase
        pulmonary alveolar pro-
           teinosis
        pulmonary artery pressure
Pap — Papanicolaou
papain
Papanicolaou's
    examination
    stain
Papaver
papaverine hydrochloride
PAP complex — peroxidase-antiperox-
        idase complex
paper
    alkannin p.
    azolitmin p.
    p. capacitor
    p. chromatography
    Congo red p.
    p. electrolysis
    p. electrophoresis
    probability p.
    p. radioimmunosorbent test

Papez circuit
papilla (pl., papillae)
    dermal p.
    lacrimal p.
    lingual p.
    neoplastic p.
    nerve p.
    renal p.
papillary
    p. adenocarcinoma
    p. adenoma
    p. adenoma of large intestine
    p. adenomatous polyp
    p. blush
    p. breast cancer
    p. carcinoma
    p. cystadenocarcinoma
    p. cystadenoma
    p. cystadenoma lymphoma-
        tosum
    p. cystic adenoma
    p. cystic tumor
    p. duct
    p. ectasia
    p. ependymoma
    p. fibroelastoma
    p. gingivitis
    p. hidradenoma
    p. hyperplasia
    p. hyperplastic nodule
    p. layer
    p. meningioma
    p. mesothelioma
    p. microcarcinoma
    p. muscle
    p. muscle dysfunction
    p. muscle syndrome
    p. necrosis
    p. pseudotumor
    p. serous carcinoma
    p. serous cystadenocarcinoma
    p. serous cystadenoma
    p. stenosis
    p. syringadenoma
    p. transitional cell carcinoma
    p. tumor
papillate
papilledema
papillitis
    anal p.
    chronic lingual p.

    necrotizing p.
    optic p.
papilloadenocystoma
papillocarcinoma
papilloma
    p. acuminatum
    basal cell p.
    p. canaliculum
    choroid plexus p.
    p. diffusum
    duct p.
    p. durum
    fibroepithelial p.
    hard p.
    hirsutoid p.
    hyperkeratotic p.
    p. inguinale tropicum
    intracanalicular p.
    intracystic p.
    intraductal p.
    inverted p.
    inverted ductal p.
    keratotic p.
    laryngeal p.
    p. molle
    mural p.
    pearly penile p.
    rabbit p.
    schneiderian p.
    Shope p.
    soft p.
    squamous p.
    squamous cell p.
    transitional cell p.
    urothelial p.
    p. venereum
    verrucous p.
    villous p.
    p. virus
papillomatosis
    p. of breast
    confluent and reticulate p.
    ductal p.
    florid oral p.
    intraductal p.
    juvenile p.
    laryngeal p.
    respiratory p.
    subareolar duct p.
papillomatous
    p. caruncle
    p. hyperplasia
papillomavirus

papillotomy
Papovaviridae
papovavirus
PAPP — para-aminopropiophenone
pappataci
        p. fever
        p. fever virus
Pappenheimer body
Pappenheim's
        lymphoid hemoblast
        stain
PAPS — phosphoadenosine diphos-
            phosulfate
        phosphoadenosine phospho-
            sulfate
        phosphoadenosylphospho-
            sulfate
Pap smear
PAP technique — peroxidase-
                antiperoxidase
                technique
Pap test
papula (papulae)
papular
        p. angiodysplasia
        p. mucinosis
        p. rosacea
papule
        Gottron's p.
        moist p.
        mucous p.
        penile p.
        prurigo p.
papuliferous
papuloerythematous
papulonecrotic
        p. tuberculid
        p. tuberculosis
papulosis
        bowenoid p.
        lymphomatoid p.
        malignant atrophic p.
papulosquamous
papulovesicular
PAPVC — partial anomalous pulmo-
             nary venous connection
papyraceous scars
PAR — pulmonary arteriolar resis-
            tance
para-aminobenzoic acid
para-aminohippuric acid
para-aminosalicylic acid
para-aortic body

para-appendicitis
parabiosis
parabiotic
parablast
parabola
Parabuthus
paracanthoma
paracanthosis
paracarcinomatous
        p. encephalomyelopathy
        p. myelopathy
paracarmine stain
paracasein
paracentesis
paracentral
        p. lobule
        p. nucleus
        p. sulcus
parachlorophenol
paracholera vibrio
Parachordodes
parachromatopsia
parachute reflex
paracoagulant
paracoagulation test
Paracoccidioides brasiliensis
paracoccidioidomycosis
paracolitis
Paracolobactrum
        P. aerogenoides
        P. arizonae
        P. coliforme
        P. intermedium
paracolon bacilli
paracolpitis
paracortical lymphoid hyperplasia
paracrine regulator
paracystitis
paracytic
paradenitis
paradichlorobenzene
paradidymis
paradoxical
        p. embolism
        p. embolus
        p. infarct
paraesophageal hiatal hernia
parafascicular nucleus
Par. aff. (pars affecta)—part affected
paraffin
        bismuth iodoform p.
        p. cancer
        p. tumor

paraffinoma
paraflocculus
parafollicular cell
paraformaldehyde
Parafossarulus
parafrenal abscess
parafuchsin
paraganglioma
 aorticosympathetic p.
 branchiomeric p.
 carotid p.
 chromaffin p.
 extra-adrenal p.
 intra-adrenal p.
 intravagal p.
 jugulotympanic p.
 parasympathetic p.
 p.-like adenoma
 medullary p.
 nonchromaffin p.
 vagal p.
paraganglion (pl., paraganglia)
paraganglionic system
paragnosis
paragonimiasis
Paragonimus
 P. africanus
 P. caliensis
 P. heterotrema
 P. kellicotti
 P. mexicanus
 P. westermani
Paragordius
 P. cintus
 P. tricuspidatus
 P. varius
paragranuloma
 Hodgkin's p.
parahemophilia
parahormone
parainfluenza
 p. antibody test
 p. viral serology
 p. virus
 p. virus antigen
 p. virus culture
 p. virus, Types 1–4
parakeratosis
 p. pustulosa
 p. scutularis
 p. variegata
paralbuminemia

paraldehyde poisoning
parallax
parallel
 p. circuit
 p. fibers
 p. grid
 p. operation
paralysis (pl., paralyses)
 p. agitans
 ascending p.
 bulbar p.
 familial periodic p.
 immunologic p.
 ischemic p.
 Landry's p.
 tick p.
 vasomotor p.
 Volkmann's p.
 Werdnig-Hoffmann p.
paralytic
 p. bladder
 p. brachial neuritis
 p. ileus
 p. shellfish poisoning
paramacular
paramagnetic electron resonance
paramammillary gray matter
paramastigote
paramecium (pl., paramecia)
Paramecium coli
paramedian lobule
paramesonephric
 p. duct
 p. rest
parameter
paramethadione
paramethasone
parametrial lymph node
parametric
 p. abscess
 p. hematocele
parametritic abscess
parametritis
parametrium (pl., parametria)
paramorphia
paramorphic
Paramphistomatoidea
paramyloid
paramyloidosis
paramyotonia congenita
paramyxovirus
paranasal sinus

paraneoplasia
paraneoplastic
    p. acrokeratosis
    p. degeneration
    p. neuropathy
    p. polyneuropathy
    p. syndrome
paranephric abscess
paranephroma
paranephros
paraneuron
para-nitrophenylic acid
para-nitrosulfathiazole
paranoia
paranoid
    p. personality
    p. reaction
    p. schizophrenia
paraortic lymph node
paraoxon
paraparesis
    tropical spastic p.
parapedesis
parapepsin
paraphenylenediamine
paraphimosis
paraphyseal cyst
Paraplast
paraplegia
parapneumonic effusion
Paraponera
parapox virus
parapraxia
paraproctitis
paraprostatitis
paraprotein
paraproteinemia
    monoclonal p.
parapsoriasis
    p. en plaque
    p. guttata
    p. lichenoides
    p. lichenoides et varioliformis
      acuta
    retiform p.
    p. varioliformis
paraquat assay
pararosanilin
pararosaniline
Parasa
Parasaccharomyces ashfordi
parasagittal meningioma

parasalpingitis
parasellar lacunae
paraseptal emphysema
parasialadenoma
parasialoma
parasite
    accidental p.
    ectozoic p.
    entozoic p.
    extracellular p.
    facultative p.
    hemic p.
    intermittent p.
    intracellular p.
    malarial p.
    metazoan p.
    obligate p.
    periodic p.
    permanent p.
    protozoan p.
    pubic p.
    p. screen
    spurious p.
    temporary p.
parasitemia
parasitic
    p. castration
    p. chylocele
    p. cyst
    p. disease
    p. ectopic pregnancy
    p. embolus
    p. fetus
    p. fibroma
    p. granuloma
    p. hemoptysis
    p. infection
    p. infestation
    p. leiomyoma
    p. thyroiditis
    p. twin
parasiticide
parasitism
parasitize
parasitoid mite
Parasitoidea
parasitologic
parasitologist
parasitology
parasol insertion
parasomnia
paraspadias

parasternal lymph node
parastriate area
parastruma
parasympathetic
    p. fiber
    p. nervous system
    p. paraganglioma
parasympatholytic
parasympathomimetic
parasynovitis
parataenial nucleus
paratenic host
paraterminal body
paratesticular
    p. fibroma
    p. fibrosarcoma
    p. histiocytoma
    p. hydrocele
    p. leiomyosarcoma
    p. lipoma
    p. liposarcoma
    p. mesothelioma
    p. neuroblastoma
    p. pseudofibroma
    p. rhabdomyosarcoma
parathion
    methyl p.
parathormone
parathyrin
parathyroid
    p. adenoma
    p. chief cell
    p. cyst
    p. extract
    p. gland
    p. hormone
    p. hormone secretion (rate)
    p. hyperplasia
    p. osteosis
    p. oxyphil cell
    p. transitional cell
    p. tumors
    p. wasserhelle cell
parathyroidectomy
parathyroidin
parathyroidoma
paratope
paratuberculous
    p. lymphadenitis
    p. pneumonia
paratyphi (*Salmonella*)
paratyphlitis

paratyphoid
    p. A and B
    p. fever
    p. immunization
paraurethral
    p. duct
    p. gland
paravaccinia
paravaginal incision
paravaginitis
paraventricular nucleus
paravirus
parchment
    p. heart
    p. skin
parectasis; parectasia
parenchyma
    hepatic p.
parenchymal infiltration
parenchymatitis
parenchymatous
    p. cell
    p. degeneration
    p. goiter
    p. keratitis
    p. mastitis
    p. neurosyphilis
parent cyst
parentage
parental generation
parenteral nutrition
paresis
    general p.
paresthesia
paretic neurosyphilis
pargyline
paries (pl., parietes)
parietal
    p. artery
    p. cancer
    p. cell
    p. cell antibody
    p. fistula
    p. gyrus
    p. lobe
    p. lobule
    p. pericardium
    p. peritoneum
    p. thrombus
parietoacanthal projection
parietography
parietomastoid suture

parieto-occipital
    p. artery
    p. fissure
    p. sulcus
parieto-orbital projection
parietotemporal projection
Paris
    classification
    green
    yellow
parity
    p. bit
    p. check
parkinsonian syndrome
parkinsonism
    idiopathic p.
    postencephalitic p.
Parkinson's facies
Park's aneurysm
Park-Williams fixative
parolfactory area
paromomycin sulfate
paromphalocele
paronychia
    herpetic p.
paroophoritic cyst
paroophoritis
paroophoron
parorchidium
parosmia
parosteal
    p. fasciitis
    p. osteoma
    p. osteosarcoma
paroosteitis
parosteosis; parostosis
parostitis
parotid
    p. abscess
    p. duct
    p. fascia
    p. gland
    p. lymph node
    p. papilla
parotidectomy
parotiditis
    postoperative p.
    punctate p.
parotitis
    infectious p.
    p. syndrome
    p. virus epidemic

parovarian cyst
parovaritis
parovirus
paroxysm
paroxysmal
    p. aciduria
    p. auricular tachycardia
    p. cold hemoglobinuria
    p. dyspnea
    p. hypertension
    p. myoglobinuria
    p. nocturnal dyspnea
    p. nocturnal hemoglobinuria
    p. ventricular tachycardia
parrot
    p. fever
    p. virus
pars (pl., partes)
    p. distalis
    p. flaccida
    p. intermedia
    p. nervosa
    p. tuberalis
part affected
parthenogenesis
parthenogenetic merogony
partial
    p. anomalous pulmonary venous connection
    p. identity pattern
    p. lipoatrophy
    p. lipodystrophy
    p. mastectomy
    p. obstruction
    p. pressure
    p. pressure of carbon dioxide
    p. pressure of nitrogen
    p. pressure of water vapor
    p. reaction of degeneration
    p. remission
    p.-thickness burn
    p. thromboplastin time
    p. thromboplastin time test
    p. trisomy
partially miscible
particle
    alpha p's
    p. beam radiotherapy
    beta p's
    carbon p's
    charged p.
    chromatin p's

p. concentration fluorescence immunoassay
Dane's p.
α-p. detector
elementary p.
p.-enhanced turbidimetric inhibition immunoassay
radioactive p's
silica p's
p. transport time
tubuloreticular p's
Zimmermann's elementary p.

particulate
p. crystalline material
p. crystalline material deposition
settled p's
suspended p's

partition
p. coefficient
oropharyngeal p.

parturition
parvicellular
parvilocular cyst
Parvobacteriaceae
parvoviral
Parvoviridae
parvovirus
Paryphostomum sufrartyfex
PAS — para-aminosalicylic acid
periodic acid-Schiff stain
pulmonary artery stenosis
PASA — para-aminosalicylic acid
PAS-C — para-aminosalicylic acid crystallized with ascorbic acid
pascal
PASM — periodic acid-silver methenamine
Passavant's bar
passenger leukocytes
passive
p. agglutination
p.-aggressive personality
p. anaphylaxis
p. Arthus reaction
p. congestion
p. cutaneous anaphylaxis
p. hemagglutination test
p. hemolysis
p. immunity
p. immunization

p. medium
p. sensitization
p. transfer
p. transport

Passovoy
defect
factor

Past. — *Pasturella*
Pasteurella
P. anapestifer
P. enterocolitica
P. haemolytica
P. multocida
P. pestis
P. pneumotropica
P. pseudotuberculosis
P. septica
P. tularensis
P. ureae

pasteurellosis
pasteurization
Pasteur's
effect
pipet
PAT — paroxysmal atrial tachycardia
patch
p. electrode
gray p.
herald p.
MacCallum's p.
mucous p.
Peyer's p's
salmon p.
shagreen p.
soldier's p's
p. test
white p.

patching
Patein's albumin
patella
patellar ligament
patent
p. ductus arteriosus
p. foramen ovale
p. urachus
paternity testing
path — pathology
pathobiology
pathogen
opportunistic p.
pathogenesis

pathogen-free
    specific p.-f.
pathogenetic
pathogenic
pathogenicity
    bacterial p.
pathognomonic
pathography
pathologic
    p. calcification
    p. cell
    p. diagnosis
    p. dislocation
    p. fracture
    p. glycosuria
    p. histology
    p. hyperplasia
    p. leukocytosis
    p. mitosis
    p. ovum
pathological anatomy
pathologist
pathology
    anatomic p.
    anatomical p.
    cellular p.
    clinical p.
    comparative p.
    dental p.
    experimental p.
    functional p.
    general p.
    geographic p.
    humoral p.
    internal p.
    medical p.
    molecular p.
    ophthalmic p.
    optical p.
    oral p.
    solidistic p.
    special p.
    speech p.
    surgical p.
pathomorphism
pathonomia; pathonomy
pathophysiologic
    p. history
    p. jaundice
pathophysiology
pathotype
pathovar

pathway
    afferent p.
    alternative p.
    alternative complement p.
    amphibolic p.
    auditory p.
    biosynthetic p.
    classical complement p.
    coagulation p.
    common p. of coagulation
    cyclooxygenase p.
    de nova p.
    efferent p.
    Embden-Meyerhof p.
    Entner-Doudoroff p.
    extrinsic p.
    final common p.
    gustatory p.
    hexose monophosphate p.
    internuncial p.
    intrinsic p.
    lipoxygenase p.
    metabolic p.
    motor p.
    olfactory p.
    pentose phosphate p.
    perforant p.
    perforating p.
    phosphogluconate oxidative p.
    reentrant p.
    sensory p.
    visual p.
pattern
    cribriform p.
    dirty fingers p.
    p. generator
    identity p.
    interference p.
    male sex chromatin p.
    mosaic p.
    partial identity p.
    polyvesicular-vitelline p.
    XX/XY sex chromosome p.
    Zellballen p.
patulous
pauciarthritis
pauciarticular
Paul-Bunnell
    antibodies
    test
Paul-Bunnell-Barrett test
Paul-Bunnell-Davidsohn test

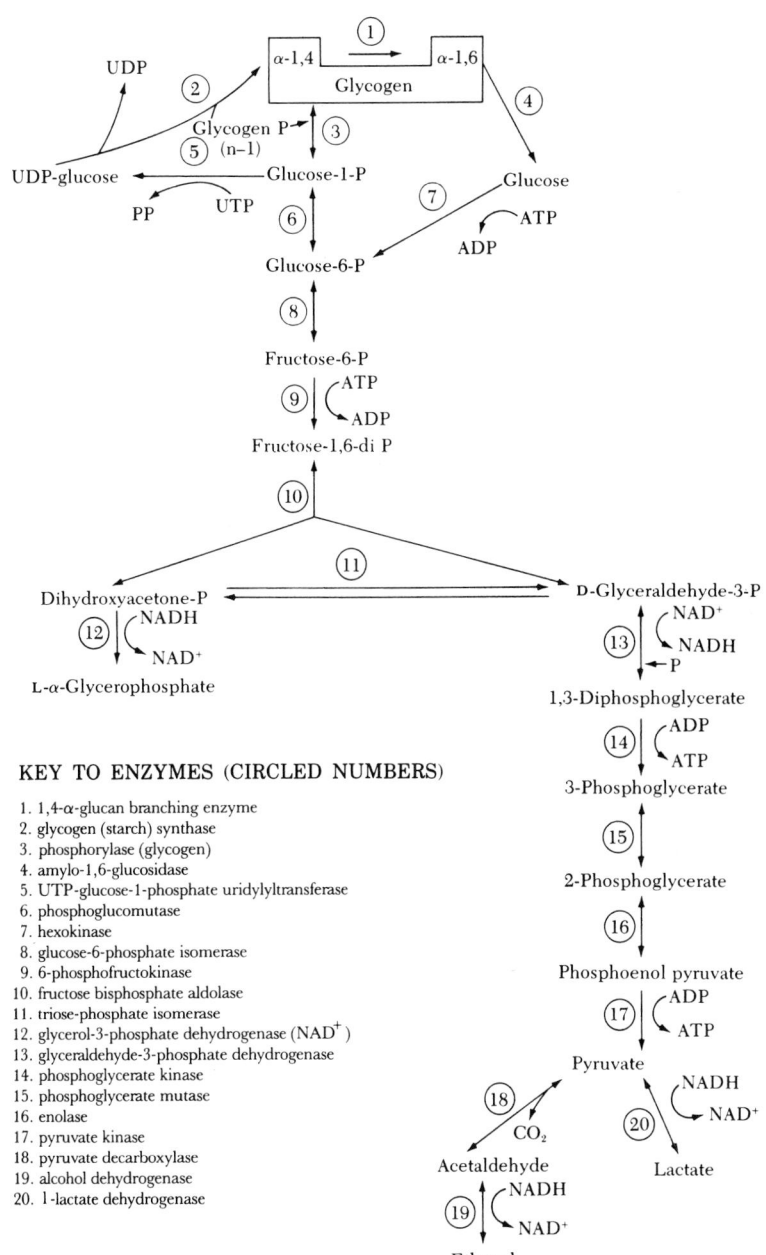

KEY TO ENZYMES (CIRCLED NUMBERS)

1. 1,4-α-glucan branching enzyme
2. glycogen (starch) synthase
3. phosphorylase (glycogen)
4. amylo-1,6-glucosidase
5. UTP-glucose-1-phosphate uridylyltransferase
6. phosphoglucomutase
7. hexokinase
8. glucose-6-phosphate isomerase
9. 6-phosphofructokinase
10. fructose bisphosphate aldolase
11. triose-phosphate isomerase
12. glycerol-3-phosphate dehydrogenase (NAD^+)
13. glyceraldehyde-3-phosphate dehydrogenase
14. phosphoglycerate kinase
15. phosphoglycerate mutase
16. enolase
17. pyruvate kinase
18. pyruvate decarboxylase
19. alcohol dehydrogenase
20. l-lactate dehydrogenase

Embden-Meyerhof pathway of glucose metabolism. (After Mazur and Harrow.) (From Dorland's Illustrated Medical Dictionary. 27th ed. Philadelphia. W. B. Saunders Company, 1988, p. 1293.)

paurometabolous
Pautrier's
    abscess
    microabscess
pavementing
Pavlov's pouch
Payr's clamp
PB — phenobarbital
    phonetically balanced
    protein binding
Pb — lead (plumbum)
PBA — pulpobuccoaxial
PBC — primary biliary cirrhosis
PBF — pulmonary blood flow
PBG — porphobilinogen
PBI — protein-bound iodine
PBI test
P-50 blood gas
P blood group
PBN — paralytic brachial neuritis
PBO — penicillin in beeswax
    placebo
PBS — phosphate-buffered saline
PBT_4 — protein-bound thyroxine
PBV — predicted blood volume
    pulmonary blood volume
PBZ — pyribenzamine
PC — pentose cycle
    phosphate cycle
        phosphatidylcholine
    phosphocreatine
    platelet concentrate
    platelet count
    portacaval
    printed circuit
    pubococcygeus
    pulmonic closure
pc — picocurie
PCA — passive cutaneous anaphy-
    laxis
PCB — paracervical block
    polychlorinated biphenyl
PcB — near point of convergence
PCC — prothrombin complex concen-
    trate
PCc — periscopic concave
PCD — phosphate-citrate-dextrose
    polycystic disease
    posterior corneal deposits
P-cell growth factor
P cells
PCF — posterior cranial fossa

PCFIA — particle concentration fluo-
    rescence immunoassay
PCG — phonocardiogram
PCH — paroxysmal cold hemoglo-
    binuria
pCi — picocurie
PCM — protein-calorie malnutrition
PCN — penicillin
PCNA — proliferating cell nuclear
    antigen
PCO_2 or pCO_2 — carbon dioxide
    pressure
P component
PCP — parachlorophenate
    pentachlorophenol
    phencyclidine
    Pneumocystis carinii
    pneumonia
PCPA — parachlorophenylalanine
PCR — plasma clearance rate
    polymerase chain reaction
PCS — portacaval shunt
pcs — preconscious
PCT — plasmacrit
    porphyria cutanea tarda
    portacaval transposition
    prothrombin consumption
    time
PCV — packed cell volume
    polycythemia vera
PCV-M — myeloid metaplasia with
    polycythemia vera
PCx — periscopic convex
PD — papilla diameter
    Parkinson's disease
    patent ductus
    phosphate dehydrogenase
    plasma defect
    prism diopter
    pulmonary disease
    pulpodistal
    pupillary distance
Pd — palladium
PDA — patent ductus arteriosus
PDAB — para-dimethylamino-benzal-
    dehyde
PDD — pyridoxine-deficient diet
PDGF — platelet-derived growth
    factor
PDH — phosphate dehydrogenase
pdl — pudendal
PDLL — poorly differentiated lympho-
    cytic lymphoma

PDP — piperidino-pyrimidine
PDT — photodynamic therapy
PE — pharyngoesophageal
phenylephrine
phosphatidylethanolamine
photographic effect
plasma exchange
pleural effusion
polyethylene
pulmonary edema
pulmonary embolism
pea
 rosary p.
peak
 absorption p.
 p. acid output
 p. broadening
 coincidence sum p.
 p. expiratory flow rate
 p. height
 iodine escape p.
 kilovolt p.
 p. kilovoltage
 p.-to-peak amplitude
 p. transmittance
pearl
 epithelial p's
 keratin p's
 Laënnec's p's
 squamous p.
 p. tumor
pearl-worker's disease
pearly penile papilloma
Pearson's coefficient
peau d'orange
PEBG — phenethylbiguanide
peccary
Pecquet's reservoir
pectenitis
pectenosis
pectin
pectinate
 p. body
 p. ligament
pectinesterase
pectineus muscle
Pectinibranchiata
Pectobacterium carotovorum
pectoral
 p. fascia
 p. lymph node
 p. muscle

pectus
 p. carinatum
 p. excavatum
 p. gallinatum
 p. recurvatum
pederin
Pediatric Oncology Group
pediatrics
pedicel
 glomerular p.
pedicellate
pedicellation
pedicle
pediculate
Pediculoides ventricosus
pediculosis
Pediculus
 P. humanus
 P. humanus capitis
 P. humanus corporis
 P. inguinalis
 P. pubis
pedigree chart
pedogenesis
pedophilia
peduncle
 cerebellar p.
 cerebral p.
 p. of flocculus
 inferior p.
 mamillary p.
peduncular nucleus
pedunculate
pedunculated
 p. leiomyoma
 p. polyp
pedunculus
peeling
PEEP — positive end-expiratory
  pressure
PEF — peak expiratory flow
PEFR — peak expiratory flow rate
PEG — pneumoencephalography
  polyethylene glycol
peg
 rete p's
PEI — phosphate excretion index
pelargonate
 zinc p.
pelargonic acid
Pel-Ebstein fever
Pelecypoda

Pelger-Huët
  anomaly
  nuclear anomaly
peliosis
  p. hepatis
  p. hepatitis
pellagra
  p. preventive
  p. sine pellagra
pelletierine
pellicle
pellicular; pelliculous
pellucid
pelvic
  p. abscess
  p. bones
  p. cellulitis
  p. endometriosis
  p. fascia
  p. girdle
  p. inflammatory disease
  p. kidney
  p. lipomatosis
  p. lymph node
  p. organs
  p. peritoneal cavity
  p. peritoneum
  p. plexus
pelvicephalography
pelvicephalometry
pelvimetry
pelvioradiography
pelviradiography
pelvirectal achalasia
pelvis (pl., pelves)
  beaked p.
  caoutchouc p.
  frozen p.
  hardened p.
  kyphoscoliotic p.
  kyphotic p.
  lordotic p.
  p. major
  p. minor
  Nägele's p.
  p. obtecta
  osteomalacic p.
  Otto p.
  Prague p.
  pseudo-osteomalacic p.
  rachitic p.
  renal p.

  Robert's p.
  Rokitansky's p.
  rostrate n.
  rubber p.
  scoliotic p.
  spider p.
  split p.
  spondylolisthetic p.
pelviureteroradiography
pelvospondylitis ossificans
Pemberton's sign
pemphigoid
  benign mucosal p.
  bullous p.
  cicatricial p.
pemphigus
  p. antibodies
  benign mucous membrane p.
  p. crouposus
  p. erythematosus
  familial benign p.
  p. foliaceus
  p. leprosus
  p. neonatorum
  ocular p.
  p. vegetans
  p. vulgaris
pen
  light p.
pen — penicillin
pencil dosimeter
pendulous heart
penetrability
penetrance
  complete p.
  incomplete p.
penetrating
  p. radiation
  p. ulcer
  p. wound
penetrometer
Penfield's method
D-penicillamine
penicillin
  p. G
  p. V
penicillinase test
penicillin-fast
penicillinosis
Penicillium
  P. barbae
  P. bouffardi

P. cyclopium
P. minimum
P. montoyai
P. notatum
P. patulum
P. spinulosum
penicillus (pl., penicilli)
penile
    p. acanthosis
    p. artery
    p. erection
    p. fascia
    p. fibromatosis
    p. horn
    p. papule
    p. plaque
    p. prosthesis
    p. shaft
    p. urethra
    p. vein
penis
    corpus cavernosum of p.
    glans of p.
    ligament of p.
    radix p.
    raphe p.
    spade p.
penitis
Penn's seroflocculation reaction
penoscrotal
    p. lymphedema
    p. transposition
pent — pentothal
pentachloroethane
pentachloronitrobenzene
pentachlorophenol
pentaene
pentaerythritol tetranitrate
pentagastrin test
Pentam 300
pentamer
pentamethyl violet
pentamidine isethionate
pentane
pentasodium tripolyphosphate
Pentastoma
    P. constrictum
    P. denticulatum
    P. taenioides
pentastomiasis
Pentastomida
Pentatrichomonas ardin delteili

pentatrichomoniasis
pentavalent
penta-X chromosomal aberration
pentazocine
    p. hydrochloride
    p. lactate
pentene
penthienate bromide
pentobarbital
pentolinium tartrate
pentolysis
pentosan
pentosazon
pentose
    p. phosphate pathway
    p. shunt
pentosealdolase
pentose-phosphate shunt
pentoside
pentosuria
    alimentary p.
    essential p.
    idiopathic p.
    primary p.
pentosyltransferase
pentoxide
    nitrogen p.
pentulose
pentylenetetrazol
PEO — progressive external ophthal-
        moplegia
PEP — phosphoenolpyruvate
        pre-ejection period
PEPP — positive expiratory pressure
        plateau
Pepper's tumor
pepsin
    p. A
    p. B
    p. C
pepsinogen
    p. assay
    plasma p.
pepsinuria
peptic
    p. cell
    p. esophagitis
    p. ulcer
peptid or peptide
    opioid p.
peptidase
    leucine amino p.
    procollagen-p.

peptide
>   atrial natriuretic p.
>   p. bond
>   C p.
>   calcitonin p.
>   calcitonin gene-related p.
>   chemotactic p.
>   corticotropin-like intermediate
>   lobe p.
>   gastrin-releasing p.
>   p. group
>   p. hormone
>   p. hydrolase
>   immunoreactive p.
>   intestinal p.
>   p. linkages
>   p. peptidohydrolase
>   phenylthiocarbamoyl p.
>   procollagen III p.
>   signal p.
>   p. synthetase
>   thymic p's
>   vasoactive p.
peptidergic nervous system
peptidoglycan
peptidyldipeptide hydrolase
Peptococcaceae
Peptococcus
>   *P. anaerobius*
>   *P. ascaccharolyticus*
>   *P. constellatus*
>   *P. magnus*
>   *P. prevotii*
peptone shock
Peptostreptococcus
>   *P. anaerobius*
>   *P. intermedius*
>   *P. lanceolatus*
>   *P. micros*
>   *P. prevotii*
>   *P. productus*
PER — protein efficiency ratio
peracetic
>   p. acid
>   p. acid-Schiff reaction
peracid
perambulating ulcer
perbromate
percentile
perception
perchlorate
>   p. discharge test
>   potassium p.

perchloric acid
perchlormethane
perchloroethane
perchloroethylene
percolate
percolation
per contiguum
per continuum
percussion
>   auscultatory p.
>   p. wave
percutaneous
>   p. renal puncture
>   p. transhepatic cholangiog-
>   raphy
>   p. umbilical blood sampling
perester
Perez's sign
perfect yeast
perfluorocarbons
perforant pathway
perforated
>   p. diverticulitis
>   p. gastric ulcer
>   p. ulcer
perforating
>   p. abscess
>   p. fasciculus
>   p. fibers of Sharpey
>   p. pathway
>   p. ulcer
>   p. wound
perforation
>   inflammatory p.
perforin
performance
>   p. testing
>   ventricular p.
performic
>   p. acid
>   p. acid reaction
>   p. acid-Schiff reaction
performin
perfusate
perfuse
perfusion
>   organ p.
>   p. pressure
>   pulmonary p.
periadenitis
periampullary cancer
periamygdaloid area

perianal
periangiocholitis
periangitis
periaortic
periaortitis
periapical
    p. abscess
    p. granuloma
periappendiceal abscess
periappendicitis decidualis
periarterial
periarteritis
    p. gummosa
    p. nodosa
    syphilitic p.
periarthritis
periarticular abscess
periaxial neuropathy
peribronchial
peribronchiolitis
peribronchitis
pericanalicular fibroadenoma
pericapillary end foot
pericardia
percardial
    p. artery
    p. cavity
    p. compression
    p. cyst
    p. effusion
    p. fluid
    p. fluid examination
    p. friction rub
    p. mesothelium
    p. sac
    p. serum
    p. tamponade
    p. tuberculosis
    p. vein
pericardiocentesis
pericardiophrenic
pericarditic
pericarditis
    acute p.
    adherent p.
    adhesive p.
    bacterial p.
    bread and butter p.
    carcinomatous p.
    caseous p.
    chronic constrictive p.
    constrictive p.

fibrinous p.
fungal p.
healed p.
hemorrhagic p.
idiopathic p.
internal adhesive p.
mediastinal p.
p. obliterans
obliterative p.
purulent p.
radiation p.
restrictive p.
rheumatic p.
serofibrinous p.
p. sicca
suppurative p.
tuberculous p.
uremic p.
p. villosa
viral p.
pericardium (pl., pericardia)
    adherent p.
    p. fibrosum
    fibrous p.
    parietal p.
    serofibrinous effusion p.
    p. serosum
    serous p.
    shaggy p.
    visceral p.
pericentral fibrosis
pericholangitis
perichondritis
    relapsing p.
perichondrium
perichondroma
perichromatin granule
pericolic
pericolitis
    p. dextra
    p. sinistra
pericolonitis
pericolpitis
pericryptal fibroblasts
pericystitis
pericystium
pericyte
    p. degeneration
    Rouget's p.
    p. of Zimmermann
pericytoma
peridesmitis

perididymitis
peridiverticulitis
periductal mastitis
periduodenitis
peridurogram
peridurography
periencephalography
perienteritis
periepithelioma
periesophageal
periesophagitis
perifocal
perifollicular
perifolliculitis
perifornical nucleus
perigastritis
periglandulitis
periglomerular cells
perihepatic
perihepatitis
    gonococcal p.
perijejunitis
perikaryon
perilymph
perilymphangitis
perilymphatic labyrinth
perimetritis
perimetrium
perimuscular fibrosis
perimyelitis
perimyelography
perimyoendocarditis
perimyositis
perimysiitis; perimysitis
perimysium (pl., perimysia)
perinatal
    p. death
    p. infection
    p. mortality rate
    p. septicemia
    p. syphilis
perinea
perineal
    p. artery
    p. nerve
perineovaginal fistula
perinephric abscess
perinephritis
perineum (pl., perinea)
    watering-can p.
perineural
    p. fibroblastoma
    p. fibrosarcoma

perineurium
perineuronal satellite cell
perinuclear
    p. cisterna
    p. space
period
    eclipse p.
    effective refractory p.
    incubation p.
    isometric p.
    latency p.
    p. of ventricular filling
    refractory p.
    relative refractory p.
periodate oxidation
periodic
    p. acid
    p. acid-Schiff method
    p. acid-Schiff reaction
    p. acid-Schiff stain
    p. acid-Schiff technique
    p. acid-Schiff test
    p. acid-silver methenamine
    p. disease
    p. edema
    p. neutropenia
    p. paralysis, familial
    p. parasite
    p. syndrome
    p. wave
periodicity
periodontal
    p. cyst
    p. disease
    p. pack
    p. tissues
periodontitis
periodontium
periodontology
perionychium
perioophoritis
perioophorosalpingitis
periorbital edema
periorchitis
    chronic proliferative p.
    p. hemorrhagica
    meconium p.
    nodular p.
periorificial lentiginosis
periosteal
    p. chondroma
    p. chondrosarcoma

p. desmoid
p. fibroma
p. fibrosarcoma
p. ganglion
p. implantation
p. osteosarcoma
p. reflex
p. sarcoma
periosteitis fibrosa
periosteoma
periosteomedullitis
periosteomyelitis
periosteophyte
periosteosis
periosteum
    alveolar p.
periostitis
periostoma; periosteoma
periostosis (pl., periostoses)
periostosteitis
periovaritis
peripancreatic
peripancreatitis
peripapillary
peripartum cardiomyopathy
peripeduncular nucleus
peripelvic lymphangioma
peripheral
    p. ameloblastoma
    p. aneurysm
    p. arterial occlusive disease
    p. arteriosclerotic occlusive
      disease
    p. blood
    p. blood preparation
    p. blood smear
    p. chemoreceptors
    p. cholangiopancreatography
    p. chondrosarcoma
    p. circulatory failure
    p. dysostosis
    p. edema
    p. giant cell granuloma
    p. lesion
    p. lobule
    p. motor structure
    p. necrosis
    p. nerve
    p. nervous system
    p. neuralgia
    p. neuroectodermal tumor
    p. neuropathy

p. odontogenic fibroma
p. perfusion scan
p. polyneuropathy
p. proteins
p. resistance
p. resistance unit
p. sensory structure
p. total resistance
p. vascular disease
p. vein plasma
periphery
periphlebitic
periphlebitis
Periplaneta
periplasm
periplasmic
periplast
peripolesis
periporitis
periportal
    p. bile ductule
    p. cardiomyopathy
    p. necrosis
periproctitis
periprostatic
periprostatitis
peripylephlebitis
perirectal abscess
perirectitis
perirenal
    p. insufflation
    p. urinoma
perisalpingo-ovaritis
perisigmoiditis
perispermatitis serosa
perisplanchnitis
perisplenic
perisplenitis
    hyaline p.
peristalsis
    reverse p.
    ureteral p.
peristaltic
    p. disorder
    p. reflex
peristasis
peristatic hyperemia
periston
peristrumous
perisynovial
peritendineum

peritendinitis
  p. calcarea
  p. serosa
peritenontitis
perithecium
perithelial
perithelioma
perithyroidal
  p. lymph nodes
  p. thymoma
perithyroiditis
peritoneal
  p. cancer
  p. cavity
  p. dialysis
  p. effusion
  p. exudates
  p. fluid
  p. fluid examination
  p. hemodialysis
  p. hernia
  p. lavage
  p. mesothelioma
  p. mesothelium
  p. sac
  p. transudate
peritoneography
  positive contrast p.
peritoneopathy
peritoneoplasty
peritoneoscopy
peritoneum
  parietal p.
peritonitis
  acute diffuse p.
  adhesive p.
  amebic p.
  bacterial p.
  bile p.
  chemical p.
  chyle p.
  circumscribed p.
  p. deformans
  diaphragmatic p.
  diffuse p.
  p. encapsulans
  fibrinous p.
  fibrocaseous p.
  gas p.
  general p.
  gonococcal p.
  localized p.

  meconium p.
  pneumococcal p.
  productive p.
  sclerosing p.
  septic p.
  tuberculous p.
peritonsillar
  p. abscess
  p. tissue
peritracheal
peritrichous
periungual fibroma
periureteral abscess
periureteritis plastica
periurethral
  p. abscess
  p. duct
  p. expansion
periurethritis
perivaginitis
perivascular cuffs
perivasculitis
perivenous encephalomyelitis
periventricular
  p. arcuate nucleus
  p. gray matter
  p. leukomalacia
perivesical
perivisceritis
perlèche
Perlmann's tumor
Perls'
  iron test
  Prussian blue stain
  reaction
permanent parasite
permanganate
  potassium p.
permeability
  p. quotient
  p. of vacuum
  vascular p.
permeable
permease
permeation
permissible exposure limits
permissive culture media
permittivity of vacuum
permselectivity
permutation
Permutit
perniciosiform

pernicious
  p. anemia
  p. anemia-type metarubricyte
  p. anemia-type prorubricyte
  p. anemia-type rubriblast
  p. leukopenia
  p. malaria
pernio (pl., perniones)
perniosis
peromelia
peroneal
  p. artery
  p. muscle
  p. muscle tendon
  p. muscular atrophy
  p. nerve
  p. vein
Peronosporales
peroral
  p. dilatation
  p. endoscopy
perosseous
peroxidase
  p.-antiperoxidase
  benzidine method for myoglo-
    bin p.
  glutathione p.
  hepatocatalase p.
  horseradish p.
  iodide p.
  p. reaction
  p. stain
  p. staining methods
peroxidase-antiperoxidase
  p.-a. complex
  p.-a. technique
peroxidation
  lipid p.
peroxide
  acyl p.
  alkyl p.
  hydrogen p.
  zinc p.
peroxisome
peroxyacetic acid
peroxyacetyl nitrate
peroxyacylnitrate
perpad — perineal pad
perpendicular fasciculus
perphenazine
per second
perseveration

persistent
  p. chronic hepatitis
  p. cloaca
  p. eosinophilia
  p. filaria
  p. generalized lymphade-
    nopathy
  p. proteinuria
  p. tolerant infection
  p. truncus arteriosus
  p. urachus
  p. viral disease
persister
personality
  compulsive p.
  cyclothymic p.
  hypomanic p.
  inadequate p.
  obsessive-compulsive p.
  paranoid p.
  passive-aggressive p.
  phobic p.
  psychopathic p.
  schizoid p.
perspiration
PERT — program evaluation and re-
    view technique
pertechnetate
Perthane
Pertik's diverticulum
Pertofrane
pertussis
  p. serology
  p. vaccine
perversion
pes (gen., pedis; pl., pedes)
  p. cavus
  p. febricitans
  p. valgus
pessary
  p. cell
  p. corpuscle
pesticemia
pesticide
  chlorinated hydrocarbon p.
  cyclodiene hydrocarbon p's
  organo-chloro p's
PET — positron-emission tomography
    pre-eclamptic toxemia
peta
petechia (pl., petechiae)
  Tardieu's petechiae

petechial
  p. angiomas
  p. hemorrhage
petechiasis
PETINIA — particle-enhanced turbidimetric inhibition immunoassay
petit mal epilepsy
PETN — pentaerythritol tetranitrate
Petragnani medium
Petri
  dish
  test
petrichloral
petriellidiosis
Petriellidium boydii
petrifaction
petrolatum
  hydrophilic p.
petroleum
  p. ether
  p. jelly
petro-occipital synchondrosis
petrosal
  p. nerve
  p. sinus
petrositis
petrosphenoidal
petrous
  p. bone
  p. ganglion
petrositis
PETT — positron emission transverse tomography
Peutz-Jeghers polyp
pexis
Peyer's patches
peyote
Pezizales
PF — peritoneal fluid
  platelet factor
pF — picofarad
P factor
PFAS — performic acid-Schiff reaction
PFC — perfluorocarbons
  plaque-forming cell
Pfeiffer-Comberg method
Pfeiffer's
  bacillus
  blood agar
  phenomenon

PFGE — pulsed field gradient gel electrophoresis
PFIB — perfluoroisobutylene
PFK — phosphofructokinase
PFO — patent foramen ovale
PFP — platelet-free plasma
PFR — peak flow rate
PFS — primary fibromyalgia syndrome
PFT — posterior fossa tumor
  pulmonary function test
PFU — plaque-forming units
PG — phosphatidylglycerol
  plasma triglyceride
  prostaglandin
  pyoderma gangrenosum
pg — picogram
PGA — pteroylglutamic acid
PGD — phosphogluconate dehydrogenase
  phosphoglyceraldehyde dehydrogenase
PGDH — phosphogluconate dehydrogenase
PGDR — plasma-glucose disappearance rate
PGH — pituitary growth hormone
PGI — potassium, glucose, and insulin
PGK — phosphoglycerate kinase
PGL — persistent generalized lymphadenopathy
P-glycoprotein
PGM — phosphoglucomutase
PGO — ponto-geniculo-occipital
PGP — postgamma proteinuria
PgR — progesterone receptor
PGTR — plasma glucose tolerance rate
PH — pharmacopeia
  prostatic hypertrophy
  pulmonary hypertension
Ph — phenyl
Ph¹ — Philadelphia chromosome
pH — hydrogen ion concentration
PHA — passive hemagglutination
  phytohemagglutinin
  pulse height analyzer
phacoanaphylactic endophthalmitis
phacoanaphylaxis
phacoid
phacolytic glaucoma
phacoma

phacomalacia
phacomatosis
    neurocutaneous p.
phacosclerosis
Phaenicia sericata
phaeohyphomycosis
phaeomycotic cyst
phage
    p. genetics
    temperate p.
    p. typing
phagedena gangrenosa
phagedenic ulcer
phage-resistant mutation
phagocyte
    alveolar p.
    endothelial p.
    globuliferous p.
    melaniferous p.
    mononuclear p.
    sessile p.
phagocytic
    p. cell immunocompetence
      profile
    p. index
phagocytoblast
phagocytolysis
phagocytolytic
phagocytosis
    induced p.
    vacuole alteration p.
phagolysis
phagolysosome
phagolytic
phagosome
phakoma
phakomatosis
phalangeal
phalanx (gen., phalangis; pl.,
    phalanges)
    tufted p.
phallitis
phalloidin
phalloncus
phallus
pH (hydrogen ion concentration) al-
    teration
phaneroplasm
phanerosis
phantom
    p. bar
    p. corpuscle
    p. four-quadrant bar

    Hine-Duley p.
    p. limb
    p. spike and wave
    p. tumor
pharmacodynamics
pharmacogenetics
pharmacokinetics
pharmacologic
pharmacology
pharmacopeia
pharyngeal
    p. aponeurosis
    p. artery
    p. auditory tube ostium
    p. blister
    p. branch
    p. calculus
    p. carcinoma
    p. cavity
    p. fibrosarcoma
    p. fornix
    p. glands
    p. gonorrhea
    p. herpes
    p. hypophysis
    p. isthmus
    p. lipoma
    p. mucous gland
    p. mucous membrane
    p. mucus
    p. muscle
    p. pouch
    p. recess
    p. submucosa
    p. tonsil
    p. tubal ostium
    p. tubercle
pharyngectasia
pharyngectomy
pharyngemphraxis
pharyngitic
pharyngitis
    atrophic p.
    croupous p.
    follicular p.
    gangrenous p.
    glandular p.
    gonococcal p.
    granular p.
    p. herpetica
    p. hypertrophica lateralis
    membranous p.

p. sicca
staphylococcal p.
streptococcal p.
viral p.
Pharyngobdellida
pharyngoconjunctival
    p. fever
    p. fever virus
pharyngocutaneous fistula
pharyngodynia
pharyngoesophageal diverticulum
pharyngogastrostomy
pharyngokeratosis
pharyngolaryngitis
pharyngolith
pharyngopalatine
pharyngoparalysis
pharyngopathy
pharyngorhinitis
pharyngoscleroma
pharyngostenosis
pharyngostoma
pharyngostomy
pharyngotonsillitis
pharyngotympanic tube
pharynx (pl., pharynges)
    oral p.
phase
    continuous p.
    p. contrast microscopy
    disperse p.
    ejection p.
    exponential p.
    G_0 p.
    G_1 p.
    G_2 p.
    inductive p.
    p. lag
    lag p.
    logarithmic p.
    M p.
    meiotic p.
    mobile p.
    moving p.
    radial growth p.
    S p.
    single p.
    stationary p.
    ventricular filling p.
    vertical growth p.
phasmid
Phasmidia

PHBB — propylhydroxybenzyl benzimidazole
Ph^1 (Philadelphia) chromosome
Phe — phenylalanine
phenacaine hydrochloride
phenacemide
phenacetin breath test
phenaceturic acid
phenaglycodol
phenanthrene
o-phenanthroline
phenazocine
phenazopyridine hydrochloride
phencyclidine assay
phendimetrazine
phene
phenelzine sulfate
phenethicillin
phenethylamine
phenoformin hydrochloride
phenindamine tartrate
phenindione
pheniramine maleate
Phenistix
    reagent strip
    test
phenmetrazine hydrochloride
phenobarbital assay
phenocopy
phenodeviant
phenogenetics
phenol
    p. coefficient
    p. liquefactum
    methyl p.
    p. salicylate
    p. sulfatase
phenolemia
phenolic esterase
phenoloxidase production test
phenolphthalein
    p. indicator
    p. test
phenolsulfonate
    zinc p.
phenolsulfonphthalein test
phenoluria
phenom; phenon
phenomenology
    Bowditch staircase p.
phenomenon (pl., phenomena)
    Arias-Stella p.

Bordet-Gengou p.
Danysz p.
Donath-Landsteiner p.
Felton p.
Gardos' p.
Hamburger's p.
Houssay's p.
Huebener-Thomsen-
    Friedenreich p.
jodbasedow p.
Kanagawa p.
Koebner's p.
LE (cell) p.
Lucio's p.
no reflow p.
Pfeiffer's p.
prozone p.
Raynaud's p.
Sanarelli-Shwartzman p.
Shwartzman's p.
second-set p.
Splendore-Hoeppli p.
vacuum p.
phenothiazine
    p. tranquilizers
    p. tranquilizers assay
phenothioxin
phenotype
    Bombay p.
    dominant p.
    Fredrickson's p.
    male p.
    McLeod p.
    murine T cell p.
    secretor p.
phenotypic
    p. adaptation
    p. variance
phenoxybenzamine hydrochloride
phenoxyethanol
phenoxypenicillin
phenprocoumon
phensuximide
phentermine
phentolamine
    p. hydrochloride
    p. mesylate
    p. test
phenyl
    p. cyclohexanol
    p. dimethyl urea
    p. mercuric acetate

p. mercuric chloride
p. mercuric salt
p. paraaminosalicylate
p. salicylate
N-phenylacetamide
phenylacetic acid
phenylacetylglutamine
phenylalanine
    p. agar
    p. assay
    p. deaminase agar slant
    p. hydroxylase deficiency
    p.-4-monooxygenase
    p. mustard
    p.-phenazone
    p. test
    p. tolerance index
phenylalanyl
phenylamine
phenylaminopropane
phenylbutazone assay
phenylcarbinol
phenyldiphenyloxadiazole
p-phenylenediamine
phenylephrine
    p. bitartrate
    p. hydrobromide
    p. hydrochloride
    p. tannate
phenylethanolamine-N-methyl trans-
    ferase
phenylethyl
    p. alcohol agar
    p. alcohol blood agar
phenylethylhydantoin
    methyl p.
phenylhydrazine anemia
phenylketonuria test
phenyllactate
    testosterone p.
phenyllactic acid
phenylmercuric
    p. nitrate
    p. triethanol ammonium
        lactate
o-phenylphenol
phenylphosphate
phenylpropanolamine
phenylpropylmethylamine
phenylpyruvate tautomerase
phenylpyruvic
    p. acid

p. acid test
p. oligophrenia
phenylpyruvicaciduria
phenylthiocarbamide
phenylthiocarbamoyl peptide
phenylthiourea
phenyltoloxamine
phenyramidol hydrochloride
phenytoin assay
pheochrome cell
pheochromoblast
pheochromoblastoma
pheochromocyte
pheochromocytoma
adrenal p.
pheomelanin
pheresis
pheromone
PHI — phosphohexose isomerase
phialide
Phialophora
P. compactum
P. dermatitidis
P. gougerotii
P. jeanselmei
P. mutabilis
P. parasitica
P. repens
P. richardsiae
P. spinifera
P. verrucosa
phialophore
phialospore
Phi body
Philip's glands
philtrum
phimosis
pH indicator
PHK — platelet phosphohexokinase
PHLA — postheparin lipolytic activity
phlebarteriectasia
phlebectasia
phlebectopia; phlebectopy
phlebemphraxis
phlebeurysm
phlebismus
phlebitic
phlebitis
adhesive p.
anemic p.
migratory p.

p. nodularis necrotisans
puerperal p.
septic p.
sinus p.
phlebogram
phlebography
phlebolite
phlebolith
phlebolithiasis
phlebometritis
phlebomyomatosis
phleborheography
phlebosclerosis
phlebostenosis
phlebothrombosis
Phlebotominae
phlebotomist
Phlebotomus
P. argentipes
P. chinensis
P. intermedius
P. macedonicum
P. noguchi
P. papatasii
P. sergenti
P. verrucarum
P. vexator
phlebotomus
p. fever
p. fever virus
phlebotomy
phlegm
phlegmasia
p. alba dolens
p. alba dolens puerperarum
cellulitic p.
p. cerulea dolens
p. dolens
p. malabarica
thrombotic p.
phlegmon
diffuse p.
emphysematous p.
gas p.
streptococcal p.
phlegmonous
p. abscess
p. adenitis
p. cellulitis
p. enteritis
p. gastritis

p. mastitis
p. ulcer
pH level
phlogocyte
phlogocytosis
phlogogenic; phlogogenous
phloridzin; phlorhizin; phlorizin
    p. diabetes
    p. glycosuria
phloroglucin
phloroglucinol
phloroglucol
phloxine B
phloxine-tartrazine stain
phlyctenular
    p. conjunctivitis
    p. keratoconjunctivitis
phlyctenule
phlyctenulosis
Phobetron
phobic
    p. personality
    p. psychoneurosis
Phocanema
phocomelia
phocomelic dwarfism
pholcodine
Phoma hibernica
phonation
phonendoscope
phonoangiography
phonoauscultation
phonocardiography
phonocatheterization
phonogram
phorate
phorbol ester
Phoridae
Phormia
phoroblast
phorocyte
phorocytosis
phosgene
phosphagen
phosphatase
    acid p.
    alkaline p.
    bisphosphoglycerate p.
    diphosphoglycerate p.
    leukocyte alkaline p.
    neutrophil alkaline p.
    placental alkaline p.

    prostatic acid p.
    protein-specific acid p.
    serum p.
    serum alkaline p.
    p. test
    total serum prostatic acid p.
    p. unit
phosphate
    acid p.
    aminohydroxypropilidene p.
    ammonium magnesium p.
    p. assay
    p. buffer
    calcium p.
    carbamoyl p.
    carbamyl p.
    creatine p.
    deoxyguanosine p.
    deoxyuridine p.
    p. diabetes
    dihydroxyacetone p.
    disodium hydrogen p.
    dolichol p.
    energy rich p.
    p. excretion index
    p. group transfer potential
    guanidine p.
    guanosine p.
    high-energy p.
    histamine acid p.
    inorganic p.
    Krebs-Ringer p.
    magnesium ammonium p.
    mercuric p.
    nicotinamide adenine dinucleotide p.
    organic p.
    potassium dihydrogen p.
    primaquine p.
    ribose 5-p.
    tribasic calcium p.
    tricresyl p.
    tri-*o*-cresyl p.
    triple p.
    tris (2,3-dibromopropyl) p.
    trisodium p.
    undecaprenol p.
    xanthosine p.
    zephiran-trisodium p.
phosphatemia
phosphatid histiocytosis
phosphatase

phosphatidate
phosphatidic acid
phosphatid-type histiocytosis
phosphatidylcholine-cholesterol acyl-
    transferase
phosphatidylethanolamine
phosphatidylglycerol
phosphatidylinositide
phosphatidylinositol 4,5-bisphosphate
1-phosphatidylinositol phosphodies-
    terase
phosphatidylserine
phosphaturia
phosphide
    zinc p.
phosphine
phosphoadenosine diphosphosulfate
phosphoadenosine phosphosulfate
3'-phosphoadenosine-5'-
    phosphosulfate
phosphoadenylate 3-nucleotidase
phosphoamidase
phosphocholine
phosphocreatine
phosphodiester
phosphodiesterase
    sphingomyelin p.
phosphoenolpyruvate
phosphoethanolamine
phosphofluoridate
    diisopropyl p.
6-phosphofructokinase
phosphofructokinase deficiency
phosphogalactose-uridyl-transferase
phosphoglucokinase
phosphoglucomutase
phosphogluconate
    p. dehydrogenase assay
    p. oxidative pathway
phosphogluconic acid
6-phospho-D-gluconolactone
phosphoglyceraldehyde
2-phospho-D-glycerate
6-phosphoglycerate
    p. dehydrogenase
    p. kinase
    p. mutase
    p. phosphomutase
phosphoglyceric acid
phosphoglycerides
phosphoglyceromutase
phosphoguanidine

phosphohexoisomerase
phosphohexokinase
phosphohexose isomerase deficiency
phosphoinositide
phosphoketolase
phosphokinase
    creatine p., B
    creatine p., MB
    serum creatine p.
phospholamban
phospholipase
    p. A
    p. A_2
    p. B
    p. C
    p. D
phospholipid
    p. assay
    p. methylation
    p. staining
    p. test
    p.-type anticoagulant
    p. vesicle
phosphomevalonate kinase
phosphomevalonic acid
5-phosphomevalonic acid
phosphomolybdate
phosphomolybdic acid
phosphomonoester
phosphomonoesterase
phosphonic acid
phosphonoacetic acid
phosphonoformate
    trisodium p.
phosphopantetheine
4'-phosphopantetheine
phosphopantothenoylcysteine syn-
    thetase
phosphoprotein
phosphopyridoxal
phosphopyruvate
    p. carboxylase
    p. hydratase (enolase)
phosphor
phosphoramide mustard
phosphorescence
phosphorescent
5-phosphoriboisomerase
phosphoribokinase
phosphoribosyl
    p.-formylglycineamidine syn-
        thetase

p.-glycineamide formyltransferase
p.-glycineamide synthetase
p.-pyrophosphate amidotrans-
ferase
phosphoribosyl-aminoimidazole
p.-a. carboxamide formyltransferase
p.-a. carboxylase
p.-a. succinocarboxamide synthetase
p.-a. synthetase
phosphoribosyl-pyrophosphatase
phosphoribosyl-pyrophosphate
phosphoribosyl-transferase
hypoxanthine p.
hypoxanthine guanine p.
nicotinamide p.
nicotinic p.
orotate p.
uracil p.
phosphoric
p. acid
p. acid test
p. diester hydrolase
p. monoester hydrolase
phosphoruria
phosphorus
p.-32
p. assay
p. isotope
nitrogen p.
yellow p.
phosphoryl
phosphorylase
p. deficiency
glycogen p.
inosine p.
p. kinase
nucleotide p.
p. phosphatase
purine nucleoside p.
uridine p.
phosphorylated thiamine
phosphorylation
oxidative p.
substrate level p.
phosphorylcholine
3-phosphoserine
phosphoserine phosphatase
phosphotransferase
creatine p.

phosphotungstate
phosphotungstic acid
p.-a. hematoxylin
p.-a. stain
phosphuria
phostex
phot (unit of illumination)
photic stimulation
photoallergen
photoallergy
photoautotroph
photoautotrophic
photocatalysis
photocatalyst
photocell
photochemical
p. reaction
p. smog
photochemistry
photochromogen
photochromogenic mycobacterium
photochromogenicity
photocoagulation
photoconductive cell
photocontact dermatitis
photoconvulsive response
photodecomposition
photodermatitis
photodetector
photodiode
photodissociation
photodynamic
photoeczematous eruption
photoelectric effect
photoelectrometer
photoelectron
photofluorography
photographic effect
photoheterotroph
photoheterotrophic
photoisomerization
photolithotroph
photolithotrophic
photoluminescence
photoluminescent
photolysis
photolytic
photometer
filter p.
flame p.
photometrazol threshold

photometric
  p. accuracy
  p. linearity
  p. reproducibility
photometry
  flame p.
photomicrograph
photomicrography
photomicroscope
photomultiplier tube
photomyoclonic response
photomyogenic response
photon
  Compton p.
  p. counting
photoorganotroph
photoorganotrophic
photoparoxysmal
photopeak detection efficiency
photophobia
photophthalmia
photopic
photopigment
photoptometer
photoreaction
photoreactivation
photoreceptor
photoresistor
photoretinitis
photoscan
photosensitive porphyria
photosensitivity
photosensitization
photostable
photosynthesis
photosynthetic organism
phototaxis
phototoxic contact dermatitis
phototoxicity
phototransduction
phototransistor
phototrophic
phototropism
phototube
photovoltaic cell
photuria
PHP — primary hyperparathyroidism
    pseudohypoparathyroidism
Phragmobasidiomycetes
Phragmobasidiomycetidae
phrenic
  p. artery
  p. vein

phrenicocolic
phrenoplegia
phrenoptosia
phrenosin
phrygian cap
phthalein test
phthalic acid
phthalocyanine dye
phthalylsulfacetamide
phthalylsulfathiazole
phthinoid
phthiriasis
Phthirus pubis
phthisic; phthisical
phthisis bulbi
phycobiliprotein
phycoerythrin
Phycomycetes
phycomycosis
phylactic
phylaxis
phyllode
phylloquinone
phylogenetic
phylogeny
phylum (pl., phyla)
phyma (pl., phymata)
phymatoid
phymatorrhysin
phymatosis
Physa
physaliferous
physaliform
physaliphore
physaliphorous
physalis
Physaloptera
    P. caucasica
    P. mordens
physalopteriasis
Physalopteridae
physical
  p. adsorption
  p. chemistry
  p. diagnosis
  p. half-life
  p. optics
  p. record
Physick's pouches
physicochemical
physics
physiochemical

physiologic; physiological
    p. albuminuria
    p. anemia
    p. chemistry
    p. dead space
    p. equilibrium
    p. hyperplasia
    p. hypertrophy
    p. hypogammaglobulinemia
    p. incompatibility
    p. jaundice
    p. leukocytosis
    p. saline solution
    p. sclerosis
    p. tremor
    p. unit
physiology
physis
physisorption
Physopsis
physostigmine
    p. salicylate
    p. sulfate
phytagglutinin
phytanic acid
phytic acid
phytin
phytoagglutinin
Phytobdella
phytobezoar
phytohemagglutinin
phytol
phytolectin
Phytomastigophora
phytomitogen
phytonadione
phytophotodermatitis
phytopneumoconiosis
phytosterol
PI — phosphatidylinositol
    protamine insulin
    protease inhibitor
    pulmonary incompetence
    pulmonary infarction
PIA — plasma insulin activity
pia-arachnitis
pia-arachnoid
pia-glia
pial terminal filament
pia mater
    p.-m. encephali
    p.-m. spinalis

pian
Piazza's test
pi bond
PICA — posterior inferior cerebellar
       artery
pica
Pichia membranaefaciens
picket cell
Pick's
      bodies
      cells
      tubular adenoma
pickwickian
    p. disease
    p. syndrome
picloram
picocurie
picofarad
picogram
picometer
picopicogram
picornavirus
picosecond
picramic acid
picrate test
picric acid
picrocarmine stain
picroformol fixative
picro-Mallory trichrome stain
picronigrosin stain
picrotoxin
PID — pelvic inflammatory disease
      plasma iron disappearance
PIDT — plasma-iron disappearance
      time
PIE — pulmonary infiltration with
      eosinophilia
      pulmonary interstitial em-
      physema
piebald skin
piecemeal necrosis
piedra
    black p.
    white p.
Piedraia hortae
PIE syndrome
piezoelectric effect
piezogenic
PIF — peak inspiratory flow
      prolactin-inhibiting factor
      proliferation inhibitory factor
PIFR — peak inspiratory flow rate

PIG-A — phosphatidyl-inositol gly-
      can class A
pigbel
pigeon
    p. breast
    p. breast deformity
    p. breeder's disease
pigment
    accumulation of p's
    anthracotic p.
    bile p's
    bilharzial deposition p.
    bilirubin p.
    calculous p.
    p. calculus
    ceroid p.
    p. cirrhosis
    deposition p., bilharzial
    deposition p., malarial
    endogenous p.
    epithelial p.
    exogenous p.
    formalin p.
    gallstone p.
    p. granules
    hematogenous p.
    hemosiderin p.
    hepatogenous p.
    p. induration of lung
    iron p.
    lipid p's
    lipofuscin p.
    malarial p.
    malarial deposition p.
    melanin p.
    melanotic p.
    minocycline-associated p.
    ochronotic p.
    pseudomelanosis p.
    respiratory p's
    retinal p's
    schistosome p.
    p. stones
    wear-and-tear p.
pigmentary
    p. cirrhosis
    p. degeneration
    p. dermatosis
    p. retinopathy
pigmentation
    arsenic p.
    bismuth p.

    exogenous p.
    hematin p.
    hematoidin p.
    hemofuscin p.
    hemoglobin p.
    iron p.
    lead p.
    lipochrome p.
    melanin p.
    porphyrin p.
    wear-and-tear p.
pigmented
    p. adenoma
    p. ameloblastoma
    p. casts
    p. dermatofibrosarcoma protu-
      berans
    p. epulis
    p. hair epidermal nevus
    p. nevus
    p. nodule
    p. pilocytic astrocytoma
    p. purpuric lichenoid derma-
      titis
    p. villonodular synovitis
    p. villonodular tenosynovitis
pigmenturia
pig skin
PII — plasma inorganic iodine
Pila
pilar
    p. cyst
    p. tumor of scalp
pile
    prostatic p.
    sentinel p.
piles
Pilidae
piliferous cyst
pilimiction
pilin
pillar
    faucial p.
pilocarpine
pilocystic
pilocytic
    p. astrocyte
    p. astrocytoma
piloid astrocytoma
piloleiomyoma
pilomatrixoma

pilonidal
  p. cyst
  p. fistula
  p. sinus
pilus (pl., pili)
  F (fertility) p.
  sex p.
piminodine esylate
pinacyanol
Pindborg tumor
pineal
  p. body
  p. corpora arenacea
  p. germinoma
  p. gland
  p. recess
  p. secretory rate
pinealocyte
pinealoma
pinene
pineoblastoma
pineocytoma
pinguecula
pink eye
"pink puffers" (emphysema)
Pinkus' fibroepithelioma
pinocytoma
pinocytosis
pinocytotic
pinosome
pinta
pinworm
pioepithelium
pion
pionemia
PIP — proximal interphalangeal
pipamazine
pipazethate hydrochloride
pipenzolate bromide
piperacetazine
piperacillin sodium
piperazine
piperidine
piperidolate hydrochloride
piperocaine hydrochloride
piperoxan hydrochloride
pipe-smoker's cancer
pipestem
  p. arteries
  p. cirrhosis
  p. fibrosis
pipethanate

pipette; pipet
  Mohr p.
PIPJ — proximal interphalangeal
    joint
pipobroman
pipradrol hydrochloride
Pirenella
piriform
  p. muscle
  p. neurons
  p. recess
Piroplasma
piroplasmosis
Pirquet's reaction
Pisano method
pisiform bone
PIT — plasma iron turnover
pit
  gastric p's
  Mantoux p.
pitch wart
pitch-worker's cancer
Pitfield's fluid
PITR — plasma iron turnover rate
pitting edema
Pittsburgh pneumonia agent
pituicyte
pituitary
  p. acidophil cell
  p. adenoma
  p. adrenocorticotropic cell
  p. alpha cell
  p. amphophil cell
  p. apoplexy
  p. basophil cell
  p. basophilia
  p. basophilism
  p. beta cell
  p. capsule
  p. cell
  p. chromophobe cell
  p. Cushing's syndrome
  p. dwarf
  p. dwarfism
  p. endocrine disorder
  p. extract
  p. failure
  p. fossa
  p. function test
  p. gigantism
  p. gland
  p. gonadotropic failure

p. gonadotropin
p. growth hormone
p. hormone
p. hypertrophic amphophil cell
p. hypothalamic axis
p. leukemia
lyophilized anterior p.
p. mammotropic cell
p. myxedema
p. pars intermedia
p. pars tuberalis
p. reserve
p. stalk
p. thyrotropic cell
p. tumor
pit viper
pityriasic
pityriasis
p. alba
p. capitis
p. lichenoides et varioliformis
acuta
p. linguae
p. pilaris
p. rosea
p. rubra
p. rubra pilaris
p. versicolor
Pityrosporon
P. orbiculare
P. ovale
P. versicolor
Pityrosporum
P. furfur
P. orbiculare
P. ovale
2-pivalyl-1,3-indandione
Pizzolato's peroxide-silver method
PK — Prausnitz-Küstner (reaction)
psychokinesis
pyruvate kinase
P-K antibody
PKU — phenylketonuria
PKU test
PKV — killed poliomyelitis vaccine
pkV or kVp — peak kilovoltage
PL — phospholipid
placebo
placental lactogen
pulpolingual
PLA — pulpolabial
pulpolinguoaxial

placebo
placenta (pl., placentas, placentae)
p. accreta
battledore p.
bilobate p.
p. circummarginata
circumvallate p.
dichorionic diamniotic p.
duplex p.
p. fenestrata
p. increta
mature abnormal p.
p. membranacea
monochorionic diamniotic p.
monochorionic monoamni-
otic p.
multilobate p.
p. multipartita
p. percreta
premature abnormal p.
prematurely separated p.
p. previa
p. spuria
p. succenturiata
p. triloba
trilobate p.
p. tripartita
twin p., dichorionic
twin p., monoamniotic
twin p., monochorionic
twin p., monochorionic diamniotic
p. twin
placental
p. alkaline phosphatase
p. and fetoplacental function
test
p. cells
p. cotyledon
p. fetal surface
p. fluids
p. fragment
p. hormone
p. lactogen
p. maternal surface
p. membrane
p. polyp
p. residual blood volume
p. spaces
p. sulfatase
p. thrombosis

p. villi
p. zone
placentation bleeding
placentitis
placentography
placentoma
placode
plagiocephaly
Plagiorchiidae
Plagiorchioidea
Plagiorchis
plague
    p. bacillus
    black p.
    bubonic p.
    hemorrhagic p.
    pneumonic p.
    septicemic p.
    p. serum
    sylvatic p.
plakoglobin
Planck's
    constant
    radiation law
plane
    auriculoinfraorbital p.
    axiobuccolingual p.
    axiomesiodistal p.
    coronal p.
    focal p.
    frontal p.
    horizontal p.
    interparietal p.
    intertubercular p.
    labiolingual p.
    mediodistal p.
    midsagittal p.
    occipital p.
    orbital p.
    parasagittal p.
    popliteal p.
    sagittal p.
    sternal p.
    sternoxiphoid p.
    symmetry p.
    transpyloric p.
    vertical p.
    p. wart
    p. xanthoma
planigraphy
planimeter
planimetry

planocyte
Planorbarius
planorbid
Planorbidae
Planorbinae
Planorbis
plant
    p. indican
    p. protease test
Plantago
plantar
    p. aponeurosis
    p. artery
    p. fibromatosis
    p. reflex
    p. vein
    p. wart
plantodorsal
planuria
planus
    atrophic lichen p.
    bullous lichen p.
plaque
    atheromatous p.
    atherosclerotic p.
    attachment p.
    cellulocutaneous p.
    dental p.
    p.-forming cell
    p.-forming units
    Hollenhorst's p.
    hyalinized p.
    McCallum's p.
    neuritic p.
    penile p.
    senile p's
    p. technique
    ureteral p.
plaques jaunes
plasm
plasma
    p. accelerator globulin
    p. activation
    adsorbed p.
    p. alteration
    antihemophilic p.
    antilymphocyte p.
    anti-*Pseudomonas* human p.
    p. bicarbonate
    blood p.
    p. blood cell
    p. blood group

p. cell
p. cell dyscrasias
p. cell granuloma
p. cell hepatitis
p. cell hyperplasia
p. cell infiltrate
p. cell leukemia
p. cell mastitis
p. cell myeloma
p. cell pneumonia
p. cell tumor
p. clearance
p. clearance rate
p. clotting time
coagulase p.
p. coagulation factor
p. defect
p. depletion
p. dyscrasia
p. exchange
p. factor X
p. fibronectin
fresh frozen p.
frozen p.
p. glucose tolerance rate
p. hemoglobin
p. hemoglobin test
p. immune factor
p. inorganic iodine
p. insulin activity
p. iodoprotein disorder
p. iron disappearance
p. iron turnover
p. iron turnover rate
p. kallikrein
p. labile factor
p. layer
p. level
lymphoid p.
p. marinum
p. membrane
normal p.
normal human p.
p. oncotic pressure
p. pepsinogen
peripheral vein p.
platelet-free p.
platelet-poor p.
platelet-rich p.
protein p.
p. protein fraction
p. proteins

p. recalcification
p. renin activity test
salted p.
p. sodium
p. stain
p. substitute
p. thrombin clot method
p. thromboplastin antecedent
p. thromboplastin antecedent
  deficiency
p. thromboplastin component
p. thromboplastin factor
p. thromboplastin factor B
p. triglyceride
p. volume
p. volume expander
plasmablast
plasmacrit test
plasmacyte
plasmacytic
  p. blood cell
  p. cells
  p. leukemia
  p. myeloma
  p. tissue
plasmacytoid
  p. lymphocyte
  p. lymphocytic lymphoma
plasmacytoma
  nasal p.
plasmacytosis
plasma expander
plasmagene
plasma-glucose disappearance rate
plasmahaut
plasma-iron disappearance time
plasmalemma
plasmalogen
plasmal reaction
plasmapheresis
plasmarrhexis
plasmatic/plasmic stain
plasmatofibrous astrocyte
plasmid
  conjugative p.
  F p.
  F' p.
  p. integration
  oligomeric p.
  R p.
  resistance p.

p. transfer
p. vector system
plasmin
    p. coagulation
    p. prothrombins conversion
      factor
plasminogen
    p. activator
    p. activator inhibitor
    p. assay
plasminokinase
plasminoplastin
plasmocrine vacuole
plasmocyte
plasmocytic leukemoid reaction
plsamocytoma
    nasal p.
Plasmodiidae
Plasmodium
    P. falciparum
    P. malariae
    P. ovale
    P. pleurodyniae
    P. vivax
    P. vivax minuta
plasmodium
    p. embolism
    exoerythrocytic p.
plasmoid humor
plasmokinin
plasmolysis
plasmolytic
plasmolyze
plasmoma
plasmon
plasmoptysis
plasmorrhexis
plasmoschisis
plasmosome
plasmotropic
plasmotropism
plasmotype
plasmozyme
plastic
    p. bronchitis
    p. corpuscle
    p. induration
    p. lymph
    p. pleurisy
    p. section stain
plasticizer

plastid
    blood p.
plate
    Abbé test p.
    alar p.
    axial p.
    blood p.
    blood agar p.
    chorionic p.
    cough p.
    counting p.
    cribriform p.
    p. culture
    epiphyseal p.
    equatorial p.
    ethmoid p.
    ethmovomerine p.
    Fresnel zone p.
    lawn p.
    lens p.
    pour p.
    spread p.
    streak p.
    subgerminal p.
    tarsal p.
    theoretical p.
    p. thrombosis
    tympanic p.
    ventrolateral p.
platelet
    p. activating factor
    p. actomyosin
    p. adhesion test
    p. adhesiveness test
    p. agglutination
    p. agglutinin
    p.-aggregating factor
    p. aggregation
    p. aggregation test
    p. aggregometer
    p. antibody
    p.-associated immunoglobulins
    p. autoantibodies
    Bizzozero's p's
    p. coagulation factor
    p. cofactor
    p. cofactor I
    p. cofactor II
    p. concentrate
    p. count
    p. defect
    p.-derived growth factor

p. factor (1, 2, 3, 4)
p.-free plasma
in vivo adhesive p.
p. isoantibodies
p.-poor blood
p.-poor plasma
p. retention test
p.-rich plasma
p. sizing
p. survival test
p. thrombosis
p. thrombus
p. tissue factor
p. transfusion
plateletpheresis
plating
platinosis
platinum
    p. chloride
    p. group
platybasia
platycyte
platyhelminth
Platyhelminthes
platykurtic
platypnea
platysma
    p. muscle
    p. musculo-cutaneous flap
PLD — platelet defect
pleated sheet
plectonemic coil
pleiotropic
    p. gene
    p. mutation
pleiotropism
pleitropy
pleochroic
pleochroism
pleochromatic
pleochromatism
pleocytosis
    mononuclear p.
pleokaryocyte
pleomorphic
    p. adenoma
    p. carcinoma
    p. lipoma
    p. liposarcoma
    p. lymphoma
    p. rhabdomyosarcoma

pleomorphism
    nuclear p.
pleonosteosis
    Leri's p.
Pleospora
plerocercoid
plerocercus
Plesiomonas shigelloides
plethora
plethysmogram
plethysmograph
plethysmography
    dynamic venous p.
    impedance p.
    strain-gauge p.
    venous occlusion p.
pleura (pl., pleurae)
pleural
    p. biopsy
    p. calculus
    p. cavities
    p. effusion
    p. exudates
    p. fibrin balls
    p. fibroma
    p. fluid
    p. fluid examination
    p. friction rub
    p. mesothelioma
    p. transudate
    p. tuberculosis
pleuralgia
pleurectomy
pleurisy
    adhesive p.
    costal p.
    dry p.
    encysted p.
    fibrinous p.
    hemorrhagic p.
    interlobular p.
    plastic p.
    productive p.
    proliferating p.
    pulmonary p.
    purulent p.
    sacculated p.
    serofibrinous p.
    serous p.
    suppurative p.
    visceral p.
    wet p.

pleuritic
pleuritis
    acute fibrinous p.
    fibrinous p.
    hemorrhagic p.
    nocardial p.
    obliterative p.
    serofibrinous p.
    suppurative p.
    tuberculous p.
    viral p.
pleuritogenous
Pleuroceridae
pleurodesis
pleurodynia
pleurography
pleurohepatitis
pleurolith
pleuropericarditis
pleuropneumonectomy
pleuropneumonia
pleuropulmonary
pleurorrhea
pleuroscopy
PLEVA — pityriasis lichenoides et
             varioliformis acuta
plexiform
    p. ameloblastoma
    p. layer
    p. neurofibroma
    p. neuroma
    p. unicystic ameloblastoma
Plexiglas
plexitis
plexogenic pulmonary arteriopathy
plexus
    Auerbach's p.
    Bonnet's p.
    brachial p.
    cavernous p.
    celiac p.
    enteric p.
    lumbar p.
    lumbosacral p.
    Meissner's nerve p.
    mesenteric p.
    myenteric p.
    pampiniform p.
    pelvic p.
    pulmonary p.
    submucosal p.

    subserosal p.
    venous p.
plica (pl., plicae)
    p. interureterica
    p. palmata
plication
Plimmer's bodies
ploidy
    nuclear p.
plot
    Scatchard p.
    Youdon p.
    Wu-Kabat p.
PLS — prostaglandin-like substance
PLT — primed lymphocyte typing
      psittacosis-lymphogranuloma
        venereum-trachoma (group)
plug
    Dittrich's p's
    hemostatic p.
    Traube's p's
plumbism
plunging goiter
pluricentric blastoma
pluriglandular adenomatosis
plurihormonal adenoma
pluripolar mitosis
pluripotent myeloid stem cell
pluripotential
    p. cells
    p. stem cells
plutonium
PLV — live poliomyelitis vaccine
      panleukopenia virus
      phenylalanine-lysine-
        vasopressin
PM — photomultiplier tube
      polymorph
      postmortem
      pulpomesial
Pm — promethium
pm — picometer
PMA — papillary, marginal, attached
        (gingivitis)
      progressive muscular atrophy
PMB — para-hydroxymercuribenzoate
      polymorphonuclear basophil
PMC — pseudomembranous colitis
PMD — primary myocardial disease
      progressive muscular dys-
        trophy
PME — polymorphonuclear eosin-
        ophil

PMF — progressive massive fibrosis
PMI — point of maximal impulse
　　　point of maximal intensity
PML — progressive multifocal leukoencephalopathy
PMM — pentamethylmelamine
PMN — polymorphonuclear neutrophil
PMR — perinatal mortality rate
　　　polymyalgia rheumatica
　　　proportionate morbidity ratio
　　　proportionate mortality ratio
PMS — phenazine methosulfate
　　　postmitochondrial supernatant
　　　pregnant mare serum
PMSG — pregnant mare serum gonadotropin
PMT — Porteus' maze test
PN — periarteritis nodosa
　　　peripheral neuropathy
　　　pneumonia
　　　positional nystagmus
　　　pyelonephritis
P_{NA} — plasma sodium
PND — paroxysmal nocturnal dyspnea
pneumarthrosis
pneumatic
pneumatinuria
pneumatocele
pneumatosis
　　　p. cystica
　　　p. cystoides intestinalis
　　　p. intestinalis cystica
pneumaturia
pneumoarthrography
pneumobacillus
　　　Friedländer's p.
pneumococcal
　　　p. bacteremia
　　　p. empyema
　　　p. infection
　　　p. meningitis
　　　p. peritonitis
　　　p. pneumonia
　　　p. polysaccharide
　　　p. sepsis
　　　p. vaccine
pneumococcemia
pneumococcosuria
pneumococcus (pl., pneumococci)

pneumoconiosis (pl., pneumoconioses)
　　　coal workers' p.
　　　rheumatoid p.
pneumocystiasis
pneumocystic
　　　p. cyst
　　　p. pneumonia
Pneumocystis
　　　P. carinii
　　　P. fluorescence
　　　P. pneumoniae
pneumocystography
pneumocystosis
pneumocyte
　　　granular p.
pneumoderma
pneumoencephalography
pneumofasciogram
pneumogenic osteoarthropathy
pneumograph
pneumography
pneumohemopericardium
pneumohemothorax
pneumohydroperitoneum
pneumohydrothorax
pneumohypoderma
pneumolith
pneumolithiasis
pneumomalacia
pneumomediastinography
pneumomediastinum
pneumonectomy
pneumonia
　　　acute gelatinous p.
　　　adenoviral p.
　　　p. alba
　　　aspiration p.
　　　atypical p.
　　　atypical primary p.
　　　bacterial p.
　　　bronchial p.
　　　caseous p.
　　　central p.
　　　chemical p.
　　　confluent p.
　　　core p.
　　　desquamative interstitial p.
　　　diffuse p.
　　　p. dissecans
　　　double p.
　　　eosinophilic p.
　　　focal p.

Friedländer's p.
fungal p.
gangrenous p.
giant cell p.
"golden" p.
Haemophilis influenzae p.
Hecht's p.
hemorrhagic p.
herpes simplex p.
hypostatic p.
inhalation p.
p. interlobularis purulenta
interstitial p.
interstitial giant cell p.
interstitial plasma cell p.
Klebsiella p.
Legionella pneumophilia p.
lipid p.
lipoid p.
lobar p.
lobular p.
Löffler's p.
Louisiana p.
metastatic p.
migratory p.
mycoplasmal p.
necrotizing p.
nocardial p.
nosocomial p.
organized p.
paratuberculous p.
Pittsburgh p. agent
plasma cell p.
pneumococcal p.
pneumocystic p.
Pneumocystis carinii p.
primary atypical p.
primary influenza virus p.
proteus p.
Pseudomonas p.
rheumatic p.
Riesman's p.
septic p.
serratia p.
staphylococcal p.
streptococcal p.
suppurative p.
p. tularemia
unresolved p.
unresolved lobar p.
uremic p.
varicella p.

viral p.
"walking" p.
wandering p.
pneumonic plague
pneumonitis
    allergic p.
    aspiration p.
    chemical p.
    desquamative interstitial p.
    hemorrhagic p.
    hypersensitivity p.
    interstitial p.
    lymphocytic interstitial p.
    lymphoid interstitial p.
    pneumocystic p.
    pulmonary p.
    radiation p.
    rheumatic p.
    uremic p.
    usual interstitial p.
    p. virus
pneumonoconiosis
pneumonocyte
pneumoperitoneum
pneumoperitonitis
pneumopleuritis
pneumopyelography
pneumoretroperitoneum
pneumoserothorax
pneumotachogram
pneumothorax
    spontaneous p.
    tension p.
    therapeutic p.
pneumotomography
    orbital p.
pneumoventriculography
pneumovirus
PNH — paroxysmal nocturnal hemo-
        globinuria
PNP — para-nitrophenol
PNPP — para-nitrophenylphosphate
PNS — peripheral nervous system
PNU — protein nitrogen unit
PO — parieto-occipital
        posterior
Po — polonium
PO_2 or pO_2 — oxygen partial pressure
        (tension)
POA — pancreatic oncofetal antigen
POB — phenoxybenzamine
pocket dosimeter

pocketed calculus
poculum
podarthritis
podedema
poditis
podocyte
    glomerular p.
podophyllin resin
podophyllotoxin
POEMS — polyneuropathy, organ-
        omegaly, endocrinop-
        athy, monoclonal
        gammopathy, and skin
        changes
poetin
POG — Pediatric Oncology Group
pOH — hydroxyl concentration
poik — poikilocyte
poikiloblast
poikilocyte
    tail p.
poikilocythemia
poikilocytosis
poikiloderma
    p. atrophicans
    p. atrophicans vasculare
    p. of Civatte
    p. congenitale
poikilodermatomyositis
poikilosmosis
poikilothrombocyte
point
    alveolar p.
    apophysiary p.
    auricular p.
    conjugate p.
    craniometric p.
    boiling p.
    end p.
    equivalent p.
    Erb's p.
    p. estimate
    freezing p.
    growing p.
    ice p.
    ignition p.
    p. of inflection
    isobestic p.
    isoelectric p.
    isoionic p.
    jugomaxillary p.
    melting p.

    p. mutation
    occipital p.
    radix p.
    refraction p.
    set p.
    supraclavicular p.
    thermal death p.
    triple p.
pointed
    p. condyloma
    p. wart
pointer
    hip p.
    p. variable
Poirier's glands
poise
Poiseuille's
    law
    space
poison
    acronarcotic p.
    industrial p.
    mitotic p.
Poison Control Center
poisoning
    alcohol p.
    anticholinergic p.
    antimony p.
    arsenic p.
    blood p.
    carbon dioxide p.
    carbon disulfide p.
    carbon monoxide p.
    carbon tetrachloride p.
    chloroform p.
    chromium p.
    cyanide p.
    cyclosporine p.
    desquamative interstitial p.
    ethyl alcohol p.
    ethylene glycol p.
    food p.
    heavy metal p.
    insecticide p.
    iron p.
    isopropyl alcohol p.
    lead p.
    lithium p.
    magnesium p.
    manganese p.
    mercuric chloride p.
    mercury p.

methanol p.
methyl alcohol p.
mushroom p.
naphthol p.
nitroaniline p.
organophosphate p.
oxygen p.
paraldehyde p.
polychlorinated biphenyl p.
Salmonella p.
scombroid p.
systemic p.
tetrachlorethane p.
thallium p.
theophylline p.
vitamin D p.
zinc p.
Poisson distribution
pokeweed mitogen
polar
    p. anemia
    p. body
    p. compound
    p. coordinates
    p. injecting filament
    p. spongioblast
polarimeter
polarimetry
polarity
polarizability
polarization
polarize
polarized light microscopy
polarizer
polarizing microscope
polarogram
polarography
poldine methylsulfate
pole
    animal p.
    vitelline p.
pol gene
polio — poliomyelitis
polioencephalitis
poliomyelitis
    acute anterior p.
    anterior acute p.
    immunization reaction p.
    p. I, II, III titer
    virus p.
    p. virus

poliovaccine
    inactivated p.
poliovirus, types I, II, III
Polistes
pollen
    p. extract
    p. grains
Pollenia
pollex (pl., pollices)
pollution
polonium
poloxalkol
poly — polymorphonuclear leukocyte
polyacrylamide gel electrolysis
polyadenitis
polyadenopathy
polyadenosis
polyadenylate tail; polyA tail
polyadenylation signal muscle
polyadenylic acid
polyagglutination
polyamide
polyamine-methylene resin
polyangiitis
polyanionic proteoglycans
polyanion precipitation
polyarteritis
    microscopic p.
    p. nodosa
polyarthritis
    p. chronica
    p. chronica villosa
    migratory p.
    p. rheumatica acute
    vertebral p.
polyarticular gout
polybasic acid
polyblast
polybrene
polybrominated biphenyl
polycarbophil
polychlorinated
    p. biphenyl assay
    p. biphenyl poisoning
polychondritis
    chronic atrophic p.
    relapsing p.
polychromasia
polychromatia
polychromatic
    p. cell
    p. erythroblast

p. erythrocyte
p. normoblast
polychromatocyte
polychromatocytosis
polychromatophil; polychromatophile
    p. cell
polychromatophilia
polychromatophilic
    p. normoblast
    p. rubricyte
polychromatosis
polychrome
    p. methylene blue
    p. methylene blue stain
polychromemia
polychromia
polychromophil
polychromophilia
polyclave
polyclonal
    p. antibody
    p. gammopathy
    p. hypergammaglobulinemia
    p. hyperglobulinemia
    p. hyperimmunoglobulinemia
    p. immunoglobulin
    p. tumor
polycyclic aromatic hydrocarbon
polycystic
    p. change
    p. disease
    p. kidney
    p. kidney disease
    p. liver
    p. liver disease
    p. ovary
    p. ovary syndrome
polycystoma
polycyte
polycythemia
    absolute p.
    compensatory p.
    familial p.
    p. hypertonica
    myelopathic p.
    relative p.
    p. rubra
    p. rubra vera
    splenomegalic p.
    spurious p.
    stress p.
    p. vera

polycytosis
polydactyly
polydeoxyribonucleotide synthetase
Polydesmus
polydipsia
polydysplasia
polydystrophia
polydystrophic dwarfism
polydystrophy
    pseudo-Hurler p.
polyelectrolyte
polyembryoma
polyembryony
polyemia
    p. aquosa
    p. hyperalbuminosa
    p. polycythaemica
    p. serosa
polyendocrine adenomatosis
polyendocrinoma
polyene antibiotics
polyenoic acid
polyester
polyether
polyethylene
    p. assay
    p. glycol
    p. glycol alkyl ester
    p. terephthalate
polyferose
polygalacturonase
polyganglionic
polygenic inheritance
polyglucosan bodies
polyglucoside
polyglutamate
    folate p.
polygon
    frequency p.
polygraphic
polygyny
polyhedral
polyhedron
polyhelminthism
polyhistiocytoma
polyhistioma
polyhydramnios
polyhydric alcohol
polyimmunoglobulin receptor
polyisoprenoid
polykaryocyte
polykaryon

polylymphocytic leukemia
polymastia
polymer
    addition p.
    condensation p.
    poly-(methylmethacrylate) p.
polymerase
    p. chain reaction
    DNA p.
    RNA p.
polymerization
polymerize
polymers
    vinyl p.
polymetaphosphate
polymethine dye
polymethylmethacrylate
poly-(methylmethacrylate) polymer
polymicrobial
polymicrogyria
polymicrolipomatosis
polymorph
polymorphic
    p. light eruption
    p. neuron
    p. reticulosis
polymorphism
    balanced p.
    restriction fragment length p.
polymorphocellular
polymorphocyte
polymorphocytic leukemia
polymorphonuclear
    p. basophil
    p. eosinophil
    p. leukocyte
    p. leukocytic infiltrate
    p. neutrophil
    p. neutrophil chemotactic
      factor
polymorphous eruption
polymyalgia
    p. arteritica
    p. rheumatica
polymyositis
polymyositis-dermatomyositis
polymyxin
    p. B sulfate
    p. E
    p. sulfate
polyneuritic-type hypertrophic muscular atrophy

polyneuritiformis
    heredopathia atactica p.
polyneuritis
    acute idiopathic p.
polyneuropathy
    arsenic p.
    arsenical p.
    carcinomatous p.
    familial amyloid p.
    paraneoplastic p.
    peripheral p.
polynuclear leukocyte
polynucleate
polynucleolar
polynucleosis
polynucleotide
    p. ligase
    p. nucleotidyltransferase
    p. phosphorylase
polyol dehydrogenase
polyolefin
polyoma
polyomavirus
polyoncosis; polyonchosis
    cutaneomandibular p.
polyorchidism
polyostotic fibrous dysplasia
polyp
    adenomatous p.
    aural p.
    bleeding p.
    bronchial p.
    cardiac p.
    cellular p.
    cervical p.
    choanal p.
    cholesterol p.
    cockscomb p.
    colonic p.
    colorectal p.
    cystic p.
    endocervical p.
    endometrial p.
    fibrinous p.
    fibroepithelial p.
    fibrous p.
    fleshy p.
    gastric p.
    gelatinous p.
    granulomatous p.
    hamartomatous p.
    hydatid p.

hyperplastic p.
inflammatory p.
juvenile p.
laryngeal p.
lipomatous p.
lymphoid p.
metaplastic p.
mucous p.
multiple p.
multiple adenomatous p's
myomatous p.
nasal p.
osseous p.
papillary adenomatous p.
pedunculated p.
Peutz-Jeghers p.
placental p.
prostatic p.
regenerative p.
retention p.
sessile p.
small intestine p.
tubular adenomatous p.
tubulovillous adenomatous p.
umbilical p.
urethral p.
vascular p.
villous adenomatous p.
polyparasitism
polypathia
polypathic
polypeptide
adrenocorticotropic p.
p. chain
cytokeratin p.
gastric inhibitory p.
p. hormone
pancreatic p.
vasoactive intestinal p.
polyphagia
polyphase anaplasia
polyphasic wave
polyphenism
polypheny
polyphosphoinositide
polyphosphoric acid
polyphyletic
p. origin
p. theory
polyphyletism
polypiform
polyplasmia

Polyplis
polyploid
polyploidy
polypnea
polypoid
p. adenocarcinoma
p. adenoma
p. cystitis
p. hyperplasia
polyposis
p. coli
familial intestinal p.
heredofamilial p.
juvenile p. syndrome
multiple intestinal p.
multiple lymphomatous p.
polypous
p. endocarditis
p. gastritis
polypropylene glycol
polypus (pl., polypi)
polypyrrylmethane
polyradiculoneuritis
polyribonucleotide
polyribosome
polysaccharide
pneumococcal p.
polyserositis
polysiloxane
methyl p.
polysinusitis
polysomaty
polysome
polysomic
polysomnogram
polysomnography
polysomy
polysorbate
polyspermy
polyspike complex
polysplenia syndrome
polystyrene
polysulfide
calcium p.
polytendinitis
polytene chromosome
polyteny
polytetrafluoroethylene (Polytef)
polythelia
polythiazide
polyunsaturated fatty acid
polyurethane

polyuria
polyuridylic acid
polyvalent
>p. antiserum
>p. serum
polyvesicular-vitelline pattern
polyvinyl
>p. alcohol
>p. alcohol fixative method
>p. chloride
polyvinylpyrrolidone
Pomatiopsis
POMP — prednisone, Oncovin, methotrexate, 6-mercaptopurine
ponceau
>p. B
>p. 2R
>p. S
Ponfick's shadow
pons (gen., pontis; pl., pontes)
>basilar p.
>decussation p.
>p. longitudinalis fasciculi
>p. nucleus
>p. reticular formation nucleus
>spinothalamic p.
>p. superficial transverse fibers
>p. superior central nucleus
>tegmental p.
>transverse p.
Pontiac fever
pontine
>p. artery
>p. nucleus
ponto-geniculo-occipital spike
pool
>circulating granulocyte p.
>gene p.
>marginal granulocyte p.
>metabolic p.
>rapidly miscible p.
>total blood granulocyte p.
>vaginal p.
pooled
>p. blood serum
>p. estimate
>p. serum
poorly differentiated carcinoma
poorly differentiated lymphocytic lymphoma
POP — plasma oncotic pressure

popliteal
>p. aneurysm
>p. artery
>p. vein
POPOP — 1,4-bis-α-(5-phenyloxazolyl)-benzene
population
>p. attributable risk
>p. biology
>p. cytogenetics
>p. genetics
>p. sample
P : O ratio
porcelain gallbladder
porcupine skin
pore
>alveolar p.
>endothelial p.
>glomerular p's
>gustatory p.
>p's of Kohn
>nuclear p.
porencephaly
>encephaloclastic p.
porfiromycin
Porges-Meier test
Porges-Salomon test
porin
pork tapeworm
porocele
Porocephalus
>*P. armillatus*
>*P. clavatus*
>*P. constrictus*
>*P. denticulatus*
porokeratosis
>actinic p.
>disseminated superficial actinic p.
>Mibelli's p.
poroma
>eccrine p.
porosis (pl., poroses)
porosity
porotic
porphin
porphobilinogen
>p. assay
>p. deaminase
>p. synthase
>p. test

porphyria
    acute intermittent p.
    congenital p.
    congenital erythropoietic p.
    p. cutanea tarda
    erythrohepatic p.
    erythropoietic p.
    p. erythropoietica
    hepatic p.
    hepatoerythropoietic p.
    hereditary p.
    latent p.
    photosensitive p.
    South African–type p.
    symptomatic p.
    variegate p.
    X p.
porphyrin
    erythrocyte p's
    free erythrocyte p.
    p. pigmentation
    p. test
porphyrinemia
porphyrinogen
porphyrinuria
porphyruria
porrigo
porta (pl., portae)
    p. hepatis
    p. renis
portacaval shunt
portal
    p. cirrhosis
    p. hypertension
    p. lymph node
    p. pyemia
    p. system
    p.-systemic encephalopathy
    p.-systemic shunt
    p. tract
    p. triad
    p. vein
    p. vein thrombosis
portasystemic
    p. encephalopathy
    p. shunt
Porter-Silber
    chromogen
    chromogen test
    reaction
Porteus' maze test
Porthetria

Portland hemoglobin
port-wine
    p.-w. mark
    p.-w. stain
pos. — positive
Posada's mycosis
position
    anatomic p.
    decubitus p.
    p. isomerism
    occipitoanterior p.
    occipitoposterior p.
    occipitotransverse p.
positive
    p. afterimage
    p. assortative mating
    p. control
    p. control enzyme induction
    p. control repression
    p. cytotaxis
    false p.
    gram-p.
    p. neutrotaxis
    p. pressure
    p. pressure breathing
    p. ray
    Rhesus factor p.
    p. stain
    weakly p.
positron
    p. annihilation
    p. beta decay
    p.-emission tomography
pos. pr. — positive pressure
post — posterior
    postmortem
postabsorptive state
postauricular
postbrachial
postcentral
    p. fissure
    p. gyrus
    p. sulcus
postchromation
postchroming
postcoital test
postductal coarctation of aorta
postencephalitic parkinsonism
posterior
    p. abdominal wall
    p. auricular artery
    p. auricular nerve

p. cerebral artery
p. chamber
p. circumflex humeral artery
p. column
p. commissure
p. communicating artery
p. corneal deposits
p. cusp
p. dislocation
p. displacement
p. external arcuate fibers
p. facial vein
p. femoral cutaneous nerve
p. forceps
p. fornix
p. fossa meningioma
p. gray column
p. horn
p. inferior cerebellar artery
p. intercostal artery
p. lateral nucleus of thalamus
p. leaflet
p. limb
p. limb bud
p. lobe of pituitary
p. lobe of prostate
p. lunate lobule
p. mediastinum
p. meningeal artery
p. papillary muscle
p. parietal artery
p. parietal gyrus
p. parolfactory area
p. pituitary
p. pituitary hormone
p. quadrangular lobule
p. quadrigeminal body
p. retromandibular vein
p. segment
p. semilunar lobule
p. sinus of Valsalva
p. spinal artery
p. subcapsular cataract
p. superior alveolar nerve
p. superior ansiform lobule
p. synechia
p. temporal artery
p. terminal vein
p. thalamic capsule
p. tibial artery
p. tibial tendon
p. tibial vein

p. tubercle
p. urethritis
p. ventral nucleus
p. wall infarct
p. wall of oropharynx
p. wall of stomach
posteroanterior
posterointermediate
    p. ventral nucleus
posterolateral
    p. artery
    p. fissure of cerebellum
    p. ventral nucleus
posteromedial
posteroventral nucleus
postgamma proteinuria
postganglionic
    p. neuron
    p. sympathetic fiber
posthemorrhagic anemia
postheparin lipolytic activity
posthepatic neuralgia
posthepatitic cirrhosis
posthitis
postholith
postinfarction
postinfectious
    p. allergic encephalitis
    p. encephalomyelitis
    p. glomerulonephritis
postirradiation
postlactation involution
postlingual fissure
postlunate fissure
postmature labor
postmaturity
postmenarcheal
postmenopausal
    p. atrophy
    p. endometrium
    p. osteoporosis
postmenstrual endometrium
postmitochondrial supernatant
postmordant
postmortem
    p. clot
    p. examination
    p. hypostasis
    p. lividity
    p. pustule
    p. suggillation
    p. thrombus

p. tubercle
p. wart
postnatal hematopoiesis
postnecrotic cirrhosis
postneonatal
postnodular fissure
post-op — postoperative
postoperative
    p. parotiditis
    p. repair
    p. shock
postpartum
    p. hemorrhage
    p. pituitary necrosis
    p. renal failure
postprandial
    p. blood sugar
    p. glucose
    p. hypoglycemia
    p. lipemia
postprimary tuberculosis
postpubertal; postpuberal
    p. hyperpituitarism
    p. hypogonadism
    p. panhypopituitarism
postpubescence
postpump syndrome
postpyknotic
postradiation
    p. dysplasia
    p. meningioma
postreceptor
postrenal
    p. albuminuria
    p. azotemia
post-traumatic hydrocephalus
postrubella syndrome
poststenotic dilatation
poststreptococcal
    p. glomerulonephritis
    p. hypersensitivity disease
postsynaptic
    p. membrane
    p. potential
post-term infant
post-transfusion
    p.-t. hepatitis
    p.-t. mononucleosis
    p.-t. thrombocytopenia
post-traumatic epilepsy
postulate
    Ehrlich's p.
    Koch's p's

postural
    p. albuminuria
    p. proteinuria
postvaccinal encephalomyelitis
post-vaccination allergic encephalitis
postzygotic
potable
Potamidae
Potamon
potassium
    p. acetate
    p. acidosis
    p. alkalosis
    p. para-aminosalicylate
    p. bicarbonate
    canrenoate p.
    carbenicillin p.
    p. channel
    p. chlorate
    p. chloride
    p. chromate
    p. citrate
    p. cyanate
    p. cyanide
    p. dichromate
    p. dihydrogen phosphate
    p. enteropathy
    p. ferrocyanide
    glucose, insulin and p.
    p. guaiacolsulfonate
    p. hydroxide
    p. hydroxide test
    p. hydroxide (KOH) test
    p. imbalance
    p. iodide
    p. isotope
    p. oxalate
    p. perchlorate
    p. permanganate
    p. phosphate
    p. salt
    p. tartrate
    p. test
    p. thiocyanate
    p. thiosulfate
    total body p.
    total exchangeable p. measurement
    p. urate crystals
    warfarin p.
    p.-42

potassium phosphate
    dibasic p.p.
    monobasic p.p.
    tribasic p.p.
potato
    p. dextrose agar
    p. node
    p. tumor of neck
potency
potential
    cervical somatosensory
      evoked p.
    corneoretinal p.
    decomposition p.
    diffusion p.
    Donnan's p.
    electric p.
    electrode p.
    end plate p.
    p. energy
    half-wave p.
    junction p.
    liquid-liquid junction p.
    membrane p.
    muscle action p.
    oxidation-reducing p.
    phosphate group transfer p.
    postsynaptic p.
    redox p.
    reduction p.
    resting membrane p.
    standard electrode p.
    standard reduction p.
    transmembrane p.
    visual evoked cortical p.
    zeta p.
potentiation
    long-term p.
potentiometer
    direct-reading p.
    null-point p.
    slide-wire p.
potentiometric titration
potentiometry
Potter-Bucky
    diaphragm
    grid
Potter sequence
potters' asthma
Potter's facies
Pott's
    abscess
    aneurysm

pouch
    branchial p.
    craniobuccal p.
    Douglas's p.
    first pharyngeal p.
    fourth pharyngeal p.
    Hunt-Lawrence p.
    Mainz's p.
    Pavlov's p.
    pharyngeal p.
    Physick's p's
    Rathke's p.
    rectouterine p.
    rectovaginal p.
    rectovesical p.
    second pharyngeal p.
    third pharyngeal p.
    vesicouterine p.
pouchitis
pour plate
povidone-iodine
Powassan's virus
power
    p. amplifier
    apparent p.
    carbon dioxide combining p.
    p. of exclusion
    p. function graph
    p. resistor
    resolving p.
    p. supply
poxvirus
PP — pancreatic polypeptide
    partial pressure
    pellagra preventive
    permanent partial
    "pink puffers" (emphysema)
    postpartum
    postprandial
    prothrombin-proconvertin
    protoporphyrin
    proximal phalanx
    pulse pressure
    pyrophosphate
PPA — phenylpyruvic acid
PPB — platelet-poor blood
    positive-pressure breathing
ppb — parts per billion
PPBS — postprandial blood sugar
PPCA — proserum prothrombin con-
      version accelerator

PPCF — plasmin prothrombin conversion factor
PPD — paraphenylenediamine
   phenyldiphenyloxadiazole
   purified protein derivative
PPF — plasma protein fraction
   purified protein fraction
PPG — protoporphyrinogen
ppg — picopicogram
PPH — postpartum hemorrhage
   primary pulmonary hypertension
   protocollagen proline hydroxylase
PPHP — pseudopseudohypoparathyroidism
PPLO — pleuropneumonia-like organism
ppm — parts per million
PPNG — penicillinase-producing *Neisseria gonorrhoeae*
PPP — pentose phosphate pathway
   platelet-poor plasma
PPR — Price precipitation reaction
PPS — pepsin
   postpump syndrome
PPT — plant protease test
Ppt or ppt — precipitate
   prepared
PPV — positive-pressure ventilation
PQ — permeability quotient
   pyrimethamine-quinine
PR — partial remission
   peripheral resistance
   prosthion
   protein
   pulse rate
Pr — praseodymium
   presbyopia
   prism
PR antigen
PRA — plasma renin activity
Prague pelvis
pralidoxime chloride
pramoxine hydrochloride
praseodymium
Prausnitz-Küstner
   antibody
   reaction
   test
prazepam
prazosin hydrochloride

PRBV — placental residual blood volume
PRC — packed red cells
PRCA — pure red cell agenesis
   pure red cell aplasia
PRD — partial reaction of degeneration
   postradiation dysplasia
preadaptation
prealbumin
   thyroxine-binding p.
preamplifier
preauricular
pre-B-cell leukemia
prebetalipoprotein
prebiventral fissure
precancer
precancerous
   p. dysplasia
   p. lesion
   p. melanosis of Dubreuilh
precarcinomatous
precentral
   p. fissure
   p. gyrus
   p. sulcus
prechroming
precipitant
precipitate
   keratitic p.
   keratotic p.
precipitating antibody
precipitation
   polyanion p.
   tuberculin p.
precipitin
   p. curve
   p. reaction
   p. test
   tube p.
precipitinogen
precision resistor
preclinical breast cancer
precocious
   p. adrenarche
   p. pseudopuberty
   p. puberty
precocity
preculminate fissure
precuneus
precursor
   ACTH-endorphin p.
   p. lesion

predaceous mite
predator
predecidual alteration
predeposit autologous transfusion
prediabetes
predictive value
predisposing cause
prednisolone
prednisone
preductal coarctation of aorta
preeclampsia
pre-eclamptic toxemia
preejection period
preeruptive
preexcitation syndrome
prefibrinolysin
preganglionic sympathetic fiber
pregnancy
    aborted ectopic p.
    ampullar p.
    corpus luteum of p.
    p. cycle
    ectopic p.
    extrauterine p.
    first trimester p.
    p. luteoma
    megaloblastic anemia of p.
    molar p.
    ovarian p.
    parasitic ectopic p.
    ruptured ectopic p.
    second trimester p.
    p. test
    third trimester p.
    toxemia of p.
    tubal p.
    p. tumor
    p. urine
    voluntary interruption of p.
pregnanediol assay
pregnanetriol
pregnant
    p. mare serum
    p. mare serum gonadotropin
pregnenolone
prehepatic hypoproteinemia
preictal
preinvasive
Preisz-Nocard bacillus
prekallikrein
prekeratin filament
prelaryngeal lymph node

preleukemia
pre-β-lipoprotein
preload
prelytic sphere
premalignant fibroepithelioma
premammary abscess
premature
    p. abnormal placenta
    p. atrial contraction
    p. climacteric
    p. contraction
    p. ejaculation
    p. infant
    p. labor
    p. menopause
    p. rupture
    p. rupture of (fetal) membranes
    p. senility syndrome
    p. separation of placenta
    p. ventricular contraction
prematurely
prematurity
premenarcheal
premenopausal
premenstrual
    p. endometrium
    p. tension
premolar
premonocyte
premorbid
premotor cortex
premyeloblast
premyelocyte
prenatal
    p. diagnosis
    p. screening
preneoplastic
prenyl groups
prenyltransferase
preoccipital notch
preoperative
preoptic nucleus
preovulatory
preparation
    allergenic protein p's
    biomechanical p.
    broken cell p.
    cell block p.
    corrosion p.
    crush p.
    cytologic filter p.

heart-lung p.
impression p.
Tzanck's p.
preparative immunofiltration
prepatellar bursitis
prepiriform area
pre-proinsulin
preprotein
prepubertal; prepuberal
    p. cryptorchidism
    p. hyperpituitarism
    p. panhypopituitarism
    p. testis
prepubescence
prepuce
    nonretractable p.
    p. of clitoris
    p. of penis
    redundant p.
    retained p.
preputial calculus
prepyloric atresia
prepyramidal fissure
prerenal
    p. albuminuria
    p. azotemia
pre-rolandic artery
presacral insufflation
presbycardia
presbycusis
presbyopia
prescription
presenile
    p. dementia
    p. spontaneous gangrene
presentation
    abnormal obstetrical p.
    antigen p.
    arm p.
    breech p.
    compound p.
    face p.
    transverse p.
    umbilical cord p.
preservative
prespermatogonia
pressor
    p. amine
    p. base
    diverticulum p.
    groove p.

p. substance
p.-volume curve
pressure
    arterial p.
    atrophy p.
    barometric p.
    carbon dioxide p.
    cerebrospinal fluid p.
    colloidal osmotic p.
    cone p.
    continuous distending p.
    p. crescent
    diverticulum p.
    end-diastolic p.
    end-systolic p.
    groove p.
    hydrostatic p.
    intracranial p.
    millimeters partial p.
    oncotic p.
    osmotic p.
    partial p.
    plasma oncotic p.
    positive p.
    pulmonary p.
    pulmonary wedge p.
    pulse p.
    screen filtration p.
    selection p.
    standard temperature and p.
    systemic arterial p.
    transpulmonary p.
    vapor p.
    venous p.
    p. volume curve
    wedged hapatic vein p.
presumptive heterophile test
presuppurative
presymphysial lymph node
presynaptic membrane
presystolic gallop
preterm infant
pretibial myxedema
pretracheal lymph node
prevalence rate
prevention
preventive
    p. medicine
    pellagra p.
previous value check
previtamin
    p. D_3
    p. H

PRF — prolactin releasing factor
PRFM — prolonged rupture of fetal
                membranes
PRH — prolactin-releasing hormone
PRI — phosphoribose isomerase
priapism
priapitis
Price-Jones curve
Price precipitation reaction
prickling sensation
prilocaine hydrochloride
primaquine
       p. phosphate
       p.-sensitive anemia
       p. sensitivity
primary
       p. active transport
       p. adrenal insufficiency
       p. African green monkey
         kidney
       p. agammaglobulinemia
       p. amenorrhea
       p. amyloidosis
       p. anemia
       p. atelectasis
       p. atypical pneumonia
       p. biliary cirrhosis
       p. carcinoma
       p. cardiomyopathy
       p. coil
       p. colors
       p. complex
       p. constriction
       p. culture
       p. endings
       p. endocardial sclerosis
       p. erythroblastic anemia
       p. extrapulmonary coccidioido-
        mycosis
       p. fibrinolysis
       p. fibromyalgia syndrome
       p. fissure
       p. glaucoma
       p. granule
       p. hyperaldosteronism
       p. hyperparathyroidism
       p. hyperplasia
       p. hyperthyroidism
       p. hypoadrenocorticism
       p. hypogammaglobulinemia
       p. immunodeficiency
       p. infertility

p. influenza virus pneumonia
p. intraosseous sarcoma
p. irritant dermatitis
p. lesion
p. lymphedema
p. lymphoma
p. lysosome
p. methemoglobinemia
p. myeloid metaplasia
p. myocardial disease
p. osteosarcoma
p. ovarian follicle
p. pentosuria
p. pulmonary hypertension
p. pyoderma
p. reference materials
p. refractory anemia
p. renal calculus
p. renal tubular acidosis
p. repair
p. sclerosing cholangitis
p. sensory neuron
p. sequestrum
p. sex character
p. somatomotor area
p. spermatocyte
p. standard
p. structure
p. synaptic cleft
p. syphilis
p. thrombocythemia
p. transcript
p. trisomy
p. tuberculosis
p. union
primate
primed lymphocyte typing
primer
primidone assay
primigravida
primipara
primitive
       p. erythroblast
       p. mesoblast
       p. neuroblastic cell
       p. neuroectodermal tumor
       p. neuroepithelial tumor
primordial
       p. dwarf
       p. germ cell
       p. ovum
       p. sex cell

primordium (pl., primordia)
primulin
principal
>p. cell
>p. focus

principle
>antianemic p.
>Fick's p.
>follicle-stimulating p.
>hematinic p.
>immediate p.
>luteinizing p.
>prothrombin-converting p.
>proximate p.
>ultimate p.
>uncertainty p.

printed circuit
P-R interval
Prinzmetal's angina
prion
Prionurus
prism
>adamantine p's
>p. degree
>Nicol p.

prismatic
pristanic acid
private antigen
privileged site
PRL — prolactin
PRM — phosphoribomutase
>preventive medicine
Pro — proline
pro — prothrombin
proaccelerin
proactivator
>C3 p. convertase
>C3 plasminogen p.

proalbumin
probabilistic
probability
>conditional p.
>p. distribution
>p. paper
>significance p.

probable error
proband
probe
>allele-specific oligonucleo-
>tide p's
>molecular hybridization p.
>nucleic acid p.

oligonucleotide p.
>radioactive p.
>viral p.

probenecid
probit transformation
proboscis
probucol
procainamide assay
procaine
>p. amide hydrochloride
>p. hydrochloride
>merethoxylline p.
>p. penicillin G

procallus
procarbazine
procarcinogen
procaryon
procaryote
procedure
>Akiyama's p.
>Anderson's p.
>Bartlett p.
>Berthelot's p.
>Camey's p.
>Cherry-Crandall p.
>Clark-Collip p.
>Cleveland p.
>concentration p's
>evacuation p's
>Faust zinc sulfate flotation p.
>Fisher's p.
>formalin-ethyl acetate p.
>formalin-zinc sulfate flota-
>tion p.
>gasometric ninhydrin p.
>helminth identification p's
>hypophysis staining p.
>Lewis p.
>Logan's p.
>Lygidakis' p.
>nylon wool adherence p.
>Ritchie formalin-ethyl ace-
>tate p.
>Silver's p.
>Tanner-Roux p.
>van Slyke amino acid p.

procentriole organizer
proceptivity
process
>acromion p.
>alveolar p.
>articular p.

caudate p.
ciliary p.
clinoid p.
p. control
coracoid p.
coronoid p.
costal p.
dendritic p.
falciform p.
foot p.
iterative p.
mastoid p.
odontoid p.
olecranon p.
pterygoid p.
spinous p.
styloid p.
Tomes' p.
transverse p.
uncinate p. of pancreas
xiphoid p.
zygomatic p.
processing
    antigen p.
    digital image p.
    image p.
    interactive p.
    RNA p.
    tissue p.
    word p.
processor
    front-end p.
processus vaginalis peritonei
prochlorperazine
    p. edisylate
    p. maleate
procidentia
procoagulant
procollagen
    p.-lysine
    p.-peptidase
    p. III peptide
    p.-proline
    p.-*N*-proteinase
procollagenase
proconvertin
proctalgia
proctatresia
proctectasia
proctencleisis; proctenclisis
proctitis
    chronic ulcerative p.

gonococcal p.
herpetic p.
idiopathic p.
p. obliterans
pseudoinfectious p.
Salmonella p.
traumatic p.
proctocele
proctoclitis
proctocolonoscopy
proctopolypus
proctoptosis
proctorrhagia
proctoscopy
proctosigmoiditis
proctosigmoidoscopy
proctostenosis
procyclidine hydrochloride
prodigiosin
prodromal
prodrome
product
    cleavage p.
    contact activation p.
    cross p.
    decay p.
    dot p.
    end p.
    fibrin/fibrinogen degrada-
        tion p's
    fibrinogen breakdown p's
    fibrinogen split p's
    fibrinolytic split p's
    fission p.
    gene p.
    ion p.
    p.-moment coefficient
    scalar p.
    solubility p.
    spallation p's
    substitution p.
    vector p.
    waste p.
production
    carbon dioxide p.
    p.-defect anemia
    excessive heat p.
    matrix p.
    pair p.
productive
    p. inflammation
    p. peritonitis
    p. pleurisy

proemial
proenzyme
proerythroblast
proerythrocyte
Professional Standards Review Organization
profibrinolysin
proficiency survey
profile
    biochemical p.
    cell volume p.
    complement p.
    fatty acid p.
    liver p.
    phagocytic cell immunocompetence p.
    test p.
profilin
progenitor cells
progeny
progeria
progeroid
progestational
    p. agents
    p. endometrium
    p. hormone
progesteroid
progesterone
    p. receptor
    p. unit
progestin
progestogen
proglottid
prognathism
prognosis
prognostic
    p. factor
    p. marker
progonoma
    p. of jaw
    melanotic p.
program
    p. evaluation and review technique
    object p.
    safety p.
    source p.
    survey p.
programming
    temperature p.
progranulocyte
progranulocytic leukemia

progravid
progressive
    p. bacterial synergistic gangrene
    p. bulbar palsy
    p. cerebellar dyssynergia
    p. coccidioidomycosis
    p. disseminated histoplasmosis
    p. emphysematous necrosis
    p. glomerulosclerosis
    p. hypocythemia
    p. lipodystrophy
    p. massive fibrosis
    p. multifocal leukoencephalopathy
    p. muscular atrophy
    p. muscular dystrophy
    p. pigmentary dermatosis
    p. pulmonary tuberculosis
    p. secondary tuberculosis
    p. shock
    p. spinal muscular atrophy
    p. staining
    p. supranuclear palsy
    p. systemic sclerosis
prohormone
proinsulin
projection
    Caldwell p.
    Fischer p.
    Towne p.
    transmandibular p.
Prokaryotae
prokaryote
prokaryotic
Proketazine
prolactin
    chorionic growth hormone p.
    p.-inhibiting factor
    p.-producing adenoma
    p. release-inhibiting hormone
    p.-releasing factor
    p.-releasing hormone
    p.-secreting tumor
    p. test
    p. unit
prolactinoma
prolan
prolapse
    mitral valve p.
    Morgagni's p.
prolapsed umbilical cord

Proleukin
proleukocyte
prolidase
proliferate
proliferating
    p. cell nuclear antigen
    p. endarteritis
    p. pleurisy
    p. systematized angioendotheli-
      omatosis
    p. trichilemmal cyst
    p. trichilemmal tumor
proliferation
    cell p.
    p. cyst
    diffuse mesangial p.
    p. inhibitory factor
    macrophage p.
    melanocytic p.
    sclerosing ductal p.
    T cell p.
proliferative
    p. arthritis
    p. bronchitis
    p. chronic arthritis
    p. cyst
    p. cystitis
    p. endometrium
    p. fasciitis
    p. fibrosis
    p. glomerulonephritis
    p. glomerulopathy
    p. inflammation
    p. intimitis
    p. mixoploid
    p. myositis
    p. retinopathy
    p. synovitis
proliferous cyst
proline
    p. dehydrogenase
    p. hydroxylase
    p. oxidase
    p. oxoglutarate dioxygenase
    p. 2-oxoglutarate dioxygenase
    procollagen-p.
prolinemia
prolinuria
prolonged
    p. bleeding time
    p. coagulation time
    p. P-R interval

    p. QRS complex
    p. rupture of fetal membranes
prolyl
prolylhydroxylase
    hepatic p.
prolymphocyte
prolymphocytic leukemia
PROM — premature rupture of
    membranes
    prolonged rupture of mem-
    branes
promastigote
promazine hydrochloride
promegakaryoblast
promegakaryocyte
promegaloblast
prometaphase banding
promethazine hydrochloride
promethestrol dipropionate
promethium
promiscuity
promoblast
promonocyte
promoter
    eosinophil stimulation p.
    tumor p.
promoting agent
promoxolane
promyelocyte
    basophilic p.
    eosinophilic p.
    neutrophilic p.
promyelocytic leukemia
pronation
pronephric glomerulus
pronephros
pronormoblast
pronucleus
proof
    constructive p.
    existence p.
pro-opiocortin
pro-opiomelanocortin
propagating thrombosis
propagation
propagule
propane
propanediolphosphate dehydrogenase
propanenitrile
propanoic acid
propanol
propantheline bromide

proparacaine
proparathyroid hormone
propenal
propenyl
propepsin
properdin
    p. assay
    p. factor A
    p. factor B
    p. factor D
    p. system
proper fasciculi
prophage
prophase
prophlogistic
prophylactic
    p. immunization
    p. mastectomy
    p. membrane
    p. serum
prophylaxis
propiolactone
propiomazine hydrochloride
propionate
    p. carboxylase
    p. metabolism
    zinc p.
Propionibacteriaceae
Propionibacterium
    P. acnes
    P. avidum
    P. granulosum
    P. lymphophilum
propionic
    p. acid
    p. acidemia
    p. aciduria
propionitrile
propionyl
    p.-coenzyme A carboxylase
    p. thiocholine
proplasia
proplasmacyte
proportional
    p. count
    p. counter
proportionate
    p. morbidity ratio
    p. mortality ratio
propositus (pl., propositi)
propoxur
propoxycaine

propoxyphene assay
propranolol
    p. assay
    p. hydrochloride
proprioceptive
proprioceptor
proprotein
proptometer
proptosis
propyl
    p. alcohol
    p. diethyl succinamate
    p. gallate
propylene
    p. dichloride
    p. glycol
propylhexedrine
propyliodone
propylthiouracil
prorenin
prorubricyte
    pernicious anemia type-p.
prosection
prosector's
    p. tubercle
    p. wart
prosencephalon
proserum prothrombin conversion accelerator
prosodemic
prosopagnosia
prosopalgia
prosopectasia
prosoplasia
prosostomate trematodes
prospective study
prostacyclin
prostaglandin
prostanoic acid
prostanoid
prostate
    p. capsule
    p. gland
    p. leukemia
    rhabdomyosarcoma of p.
    p.-specific acid phosphatase
    p.-specific anticoagulation
    p.-specific antigen
    p.-specific glycoprotein
prostatectomy
prostatic
    p. acid phosphatase

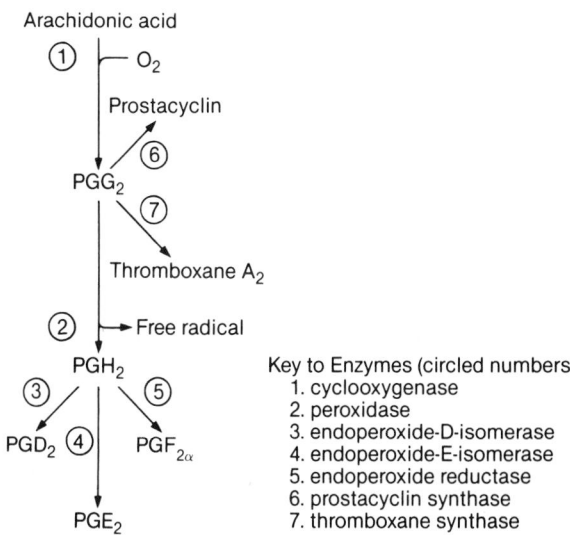

Arachidonic acid

Key to Enzymes (circled numbers):
1. cyclooxygenase
2. peroxidase
3. endoperoxide-D-isomerase
4. endoperoxide-E-isomerase
5. endoperoxide reductase
6. prostacyclin synthase
7. thromboxane synthase

The cyclooxygenase pathway of prostaglandin synthesis. (From Dorland's Illustrated Medical Dictionary, 27th ed. Philadelphia, W.B. Saunders Company, 1988, p. 1367.)

p. acinus
p. adenocarcinoma
p. adenoma
p. antibacterial factor
p. calculus
p. cancer
p. capsule
p. carcinoma
p. chips
p. cyst
p. duct
p. gland
p. granuloma
p. hyperplasia
p. hypertrophy
p. leukemia
p. muscle
p. pile
p. polyp
p. secretion
p. stones
p. tumor
p. urethra
p. utricle

prostatism
prostatitis
    allergic p.
    bacterial p.
    chronic p.
    eosinophilic p.
    gonococcal p.
    granulomatous p.
prostatocystitis
prostatodynia
prostatography
prostatolith
prostatomegaly
prostatovesiculitis
prosthesis
    antireflux p.
    cardiac p.
    facial p.
    penile p.
    Starr-Edwards p.
prosthetic
    p. group-labeled immunoassay
    p. obturator
    p. reconstruction

prosthion
prostration
    heat p.
prot — protein
protactinium
protaminase
protamine
    p. insulin
    p. sulfate
    p. sulfate test
    p. titration test
    p. zinc
    p. zinc insulin
protan
protanomaly
protanopia
Protargol
protease
    p. inhibitor
    slow-moving p.
protection
    radiation p.
protective protein
protector
Proteeae
proteidin
    pyocyanase p.
protein
    AA (amyloid A) p.
    AC p.
    accumulation of p.
    actin-binding p.
    acyl carrier p's
    AL p.
    β_{12} amyloid p.
    Bence Jones p.
    p. binding
    bone Gla p.
    bone morphogenetic p.
    p.-bound iodine assay
    p.-bound iodine 131 test
    p. breakdown
    p. buffer
    p. C antigen
    p.-calorie nutrition
    carrier p.
    catabolite activator p.
    p. channel
    chromogranin p.
    conjugated p.
    contractile p.
    copper storage p.

corticosteroid-binding p.
C-reactive p.
cytotoxic cell p.
p. deficiency anemia
p. denaturation
derived p.
dietary p.
p. efficiency ratio
p. electrolyte
p. electrophoresis
p.-energy malnutrition
eosinophil p.
eosinophil cationic p.
fibrous p's
G p.
glial fibrillary acidic p.
globular p.
guanyl-nucleotide-binding p.
heat-shock p.
high p.
p. hormone
p. hydrolysate
immune p.
integral p's
iron-sulfide p.
p. kinase, A and C
Kolmer's test with Reiter p.
lenticular p's
leukocyte adhesion p.
liver membrane p.
liver specific p.
p.-losing enteropathy
M p.
major basic p.
membrane-control p.
mild silver p.
mitotic-control p.
muscle contractile p.
myelin p.
myelin basic p.
myeloma p.
net dietary p.
neurofilament p.
p. nitrogen unit
nonhistone chromosomal p.
peripheral p's
p. plasma
plasma p's
protective p.
oncofetal p.
oncogenic p.
p. quotient

R p.
reactive p.
p. receptor
respiratory p.
retinol-binding p.
ribosomal P p.
p. S
S-100 p.
SAA p.
p. separation methods
p. shock
simple p.
sterol carrier p's
stress p.
structural p.
p. synthesis
Tamm-Horsfall p.
p. test
thyroxine-binding p.
total p.
total serum p.
transport p.
uncoupling p.
unwinding p.
Y p.
zinc finger p.
proteinase
    Bothrops atrox serine p.
    procollagen-*N*-p.
    Staphylococcus aureus neutral p.
proteinemia
proteinosis
    alveolar p.
    lipid p.
    lipoid p.
    pulmonary alveolar p.
proteinuria
    asymptomatic p.
    Bence Jones p.
    functional p.
    gestational p.
    glomerular p.
    intermittent p.
    isolated p.
    nonisolated p.
    orthostatic p.
    overflow p.
    persistent p.
    postgamma p.
    postural p.
    transient p.
    tubular p.

proteoclastic
proteoglycan
    polyanionic p.
proteolipid
proteolysis
proteolytic enzyme
Proteomyces
proteose peptone media
proteosuria
Proteus
    P. inconstans
    P. mirabilis
    P. morganii
    P. OX-K, OX-2, OX-19
    P. rettgeri
    P. stuartii
    P. vulgaris
proteus
    p. group
    p. pneumonia
prothipendyl hydrochloride
prothoracicotropic hormone
prothrombase
prothrombin
    p. accelerator
    p. activator
    p. complex
    p. consumption test
    p. consumption time
    p. conversion factor
    p.-converting principle
    p. deficiency
    p.-proconvertin test
    p. test
    p. time
    p. time test
prothrombinase
prothrombinogen
prothrombinogenic
prothrombinopenia
prothrombokinase factor
prothymocyte
proticity
protic solvent
protirelin
protist
Protista
protium
protoanemonin
Protobacterieae
protoblast
protocatechuate oxygenase

protocol
  Abraham's p.
  p. 019
  Stanford p.
protocoproporphyria hereditaria
protodiastolic gallop
protoerythrocyte
protohemin IX
protokylol hydrochloride
protoleukocyte
protometrocyte
proton
  p. acceptor
  p. acid
  p. donor
  p.-motive hypothesis
  p. pump
  p. tautomer
protonephridium
proto-oncogene
protoplasm
protoplasmic
  p. astrocyte
  p. astrocytoma
  p. bridge
  p. streaming
protoplasmolysis
protoplast fusion
protoporphyria
  erythrohepatic p.
  erythropoietic p.
protoporphyrin
  p. assay
  erythrocyte p.
  p. IX
  zinc p.
protoporphyrinogen oxidase
protoporphyrinuria
Prototheca
  P. ciferrii
  P. filamenta
  P. portoricensin
  P. segbwema
  P. wickerhamii
  P. zopfii
protothecosis
prototype
protoveratrine A and B
Protozoa
protozoal
  p. dysentery

p. enterocolitis
p. infection
protozoan
  p. infection
  p. parasite
protozoon (pl., protozoa)
  intestinal p.
protozoophage
protransglutaminase
protriptyline assay
protrude
protrusio acetabuli
protrusion
protuberance
  external occipital p.
  internal occipital p.
proud flesh
pro-UK — prourokinase
Providencia
  P. alcalifaciens
  P. providenciae
  P. stuartii
proviral
provirus
provisional callus
provitamin
  p. A
  p. carotenoids
  p. D_2
  p. D_3
provocation
provocative
  p. chelation test
  p. diagnosis
  p. test
  p. Wassermann test
prowazekia
Prower factor
prox — proximal
proximal
  p. convoluted renal tubule
  p. histidine
  p. radioulnar joint
  p. tibiofibular joint
  p. tubule
proximate
  p. cause
  p. principle
prozone phenomenon
PRP — pityriasis rubra pilaris
  platelet-rich plasma

PRPP — phosphoribosylpyrophos-
        phate
P-R segment
PRT — phosphoribosyltransferase
PRU — peripheral resistance unit
prune
        p. belly
        p. belly syndrome
prune-juice
        p.-j. expectoration
        p.-j. sputum
prurigo
        p. nodularis
        p. papule
pruritus
        p. ani
        scrotal p.
        p. vulvae
Prussian blue
        P.-b. reaction
        P.-b. stain
prussiate
prussic acid
PS — periodic syndrome
        phosphatidylserine
        population sample
        Porter-Silber (chromogen)
        prescription
        pulmonary stenosis
        pyloric stenosis
P/S — polyunsaturated-to-saturated
        fatty acids ratio
Ps. — Pseudomonas
ps — per second
        picosecond
PSA — polyethylene sulfonic acid
        prostate-specific anticoagu-
           lation
        prostate-specific antigen
psammocarcinoma
Psammolestes
psammoma bodies
psammomatous meningioma
psammosarcoma
PSC — Porter-Silber chromogen
        posterior subcapsular cataract
PSD — peptone-starch-dextrose
PSE — portal systemic encepha-
        lopathy
Pselaphephilia
pseudacromegaly
pseudalbuminuria

Pseudallescheria boydii
pseudallescheriasis
Pseudamphistomum truncatum
pseudarthrosis
pseudinoma
pseudoacanthosis
pseudoacanthosis nigricans
pseudoachondroplasia
pseudoachrondroplastic spondyloepi-
        physial dysplasia
pseudoacini
pseudoagglutination
pseudo-ainhum
pseudoalbuminuria
pseudoaldosteronism
pseudoalleles
pseudoanemia
pseudoaneurysm
pseudoangiosarcoma
        Masson's p.
pseudoarthrosis
pseudobacillus
pseudobacterium
pseudobulbar palsy
pseudocarcinomatous hyperplasia
pseudocartilaginous
pseudocast
pseudocholesteatoma
pseudocholinesterase deficiency
pseudochromhidrosis
pseudochylous
        p. ascites
        p. effusion
pseudochyluria
pseudocirrhosis
pseudoclear nucleus
pseudocolloid
pseudocoxalgia
pseudocyesis
pseudocylindroid
pseudocyst
        adrenal p.
        mesenteric p.
        pancreatic p.
pseudodecidual
pseudodiploid
pseudodiverticulum
pseudoencapsulated
pseudoephedrine hydrochloride
pseudoepitheliomatous
        p. balanitis
        p. hyperplasia

pseudoerysipelas
pseudoexfoliation
pseudofibroma
     paratesticular p.
pseudo-Gaucher cell
pseudogene
pseudoglioma
pseudoglobulin
pseudoglomerulus
pseudoglucosazone
Pseudogordius
pseudogout
pseudogranulomatous thyroiditis
pseudogynecomastia
Pseudohazis
pseudohematuria
pseudohermaphrodism
pseudohermaphroditism
pseudohernia
pseudoheterotopia
pseudo-Hurler polydystrophy
pseudohydronephrosis
pseudohyperkalemia
pseudohyperparathyroidism
pseudohyperplasia
pseudohypertriglyceridemia
pseudohypertrophic
pseudohypertrophy
pseudohyphae
pseudohyponatremia
pseudohypoparathyroidism
pseudoinfectious proctitis
pseudointraligamentous
pseudoisochromatic
pseudoleukemia
pseudolipoma
pseudolithiasis
pseudolobule
pseudolymphocyte
pseudolymphoma
     ocular p.
     Spiegler-Fendt p.
pseudomalignancy
pseudomamma
pseudomelanoma
pseudomelanosis
     p. coli
     p. pigment
pseudomembrane
pseudomembranous
     p. acute inflammation
     p. bronchitis

     p. colitis
     p. enterocolitis
     p. gastritis
     p. inflammation
     p. trigonitis
pseudomonad
Pseudomonadaceae
Pseudomonadales
Pseudomonadineae
Pseudomonas
     P. acidovorans
     P. aeruginosa
     P. alcaligenes
     P. cepacia
     P. diminuta
     P. eisenbergii
     P. fluorescens
     P. fragi
     P. kingii
     P. mallei
     P. maltophilia
     P. multivorans
     P. nonliquefaciens
     P. paucimobilis
     P. pseudoalcaligenes
     P. pseudomallei
     P. putida
     P. putrefaciens
     P. pyocyanea
     P. pyrrocinia
     P. stutzeri
     P. syncyanea
     P. testosteroni
     P. viscosa
pseudomonas
     p. bronchopneumonia
     p. pneumonia
     p. vasculitis
Pseudomonilia
pseudomucinous
     p. cyst
     p. cystadenocarcinoma
     p. cystadenoma
     p. degeneration
pseudomycelia
pseudomyiasis
pseudomyxoma peritonei
pseudoneoplasm
pseudoneuroma
pseudoneurotic schizophrenia
pseudoneutropenia
pseudo-osteomalacia pelvis

pseudo-osteomalacic
pseudoparakeratosis
pseudoparaproteinemia
pseudo-Pelger anomaly
pseudoperiodic
pseudoperoxidase
pseudophlegmon
    Hamilton's p.
Pseudophyllidea
pseudophyllidean
pseudoplatelet
pseudopod
pseudopodium (pl., pseudopodia)
pseudopolycythemia
pseudopolydystrophy
pseudopolyp
pseudopolyposis
pseudoprimary hyperaldosteronism
pseudo-pseudohypoparathyroidism
pseudopuberty
    precocious p.
pseudopyloric metaplasia
pseudopyogenic granuloma
pseudoreaction
pseudoreplica
pseudorheumatism
pseudorosette
    Homer-Wright p.
pseudosarcoma
pseudosarcomatous
    p. factor
    p. fasciitis
    p. metaplasia
pseudosclerosis
    Jakob-Creutzfeldt p.
    Westphal-Strümpell p.
pseudostoma (pl., pseudostomas,
    pseudostomata)
pseudostratified
pseudothalidomide syndrome
Pseudothelphusa
pseudothrombocytopenia
pseudothyroiditis
    malignant p.
pseudotrichinosis; pseudotrichiniasis
pseudotruncus arteriosus
pseudotubercle
pseudotuberculosis bacillus ✳
pseudotuberculous thyroiditis
pseudotubular degeneration
pseudotumor
    fibrous p.

✳ *Corynebacterium*

    inflammatory p.
    papillary p.
pseudouridine excretion
pseudovacuole
pseudovaginal perineoscrotal hypo-
    spadias
pseudoxanthoma
    p. cell
    p. elasticum
PSG — peak systolic gradient
    polysomnogram
    presystolic gallop
PSGN — poststreptococcal glomerulo-
    nephritis
p.s.i. — pounds per square inch
psilocin
psilocybin
psittacosis
    p. titer
    p. virus
psittacosis-lymphogranuloma vene-
    reum-trachoma (group)
psoas
    p. abscess
    p. muscle
psorenteritis
psoriasiform dermatitis
psoriasis
    p. arthropica
    exfoliative p.
    generalized pustular p. of Zam-
    busch
    pustular p.
    p. vulgaris
psoriatic arthritis
Psorophora
PSP — periodic short pulse
    phenolsulfonphthalein
    positive spike pattern
    progressive supranuclear palsy
PSRO — Professional Standards Re-
    view Organization
PSS — physiological saline solution
    progressive systemic sclerosis
p21 staining
PST — penicillin, streptomycin and
    tetracycline
psychalgia
psychataxia
psychiatric
psychiatry
psychoacoustics

psychoendocrinology
psychogenic
psychology
psychomotor
        p. epilepsy
        p. variant
psychoneuroimmunology
psychoneurosis
        anxiety p.
        obsessive-compulsive p.
        phobic p.
psychoneurotic
psychopathic
        p. inferiority
        p. personality
psychosexual
psychosin
psychosis (pl., psychoses)
        affective p.
        involutional p.
        Korsakoff's p.
        manic-depressive p.
        puerperal p.
        schizophrenic p.
psychosomatic
psychotropic
psychrophile
psychrophilic bacterium
psyllium
        p. hydrophilic mucilloid
        Spanish p.
PT — parathyroid
        paroxysmal tachycardia
        pneumothorax
        prothrombin time
PTA — persistent truncus arteriosus
        phosphotungstic acid
        plasma thromboplastin ante-
            cedent
        post-traumatic amnesia
PTAH — phosphotungstic acid hema-
            toxylin
PTB — patellar tendon-bearing
PTC — percutaneous transhepatic
            cholangiography
        phenylthiocarbamide
        phenylthiocarbamoyl
        plasma-thromboplastin com-
            ponent
PTE — parathyroid extract
        pulmonary thromboembolism

PTED — pulmonary thromboembolic
            disease
pteridine
pterin
pterion
pteroic acid
pteroylglutamic acid
pteroyl monoglutamic acid
pteroylpolyglutamate
pterygium
        p. coli
        congenital p.
        p. syndrome
pterygoid
        p. chest
        p. muscle
pterygomandibular
pterygomaxillary
pterygopalatine
        p. fossa
        p. ganglion
        p. nerve
Pterygota
PTF — plasma thromboplastin factor
PTFE — polytetrafluoroethylene
PTH — parathormone
        parathyroid hormone
        post-transfusion hepatitis
PTHS — parathyroid hormone secre-
            tion (rate)
PTI — persistent tolerant infection
PTM — post-transfusion mononu-
            cleosis
PTMA — phenyltrimethylammonium
ptomaine
ptomainemia
ptomatine
ptosed
ptosis (pl., ptoses)
ptotic organ
PTP — post-tetanic potentiation
        post-transfusion purpura
PTR — peripheral total resistance
PTS — para-toluenesulfonic acid
PTT — partial thromboplastin time
        particle transport time
PTU — propylthiouracil
PTX — parathyroidectomy
ptyalin
ptyalism
ptyalocele

PU — peptic ulcer
     pregnancy urine
Pu — plutonium
pubarche
puberty
     delayed p.
     precocious p.
pubic
     p. louse
     p. parasite
     p. symphysis
     p. tuberosity
pubis
public
     p. antigens
     p. specificity
Puchtler's
     alkaline Congo red method
     Sirius red method
Puchtler-Sweat
     stain for basement membranes
     stain for hemoglobin and hemo-
       siderin
PUD — pulmonary disease
pudendal
     p. artery
     p. hematocele
     p. nerve
     p. plexus
     p. vein
     p. venous plexus
pudendum (pl., pudenda)
     p. femininum
     p. muliebre
PUE — pyrexia of unknown etiology
puerpera
puerperal
     p. eclampsia
     p. mastitis
     p. osteomalacia
     p. phlebitis
     p. sepsis
     p. septicemia
     p. thrombosis
puerperium
PUFA — polyunsaturated fatty acid
pul — pulmonary
Pulex irritans
Pulicidae
pullorin
Pullularia pullulans
pullulate

pulmolith
pulmonary
     p. adenomatosis
     p. airway disease
     p. alveolar macrophage
     p. alveolar microlithiasis
     p. alveolar proteinosis
     p. alveolus
     p. anthracosis
     p. arteriovenous fistula
     p. artery
     p. artery hypertension
     p. artery stenosis
     p. atresia
     p. blastoma
     p. blastomycosis
     p. blood flow
     p. bulla
     p. candidiasis
     p. capillary blood volume
     p. carcinosis
     p. circulation
     p. coccidioidomycosis
     p. congestion
     p. cyst
     p. disease
     p. distomiasis
     p. docimasia
     p. dysmaturity syndrome
     p. edema
     p. embolism
     p. emphysema
     p. eosinophilia
     p. fibrosis
     p. fistula
     p. function test
     p. glomangiosis
     p. hamartoma
     p. heart disease
     p. hemorrhage
     p. hemosiderosis
     p. histoplasmosis
     p. hypertension
     p. hypoplasia
     p. hypostasis
     p. incompetence
     p. infarct
     p. infarction
     p. infiltration and eosinophilia
     p. insufficiency
     p. interstitial emphysema
     p. leukemia

p. ligament
p. lymph node
p. nodulosis
p. osteoarthropathy
p. pancreas
p. perfusion
p. perfusion scan
p. pleurisy
p. plexus
p. pneumonitis
p. pressure
p. sarcoidosis
p. stenosis
p. surfactant
p. thromboembolic disease
p. thromboembolism
p. tissue resistance
p. trunk
p. tuberculosis
p. valve
p. vascular resistance
p. vascular sclerosis
p. vein
p. venous congestion
p. ventilation
p. wedge pressure

pulmonic
p. ring
p. valve

pulmonic valve
p.v. anterior cusp
p.v. commissure
p.v. cusp

pulmonitis
pulmonology
pulp
p. gangrene
putrescent p.
vertebral p.

pulpar cell
pulpefaction
pulpiform
pulpitis
putrescent p.

pulpy testis
pulsating
p. empyema
p. metastases

pulsation
pulse
alternating p.
anacrotic p.

bigeminal p.
bisferiens p.
carotid p.
Corrigan's p.
p. deficit
dicrotic p.
p. height analyzer
irregular p.
jugular venous p.
p. oximetry
paradoxical p.
p. pressure
Quincke's p.
p. rate

pulsed field gradient gel electrophoresis
pulseless disease
pulsion diverticulum
pulsus (pl., pulsus)
p. parvus
p. tardus

pultaceous
pulvinar
p. nucleus
p. thalami

pump
calcium p.
cardiac balloon p.
electrogenic p.
infusion p.
perfusion p.
peristaltic p.
proton p.
sodium-potassium p.

punch biopsy
punctate
p. basophilia
p. keratoderma
p. parotiditis

punctation
Schüffner's p.

punctiform extravasation
punctum (pl., puncta)
puncture
femoral p.
lumbar p.
percutaneous renal p.

Puntius
PUO — pyrexia of unknown origin
pupil
Adie's p.
Argyll Robertson p.

bounding p.
tonic p.
pupillary membrane
pure
    chemically p.
    p. chemotasis
    p. culture
    p. red cell agenesis
    p. red cell anemia
    p. red cell aplasia
purification
    affinity p.
purified protein derivative
puriform
purinase
purine
    p. antimetabolite
    p. bases
    p. bodies test
    p. nucleoside phosphorylase
    p. and pyrimidine bases
purinemia
purity
    optical p.
    radiochemical p.
    radionuclidic p.
Purkinje's
    cells
    fibers
    neurons
puromucous
purple
    bromocresol p.
purpura
    allergic p.
    anaphylactoid p.
    p. angioneurotica
    p. annularis telangiectodes
    autoimmune thrombocytope-
        nic p.
    fibrinolytic p.
    p. fulminans
    p. hemorrhagica
    Henoch's p.
    Henoch-Schönlein p.
    hypergammaglobulinemic p.
    hyperglobulinemic p.
    idiopathic thrombocytope-
        nic p.
    immunologic thrombocyto-
        penic p.
    nonthrombocytopenic p.

post-transfusion p.
    Schönlein's p.
    Schönlein-Henoch p.
    testicular p.
    thrombocytopenic p.
    thrombotic thrombocytope-
        nic p.
    Waldenström's p.
purpuric
purpuriferous
purpurigenous
purpurin
purpurinuria
purpuriparous
purulence; purulency
purulent
    p. inflammation
    p. pachymeningitis
    p. pericarditis
    p. pleurisy
    p. synovitis
puruloid
pus
    blue p.
    p. bonum et laudabile
    p. cell
    cheesy p.
    p. corpuscle
    curdy p.
    green p.
    ichorous p.
    sanious p.
pustular
    p. bacterid
    p. inflammation
    p. psoriasis
pustule
    malignant p.
    postmortem p.
    spongiform p. of Kogoj
putamen
putrefaction
putrescent
    p. pulp
    p. pulpitis
putrescine
putrid throat
putty kidney
PV — peripheral vascular
    peripheral vein
    peripheral vessels
    plasma volume

polycythemia vera
portal vein
P & V — pyloroplasty and vagotomy
PVA — polyvinyl alcohol
PVA fixative method
PVA lacto-phenol medium
PVC — polyvinyl chloride
    postvoiding cystogram
    premature ventricular con-
      traction
    pulmonary venous congestion
PVD — peripheral vascular disease
PVF — portal venous flow
PVM — pneumonia virus of mice
PVP — penicillin V potassium
    peripheral vein plasma
    polyvinylpyrrolidone
    portal venous pressure
PVR — peripheral vascular resistance
    pulmonary vascular resistance
PVS — premature ventricular systole
PVT — paroxysmal ventricular tachy-
      cardia
    portal vein thrombosis
PW — posterior wall
PWA — person with AIDS
P wave
PWB — partial weight-bearing
PWI — posterior wall infarct
PWM — pokeweed mitogen
Px — pneumothorax
PXE — pseudoxanthoma elasticum
pyarthrosis
pycno-; pykno-
pyelectasis; pyelectasia
pyelitic
pyelitis
    p. cystica
    p. glandularis
pyelocaliectasis
pyelocystitis
pyelofluoroscopy
pyelogram
    intravenous p.
    retrograde p.
pyelography
pyelonephritic kidney
pyelonephritis
    acute p.
    ascending p.
    chronic p.
    obstructive p.

    reflux-associated p.
    xanthogranulomatous p.
pyelophlebitis
pyeloureterectasis
pyemia
    cryptogenic p.
    portal p.
pyemic
    p. abscess
    p. embolism
Pyemotes
Pyemotidae
pyesis
pygomelus
pygopagus
pyknocyte
pyknocytoma
pyknodysostosis
pyknomorphous
pyknosis
pyknotic index
pylemphraxis
pylephlebectasis; pylephlebectasia
pylephlebitis
pylethrombophlebitis
pylethrombosis
pyloric
    p. antrum
    p. Brunner's glands
    p. cap
    p. glands
    p. lymph node
    p. sphincter
    p. stenosis
pyloristenosis
pyloritis
pyloroduodenitis
pyloroplasty
    Mikulicz's p.
pyloroptosis; pyloroptosia
pyloroscopy
pylorospasm
pylorostenosis
pylorus-preserving resection
pyocele
pyocelia
pyocin
pyocolpocele
pyocolpos
pyocyanase
pyocyanic
pyocyanin

pyocyanogenic
pyocyst
pyocyte
pyoderma
    chancriform p.
    p. gangrenosum
    primary p.
    secondary p.
    streptococcal p.
pyodermatitis
pyodermatosis
pyogen
pyogenesis
pyogenic; pyogenetic
    p. bacterium
    p. cocci infection
    p. fever
    p. granuloma
    p. membrane
    p. meningitis
    p. osteomyelitis
    p. sacroiliitis
    p. salpingitis
pyogenous
pyohemia
pyoid
pyometra
pyometritis
pyomyoma
pyomyositis
pyonephritis
pyonephrolithiasis
pyonephrosis
pyopericarditis
pyopericardium
pyoperitoneum
pyoperitonitis
pyopoiesis
pyopoietic
pyopyelectasis
pyorrhea
pyosalpinx
pyosemia
pyosepticemia
pyosis
pyospermia
pyostatic
pyothorax
pyoureter
pyoverdin
pyoxanthin
pyoxanthose

pyramid
    renal p.
pyramidal
    p. cell
    p. decussation
    p. lobe
    p. neuron
    p. tract
pyran
pyranose
pyranoside
pyrantel pamoate
pyrathiazine
pyrazinamide
pyrazofurin
Pyrazus
pyrenemia
Pyrenochaeta romeroi
pyrethrin
pyrethrum
pyrexia
pyridine
    p. aldoxime methiodide
    alum-precipitated p.
    p. nucleotide
pyridostigmine bromide
pyridoxal
    p. kinase
    p. phosphate
pyridoxal-5′-phosphate
pyridoxamine
pyridoxic acid
pyridoxine-responsive anemia
pyriform sinus
pyrilamine maleate
pyrimethamine assay
pyrimethazine
pyrimidine
    p. analog
    p. bases
    p. biosynthesis
    p.-5′-nucleotidase
pyrithione zinc
pyrocatechol
pyrogallic acid
pyrogallol
pyrogallolphthalein
pyrogen
    endogenous p.
pyrogenic
pyroglobulin
pyroglobulinemia

pyroglutamase
pyroglutamate hydroxylase
pyroglutamicaciduria
pyrolysis
pyronin; pyronine
     p. B
     p. G
     p. Y
pyroninophilia
pyroninophilic
pyrophosphatase
     inorganic p.
     nucleotide p.
pyrophosphate
     calcium p.
     inorganic p.
pyrophosphohydrolase
pyrophosphokinase
pyrophosphomevalonate decarboxylase
pyrophosphoric acid
pyrophosphorylase
     nicotinamide mononucleo-
     tide p.
pyrophosphotransferase
pyropoikilocytosis
pyroracemic acid
pyrrobutamine phosphate
pyrrol; pyrrole
     p. blue

     p. cell
     p. ring
pyrrolia
pyrrolidone carboxylate
pyrrolidonyl aminopeptidase test
1-pyrroline-5-carboxylate dehydro-
     genase
pyrroline-5-carboxylate reductase
pyruvate
     p. carboxylase
     p. decarboxylase
     p. dehydrogenase
     p. kinase
     p. kinase assay
     p. kinase deficiency
     p. phosphokinase
pyruvic acid
pyrvinium
     p. chloride
     p. pamoate
Pythiaceae
pythium insidium
pythogenesis
pythogenic; pythogenous
pyuria
PZ — pancreozymin
PZA — pyrazinamide
PZ-CCK — pancreozymin cholecysto-
     kinin
PZI — protamine zinc insulin

Q — coulomb (electric quantity)
Q_{10} — temperature coefficient
q — long arm of a chromosome
Qa antigen
Q_B — total body clearance
Q-banding stain
QC — quality control
     quinine-colchicine
Q-enzyme
QF — quality factor
Q fever titer
q.n.s. — quantity not sufficient
QO_2 or qO_2 — oxygen quotient
QP — quanti-Pirquet reaction
Q. prep
QRS complex

QRZ — wheal reaction time
q.s. — sufficient quantity
quadrangular ligament
quadrant
quadrat
quadrate muscle
quadribasic
quadriceps
     q. femoris muscle
     q. tendon
quadriceptor
quadricuspid
quadrigeminal
quadriplegia
quadripolar
quadriradial

quadrivalent
qualitative analysis
quality
    q. control
    q. control chart
    q. factor
quanta
quantasome
quantatrope
quantile
quantimeter
quanti-Pirquet reaction
quantitation
    fecal fat t.
    q. test
quantitative
    q. analysis
    q. hypertrophy
    q. inheritance
    q. precipitin reaction
quantity
    q. not sufficient
    sufficient q.
quantotrope
quantum (pl., quanta)
    q. limit
    q. yield
quarantine
quartile
quark
QUART — quadrantectomy, axillary
               dissection, and radio-
               therapy
quartan
    q. fever
    q. malaria
quartile
quartz
quasicontinuous inheritance
quasidiploid
quasidominance
quasidominant inheritance
quassation
quaternary structure
quazodine
Queckenstedt's test
Queensland tick typhus
Quellung
    reaction
    test
quenching
    fluorescence q.

quercetin
Quetelet index
queue
Queyrat's erythroplasia
QUICHA — quantitative inhalation
              of challenge appa-
              ratus
quicksilver
Quick's
    method
    test
quiescent
quinacrine
    q. banding
    q. chromosome banding stain
    q. hydrochloride
    q. stain
quinaldine red
quinaldinic acid
quinate dehydrogenase
Quincke's
    edema
    pulse
quinestrol
quinethazone
quingestanol acetate
quinhydrone electrode
quinic acid
quinidine assay
quinine
    q. assay
    q. carbacrylic resin
    q. carbacrylic resin test
    q.-colchicine
    q. hydrochloride
    q. sulfate
Quinlan's test
quinoid
quinoline dye
quinolinic acid
quinology
quinone
    q.-oxime benzoyl hydrazine
    q. reductase
quinovose
quinquecuspid
quinquevalent
quinsy
quintisternal
quisqualic acid
quotidian
    q. fever
    q. malaria

quotient
    albumin q.
    blood q.
    caloric q.
    cerebral glucose
      oxygen q.
    circadian q.
    oxygen q.
    permeability q.
    protein q.
    rachidian q.
    reaction q.
    respiratory q.
Q wave

R

R — Behnken's (roentgen ray) unit
    organic radical
    Rankine (scale)
    Réaumur (scale)
    rectal
    regression coefficient
    respiration
    Rinne's test
    roentgen
    rough colony
R. — *Rickettsia*
R_A — airway resistance
R_x — prescription
RA — refractory anemia
    renal artery
    rheumatoid arthritis
    right atrial
Ra — radium
rabbetting
    Watanabe heritable hyperlipid-
      emic r.
rabbit
    r. antidog-thymus serum
    r. antimouse-thymocyte
      (serum)
    r. antirat-lymphocyte serum
    r. aorta-contracting substance
    r. blood agar
    r. fever
    r. fibroma
    r. kidney
    r. papilloma
    r. test
rabies
    r. immune globulin
    r. virus
RA (ragocyte) cell
racemase

racemate
racemic
    r. mixture
    r. modification
racemization
racemose
    r. adenoma
    r. aneurysm
    r. glands
    r. hemangioma
racephedrine
rachianesthesia
rachidean quotient
rachidial
rachigraph
rachiometer
rachis
rachischisis
rachitic
    r. pelvis
    r. rosary
rachitis
    r. fetalis
    r. fetalis annularis
    r. fetalis micromelica
    r. intrauterina
    r. uterina
racquet hypha
RAD — right axis deviation
rad — radial
    radiation-absorbed dose
    radiation-absorbed unit
radar
Radford nomogram
radial
    r. artery
    r. aplasia-thrombocytopenia
      syndrome

r. excision
r. growth phase
r. immunodiffusion
r. partition immunofluorometric assay
r. scar
r. sclerosing lesion
r. styloid tendovaginitis
r. symmetry
r. vein
radian
radiant energy
radiation
r.-absorbed dose
acoustic r.
adaptive r.
alpha r.
r. anemia
background r.
beta r.
braking r.
Cerenkov r.
r. chimera
chromatic r.
r. colitis
cosmic r.
corpuscular r.
r. counter
r. cystitis
r. damage
r. dermatitis
r. dermatosis
r. dose
r. effects
electromagnetic r.
r. fibroblasts
gamma r.
r. gastritis
Gratiolet r.
r. hazard
heterogeneous r.
homogeneous r.
Huldshinsky's r.
r. illness
r.-induced mutation
infrared r.
r. injury
interstitial r.
ionizing r.
magnetic r.
r. measuring units
mitogenic r.

monochromatic r.
monoenergetic r.
r. myelitis
r. myelopathy
r. necrosis
r. nephritis
nonionizing r.
occipitothalamic r.
optic r.
penetrating r.
r. pericarditis
r. pneumonitis
r. protection
pyramidal r.
r. reaction
r.-related hyperthyroidism
r.-related hypothyroidism
r.-related thyroiditis
r. response
r. sickness
tegmental r.
thalamic r.
thalamotemporal r.
r. therapy
total body r.
ultraviolet r.
radiative capture
radical
acid r.
alcohol r.
free r.
r. mastectomy
organic r.
r. scavenger
toxic oxygen r's
radicular cyst
radiculitis
radiculoganglionitis
radiculomedullary
radiculomeningomyelitis
radiculomyelopathy
radiculoneuropathy
radiculopathy
radioactive
r. concentration
r. constant
r. copper test
r. decay
r. drug
r. elements
r. equilibrium
r. gold

r. iodide uptake test
r. iodinated human serum albumin
r. iodinated serum albumin
r. iodine implants
r. iodine test
r. iodine-131 uptake
r. iodine uptake test
r. iridium implant
r. probe
r. tracer
r. waste
radioactivity
radioallergosorbent test
radioanaphylaxis
radioassay
radioautography
radiobiology
radiocarcinogenesis
radiocarpal
    r. joint
    r. ligament
radiochemical analysis
radiochroism
radiochromatogram
radiocinematograph
radiocystitis
radiodense
radiodensity
radiodermatitis
radioencephalogram
radioencephalography
radioenzymatic assay
radiogold colloid
radiograph
    Fab (formalin ammonium bromide) r.
    Fc r.
    homogeneously staining r's
radiographic media crystals
radiography
    stereoscopic r.
radioimmunity
radioimmunoassay
    r. automation
    solid-phase r.
radioimmunodiffusion
radioimmunoelectrophoresis
radioimmunoprecipitation assay
radioimmunosorbent test
radioiodinated
    r. fatty acid
    r. serum albumin

radioiodination
    lactoperoxidase r.
radioiodine
radioiron
    multidrug r.
    multiple drug r.
radioisotope
radioisotopic
    r. culture
    r. immunoassay
radiokymography
radiolabeled
radiolabeling
radioligand assay
radiologic
radiologist
radiology
radiolucency
radiolucent
radiolysis
radiometer
radiometry
radiomimetic
radiomutation
radionecrosis
radionuclide
radionuclidic
radiopacity
radiopaque medium
radiopathology
radiopharmaceutical
radiophosphorus
radiopulmonography
radioreceptor assay
radiorenography
radioresistant
radioresponsiveness
radioscopic
radioscopy
radiosensitivity test
radiosialography
radiostereoscopy
radiostrontium
radiotelemetry
radiotellurium
radiotherapy
    adjuvant r.
    interstitial r.
    intracavitary r.
    involved field r.
    particle beam r.
radiotoxemia

radiotracer
radiotropic
radioulnar joint
radio waves
radium
    r. implant
    r. isotope
    r. necrosis
    r. therapy
radius (pl., radii)
    r. of resolution
    r. of view
    oncogenous r.
    thrombocytopenia with absence of r.
radix (pl., radices)
radon implant
RADTS — rabbit anti–dog thymus serum
RAE — right atrial enlargement
RAF — rheumatoid arthritis factor
raffinose
ragged red fibers
ragocyte
ragweed
RAH — right atrial hypertrophy
RAI — radioactive iodine
RAI
    scan
    scan uptake
    test
Raillietina
    R. celebensis
    R. demerariensis
Rainier hemoglobin
raised colony
RAIU — radioactive iodine uptake
Raji
    cell
    cell assay
    cell radioimmune assay
rale
RA latex fixation test
RAM — random-access memory
Raman spectroscopy
Rambourg's
    chromic acid–phosphotungstic acid stain
    periodic acid–chromic methenamine–silver stain
ramex
Ramon flocculation

Ramsden's eyepiece
RAMT — rabbit antimouse thymocyte (serum)
ramus (pl., rami)
    r. communicans
    dorsal r.
    ventral r.
    white r.
rancid
rancidification
rancidity
random
    r. access
    r.-access memory
    r. analytical variability
    r. breeding
    r. coil
    r. error
    r. genetic drift
    r. mating
    r. number
    r. number generator
    r. plasma glucose test
    r. sample
    r. urine specimen
    r. variable
randomization
randomized
random sample
    muliple stage r.s.
    simple r.s.
    stratified r.s.
Raney nickel
range
    r. of motion
    semiinterquartile r.
ranine tumor
ranitidine hydrochloride
rank
    r. correlation coefficient
    r. sum test
ranked data
Ranke's formula
Rankine
    temperature scale
    thermometer
Rankin's clamp
ranula pancreatica
ranular cyst
Ranvier's node
RAO — right anterior oblique
Raoult's law

RAP — right atrial pressure
rapeseed oil
raphe
rapid
>r. duodenal intubation
>r. eye movement
>r. lysis mutation
>r. plasma reagin test
>r. recompression
>r. streptococcal antigen test

rapidly
>r. miscible pool
>r. progressive glomerulone-
>phritis
>r. adapting receptor

Rapoport's test
Rapoport-Luebering
>cycle
>shunt

Rappaport's classification
rare earth elements
rarefaction
RARLS — rabbit antirat lymphocyte
>serum
RARS — refractory anemia with
>ringed sideroblasts
RAS — renal artery stenosis
ras oncogene
rash
>academy r.
>black currant r.
>butterfly r.
>heliotrope r.
>hydatid r.

Rasmussen's aneurysm
raspberry tongue
RAST — radioallergosorbent test
rat
>r.-bite fever
>r.-line test
>r. ovarian hyperemia (test)
>r. tapeworm
>r. thymus antiserum
>r. unit
>r. virus

rate
>acid-secretion r.
>adjusted r.
>age-adjusted r.
>age-specific r.
>aldosterone excretion r.
>aldosterone secretion r.

>aldosterone secretory r.
>amebic prevalence r.
>attack r.
>basal metabolic r.
>birth r.
>bone formation r.
>case fatality r.
>cause-specific death r.
>cerebral cortex perfusion r.
>cerebral metabolic r.
>circulation r.
>r. constant
>corrected sedimentation r.
>cortisol production r.
>cortisol secretion r.
>count r.
>crude r.
>death r.
>decay r.
>dose r.
>error r.
>erythrocyte sedimentation r.
>estradiol production r.
>failure r.
>fatality r.
>fetal death r.
>flotation r.
>flow r.
>glomerular filtration r.
>growth r.
>incidence r.
>infant mortality r.
>intrauterine growth r.
>maternal mortality r.
>maximal midflow r.
>metabolic clearance r.
>r. meter
>mobidity r.
>mortality r.
>mutation r.
>neonatal mortality r.
>output exposure r.
>perinatal mortality r.
>pineal secretory r.
>plasma clearance r.
>plasma-glucose disappear-
>ance r.
>plasma-glucose tolerance r.
>plasma iron turnover r.
>prevalence r.
>pulse r.
>reaction r.

red cell iron turnover r.
relative survival r.
renin-release r.
respiration r.
Rourke-Ernstein sedimentation r.
secondary attack r.
secretion r.
sedimentation r.
somnolent metabolic r.
specific r.
sporozoite r.
standardized r.
testosterone production r.
time-kill r.
Westergren's sedimentation r.
Wintrobe's sedimentation r.
work metabolic r.
zeta sedimentation r.
RATHAS — rat thymus antiserum
Rathke's
   cleft cyst
   pouch
   pouch tumor
rating
   reactivity hazard r's
ratio
   a/A r.
   acid-base r.
   activity r.
   ADP/ATP (adenosine diphos-
      phate/adenosine triphos-
      phate) r.
   albumin-globulin r.
   ALT/AST (alanine aminotrans-
      ferase/antilymphocytic se-
      rum) r.
   amniotic fluid lecithin/sphingo-
      myelin r.
   amylase-creatinine clearance r.
   base r.
   blood urea nitrogen/creati-
      nine r.
   body hematocrit–venous hema-
      tocrit r.
   bound-free r.
   branching r.
   carpometacarpal r.
   cholesterol-phospholipid r.
   common mode rejection r.
   conduction r.
   conversion r.

corticomedullary r.
crude mortality r.
De Ritis r.
distribution r.
epinephrine:norepinephrine r.
granulocyte-erythroid r.
helper-suppressor cell r.
insulin-to-glucose r.
ketogenic-antiketogenic r.
lactate-pyruvate r.
left-to-right r.
L/S (lecithin-
   sphingomyelin) r.
mean diameter-thickness r.
monocyte-lymphocyte r.
myeloid-erythroid r.
net protein r.
nuclear-cytoplasmic r.
oil-water r.
packing r.
polyunsaturated-to-saturated
   fatty acids r.
proportionate morbidity r.
proportionate mortality r.
protein efficiency r.
resin-uptake r.
reversed albumin-globulin r.
r. scale
selectivity r.
standard morbidity r.
standard mortality r.
testosterone-to-estradiol r.
therapeutic r.
thyroid-to-serum r.
urine-plasma r.
urine-serum osmolality r.
U/S osmal r.
ventilation-perfusion r.
zeta sedimentation r.
rat-tail maggot
Rattus
RATx — radiation therapy
Rauwolfia serpentina
ray
   alpha r.
   beta r.
   cathode r.
   corresponding r.
   cosmic r.
   delta r.
   erythema-producing r's
   fluorescent r's

gamma r.
Goldstein's r's
grenz r's
infrared r.
medullary r's
monochromatic r.
necrobiotic r.
positive r.
refracted r.
roentgen r.
titanium r.
ultraviolet r.
W r's
x r's
Raynaud's phenomenon
razoxane
RB — respiratory bronchiole
Rb — rubidium
RBA — rose bengal antigen
R-banding stain
RBB — right bundle branch
RBBB — right bundle branch block
rbc or RBC — red blood cell
      red blood count
RBC/hpf — red blood cells per high
          power field
RBCM — red blood cell mass
RBCV — red blood cell volume
RBE — relative biological effec-
      tiveness
RBF — renal blood flow
RBL — Reid's base line
RBP — retinol-binding protein
RC — red cell
      red cell casts
      retrograde cystogram
RCA — right coronary artery
RCBV — regional cerebral blood
        volume
RCC — red cell count
RC circuit
RCD — relative cardiac dullness
RCF — red cell folate
      relative centrifugal force
RCM — red cell mass
      right costal margin
R (rough) colony
RCR — respiratory control ratio
RCS — reticulum cell sarcoma
RCV — red cell volume
RD — Raynaud's disease
      reaction of (to) degeneration

      resistance determinant
      respiratory disease
      right deltoid
      right dorsoanterior
rd — rutherford
RDE — receptor-destroying enzyme
RDI — rupture-delivery interval
rDNA — ribosomal DNA
        recombinant DNA
RDP — right dorsoposterior
RDS — respiratory distress syndrome
RDW — red-cell distribution width
RE — radium emanation
      regional enteritis
      reticuloendothelial
Re — rhenium
REA — radioenzymatic assay
reabsorb
reabsorption
react
reactance
      capacitive r.
      inductive r.
reactant
      acute phase r's
      limiting r.
reaction
      acid r.
      acrosome r.
      acute phase r.
      addition r.
      alkaline r.
      allergic r.
      alloxan-Schiff r.
      amphoteric r.
      anaphylactoid r.
      anoxia r.
      antigen-antibody r.
      antigen-antiglobulin r.
      antiglobulin r.
      antitryptic r.
      argentaffin r.
      Arias-Stella r.
      Arthus r.
      associative r.
      autoimmune r.
      azo-coupling r.
      Bauer r.
      Bence Jones r.
      Berthelot r.
      biuret r.
      Bloch's r.
      blocking antibody r.

Brand-Legal nitroprusside r.
Burchard-Liebermann r.
cachexia r.
Carr-Price r.
chain r.
chemical r.
chloroacetate esterase r.
cholera-red r.
Christeller r.
chromaffin r.
clot r.
conglutination r.
contrast media r.
cross r.
cutaneous r.
cytokeratin r.
dark r's
r. of degeneration
delayed hypersensitivity r.
diacetyl r.
diazo r.
digitonin r.
Dold's r.
dopa r.
Edman r.
Ehrlich's r.
Ehrlich's aldehyde r.
Ehrlich's benzaldehyde r.
Ehrlich's diazo r.
elimination r.
endergonic r.
endogenous antigen–cell-
   bound antibody r.
endogenous antigen–circulating antibody r.
endogenous antigen–trans-
   ferred antibody r.
endogenous antigen–trans-
   ferred cell-bound antibody r.
enthalpy of r.
eosinophilic leukemoid r.
erythrocyte sedimentation r.
exergonic r.
false-negative r.
false-positive r.
Felix-Weil r.
Fenton r.
Fernandez r.
ferric chloride r. of epinephrine
Feulgen r.
first-order r.

flocculation r.
foreign body r.
Frei-Hoffman r.
Freund's r.
fuchsinophil r.
Fujiwara r.
furfurol r.
generalized Sanarelli-Shwartzman r.
generalized Shwartzman r.
Gerhardt's r.
giant cell r.
glycine-arginine r.
graft-versus-host r.
graft-versus-host disease r.
Gruber-Widal r.
GVH (graft-versus-host) r.
Haber-Weiss r.
hemoclastic r.
Henle's r.
Herxheimer's r.
heterophil antigen r.
high-altitude r.
hypersensitivity r.
id r.
immunoprecipitin r.
incompatible blood transfusion r.
indophenol r.
inflammatory r.
r. intermediate
intradermal r.
iodate r. of epinephrine
iodine r. of epinephrine
irreversible r.
Jaffe's r.
Jarisch-Herxheimer r.
Jones-Mote r.
Klein's r.
Kveim r.
Langhans's type of giant cell r.
Legal nitroprusside r.
lepromin r.
leukemoid r.
Liebermann-Burchard r.
light r.
Marchi's r.
Mazzotti r.
Meinicke turbidity r.
Mitsuda's r.
mixed agglutination r.
mixed lymphocyte r.

Nadi r.
Nagler's r.
Neisser's r.
neutrophilic leukemoid r.
Nickerson-Kveim test r.
ninhydrin r.
ninhydrin-Schiff r.
nitritoid r.
oxidase r.
oxidation-reduction r.
Pandy's r.
PAS (periodic acid–Schiff) r.
passive Arthus r.
Penn's seroflocculation r.
peracetic acid-Schiff r.
performic acid r.
performic acid-Schiff r.
periodic acid-Schiff r.
Perls's r.
peroxidase r.
photochemical r.
Pirquet's r.
PK (Prausnitz-Küstner) r.
plasmal r.
polymerase chain r.
Porter-Silber r.
Prausnitz-Küstner r.
precipitin r.
Price precipitation r.
Prussian blue r.
quanti-Pirquet r.
quantitative precipitin r.
Quellung r.
r. quotient
radiation r.
r. rate
reagin r.
redox r.
rheumatoid factor r.
Sakaguchi's r.
Schmorl's r.
Schultz-Dale r.
Schultz's r.
second-order r.
sedimentation r.
Shwartzman's r.
sigma r.
Stammler's r.
streptococcal toxin immunization r.
substitution r.
Szent-Györgyi r.

tetanus toxin immunization r.
thermoprecipitin r.
r. time
r. to degeneration
transferred antigen–cell-bound antibody r.
transferred antigen–transferred antibody r.
transfusion r.
Treponema pallidum immobilization r.
triketohydrindene r.
tuberculin r.
typhoid immunization r.
Voges-Proskauer r.
Wassermann r.
Weidel's r.
Weil-Felix r.
Weinberg's r.
Widal's r.
Yorke's autolytic r.
zero-order r.
Zimmermann's r.
reactivation
  dark r.
  r. tuberculosis
reactive
  r. arthropathy
  r. dermatitis
  r. eosinophilia
  r. hyperemia
  r. hyperemia blood flow
  r. hypoglycemia
  r. leukocytosis
  r. lymphadenitis
  r. lysis
  r. material
  r. protein
  r. systemic amyloidosis
  weakly r.
reactivity
  r. hazard ratings
  lymphoid r.
reactone red test
reactor
  biologic false-positive r.
  nuclear r.
readability
reader
  mark sense r.
reading frame
readout

readthrough
read-write memory
reagent
    acetic anhydride–acetic acid–
      sulfuric acid r.
    Benedict-Hopkins-Cole r.
    Benedict's r.
    Berthelot's r.
    Bial's r.
    chlorous acid r.
    Cleland's r.
    Coleman-Schiff r.
    diazo r.
    Drabkin's r.
    Edlefsen's r.
    Ehrlich's r.
    Ellman r.
    Esbach's r.
    Exton's r.
    Folin-Ciocalteu r.
    Fouchet's r.
    Frohn's r.
    furfural r.
    Girard's r.
    gold chloride r.
    r. grade
    Günzberg's r.
    Hahn's oxine r.
    Hammarsten's r.
    Hanker-Yates r.
    Ilosvay r.
    iron salt–sulfuric acid r.
    Izar's r.
    Kasten's fluorescent Schiff r's
    Kober's r.
    Kovács' r.
    Lloyd's r.
    Mandelin's r.
    Marme's r.
    Marquis's r.
    maximum impurities r's
    Mecke's r.
    Millon's r.
    Nessler's r.
    Nichols's r.
    Rosenthaler-Turk r.
    Sanger's r.
    Schaer's r.
    Scheibler's r.
    Schiff's r.
    Selivanoff's (Seliwanow's) r.
    Sickledex r.

    r. strip
    Sulkowitch's r.
    p-toluenesulfonic acid r.
    Trinder's r.
    Voges-Proskauer r.
reagin
    r. reaction
    r. test
reaginic antibody
real
    r. number
    r. time
    r.-time clock
reanneal
reassociation
    DNA r.
Réaumur
    scale
    thermometer
Rebuck's skin window technique
recalcification time
recall antigen
recanalization
receiver operating characteristic
recent
    r. embolus
    r. infarct
    r. thrombus
receptoma
receptor
    acetylcholine r's
    adrenergic r's
    alpha r.
    alpha-adrenergic r.
    γ-aminobutyric acid r's
    androgen r.
    antigenic binding r.
    beta r.
    C3a, C5a r.
    cell surface r.
    cholinergic r.
    cold r.
    complement r., 1, 2, 3, 4
    contiguous r.
    cutaneous r.
    r.-destroying enzyme
    dominant r.
    estradiol r.
    estrogen r.
    Fc (cell surface) r's
    GABA (γ-aminobutyric
      acid) r's

gustatory r.
hair follicle r's
homing r.
hormone r.
insulin r's
joint r.
juxtapulmonary-capillary r.
muscle r.
nonadapting r.
olfactory r.
opiate r.
opioid r.
orphan r.
paciniform r's
pain r.
polyimmunoglobulin r.
progesterone r.
protein r.
rapidly adapting r.
sensory r.
sessile r.
slowly adapting r.
soluble interleukin-2 r's
stretch r.
tacile r.
T-cell antigen r's
thermal r.
touch r.
transferrin r.
vibration r.
visual r.
volume r's
warmth r.
recess
    duodenojejunal r.
    facial r.
    lateral r.
recessive
    r. abetalipoproteinemia
    r. character
    r. enzymatic deficiency
    r. gene
    r. inheritance
recessus (pl., recessi)
recipient
reciprocal
    r. genes
    r. translocation
recirculation
    lymphocyte r.
Recklinghausen's tumor
recognin

recognition
    antigen r.
    cognate r.
    r. factor
recombinant
    r. DNA analysis
    r. erythropoietin
recombination
    r. frequency
    high-frequency r.
    meiotic r.
Recombivax HB
reconstruction
    breast r.
    prosthetic r.
record
    logical r.
    medical r.
    physical r.
recorder
recording
    r. electrode
    r. thermometer
recovery
    Elkind's r.
recrudescent
    r. fever
    r. typhus
rectal
    r. ampulla
    r. artery
    r. crypt of Lieberkühn
    r. gonorrhea
    r. lumen
    r. mucous membrane
    r. mucus
    r. muscularis propria
    r. solitary nodule
    r. submucosa
    r. vein
rectification
rectifier
    bridge r.
    full-wave r.
    half-wave r.
    silicon-controlled r.
rectilinear scanner
rectitis
rectoabdominal
rectocele
rectocolitis
rectolabial fistula

rectosigmoid colon
rectostenosis
rectourethral fistula
rectouterine
rectovaginal
    r. fistula
    r. septum
rectovesical
    r. fistula
    r. pouch
    r. septum
rectovestibular fistula
rectovulvar fistula
rectum
recurrence risk
recurrent
    r. albuminuria
    r. artery
    r. carcinoma
    r. cystitis
    r. inflammation
    r. laryngeal nerve
    r. upper respiratory tract in-
        fection
recurring
    r. digital fibromas of childhood
    r. hemorrhage
recursion
recursive
    r. definition
    r. subroutine
red
    alizarin r.
    r. atrophy
    r. blood cell
    r. blood cell count
    r. blood cell enzyme deficiency
    r. blood cell mass
    r. blood cell morphology
    r. blood cells per high power
        field
    r. blood cell survival
    r. blood cell urinary cast
    r. blood cell volume
    r. blood count
    r. bugs (itch mites)
    calcium r.
    r. cell
    r. cell aplasia
    r. cell casts
    r. cell count
    r. cell diapedesis

    r. cell distribution width
    r. cell folate
    r. cell fragility
    r. cell fragmentation syndrome
    r. cell index
    r. cell iron turnover rate
    r. cell lysis
    r. cell mass
    r. cell survival test
    r. cell volume
    chlorophenol r.
    Congo r.
    r. corpuscle
    r. degeneration
    r. hepatization
    r. induration
    r. infarct
    r. infarction
    r. mite
    r. neurons
    r. nucleus
    oil r.
    Sirius r.
    r. squill
    r. test
    r. thrombus
    r. urine
    r. venous blood
redox
    r. couple
    r. indicator
    r. potential
    r. reaction
reduce
reduced
    r. glutathione
    r. hematin
    r. hemoglobin
    r. nicotinamide-adenine dinu-
        cleotide
reducing
    r. agent
    r. substances
    r. sugar
reductant
reductase
    acetoacetyl-CoA r.
    5-alpha r.
    biliverdin r.
    cytochrome b_5 r.
    dihydrofolate r.
    dihydropteridine r.

folate r.
glutathione r.
lysine ketoglutarate r.
lysine-2-oxoglutaryl r.
methemoglobin r.
NADH-cytochrome b_5 r.
NADH-dependent methemo-
    globin r.
4-oxoproline r.
pyrroline-5-carboxylate r.
ribonucleotide r.
ubiquinone r.
L-xylulose r.
reduction
    r. division
    r. potential
    tetrazolium r.
redundancy
    ureteral r.
reduplication
Reduviidae
reduviid bugs
Reduvius
Reed cells
reed relay
Reed-Sternberg
    cells
    giant cell
reentrant pathway
reentry
Reese dermatome
Reese-Ecker
    fluid
    method
Rees's culture medium
REF — renal erythropoietic factor
reference
    common r.
    r. distribution
    r. electrode
    r. interval
    laboratory r.
    r. method
    r. strain
    r. values
referent value
reflecting microscope
reflection
    angle of r.
    Bragg r.
    diffuse r.

specular r.
total internal r.
reflex
    accommodation r.
    Achilles r.
    antigravity r's
    audiocular r.
    autonomic r.
    axon r.
    Babinski's r.
    Bainbridge's r.
    baroreceptor r.
    Bezold-Jarisch r.
    Bezold's r.
    brachioradialis r.
    brain stem r's
    bulbospongiosus r.
    carotid sinus r.
    ciliospinal r.
    closed loop r.
    cochleopupillary r.
    conditioned r.
    corneal r.
    cough r.
    cremasteric r.
    crossed adductor r.
    crossed extension r.
    Cushing's r.
    enterogastric r.
    esophagosalivary r.
    extensor plantar r.
    flexion r.
    flexor plantar r.
    gag r.
    H r.
    Hering-Breuer r.
    Hoffmann's r.
    hypogastric r.
    increased flexion r.
    increased stretch r.
    ischemic r.
    labyrinthine r.
    light r.
    mass r.
    micturition r.
    monosynaptic r.
    neck r's
    oculocardiac r.
    oculocephalic r.
    oculovestibular r.
    open loop r.
    orienting r.

palmar r.
parachute r.
patellar tendon r.
periosteal r.
peristaltic r.
polysynaptic r.
pupillary r.
Roger's r.
scratch r.
spinal r.
stretch r.
suckling r.
testicular compression r.
viscerotrophic r.
withdrawal r.

reflux
    r.-associated pyelonephritis
    r. esophagitis
    hepatojugular r.
    r. nephropathy
    vesicoureteral r.

refract

refracted
    r. light
    r. ray

refracting medium

refraction
    angle of r.
    double r.
    index of r.

refractive index

refractometer

refractory
    r. anemia
    r. cytopenia
    r. leukemia
    r. normoblastic anemia
    r. period
    r. sideroblastic anemia

REG — radioencephalogram

Regan isoenzyme

Regan-Lowe agar

Regaud's
    fixative
    tumor

regeneration
    atypical r.
    compensatory r.
    epimorphic r.
    morphallactic r.

regenerative
    r. blood shift

r. endometrium
r. polyp

region
    antigen-binding r.
    complementarity-determining r.
    critical r.
    framework r.
    hinge r.
    homogeneously staining r.
    inguinal r.
    J r.
    sacrococcygeal r.
    variable r.

regional
    r. cerebral blood volume
    r. colitis
    r. enteritis
    r. enterocolitis
    r. ileitis

register
    index r.
    shift r.

registry
    tumor r.

Regitine

regressing atypical histiocytosis

regression
    r. analysis
    r. coefficient
    r. curve
    least squares r.
    r. line
    linear r.

regressive staining

regulated area

regulation
    genetic r.
    lipolysis r.
    transacting transcriptional r.

regulator
    current r.
    r. gene
    paracrine r.
    voltage r.

regulatory
    r. albuminuria
    r. gene
    r. sequence

regurgitation
    cardiac valvular r.
    r. jaundice
    mitral r.

rehabilitation
Rehfuss's test
rehydration
Reid's
    base line
    index
Reil's limiting sulcus
Reiner's D-xylose absorption test
reinfection tuberculosis
Reinke's
    crystalloids
    crystals
reinnervation
Reinsch's test
Reissner's
    fiber
    membrane
Reiter's protein complement-fixation
    test
Reitland-Franklin unit
rejected
    total graft area r.
rejection
    acute cellular r.
    chronic allograft r.
    graft r.
    homograft r.
    hyperacute r.
    r. vasculitis
rejuvenescence
relapse
relapsing
    r. febrile nodular panniculitis
    r. fever
    r. pancreatitis
    r. perichondritis
    r. polychondritis
relation
    Duane-Hunt r.
    equivalence r.
    Frank-Starling r.
    length-tension r.
relationship
    host-parasite r.
relative
    r. biological effectiveness
    r. cardiac volume
    r. centrifugal force
    r. erythrocytosis
    r. fluorescence
    r. frequency
    r. hepatic dullness

    r. leukocytosis
    r. molecular mass
    r. polycythemia
    r. refractory period
    r. retention time
    r. sensitivity
    r. specific activity
    r. specificity
    r. standard deviation
    r. survival rate
    r. value index
relaxation
    isovolumetric r.
    isovolumic r.
relaxin
relaxing response
relay
    mercury-wetted r.
    reed r.
release
    renin r.
releasing
    r. factor
    r. hormone
REM — rapid eye movement
         roentgen-equivalent—man
REM latency
remission
    partial r.
remittent
    r. malaria
    r. malarial fever
remnant
    chylomicron r's
    Cloquet's canal r.
    r. hyperlipidemia
    mesonephric r.
    sinus venosus r.
remodeling
    bone r.
REMP — roentgen-equivalent—man
         period
ren (pl., renes)
    r. mobilis
    r. unguliformis
renal
    r. adenocarcinoma
    r. adenoma
    r.-adrenal axis
    r. agenesis
    r. aminoaciduria
    r. amyloidosis

r. area cribrosa
r. artery
r. artery stenosis
r. azotemia
r. biopsy
r. blastema
r. blockade
r. calculi
r. calculus
r. calyx
r. cancer
r. capsuloma
r. carbuncle
r. carcinosarcoma
r. cast
r. cell carcinoma
r. clearance
r. colic
r. columns
r. corpuscle
r. cortex
r. cortical abscess
r. cortical adenoma
r. cortical interstitial tissue
r. cortical necrosis
r. cortical pancreas
r. cyst
r. cystic disease
r. diabetes
r. dysplasia
r. edema
r. embryoma
r. erythropoietic factor
r. failure
r. failure index
r. function study
r. glucosuria
r. glycosuria
r. hematuria
r. hemorrhage
r. hypertension
r. hypoplasia
r. hypoxia
r. infarct
r. infarction
r. insufficiency
r. interstitium
r. leiomyosarcoma
r. medulla
r. medullary ductal ectasia
r. medullary fibroma
r. medullary interstitial tissue

r. medullary necrosis
r. neoplasm
r. oncocytoma
r. osteodystrophy
r. papilla
r. papillary necrosis
r. parenchymal cyst
r. pelvic cavity
r. pelvic washing
r. pelvis
r. plasma flow
r. pressor substance
r. pyramid
r.-retinal dysplasia
r. rickets
r. salt washing
r. scarring
r. sinus
r. stones
r. threshold
r. threshold for glucose
r. toxicity
r. transplantation
r. tuberculosis
r. tubular acidosis
r. tubular basement membrane
r. tubular neck
r. tubular osteomalacia
r. tubules
r. tumors
r. vascular resistance
r. vein
r. vein renin activity
r. vein renin concentration
r. vein thrombosis
r. venous renin assay
r. vessels
renaturation
    DNA r.
reniform
renin
    r.-aldosterone axis
    r.-angiotensin-aldosterone axis
    r. release
    r.-release rate
    r.-sodium profiling
reninism
    primary r.
rennin
Renografin
renogram
renography

renomedullary interstitial cell tumor
renomegaly
renotropic
renovascular hypertension
Renshaw cell
reoviral infection
Reovirus
reovirus. types 1, 2, and 3
reoxidation
reoxygenation
REP — roentgen equiv-
       alent—physical
repair
    density-dependent r.
    DNA r.
    fibrous r.
    postoperative r.
    primary r.
    secondary r.
reparative
    r. giant cell granuloma
    r. granuloma
repeatability
    wavelength r.
repeated DNA sequences
repeats
    interspersed r.
    variable number tandem r.
reperfusion
repetitive stimulation
replacement
    aortic valve r.
    r. fibrosis
    fibrous r.
replenisher
replica
replication
    r. and transfer
    r. cycle
    DNA r.
    r. fork
replicon
repolarization
repressed gene
repression
    catabolite r.
    end-product r.
    enzyme r.
    negative control r.
    positive control r.
repressor gene

reproducibility
    photometric r.
reproduction
    asexual r.
    sexual r.
reproductive
reptilase fibrin
Reptilia
repullulation
repulsion
RER — rough endoplasmic reticulum
RES — reticuloendothelial system
resazurin
rescinnamine
rescue
    marker r.
resectability factor
resection
    gastric r.
    pylorus-preserving r.
    transurethral r.
    wedge r.
    Whipple's r.
resectoscopy
reserpine
reserve
    adrenocorticotropic hormone r.
    r. cell
    r. cell carcinoma
    r. cell hyperplasia
    contractile r.
reservoir
    chromatin r.
    r. host
    Koch's ileostomy r.
    r. of virus
    Ommaya's r.
    Pecquet's r.
reset
residual
    r. abscess
    r. body
    r. carcinoma
    r. urine
residue
    methanol-extruded r.
    spill r.
resin
    anion-exchange r.
    cation-exchange r.
    cholestyramine r.
    epoxy r.

Harleco synthetic r.
ion-exchange r.
podophyllin r.
polyamine-methylene r.
quinine carbacrylic r.
r. uptake
r.-uptake ratio
resistance
cardiovascular-renal cerebrovascular r.
cross-r.
r. determinant
electrode r.
r. factor
r.-inducing factor
internal r.
peripheral r.
peripheral total r.
r. plasmid
pulmonary tissue r.
pulmonary vascular r.
renal vascular r.
systemic r.
systemic vascular r.
r. thermometer
total r.
total peripheral r.
total pulmonary vascular r.
r. to venous return
r. transfer factor
r. unit
vascular r.
resistivity
resistor
carbon r.
carbon-film r.
r. color code
composition r.
power r.
precision r.
trimming r.
variable r.
wire-wound r.
resolution
energy r.
limit of r.
radius of r.
spectral r.
resolve
resolvent
resolving
r. power
r. time

resonance
electron paramagnetic r.
electron spin r.
r. fluorescence
r. line
nuclear magnetic r.
resonator
Oudin's r.
resorbed
resorcin
resorcin-fuchsin stain
resorcinol
r. monoacetate
r. phthalic anhydride
r. test
resorcinolphthalein sodium
resorption
bone r.
lacunar r.
osteoclastic r.
Resource Conservation and Recovery
Act
respiration
aerobic r.
anaerobic r.
artificial r.
Cheyne-Stokes r.
cogwheel r.
interrupted r.
Kussmaul's r.
r. rate
respirator
Drinker r.
respiratory
r. acidosis
r. alkalosis
r. apparatus
r. bronchiole
r. burst
r. chain
r. disorder
r. distress syndrome
"r. enteric orphans"
r. epithelium
r. exanthematous virus
r. exchange ratio
r. failure, acute
r. failure, chronic
r. fluids
r. illness
r. infection virus
r. insufficiency

r. mucosa
r. papillomatosis
r. pigments
r. protein
r. quotient
r. rate disorder
r. rhythm disorder
r. scleroma
r. sound
r. spaces
r. syncytial virus
r. syncytial virus antibody tests
r. syncytial virus antigen
r. syncytial virus antigen test
r. syncytial virus culture
r. syncytial virus serology
r. syndrome
r. system
r. tract fluid
r. tract infection
r. undulation
r. viral disease

respirometer
Wright r.

response
anamnestic r.
autoimmune r.
cell-mediated immune r.
cold r., paradoxical
galvanic skin r.
host r.
humoral immune r.
IgM r.
immune r.
logarithmic r.
orienting r.
photomyoclonic r.
radiation r.
relaxing r.
reticulocyte r.
sensitization r.
spectral r.
stringent r.
total r.

responsibility

rest
aberrant r.
adrenal r.
cartilaginous r.
embryonal r.
epithelial r.
Erdheim r.

Marchand's r.
mesonephric r.
müllerian r.
paramesonephric r.
thyroid r's
Walthard's cell r's
wolffian r.

restiform

resting
r. cell
r. membrane potential

restitope

restricted access laboratory

restriction
r. endonuclease
r. enzymes
r. fragment
r. fragment length polymorphism
r. map
MHC (major histocompatibility complex) r.

restrictive
r./infiltrative cardiomyopathy
r. pericarditis
r. pulmonary disease

resuscitation
cardiopulmonary r.

retained
r. foreign body
r. placental fragment
r. prepuce
r. products of conception
r. testis

retardation
growth r.
mental r.
psychomotor r.

rete (pl., retia)
acromial r.
articular r.
calcaneal r.
r. cell tumor
r. cyst of ovary
r. of patella
r. ovarii
r. pegs
r. ridges
r. testis carcinoma
r. vasculosum
r. venosum

retethelioma

retention
- r. content
- r. cyst
- r. fluid
- r. gas
- r. index
- r. jaundice
- r. meconium
- mucus r.
- r. mucus
- r. polyp
- r. time: absolute, corrected, relative
- urinary r.
- r. volume

retic. — reticulocyte

reticular
- r. activating system
- r. cell
- r. cell carcinoma
- r. colliquation
- r. degeneration
- r. dysgenesis
- r. erythematous mucinosis
- r. formation
- r. keratitis
- r. lamina
- r. layer
- r. lymphoblast
- r. lymphocyte
- r. membrane of cochlear duct
- r. nucleus of thalamus
- r. substance
- r. tissue

reticulated corpuscle

reticulating colliquation

reticulation

reticulatum
- atrophoderma r.

reticulin
- r. fibril alteration
- r. M
- r. staining

reticulocyte
- r. count
- r. production index
- r. response
- shift r.
- stress r.

reticulocytic
- r. marrow
- r. production index

reticulocytogenic

reticulocytopenia

reticulocytosis

reticuloendothelial
- r. blockade
- r. cell
- r. cell hyperplasia
- r. sarcoma
- r. system

reticuloendothelioma

reticuloendotheliosis
- leukemic r.
- systemic r.

reticulohistiocytic granuloma

reticulohistiocytoma

reticulohistiocytosis
- multicentric r.

reticuloid
- actinic r.

reticuloma

reticulopenia

reticulosarcoma

reticulosis
- hemophagocytic r.
- histiocytic medullary r.
- leukemic r.
- lipomelanic r.
- malignant midline r.
- medullary r.
- medullary histiocytic r.
- midline malignant r.
- myeloid r.
- pagetoid r.
- polymorphic r.

reticulospinal

reticulotomy

reticulum (pl., reticula)
- agranular endoplasmic r.
- r. cell carcinoma
- r. cell hyperplasia
- r. cell lymphosarcoma
- r. cells
- r. cell sarcoma
- endoplasmic r.
- granular r.
- granular endoplasmic r.
- sarcoplasmic r.
- stellate r.
- r. thymic cell

retiform parapsoriasis

retina
- coarctate r.

horizontal cell of r.
spotted r.
retinaculum (pl., retinacula)
    retinacula cutis
    r. extensorum
    r. flexorum
retinal
    all-*trans*-r.
    r. angiomatosis
    r. anlage tumor
    r. aplasia
    r. artery
    11-*cis*-r.
    r. detachment
    r. embolism
    r. hemangioblastoma
    r. hemorrhage
    r. microaneurysm
    r. pigments
    r.-renal dysplasia
    r. vein
retinene isomerase
retinitis
    cytomegalovirus r.
    r. pigmentosa
    r. proliferans
retinoblastic teratoma
retinoblastoma
    endophytic r.
    r. endophytum
    exophytic r.
    r. exophytum
    intraocular r.
retinochoroidal
retinochoroiditis
retinocytoma
retinography
retinoic acid
retinoid
retinol
retinol-binding protein
retinoma
retinopathy
    arteriosclerotic r.
    circinate r.
    diabetic r.
    hypertensive r.
    leukemic r.
    pigmentary r.
    proliferative r.
    rubella r.
retinoscopy

retinothalamic projection fibers
retinotopic
retinyl
retoperithelium
retort
Retortamonas intestinalis
retothelioma
retractile testis
retraction
    clot r.
    massive vitreous r.
retrieval
    information r.
retrobulbar
    r. abscess
    r. neuropathy
retrocaval ureter
retrocecal abscess
retrocolic hernia
retroduodenal
retroflexion
retrograde
    r. cancer
    r. embolism
    r. intussusception
    r. pyelogram
retrohyoid bursa
retrolental fibroplasia
retrolenticular
retromammary mastitis
retromandibular
retroperitoneal
    r. fibromatosis
    r. fibrosis
    r. gas insufflation
    r. liposarcoma
retroperitoneum
retroperitonitis
    idiopathic fibrous r.
    sclerosing r.
retropharyngeal
    r. abscess
    r. lymph nodes
retroplasia
retrospective study
retrosternal
    r. goiter
    r. hernia
retrotracheal
retrourethral catheterization
retrouterine hematocele
retroversion

Retrovir
retroviral
    r. oncogenes
    r. virus disease
Retroviridae
retrovirus
    AKT8 r.
    C-type r.
    lymphotropic r.
Rettgerella rettgeri
return
    resistance to venous r.
Reuss's
    formula
    test
reverberating circuit
reverberation
Reverdin's needle
reverse
    r. agglutination
    r. banding
    r. bias
    r. cholesterol transport
    r. endocytosis
    r. genetics
    r. grouping
    r. immunoelectrophoresis
    r. mutation
    r. osmosis
    r. passive hemagglutination
    r. peristalsis
    r. transcriptase
    r. transcription
    r. triiodothyronine
reversed albumin-globulin ratio
reversible calcinosis
revision
    fusiform skin r.
revivescence
revolutions per minute
Reynold's number
RF — Reitland-Franklin (unit)
    relative fluorescence
    releasing factor
    rheumatic fever
    rheumatoid factor
RFA — right femoral artery
    right frontoanterior
R (R plasmid) factor
RFB — retained foreign body
RFI – renal failure index

RFLA — rheumatoid factor–like
    activity
RFLP — restriction fragment length
    polymorphism
RFP — right frontoposterior
RFS — renal function study
RFT — right frontotransverse
RG — right gluteal
Rg^a antigen
RH — reactive hyperemia
    relative humidity
    releasing hormone
Rh — Rhesus (factor)
    rhodium
rh — rheumatic
Rhabdiasoidea
Rhabditata
Rhabditida
rhabditiform larva
Rhabditis hominis
rhabdocyte
rhabdoid
    r. sarcoma
    r. tumor
Rhabdomonas
rhabdomyoblast
    multinucleated r.
    spider cell r.
    syncytial r.
rhabdomyoblastic
rhabdomyoblastoma
rhabdomyochondroma
rhabdomyolysis
    acute recurrent r.
    familial paroxysmal r.
    idiopathic paroxysmal r.
rhabdomyoma
rhabdomyomyxoma
rhabdomyosarcoma
    alveolar r.
    botryoid r.
    cordal r.
    embryonal r.
    r. of prostate
    orbital r.
    paratesticular r.
    pleomorphic r.
    vaginal r.
rhabdomyosarcomatous nephro-
    blastoma
rhabdosarcoma
rhabdovirus
rhagades

rhagadiform
Rh agglutinin
rhagiocrine cell vacuole
rhamnulokinase
Rh antibody
Rh antigen incompatibility
RHBF — reactive hyperemia blood
　　　flow
Rh blocking test
Rh blood group
RHD — relative hepatic dullness
　　　rheumatic heart disease
Rh_0D
　　antigen
　　immune globulin
　　typing
rhegmatogenous retinal detachment
rhenium
rheobase
rheostat
rheostosis
rhestocythemia
rhesus monkey kidney
rheum. — rheumatic
rheumatic
　　r. arteritis
　　r. arthralgia
　　r. carditis
　　r. disease
　　r. endocarditis
　　r. endocartitis
　　r. factor
　　r. fever
　　r. heart disease
　　r. myocarditis
　　r. nodule
　　r. pericarditis
　　r. pneumonia
　　r. pneumonitis
　　r. valvulitis
rheumatid
rheumatism
　　articular r.
　　chronic r.
　　gonorrheal r.
　　Heberden's r.
　　inflammatory r.
　　Macleod's capsular r.
　　muscular r.
　　nodose r.
　　palindromic r.
　　tuberculous r.
rheumatismal

rheumatoid
　　r. agglutinator
　　r. aortitis
　　r. arteritis
　　r. arthritis
　　r. arthritis factor
　　r. disease
　　r. episcleritis
　　r. factor
　　r. factor–like activity
　　r. factor reaction
　　r. factor tests
　　r. heart disease
　　r. nodule
　　r. pneumoconiosis
　　r. scleritis
　　r. spondylitis
　　r. vasculitis
rheumatologic
Rh immunization
rhinal
Rh incompatibility
rhinencephalon
rhinitis
　　allergic r.
　　atrophic r.
　　fetid r.
　　r. sicca
　　vasomotor r.
　　viral r.
rhinoantritis
rhinocerebral mucormycosis
Rhinocladium
rhinocleisis
rhinoentomophthoromy-
　　cosis
Rhinoestrus
rhinofacial zygomycosis
rhinolaryngitis
rhinonasopharyngitis
rhinonecrosis
rhinopharyngitis mutilans
rhinopharyngocele
rhinophycomycosis
rhinophyma
rhinopneumonitis
　　equine r.
rhinorrhea
rhinoscleroma bacillus
rhinosporidiosis
Rhinosporidium seeberi
rhinotracheitis
　　infectious bovine r.

rhinovirus
Rhipicentor
Rhipicephalus sanguineus
Rh isoantigen
Rh isoimmunization syndrome
Rhizobiaceae
Rhizobium
Rhizoglyphus parasiticus
rhizoid
rhizomelia
Rhizomucor pusillus
Rhizopoda
Rhizopodea
Rhizopus
  R. arrhizus
  R. equinus
  R. niger
  R. nigricans
  R. oryzae
  R. prolixus
  R. rhizopodoformis
rhizotomy
RHL — right hepatic lobe
RHLN — right hilar lymph node
rhm — roentgen (per) hour (at one)
  meter
Rh neg. — Rhesus factor negative
Rh-negative cells
rho (rank correlation coefficient)
  Spearman's r.
rhodamine
  r. B
  r. isothiocyanate
rhodanile blue
Rhodesian trypanosomiasis
rhodium
Rhodnius prolixus
Rhodococcus
  R. bronchialis
  R. equi
Rhodophyllus sinuatus
rhodopsin
Rhodotorula
  R. mucilaginosa
  R. rubra
rhodotorulosis
rho factor
RhoGAM vaccine
rhombencephalon
rhombic lip
rhomboid
  r. fossa

Michaelis's r.
  r. muscle
  r. nucleus
rhombomere
Rhombomys
rhonchus (pl., rhonchi)
rhopheocytosis
Rh pos. — Rhesus factor positive
Rh type
rhythm
  Berger's r.
  bigeminal r.
  cardiac r.
  circadian r.
  gallop r.
  isochronal r.
  junctional r.
  metachronal r.
  respiratory r.
  sinoatrial r.
rhytidosis
RI — refractive index
  regional ileitis
  respiratory illness
RIA — radioimmunoassay
ribavirin
Ribbert's theory
riboflavin
  r. deficiency
  r. kinase
  r. loading test
  r. phosphate
  r. unit
  r.-5′-phosphate
ribokinase
ribonuclease
  r. A
  alkaline r.
  r. I
  pancreatic r.
ribonucleic acid (*see also* RNA)
ribonucleoprotein
  r. complex
  small nuclear r.
ribonucleoside
  xanthine r.
ribonucleoside-5′-phosphate
  thymine r.
ribonucleotide
  glycinamide r.
  nicotinate r.
  r. reductase

riboprine
ribopyranose
ribose
     5-P-r. isomerase
     r.-1-phosphate
     r.-5-phosphate
ribosephosphate
     r. isomerase
     r. pyrophosphokinase
ribosomal
     r. DNA
     r. P protein
     r. RNA
ribosome
ribosome-lamella complex
ribosuria
ribosylnicotinamide kinase
ribothymidylic acid
ribulokinase
ribulose-5-phosphate
ribulose phosphate epimerase
rice body
Richet's aneurysm
Richter's hernia
ricin
ricinoleic acid
rickets
     acute r.
     celiac r.
     hemorrhagic r.
     renal r.
     vitamin D–dependent (types I, II) r.
     X-linked hypophosphatemic r.
Rickettsia
     R. *akamushi*
     R. *akari*
     R. *australis*
     R. *burnetii*
     R. *canis*
     R. *conorii*
     R. *diaporica*
     R. *mooseri*
     R. *muricola*
     R. *nipponica*
     R. *orientalis*
     R. *pavlovskii*
     R. *pediculi*
     R. *prowazekii*
     R. *quintana*
     R. *rickettsii*
     R. *sibirica*

     R. *tsutsugamushi*
     R. *typhi*
     R. *wolhynica*
Rickettsiaceae
rickettsia (pl., rickettsiae)
rickettsial
     r. infection
     r. vasculitis
rickettsialpox
Rickett's organism
RID — radial immunodiffusion
Rideal-Walker
     coefficient
     method
ridge
     genital r.
     interpapillary r's
     meningioma of the sphenoid r.
     rete r's
     truncus arteriosus r.
     urogenital r.
riding embolism
Riedel's
     lobe
     struma
     thyroiditis
Rieder
     cell leukemia
     cells
Rieder's lymphocyte
Riehl's melanosis
Riesman's pneumonia
RIF — right iliac fossa
RIFA — radioiodinated fatty acid
rifabutine
rifamide
rifampicin
rifampin
rifamycin
rifomycin
Rift Valley fever
Rift Valley fever virus
right
     r. anterior oblique
     r. atrial enlargement
     r. atrial hypertrophy
     r. axis deviation
     r. bundle branch block
     r.-handed α-helix
     r. ovarian vein syndrome
     r. posterior oblique
     r.-sided aortic arch

r.-sided ductus arteriosus
r. ventricular enlargement
r. ventricular hypertrophy
r. ventricular hypoplasia
r. ventricular infarction
rigidity
decerebrate r.
lead-pipe r.
muscular r.
nuchal r.
rigor mortis
rigorous
RIHSA — radioactive iodinated human serum albumin
rim
"endo-ecto cytoplasmic" r.
Rimini's test
rimming
Rindfleisch's cells
ring
aromatic r.
Balbiani's r's
Bandl's r.
Cannon's r.
r. chromosome
contractile r.
corrin r.
r. counter
r. fibers
inguinal r.
Kayser-Fleischer r's
Liesegang r's
mitral r.
pyrrol r.
Schatzki's r.
r. sideroblasts
signet r.
vascular r.
Waldeyer's tonsillar r.
ring-chain tautomer
ringed sideroblast
Ringer's
lactate solution
solution
ring-wall lesion
ringworm
gray-patch r.
Rinne's test
Riolan's muscle
RIP — radioimmunoprecipitation
ripening

ripple
r. counter
r. factor
r. voltage
RISA — radioactive iodinated serum albumin
risk
r. factor
population-attributable r.
recurrence r.
RIST — radioimmunosorbent test
ristocetin
r. aggregation test
r. cofactor
RITC — rhodamine isothiocyanate
Ritchie formalin-ethyl acetate procedure
Ritter-Oleson technique
RIU — radioactive iodine uptake
riziform
RK — rabbit kidney
right kidney
RKY — roentgen kymography
RLC — residual lung capacity
RLF — retrolental fibroplasia
RLL — right lower lobe
RLN — recurrent laryngeal nerve
R-loop
RLP — radiation-leukemia-protection
RLQ — right lower quadrant
RLS — Ringer's lactate solution
RM — radical mastectomy
respiratory movement
RMA — right mentoanterior
RMK — rhesus monkey kidney
RML — right middle lobe
RMP — rapidly miscible pool
right mentoposterior
RMS — root-mean-square
RMSF — Rocky Mountain spotted fever
RMT — retromolar trigone
right mentotransverse
RMV — respiratory minute volume
Rn — radon
RNA — ribonucleic acid
RNA
heterogeneous nuclear RNA
messenger RNA
RNA nucleotidyltransferase
RNA oncogenic viruses
RNA polymerase

ribosomal RNA
small nuclear RNA
soluble RNA
RNA splicing
RNA transcription
transfer RNA
RNA virus
RNA-driven hybridization
RNA-RNA hybridization
RNase — ribonuclease
RND — radical neck dissection
RNP — ribonucleoprotein
RNP complex
Ro antigen
RO — Ritter-Oleson (technique)
ROA — right occipitoanterior
robertsonian translocation
Robert's pelvis
Robson's staging system
robust
ROC — receiver operating character-
    istic
roccellin
Rochalimaea quintana
Roche cutoff
rocker microtome
rocket immunoelectrophoresis
Rocky Mountain spotted fever
Rocky Mountain spotted fever anti-
    body tests
Rocky Mountain spotted fever se-
    rology
rod
    Auer's r.
    r. body myopathy
    r. cells myopathy
    gram-negative r's
    r. neutrophil
rodenticide
rodent ulcer
Rodrigues' aneurysm
roentgen
    r. intoxication
    r. rays
roentgenkymography
roentgenogram
roentgenography
roentgenology
roentgenoscopy
Roger
    antigen
    maladie de R.

Roger's
    antigen
    reflex
    test
ROH — rat ovarian hyperemia (test)
Rokitansky-Aschoff sinus
Rokitansky's pelvis
rolandic epilepsy
Rolando's fissure
roll
    iliac r.
    r. tube technique
Roller's nucleus
Rollet's stroma
rolling hernia
ROM — range of motion
    rupture of membranes
Romaña's sign
Romanowsky's
    blood stain
    stain
Romberg's trophoneurosis
Rommelaere's sign
ronnel
root
    belladonna r.
    bitter r.
    cochlear r.
    facial r.
    r.-mean-square
    motor r.
    sensory r.
ROP — right occipitoposterior
ropalocytosis
Ropes test
rosacea
    granulomatous r.
    r.-like tuberculid
    lupoid r.
    papular r.
rosanilin dyes
rosaniline
rosary
    r. pea
    rachitic r.
rosea-like
rose bengal
    r.-b. antigen
    r.-b. radioactive (^{131}I) test
    r.-b. sodium
    r.b. test
Rose-Bradford kidney

Rosenbach-Gmelin test
Rosenbach's test
Rosenfield system
Rosenmüller's
        fossa
        lymph node
Rosenthaler-Turk reagent
Rosenthal's
        fibers
        vein
roseola
        r. infantum
        r. infantum virus
        r. vaccination
Rose's test
rosette
        E, EA, EAC r.
        Flexner-Wintersteiner r.
        r.-forming cells
        Homer Wright r.
        malarial r.
rosetting
Rose-Waaler test
p-rosolic acid
Ross-Jones test
rostral
        r. displacement
        r. lamina, corpus callosum
rostrate pelvis
rostrum (pl., rostra)
        r. corpus callosi
        r. sphenoidale
ROT — right occipitotransverse
rotamer
rotary microtome
rotation
        axis of r.
        r. flap
        optical r.
        specific r.
        wheel r.
rotavirus serology
rotenone
Rothera's nitroprusside test
Rothera's test
Rothia
Roth's spots
rotoxamine
Rotter's
        node
        test
rot value

Rouget's
        bulb
        cell
        pericyte
rough
        r. bacterium
        r. colony
        r. endoplasmic reticulum
rough-smooth variation
Roughton-Scholander
        apparatus
        syringe
rouleau (pl., rouleaux) formation
round
        r. atelectasis
        r. cell inflammation
        r. cell liposarcoma
        r. cell sarcoma
rounding
roundworm
        intestinal r.
Rourke-Ernstein sedimentation rate
Rous
        sarcoma
        sarcoma virus
        test
        tumor
routine
        r. test dilution
        trace r.
Rouviere's node
Roux-en-Y
        anastomosis
        limb
Roux's
        bottle
        stain
rovamycin
Rowntree and Geraghty's test
RP — reactive protein
        refractory period
        resting pressure
        retrograde pyelogram
Rp — pulmonary resistance
RPA — right pulmonary artery
RPCF — Reiter protein complement-
                fixation
RPCFT — Reiter protein
                complement-fixation
                test
RPE — retinal pigment epithelium
RPF — renal plasma flow

RPG — retrograde pyelogram
RPGN — rapidly progressive glomeru-
lonephritis
RPI — reticulocytic production index
RPK — ribosephosphate kinase
rpm — revolutions per minute
RPND — retroperitoneal lymph node
dissection
RPO — right posterior oblique
RPR — rapid plasma reagin (test)
R protein
RPS — renal pressor substance
RPV — right pulmonary veins
RQ — respiratory quotient
RR — radiation response
relative response
renin release
respiratory rate
response rate
RRA — radioreceptor assay
RR (relative risk) factor
RR-HPO — rapid recompres-
sion–high pressure
oxygen
rRNA — ribosomal RNA
RRP — relative refractory period
RRR — renin-release rate
RS — Reed-Sternberg cell
respiratory syncytial
RSA — relative specific activity
reticulum cell sarcoma
right sacroanterior
RSB — right sternal border
RSC — rested-state contraction
RScA — right scapuloanterior
RScP — right scapuloposterior
RSD — relative standard deviation
RSP — right sacroposterior
RSR — regular sinus rhythm
RST — radiosensitivity test
right sacrotransverse
RSV — respiratory syncytial virus
right subclavian vein
Rous sarcoma virus
R-S (rough-smooth) variation
RSV culture
RS (Rous sarcoma) virus
RT — reaction time
room temperature
rT_3 — reverse triiodothyronine
RTA — renal tubular acidosis
RTD — routine test dilution

RTF — replication and transfer
resistance transfer factor
respiratory tract fluid
RU — rat unit
resistance unit
retrograde urogram
Ru — ruthenium
rub
pericardial friction r.
pleural friction r.
pleural-pericardial friction r.
rubber pelvis
rubeanic acid
rubella
r. antibody tests
congenital r. syndrome
r. HI test
r. retinopathy
r. serology
r. virus
r. virus culture
rubeola
r. serology
r. virus
rubescent
rubidium
rubidomycin
rubin
Rubin's test
rubivirus
Rubner's lactose test
rubor
rubredoxin
rubriblast
pernicious anemia–type r.
rubricyte
polychromatophilic r.
rubrospinal
rubrum
r. Congo
r. scarlatinum
ruby spots
rudimentary
r. finger
r. lung
r. structure
r. testis syndrome
r. uterus, male
Ruffini's
corpuscle
ending
ruga (pl., rugae)

RUL — right upper lobe
rule
        Bayes's r.
        Cahn-Ingold-Prelog sequence r's
        Clark r.
        Clark's r.
        Goriaew's r.
ruling
        Neubauer r.
rump
        crown r.
Rumpel-Leede test
Runeberg's
        anemia
        formula
running fit
runt disease
Runyon's
        classification
        group
rupture
        r.-delivery interval
        inflammatory r.
        r. of membranes
        premature r.
ruptured
        r. aneurysm
        r. ectopic pregnancy
        r. myocardial infarct
        r. umbilical cord
RUQ — right upper quadrant
RUR — resin-uptake ratio
RURTI — recurrent upper respiratory tract infection
Rusconi's anus

Russell-Crooke cell
Russell's
        bodies
        unit
        viper venom
        viper venom time
Russian spring-summer encephalitis virus
Russula emetica
rusty sputum
ruthenium red
rutherford
Rutherford scattering
rutidosis
RV — rat virus
        residual volume
        respiratory volume
        right ventricle
        rubella virus
RVB — red venous blood
RVD — relative vertebral density
RVE — right ventricular enlargement
RVEDP — right ventricular end-diastolic pressure
RVH — right ventricular hypertrophy
RVI — relative value index
RVR — renal vascular resistance
        resistance to venous return
RVRA — renal vein renin activity
RVRC — renal vein renin concentration
RVT — renal vein thrombosis
RV (residual volume) time
R wave
ryania
Rye classification

S — sacral
        serum
        smooth (colony)
        soluble
        spherical lens
        sulfur
        supravergence
        Svedberg's unit

        Svedberg's unit of sedimentation coefficient
S. — *Salmonella*
        Schistosoma
        Spirillum
        Staphylococcus
        Streptococcus
s — second, seconds

SA — salicylic acid
    sarcoma
    secondary amenorrhea
    secondary anemia
    serum albumin
    sinoatrial
    Stokes-Adams
    surface area
SAA protein
SAB — significant asymptomatic bacteriuria
sabadilla
saber
    s. shin
    s. tibia
Sabethes
Sabhi agar
Sabin
    megaloblast of S.
    vaccine
Sabin-Feldman dye test
Sabouraud's dextrose agar
sac
    aneurysmal s.
    endolymphatic s.
    lacrimal s.
    pericardial s.
saccharase
saccharephidrosis
saccharic acid
saccharide
    O-linked s.
saccharin
saccharoid
saccharometer
Saccharomonospora viridis
Saccharomyces
    S. *albicans*
    S. *anginae*
    S. *apiculatus*
    S. *cantliei*
    S. *capillitii*
    S. *carlsbergensis*
    S. *cerevisiae*
    S. *coprogenus*
    S. *epidermica*
    S. *galacticolus*
    S. *glutinis*
    S. *hominis*
    S. *lemonnieri*
    S. *mellis*
    S. *mycoderma*

    S. *neoformans*
    S. *pastorianus*
saccharomyces
    Busse's s.
saccharomycosis
L-saccharopine
saccharopine dehydrogenase
saccharopinemia
saccharopinuria
Saccharopolyspora rectivirgula
saccharorrhea
saccharosuria
Saccomanno's fixative
saccular
    s. aneurysm
    s. bronchiectasis
    s. gland
sacculated
    s. aneurysm
    s. pleurisy
saccule
saccus
SACD — subacute combined degeneration
Sachs-Georgi test
sacral
    s. artery
    s. bursa
    s. lymph node
    s. myotome
    s. nerve
    s. plexus
    s. region
    s. spinal cord
    s. vein, lateral
    s. vertebra of intervertebral disc
sacralization
    lumbar vertebra s.
sacrococcygeal
    s. joint
    s. region
    s. teratoma
sacroiliac joint
sacroiliitis
    pyogenic s.
sacrum
saddle
    s. embolism
    s. embolus
    s. nose deformity
Saenger's macula

safety
>   s. glasses
>   s. program
>   s. shower

safflower oil

safranin O

safranophil; safranophile

safrol

SAG — Swiss-type agammaglobuli-
    nemia

sagittal
>   s. sinus
>   s. suture

sago spleen

SAH — subarachnoid hemorrhage

Sahli's method

SAIDS — simian AIDS

sailor's skin

Saint (*see entries under* St.)

Sakaguchi reaction

Saksenaeaceae

Saksenaea vasiformis

sal — saline
>   saliva

salicylamide

salicylanilide

salicylate
>   carbazochrome s.
>   s. isoamyl
>   s. level
>   methyl s.
>   s. phenyl
>   physostigmine s.

salicylic acid test

salicylism

salicylsalicylic acid

salicylsulfonic acid

salicyluric acid

salimeter

saline
>   s. agglutination test
>   s. agglutinin
>   s. antibody
>   s. infusion
>   physiologic s.
>   s. technique

saline solution
>   physiologic s.s.

salinometer

Salisbury common cold virus

saliva

salivary
>   s. amylase
>   s. calculus
>   s. corpuscle
>   s. fistula
>   s. gland
>   s. gland capsule
>   s. gland tumors
>   s. gland virus
>   s. gland virus disease
>   s. virus

Salk vaccine

Salmonella
>   *S. arizonae*
>   *S. choleraesuis*
>   *S. derby*
>   *S. enteritidis*
>   *S. enteritidis* serotype *agona*
>   *S. enteritidis* serotype *heidelberg*
>   *S. enteritidis* serotype *hirschfeldii*
>   *S. enteritidis* serotype *infantis*
>   *S. enteritidis* serotype *monte-
>   video*
>   *S. enteritidis* serotype *newport*
>   *S. enteritidis* serotype *para-
>   typhi* A
>   *S. enteritidis* serotype *schott-
>   mülleri*
>   *S. enteritidis* serotype *typhi-
>   murium*
>   *S. gallinarum*
>   *S. hirschfeldii*
>   *S. indiana*
>   *S. infantis*
>   *S. minnesota*
>   *S. montevideo*
>   *S. muenchen*
>   *S. newington*
>   *S. oranienburg*
>   *S. paratyphi*, A, B, C
>   *S. schottmülleri*
>   *S. sendai*
>   *S. thompson*
>   *S. typhi*
>   *S. typhimurium*
>   *S. typhisuis*
>   *S. typhosa*
>   *S. virginia*

salmonella (pl., salmonellae)
>   s. agglutinins
>   s. group
>   s. poisoning

s. proctitis
s. serogroup D
Salmonella-Shigella
Salmonella-Shigella agar
Salmonella titer
Salmonella typhimurium
salmonellosis
salmon patch
salpingioma
salpingitis
    chronic interstitial s.
    follicular s.
    foreign body s.
    gonococcal s.
    gonorrheal s.
    s. isthmica nodosa
    pyogenic s.
    suppurative s.
    tuberculous s.
salpingo-oophorectomy
salpingo-oophoritis
    gonococcal s.
salpingoperitonitis
salpingopharyngeus muscle
salpinx
    s. auditiva
    s. uterina
salsalate
salt
    s. agglutination
    s. antagonism
    bile s's
    s. bridge
    calcium s's
    diazonium s.
    s. dye
    hexazonium s's
    s. loading
    s.-losing crisis
    mercuric s.
    tetrazolium s's
    tetrazonium s's
    s.-washing
saltation
Saltatoria
saltatory conduction
salted
    s. plasma
    s. serum
salting-in
salting-out
saluresis

saluretic
salvage mastectomy
salvarsanized serum
Salvia
    S. horminium
    S. sclarea
Salzman method
SAM — sulfated acid mucopolysac-
        charide
samarium
sample
    s. correlation coefficient
    s. distribution
    s. interaction
    population s.
    random s.
    s. steady state
sampler
sampling
    percutaneous s.
    umbilical blood s.
Sanarelli-Shwartzman phenomenon
sand
    brain s.
    s. granules
    intestinal s.
    urinary s.
sandal foot
sandalwood oil
sandfly
    s. fever
    s. fever virus
Sandford's test
Sandimmune
sandpaper gallbladder
S and s antigens
sandwich immunoassay
Sanger's reagent
sanguifacient
sanguiferous
sanguification
sanguineous
    s. cyst
    s. infiltration
sanguinolent
sanguinopurulent
sanguis
sanguivorous myiasis
sanies
saniopurulent
sanioserous
sanious pus

sanitary bacteriology
sanitization
San Joaquin fever
San Joaquin Valley fever
SA node
santal oil
santonin
Santorini's
    cartilage
    duct
    fissure
SAP — serum alkaline phosphatase
    systemic arterial pressure
sap
    cell s.
saphenous
    s. nerve
    s. vein
saponifiable fraction
saponification
saponin
    steroid s.
    triterpenoid s.
Sappinia diploidea
sapremia
saprobe
saprol
sapronosis
saprophyte
Saprospira
saramycetin
Sarcina
sarcina (pl., sarcinae)
sarcocele
sarcocyst
sarcocystin
Sarcocystis
sarcocyte
Sarcodina
sarcogenic cells
sarcoid
    Boeck's s.
    Darrier-Roussy s.
    s. granuloma
    granuloma s.
    Spiegler-Fendt s.
sarcoidal granuloma
sarcoidosis
    hypercalcemic s.
    pulmonary s.
sarcolemma

sarcoma (pl., sarcomas, sarcomata)
    Abernethy's s.
    alveolar s.
    alveolar soft part s.
    ameloblastic s.
    avian s.
    botryoid s.
    s. botryoides
    cerebellar s.
    clear cell s.
    endometrial stromal s.
    endothelial s.
    epithelioid s.
    Ewing's s.
    fascicular s.
    giant cell s.
    granulocytic s.
    s. growth factor
    hemangioendothelial s.
    Hodgkin's s.
    immunoblastic s.
    Jensen's s.
    juxtacortical osteogenic s.
    Kaposi's s.
    Kupffer's cell s.
    leukocytic s.
    lymphangioendothelial s.
    lymphatic s.
    lymphosarcoma-reticulum
      cell s.
    mast cell s.
    medullary s.
    meningeal s.
    mesothelial s.
    multiple hemorrhagic s.
    multiple idiopathic hemor-
      rhagic s.
    multipotential primary s. of
      bone
    myeloblastic granulocytic s.
    myelogenic s.
    myeloid s.
    neurogenic s.
    osteogenic s.
    periosteal s.
    reticuloendothelial s.
    reticulum cell s.
    rhabdoid s.
    round cell s.
    Rous s.
    small cell s.
    soft tissue s.

spindle cell s.
stromal s.
synovial s.
telangiectatic osteogenic s.
undifferentiated s.

Sarcomastigophora
sarcomatoid
  s. carcinoma
  s.-type mesothelium
  s. variant
sarcomatosis
  meningeal s.
sarcomatous
sarcomere
Sarcophaga
  S. carnaria
  S. dux
  S. fuscicauda
  S. haemorrhoidalis
  S. nificornis
  S. rubicornis
Sarcophagidae
sarcoplasm
sarcoplasmic reticulum
Sarcoptes scabiei
sarcoptic mange
Sarcoptidae
sarcoptidosis
sarcosine
  s. dehydrogenase
  s. oxidase
sarcosinemia
sarcosinuria
sarcosis
Sarcosporidia
sarcosporidiosis
sarcostosis
sarcotic
sargramostim
sartorius muscle bursa
SAS — supravalvular aortic stenosis
sat — saturated
satellite
  s. abscess
  s. cell
  s. colony
  s. DNA
  s. metastasis
  nucleolar s.
satellitosis
satiety center

saturated
  ambient temperature and pressure, s.
  body temperature, ambient pressure, s.
  s. calomel electrode
  s. fatty acids
  s. hydrocarbon
  s. phosphatidylcholine
  s. solution
  s. solution of potassium iodide
saturation
  s. analysis
  s. current
  s. hybridization
  s. index
  iron s.
  s. limit
  oxygen s.
  transferrin s.
saturnina
  arthralgia s.
saturnine gout
satyriasis
Saundby's test
sauriasis
sauriderma
sauriosis
sauroderma
sausage fingers
sawtooth wave
SB — serum bilirubin
  sternal border
Sb — antimony (stibium)
$SbCl_3$ — antimony trichloride
SBE — subacute bacterial endocarditis
SBF — splanchnic blood flow
SBN — single-breath nitrogen (test)
Sb_2O_3 — antimony trioxide
Sb_2O_5 — antimony pentoxide
Sb_4O_6 — antimony trioxide
SBP — systemic blood pressure
  systolic blood pressure
SBTI — soybean trypsin inhibitor
SC — closure of the semilunar valves
  sacrococcygeal
  sickle cell
  sternoclavicular
  subcutaneous
  succinylcholine
Sc — scandium

scabies
>Norwegian s.
scala (pl., scalae)
>s. tympani
>s. vestibuli
scalar product
scalded skin syndrome
scale
>absolute s.
>absolute temperature s.
>Baumé's s.
>Benois' s.
>Celsius s.
>Celsius temperature s.
>centigrade s.
>centigrade temperature s.
>customary temperature s.
>Fahrenheit temperature s.
>Gaffky s.
>gray s.
>Hamilton Rating s.
>hydrometer s.
>interval s.
>Karnofsky performance s.
>Kelvin temperature s.
>Rankine's temperature s.
>ratio s.
>Réaumur s.
scalene
>s. lymph node
>s. muscles
>s. node biopsy
>s. region
scalenus anticus syndrome
scaler
scaler-timer
scalloping
scalp
>gyrate s.
scan
>bilirubin s.
>bone s.
>bone marrow s.
>brain s.
>CT (computed tomography) s.
>dot s.
>gallium s.
>s. information density
>kidney s.
>krypton s.
>liver s.

lung s.
>pulmonary perfusion s.
>pulmonary ventilation s.
>RAI s.
>RISA s.
>spleen s.
>technetium s.
scandium
Scanlon mastectomy
scanner
>EMI s.
>optical s.
scanning
>s. electron microscope
>fluorescent s.
>gallium s.
>s. sequence
scanography
scaphocephaly
scaphoid
>s. bone
>s. facies
scapula (pl., scapulae)
scapular
scar
>s. cancer
>s. carcinoma
>hypertrophic s.
>papyraceous s's
>radial s.
scarabiasis
scarlatinal nephritis
scarlatiniform
scarlet
>Biebrich s.
>s. fever
>s. G
>s. R
>s. red
>s. red sulfonate
>water-soluble s.
Scarpa's ganglion
scarring
>renal s.
scarry shrunken kidney
SCAT — sheep cell agglutination test
Scatchard
>equation
>plot
scatemia
scatologic
scatology

scatoma
scatoscopy
scatter diagram
scattergram
scattering
    elastic s.
    inelastic s.
    Rutherford s.
scatterplot
Scaurus
scavenger
    s. cell
    radical s.
SCC — squamous cell carcinoma
SCD — subacute combined degener-
        ation
    sudden cardiac death
    sudden coronary death
ScDA — scapulodextra anterior
ScDP — scapulodextra posterior
SCE — saturated calomel
      electrode
Scedosporium apiospermum
SCG — serum chemistry graft
SCH — succinylcholine
Schaedler's blood agar
Schaeffer-Fulton stain
Schaer's reagent
Schäffer's test
Schales and Schales method for
chloride
Schamberg's dermatitis
scharlach red
Schatzki's ring
Schaudinn's fixative
Schaumann's
    bodies
    lymphogranuloma
Scheibler's reagent
Scheloribates
schematic
scheme
    decay s.
    Kauffmann-White s.
Scheuermann's juvenile kyphosis
Schick's test
Schiff's
    base
    biliary cycle
    reagent
Schiller-Duval bodies
Schiller's test

Schilling's
    blood count
    index
    leukemia
    test
    type of monocytic leukemia
Schirmer's test
schistocelia
schistocystic hemolytic anemia
schistocystis
schistocyte
schistocytosis
schistomula
Schistosoma
    S. haematobium
    S. intercalatum
    S. japonicum
    S. mansoni
    S. mekongi
schistosomal
    s. bladder cancer
    s. miracidium
    s. ovum
Schistosomatidae
Schistosomatoidea
schistosome
    s. cercarial dermatitis
    s. granuloma
    s. pigment
schistosomiasis
    genitourinary s.
    Manson's s.
    s. serological test
    toxemic s.
schistosomicidal
schistosomicide
schizoaffective schizophrenia
Schizoblastosporion
schizocyte
schizocytosis
schizogony
schizoid
schizomycete
schizont
Schizophora
schizophrenia
    acute undifferentiated s.
    catatonic s.
    chronic undifferentiated s.
    hebephrenic s.
    paranoid s.
    pseudoneurotic s.

schizoaffective s.
simple s.
schizophrenic psychosis
schizophreniform
Schizophyllum commune
Schizosaccharomyces
Schlemm's canal
Schmidt-Lantermann segment
Schmitz's bacillus
Schmorl's
    bacillus
    ferric-ferricyanide reduction
        stain
    nodule
    picrothionin stain
    reaction
schneiderian papilloma
Schneider's carmine
Schoemaker's gastroenterostomy
Schoenheimer-Sperry method
Schönbein's test
Schönlein-Henoch purpura
Schönlein's purpura
Schridde's cancer hairs
Schüffner's
    dots
    granules
    punctation
    stippling
Schultz-Dale
    reaction
    test
Schultz's
    reaction
    stain
    triad
Schumm's test
schwannoma
    acoustic s.
    malignant s.
Schwann-cell tumor
Schwann's
    cell
    sheath
    white substance
Schwartz leukemia virus
Schwartzman (*see* Shwartzman)
Schwarz's test
Schweninger-Buzzi anetoderma
Scianna
    antigen
    blood group system

sciatica
sciatic nerve
SCID — severe combined immunode-
        ficiency
science
    applied s.
    theoretical s.
scientific notation
scillaren
scilliroside
scimitar sign
scintigram
scintigraphy
scintillation
    s. camera
    s. count
    s. counter
    s. crystal
    s. technique
scintillator
    liquid s.
scintiphotograph
scintiscanning
scirrhosity
scirrhous
    s. cancer
    s. carcinoma
scirrhus
SCJ — squamocolumnar junction
SCK — serum creatine kinase
Scl-70 antibody
ScLA — scapulolaeva anterior
sclera (pl., sclerae)
    lamina cribrosa sclerae
scleradenitis
scleratogenous
scleredema adultorum
sclerema
    s. adiposum
    s. neonatorum
scleriasis
scleritis
    rheumatoid s.
scleroatrophy
sclerodactylia calcinosis cutis
sclerodactyly
scleroderma
    s. antibody
    localized s.
sclerodermatitis
sclerodermatous
sclerogenous; sclerogenic

scleroid
scleroma
 respiratory s.
scleromalacia
scleromyxedema
sclero-oophoritis
sclerosal
sclerose
sclerosing
 s. adenosis
 s. carcinoma
 s. cholangitis
 s. ductal proliferation
 s. epithelial hamartoma
 s. epithelial neoplasm
 s. hemangioma
 s. histoplasmosis
 s. hyaline necrosis
 s. inflammation
 s. keratitis
 s. lipogranuloma
 s. lymphosarcoma
 s. mediastinitis
 s. myeloma
 s. osteitis
 s. panencephalitis
 s. peritonitis
 s. retroperitonitis
 s. sinusitis
sclerosis (pl., scleroses)
 amyotrophic lateral s.
 arterial s.
 arteriocapillary s.
 arteriolar s.
 bone s.
 cardiac s.
 s. corii
 s. cutanea
 disseminated s.
 endocardial s.
 glomerular s.
 idiopathic hypercalcemic s.
 lobar s.
 medial calcific s.
 menstrual s.
 Mönckeberg's s.
 Mönckeberg's medial s.
 multiple s.
 nodular s.
 ovulational s.
 physiologic s.
 primary endocardial s.

 progressive systemic s.
 pulmonary vascular s.
 subacute combined s.
 systemic s.
 tuberous s.
 unicellular s.
 vascular s.
 venous s.
sclerostenosis
sclerotic
 s. bodies
 s. gastritis
 s. kidney
 s. stomach
sclerotium
sclerotylosis
sclerous
ScLP — scapulolaeva posterior
SCM — Society of Computer Medicine
SCN — solid cell nests
scolecoid
scolex (pl., scoleces)
scolices
scoliosis
scoliotic pelvis
S (smooth) colony
Scolopendra
scombroid poisoning
scop — scopolamine
scopolamine
scopometer
Scopulariopsis
 S. americana
 S. aureus
 S. blochi
 S. brevicaulis
 S. cinereus
 S. koningi
 S. minimus
scopulariopsosis
scorbutic
 s. anemia
 s. dysentery
 s. gingivitis
score
 Gleason's s.
 initial prognostic s.
 lod (logarithm of the odds) s.
 standard s.
 Z s.
Scorpio

Scorpiones
Scotch tape method
scotochromogen
scotochromogenic
scotoma (pl., scotomata)
scotopic
Scott's tap water substitute
SCPK — serum creatine phospho-
                kinase
SCR — silicon-controlled rectifier
scrape
scraper
    cervical s.
scratch
    s.-pad memory
    s. reflex
    s. test
screen
    amino acid s.
    s. burn
    s. filtration pressure
screening
    automated multiphasic s.
    biochemical s.
    cytologic s.
    drug s.
    genetic s.
    multiphasic s.
    neonatal s.
    prenatal s.
    s. test
screw-worm
scrobiculate
scrofula
scrofuloderma
    s. gummosa
    tuberculous s.
    ulcerative s.
    verrucous s.
scrofulotuberculosis
scrofulous ophthalmia
scroll ear
scrotal
    s. edema
    s. erythrasma
    s. fat necrosis
    s. gangrene
    s. hematocele
    s. itching
    s. mass
    s. nevoxanthoendothelioma
    s. pruritus

    s. raphe
    s. septum
    s. spleen
scrotitis
scrotum (pl., scrota, scrotums)
    accessory s.
    bifid s.
    lymph s.
    watering-can s.
scrub typhus
SCS — silicon-controlled switch
SCT — sex chromatin test
       staphylococcal clumping test
scum
scurvy
    land s.
Scutigera
scybalum (pl., scybala)
SD — septal defect
    serologically defined
    serum defect
    spontaneous delivery
    standard deviation
    streptodornase
S/D — systolic to diastolic
SDA — sacrodextra anterior
      specific dynamic action
SD antigen
Sd^a antigen
S-D curve — strength-duration curve
SDE — specific dynamic effect
SDH — serine dehydrase
      sorbitol dehydrogenase
      succinate dehydrogenase
SDM — standard deviation of the
       mean
SDP — sacrodextra posterior
SDS — sodium dodecyl sulfate
      sudden death syndrome
SDS-gel
    S.-g. electrophoresis
    S.-g. filtration chromatography
SDT — sacrodextra transversa
SE — standard error
    Starr-Edwards (prosthesis)
Se — selenium
sea-blue
    s.-b. histiocyte
    s.-b. histiocytic disease
seal
    hermetic s.
sealed envelope technique

sealing
    impulse s.
seam
    osteoid s.
Seattle classification
seatworm
sea urchin granuloma
sebaceous
    s. adenocarcinoma
    s. adenoma
    s. carcinoma
    s. cyst
    s. epithelioma
    s. gland
    s. horn
    s. hyperplasia
    s. nevus
    s. tubercle
sebolith
seborrhea
seborrheic
    s. dermatitis
    s. keratosis
    s. verruca
    s. wart
sebum
secobarbital
second
    s. cranial nerve
    cycles per s.
    s. degree
    s. degree burn
    s. degree frostbite
    s. degree heart block
    s. degree radiation injury
    s. filial generation
    kilocycles per s.
    s.-order reaction
    s.-set graft rejection
    s.-set phenomenon
    vibration s's
secondary
    s. active transport
    s. agammaglobulinemia
    s. amenorrhea
    s. amyloidosis
    s. anemia
    s. antibody deficiency
    s. atelectasis
    s. attack rate
    s. buffer
    s. buffering

    s. carcinoma
    s. cardiomyopathy
    s. coccidioidomycosis
    s. coil
    s. constriction
    s. culture
    s. degeneration
    s. dextrocardia
    s. endings
    s. fixation
    s. glaucoma
    s. granule
    s. hyperaldosteronism
    s. hyperparathyroidism
    s. hyperplasia
    s. hypertension
    s. hyperthyroidism
    s. hypertrophic osteoar-
        thropathy
    s. hypoadrenocorticism
    s. hypogammaglobulinemia
    s. hypothyroidism
    s. immunodeficiency
    s. infertility
    lacrimal s.
    s. lymphoma
    s. lysosome
    s. methemoglobinemia
    s. myeloid metaplasia
    s. osteosarcoma
    s. pulmonary hemosiderosis
    s. pyoderma
    s. reference materials
    s. refractory anemia
    s. renal calculus
    s. renal tubular acidosis
    s. repair
    s. sensory neuron
    s. sequestrum
    s. sex character
    s. structure
    s. synaptic cell
    s. syphilis
    s. thrombus
    s. trisomy
    s. tuberculosis
    s. union
    s. x-rays
secretin stimulation test
secretinase
secretion
    cervical s.

        gastric s.
        oxytocin s.
        s. rate
        tracheobronchial s.
        transport and s.
secretor
        s. factor
        s. gene
        s. phenotype
        s. status
        s. trait
secretory
        s. alteration
        s. breast cancer
        s. canaliculus
        s. capillaries
        s. carcinoma
        s. cell
        s. component
        s. compound
        s. cyst
        s. endometrium
        s. granule
        s. immunoglobulin A
        s. otitis media
        s. vagina
section
        capture cross s.
        cesarean s.
        s. cutting
        s. freeze substitution technique
        frozen s.
        thin s.
        ultrathin s.
sectioning
        Albert-Linder bone s.
secular equilibrium
SED — skin erythema dose
        spondyloepiphyseal dysplasia
sedation
sedative
sediment
        crystals in urine s.
        stained urinary s.
        telescoped s.
        urinary s.
        urine s.
sedimentate
sedimentation
        s. coefficient
        s. equilibrium
        erythrocyte s.

        s. index
        s. rate
        s. reaction
        s. techniques
        s. test
        velocity-diffusion s.
sedimentation rate
        Rourke-Ernstein s.r.
        Westergren's s.r.
        Wintrobe's s.r.
        zeta s.r.
sedimentator
sedimented red cells
sedimentometer
sedimentum lateritium
sedoheptulokinase
sedoheptulose-7-phosphate
sed rate — sedimentation rate
SEE — standard error of estimate
SEG — sonoencephalogram
seg — segmented (leukocyte)
segment
        bronchopulmonary s.
        cranial s's
        frontal s.
        hepatic s's
        inferior s.
        initial s.
        interannular s.
        internodal s.
        lateral s.
        s. long-spacing (collagen)
        medullary s.
        mesoblastic s.
        neural s.
        occipital s.
        Okazaki's s's
        pairing s.
        P-R s.
        protovertebral s.
        pubic s.
        renal s's
        rivinian s.
        sacral s.
        Schmidt-Lantermann s.
        spinal s.
        S-T s.
        uterine s.
segmental
        s. bronchus
        s. cystic disease
        s. demyelination

s. enteritis
s. glomerulonephritis
s. mastectomy
segmentation sphere
segmented
s. cell
s. granulocyte
s. hyalinizing vasculitis
s. leukocyte
s. neutrophil
Segmentina
Segmentininae
segregation
segs — segmented neutrophils
Seitz's filter
seizure
jacksonian motor s.
Selas filter
Seldinger's
needle
technique
selectin
selection
s. against dominant mutations
s. against heterozygotes
s. against homozygotes
s. against recessive mutations
coefficient of s.
directional s.
natural s.
s. pressure
selective
s. medium
s. stain
selectivity ratio
selenite broth
selenium
s.-75
s. assay
s. deficiency
s. isotope
s. sulfide
selenocyte
selenoid body
selenomethionine
self-absorption
self-dose
selfing
self-tolerance
immunologic s.
Selivanoff's (Seliwanow's)
reagent
test

sellar
sella turcica
SEM — scanning electron microscope
standard error of the mean
semantics
semeiography
semen
s. analysis
s. examination
hyaluronidase unit for s.
semenuria
semialdehyde
glutamate s.
glutamic-γ-s.
succinate s.
semiapochromatic objective
semicarbazide hydrochloride
semicircular
s. canal
s. duct
semiconductor
s. device
extrinsic s.
intrinsic s.
semidominance
semidrying oil
semiinterquartile range
semilethal mutation
semilunar
s. cartilage
s. ganglion
seminal
s. colliculus
s. duct
s. fibrinolysin
s. fluid
s. vesicle cells
s. vesicle lumen
s. vesicle mucosa
seminiferous
s. cord
s. epithelium
s. tubule
s. tubule dysgenesis
seminoma
anaplastic s.
s. cells
classical s.
s. in situ
spermacytic s.
spermatocytic s.
seminomatous

seminuria
semipermeable membrane
semipronation
semiquantitative analysis
semiquinone
semisupination
semitendinous muscle
Semliki Forest virus
Sendai virus
seneciosis
senescence
senescent erythrocyte antigen
Sengstaken-Blakemore tube
senile
    s. arteriosclerosis
    s. atrophy
    s. cardiac amyloidosis
    s. cataract
    s. cerebral amyloidosis
    s. cystic endometrial atrophy
    s. degeneration
    s. dementia
    s. dwarfism
    s. ectasia
    s. elastosis
    s. emphysema/hyperinflation
    s. endometrium
    s. fibroma
    s. hemangioma
    s. hip disease
    s. involution
    s. keratoderma
    s. keratoma
    s. keratosis
    s. melanoderma
    s. nephrosclerosis
    s. osteomalacia
    s. osteoporosis
    s. plaques
    s. sebaceous hyperplasia
    s. wart
senility
senna
sennoside
sensation
    burning s.
    prickling s.
    somatic s's
    tactile s.
    tingling s.
    vestibular s.
    vibration s.

sense strand
sensibility
    epicritic s.
    protopathic s.
sensitivity
    antibiotic s.
    contact s.
    culture and s.
    diagnostic s.
    electrode s.
    primaquine s.
    relative s.
sensitization
    active s.
    cross-s.
    passive s.
    s. response
sensitizing dose
sensor
sensorimotor neuropathy
sensorineural dysfunction
sensorium commune
sensory
    s. afferent system
    s. aphasia
    s. association area
    s. epithelium
    s. ganglion
    s. neuron
    s. nucleus
    s. pathway
    s. radicular neuropathy
    s. receptor
    s. root
    s. structure
    s. transduction
sentinel
    s. animal
    s. gland
    s. node
    s. pile
    s. tag
SEP — sensory evoked potential
    somatosensory evoked potential
    systolic ejection period
separating medium
separation
    Ficoll-Hypaque s.
separatory funnel
Sephadex
Sepharose

Sepracell-MN
Sepsidae
sepsis (pl., sepses)
    intestinal s.
    s. lenta
    pneumococcal s.
    puerperal s.
septa
septal
    s. bladder
    s. cartilage
    s. defect
    s. fibrosis of liver
    s. hypertrophy
    s. leaflet of tricuspid valve
    s. mucoperichondrial flap
    s. papillary muscle
septal defect
    atrial s.d.
    interatrial s.d.
    interventricular s.d.
    ventricular s.d.
septate
    s. cervix
    s. uterus
    s. vagina
septation
septemia
septic
    s. abortion
    s. arthritis
    s. bursitis
    s. embolus
    s. endocarditis
    s. fever
    s. infarct
    s. infarction
    s. intoxication
    s. knee
    s. necrosis
    s. peritonitis
    s. phlebitis
    s. pneumonia
    s. shock
septicemia
    acute fulminating meningococ-
       cal s.
    anthrax s.
    Bacteroides s.
    Campylobacter s.
    cryptogenic s.
    meningococcal s.

    perinatal s.
    puerperal s.
    staphylococcal s.
    streptococcal s.
    typhoid s.
septicemic
    s. abscess
    s. plague
SeptiChek blood culture system
septicopyemia
septicopyemic
Septra
septum (pl., septa)
    alveolar s.
    atrial s.
    atrioventricular s.
    deviated s.
    interatrial s.
    intermuscular s.
    interventricular s.
    nasal s.
    orbital s.
    s. pellucidum
    s. primum
    rectovaginal s.
    rectovesical s.
    scrotal s.
    s. secundum
    s. spurium
    tracheoesophageal s.
    s. transversum
    urorectal s.
    ventricular s.
seq — sequela
    sequestrum
sequela (pl., sequelae)
sequence
    complement s.
    consensus s.
    insertion s.
    intervening s.
    s. ladder
    oligohydramnios s.
    Potter s.
    regulatory s.
    repeated DNA s's
    scanning s.
    Shine-Dalgarno s.
    signal s.
    termination s.
sequential
    s. access

s. analysis
s. determinant
s. multichannel autoanalyzer
sequester
sequestered antigen
sequestral
sequestration
s. bronchopneumonia
bronchopulmonary s.
s. cyst
s. dermoid
sequestrum (pl., sequestra)
primary s.
secondary s.
tertiary s.
SER — smooth endoplasmic reticulum
systolic ejection rate
seralbumin
Sereny test
serial
s. data transmission
s. dilution
s. operation
s. protamine sulfate test
s. thrombin time
Sericopelma communis
series (pl., series)
s. circuit
erythrocytic s.
gastrointestinal s.
granulocytic s.
homologous s.
lymphocytic s.
lymphoid s.
monohistiocytic s.
myeloid s.
thrombocytic s.
serine
s. deaminase
L-s. dehydratase
s. hydroxymethyltransferase
serocolitis
seroconversion
serocystic
serodiagnosis
serodiagnostic syphilis
seroenteritis
serofibrinous
s. effusion
s. inflammation
s. pericarditis

s. pleurisy
s. pleuritis
serologic
s. reaction
s. test for syphilis
serologically
s. defined
s. defined antigen
serological tumor markers
serology
bacterial s.
mycoplasmal s.
sporotrichosis s.
s. test
seroma
seromucoid
acid s.
α_1-seromucoid
seromucous gland
seronegative
serophilic
seropositive
seropositivity
seroprevalence
seropurulent
seropus
seroreversion
serosa
appendiceal s.
colonic s.
duodenal s.
gallbladder s.
gastric s.
polyemia s.
small intestinal s.
tubal s.
urinary bladder s.
uterine s.
serosamucin
serosanguineous effusion
serositis
multiple s.
serosity
serosynovial
serosynovitis
serotherapy
serothorax
serotonergic
serotonin assay
serotype
serotyping

serous
- s. acute inflammation
- s. acute synovitis
- s. atrophy
- s. cell
- s. cyst
- s. cystadenocarcinoma, papillary
- s. cystadenoma, papillary
- s. cystoma
- s. effusion
- s. fluid
- s. gland
- s. infiltration
- s. inflammation
- s. otitis media
- s. pleurisy
- s. tumor

serozyme

serpent
- s. infection
- s. worm

serpentine aneurysm

serpiginosum
- angioma s.

serpiginous
- s. keratitis
- s. ulcer

"serpin"

serrate

Serratia
- *S. indica*
- *S. kiliensis*
- *S. liquefaciens*
- *S. marcescens*
- *S. piscatorum*
- *S. plymuthica*
- *S. proteamaculans*
- *S. rubidaea*

Serratieae

serratus
- s. anterior muscle
- s. posterior muscle

Sertoli-Leydig cell tumor

Sertoli's
- cell
- cell junction
- cell nodule
- cell tumor

serum (pl., serums, sera)
- s. accelerator
- s. accelerator globulin

s. agar
aged s.
s. agglutinin
s. albumin
s. alkaline phosphatase
s. alkaline phosphatase test
s. amylase
s. amyloid A. component
s. amyloid P. component
anallergenic s.
anticholera s.
anticomplementary s.
antidiphtheric s.
antihepatic s.
antihuman lymphocyte s.
antilymphocyte s.
antimacrophage s.
antimeningococcus s.
anti–mouse lymphocyte s.
antineutrophilic s.
antipertussis s.
antiplague s.
antiplatelet s.
antipneumococcus s.
antirabies s.
antireticular cytotoxic s.
antiscarlatinal s.
antistaphylococcus s.
antistreptococcus s.
antitetanic s.
antithymocyte s.
antityphoid s.
antivenomous s.
s. bactericidal test
s. bilirubin
blood s.
s. chemistry graft
convalescent s.
Coombs' s.
s. creatine kinase
s. creatine phosphokinase
s. creatinine
cytotrophic s.
s. defect
despeciated s.
s. diagnosis
endotheliolytic s.
s. enzyme
equine antihuman lymphoblast s.
s. equinum
s. estriol

fetal bovine s.
s. globulin
s. globulin test
s. glutamate oxaloacetate transaminase
s. glutamate pyruvate transaminase
s. glutamic-oxaloacetic transaminase
s. glutamic-pyruvic transaminase
glycerin blood s.
guinea pig anti-insulin s.
s. hepatitis
s. hepatitis antigen
s. hepatitis virus
hereditary erythroblastic multinuclearity s.
hereditary erythrocytic multinuclearity s.
heterologous s.
hog cholera s.
homologous s.
horse s.
human s.
s. hydroxybutyrate dehydrogenase
hyperimmune s.
icteric s.
immune s.
inactivated s.
inactivated leukocytolytic s.
s. inhibitor
s. intoxication
s. iron
s. isocitric dehydrogenase
lactescent s.
s. lactic dehydrogenase
leukocytolytic s.
s. lipase
s. lipoprotein
Löffler's blood s.
motile s.
muscle s.
s. nephritis
nephrotoxic s.
normal blood s.
normal horse s.
normal human s.
normal rabbit s.
normal reference s.
s. osmolality

pericardial s.
s. phosphatase
plague s.
polyvalent s.
pooled s.
pooled blood s.
s. precipitable iodine
pregnant mare s.
prophylactic s.
s. protein-bound iodine
s. protein electrophoresis *
s. prothrombin conversion accelerator
s. prothrombin conversion accelerator deficiency
s. prothrombin conversion accelerator factor
s. prothrombin time
rabbit antidog-thymus s.
rabbit antirat-lymphocyte s.
salted s.
salvarsanized s.
s. shock
s. sickness
streptococcus s.
s. thrombotic accelerator
thyrotoxic s.
s. urate level
s. urea nitrogen
s. uric acid
veronal-buffered saline : fetal bovine s.
serumal
servomechanism
servomotor
seryl
seryl-RNA-synthetase
sesame oil
sesamoid bone
sesquioxide
        chromium s.
sesquiterpene
sessile
        s. hydatid
        s. phagocyte
        s. polyp
SET — systolic ejection time
set-point
settled particulates
seven-segment display
seventh cranial nerve
severe

*serum proteins lettered as Greek letters

severely subnormal
Severinghaus electrode
sex
        s. cell
        s. chromatin
        s. chromatin test
        s. chromosome
        s.-conditioned character
        s. cords
        s. cord–stromal tumor
        s. cord tumor, undifferentiated
        s. determination
        s. differentiation
        heterogametic s.
        homogametic s.
        s. hormone
        s. hormone-binding
        s.-limited character
        s.-limited gene globulin
        s.-linked character
        s.-linked gene
        s.-linked inheritance
        s. pilus
        primordial s. cell
        s. reversal
        s.-reversed mutation
        s. steroid
sexduction
sexivalent
sexual
        s. deviation
        s. exhibitionism
        s. impotence
        s. maturation
        s. perversion
        s. reproduction
        s. transmission
sexually transmitted disease
Sézary-Lutzner cells
Sézary's
        cells
        erythroderma
        lymphoma
        reticulosis
SF — scarlet fever
        spinal fluid
Sf — Svedberg's flotation unit
S factor
SFD — skin-film distance
SFEMG — single-fiber electromy-
        ography

SFP — screen filtration pressure
        spinal fluid pressure
SFS — split function study
SG — serum globulin
        skin graft
        specific gravity
S-G — Sachs-Georgi (test)
SGA — small for gestational age
SGOT — serum glutamic-oxaloacetic
        transaminase
SGP — serine glycerophosphatide
SGPT — serum glutamic-pyruvic
        transaminase
SGV — salivary gland virus
SH — serum hepatitis
        sex hormone
        sinus histiocytosis
        sulfhydryl
shadow
        s.-casting
        s. cells
        s. corpuscle
        Gumprecht's s's
        s. nucleus
        Ponfick's s.
Shaffer-Hartmann method
shaft
        penile s.
shaggy pericardium
shagreen
        s. patch
        s. skin
shake
        s. culture
        s. test
Sharpey's perforating fibers
SHB or SHb — sulfhemoglobin
SHBD — serum hydroxybutyrate de-
        hydrogenase
Shea-Anthony antral balloon
sheath
        carotid s.
        rectus s.
        Schwann's s.
        tendon s.
sheep
        s. blood agar
        s. cell agglutination test
        s. erythrocyte
        s. liver fluke
        s. red blood cells
        s. red cells

sheet
>beta pleated s.
>material safety data s.

shell
>diffusion s.
>s. nail

Sherman-Bourquin unit of vitamin B$_2$

Sherman-Munsell unit

Sherman's unit

SHG — synthetic human gastrin

shield
>chloride s.
>gonadal s.
>syringe s.
>tabletop s.

shielding

shift
>antigenic s.
>bathochromic s.
>chemical s.
>chloride s.
>s. counter
>hyperchromic s.
>hypochromic s.
>hypsochromic s.
>isohydric s.
>regenerative blood s.
>s. register
>s. reticulocyte
>Stokes' s.

Shiga's
>bacillus
>toxin

Shigella
>S. *alkalescens*
>S. *ambigua*
>S. *arabinotarda* Type A, B
>S. *boydii*
>S. *ceylonensis*
>S. *dispar*
>S. *dysenteriae*
>S. *etousae*
>S. *flexneri*
>S. *madampensis*
>S. *newcastle*
>S. *paradysenteriae*
>S. *parashigae*
>S. *schmitzii*
>S. *shigae*
>S. *sonnei*
>S. *wakefield*

shigellosis

Shihabi-Bishop method

shikimate dehydrogenase

Shimoda's blood group system

shin
>saber s.

Shine-Dalgarno sequence

Shiner's tube

shingles

Shinowara-Jones-Reinhard unit

"ship's wheel" image

shirt-stud abscess

shivering thermogenesis

SHO — secondary hypertrophic osteoarthropathy

shock
>anaphylactic s.
>anaphylactoid s.
>s. artifact
>bacterial s.
>cardiogenic s.
>colloid s.
>compensated s.
>decompensated s.
>endotoxic s.
>endotoxin s.
>faradic s.
>gram-positive s.
>hemoclastic s.
>hemodynamic s.
>hemorrhagic s.
>histamine s.
>hypoglycemic s.
>hypotensive s.
>hypovolemic s.
>insulin s.
>irreversible s.
>s. lung
>micro s.
>neurogenic s.
>osmotic s.
>peptone s.
>progressive s.
>protein s.
>septic s.
>serum s.
>thyrotoxin s.
>toxic s.
>traumatic s.
>vasogenic s.

Shone's anomaly

Shope's
    fibroma
    papilloma
short
    s. circuit
    s. incubation hepatitis
shortened
    s. bleeding time
    s. coagulation time
shortening
    abnormal s.
shotty breast
shoulder
    frozen s.
    s. ligament
shower
    safety s.
Shrapnell's membrane
shudder
shuffling gait
shunt
    anatomic s.
    arteriovenous s.
    hexose monophosphate s.
    Israels' s.
    pentose s.
    pentose-phosphate s.
    physiologic s.
    portacaval s.
    portal-systemic s.
    portosystemic s.
    Rapoport-Luebering s.
    venous-to-arterial s.
shunting
    cardiac s.
Shwartzman's
    phenomenon
    reaction
SI — International System of Units
    sacroiliac
    saturation index
    serum iron
    soluble insulin
    stroke index
sialadenitis
    bacterial s.
    obstructive s.
sialadenoma papilliferum
sialadenoncus
sialadenosis
sialic acid
sialidase digestion

sialoadenitis
    suppurative s.
sialocele
sialoglycoconjugate
sialoglycoprotein
sialography
sialolithiasis
sialometaplasia
    necrotizing s.
sialomucin
sialophorin
sialorrhea
sialyloligosaccharide
Siamese twins
Sia test
Sibine
Sibley-Lehninger unit
sibling species
sib pair analysis
sibship
Sicariidae
sicca
    s. complex
    s. syndrome
siccant
siccative
siccolabile
siccostabile; siccostable
SICD — serum isocitric dehydro-
    genase
sickle cell
    s.c. anemia
    s.c. C disease
    s.c. crisis
    s.c. disease
    s.c. hemoglobin
    s.c. hemoglobin C disease
    s.c. nephropathy
    s.c. test
    s.c. thalassemia
    s.c. β-thalassemia
    s.c.-thalassemia disease
    s.c. trait
sickled cell
Sickledex reagent
sicklemia
sickling test
sickness
    African sleeping s.
    decompensation s.
    decompression s.
    green s.

Jamaican vomiting s.
radiation s.
serum s.
sleeping s.
SID — sudden infant death
side-chain theory
side effect
sideramine
sideroachrestic anemia
Siderobacter
sideroblast
 ringed s.
sideroblastic anemia
Siderocapsa
Siderocapsaceae
siderochrome
Siderococcus
siderocyte stain
siderocytic granule
sideroderma
siderofibrosis
siderofibrotic nodules
siderogenous
sideromycin
sideropenia
sideropenic
 s. anemia
 s. dysphagia
siderophage
siderophagocytosis
siderophil; siderophile
siderophilin
siderophilous
siderophore
siderosilicosis
siderosis
 Bantu s.
siderosome
siderotic
 s. granule
 s. nodules
SIDS — sudden infant death syndrome
sieve
 molecular s.
sievert
Siggaard-Andersen
 alignment nomogram
 nomogram
sigma
 s. bond

s. reaction
s. rhythm
sigmavirus
sigmoid
 s. artery
 s. colon
 s. colon mesentery
 s. kidney
 s. mesocolon
 s. sinus
sigmoiditis
sigmoidoscopy
sigmoidovesical fistula
Sigmund's glands
sign
 Auspitz s.
 crescent s.
 Babinski's s.
 Bamberger's s.
 Blumberg's s.
 Brudzinski's s.
 Bryce's s.
 Chaddock's s.
 Chvostek's s.
 Courvoisier's s.
 Cullen's s.
 Darier's s.
 dimple s.
 Ewart's s.
 Goodell's s.
 groove s.
 Hegar's s.
 Heryng's s.
 Higoumenakia s.
 Kernig's s.
 Kussmaul's s.
 Küstner's s.
 Leser-Trélat s.
 Lhermitte's s.
 Nikolsky's s.
 Pemberton's s.
 Perez's s.
 Romaña's s.
 Rommelaere's s.
 scimitar s.
 string s.
 Tinel's s.
 trolley-track s.
 Trousseau's s.
 Unschuld's s.
 Verril's s.
 Vierra's s.

vital s's
Yergason's s.

signal
    analog s.
    common mode s.
    deflection s.
    s. level
    s. nociceptor
    s. node
    s. peptide
    s. sequence
    s.-to-noise ratio

signature

signed
    s. magnitude
    s. rank test

signet
    s. cell carcinoma
    s. ring adenocarcinoma
    s. ring carcinoma
    s. ring cell adenoma
    s. ring cell carcinoma
    s. ring cell lymphoma

significance
    s. level
    s. probability
    test of s.

significant
    s. asymptomatic bacteriuria
    s. digits
    not statistically s.
    statistically s.

SIJ — sacroiliac joint
silane
silanization
Silastic implant
silent
    s. mutation
    s. myocardial infarction

silhouette
    cardiac s.

silica
    s. gel
    s. particles

silicate
silicatosis
silicic acid
silicofluoride salt
silicon
    colloidal s. dioxide
    s.-controlled rectifier
    s.-controlled switch

    s. dioxide
    s. granuloma

silicone
siliconoma
silicoproteinosis
silicosis
    accelerated s.

silo-fillers' lung
silver
    s.-ammoniacal silver stain
    s. cell
    s. impregnation
    methenamine s.
    mild s. protein
    s. nitroprusside test
    s. protein stain
    s./silver chloride electrode
    s. stain
    s. sulfadiazine

silver nitrate
    Barnett-Bourne acetic alcohol
        s.n.
    s.n. test

Silver-Russell dwarfism
Silver's procedure
silvex
silyation
silylation
Simbu
    hepatitis
    virus

simethicone
simian
    s. AIDS
    s. crease
    s. sarcoma virus
    s. T-cell leukemia virus-III
    s. virus

simian immunodeficiency virus (SIV)
Simmonds' cachexia
Simmons' citrate agar
Simon's
    foci
    septic factor

simple
    s. allotype
    s. asphyxiant
    s. atrophy
    s. cyst
    s. fracture
    s. goiter
    s. hypertrophy

s. lymphangiectasis
s. mastectomy
s. microscope
s. necrosis
s. protein
s. pulmonary eosinophilia
s. random sample
s. ulcer
s. urethritis
simplex
    herpes s.
    hidroacanthoma s.
Sims-Huhner test
simulated hypertrophy
simulation
Simuliidae
Simulium
sincalide
Sindbis virus
sine wave
Singer-Blom stoma valve
Singer's node
single
    s.-blind
    s.-breath nitrogen test
    s. chain-urokinase-like plasmin-
      ogen activator
    s.-diffusion test
    s.-dimension electroimmunodif-
      fusion
    s.-human leukocyte antigen
    s.-phase
sinistrocardia
    isolated s.
sink
    heat s.
sinoatrial
    s. block
    s. node
    s. rhythm
sinopulmonary
sinus (pl., sinus, sinuses)
    accessory s.
    Aschoff-Rokitansky s.
    s. bradycardia
    branchial cleft s.
    cavernous s.
    circular s.
    s. confluens
    dermal s.
    draining s.
    dural s.

ethmoid s.
frontal s.
frontoethmoid s.
s. histiocytosis
s. histiocytosis with massive
    lymphadenopathy
inferior petrosal s.
inferior sagittal s.
inflammatory s.
lactiferous s.
marginal venous s.
maxillary s.
occipital s.
paranasal s.
s. phlebitis
pilonidal s.
pyriform s.
s. rectus
renal s.
Rokitansky-Aschoff s.
sigmoid s.
sphenoid s.
sphenoparietal s.
straight s.
superior petrosal s.
superior sagittal s.
s. tract, inflammatory
transverse s.
urachal s.
urachal umbilical s.
urachal-vesical s.
urogenital s.
Valsalva's posterior s.
s. venosus
s. venosus remnants
sinusitis
    necrotizing granulomatous s.
    sclerosing s.
    staphylococcal s.
    viral s.
sinusoid
    hepatic s.
    s. lymph node
sinusoidal
    s. capillaries
    s. dilatation
    s. endothelial cell
sinuspiral
Siperstein criteria
Siphonaptera
Siphunculina
sirenomelia

Sirius
    red
    red 4B
SIRS — soluble immune response sup-
        pressor
SISI — short-increment sensitivity
        index
sister chromatids
Sister Joseph's nodule
Sisyrosea
site
    allosteric s.
    antigen-binding s.
    implantation s.
    privileged s.
β-sitosterolemia
sitosterols
situs inversus totalis
SI (Système Internationale d'Unités)
    unit
SIV — simian immunodeficiency
        virus
sixth
    s. cranial nerve
    s. venereal disease
size-exclusion chromatography
Sjögren's antibodies
SJR — Shinowara-Jones-Reinhard
        (unit)
SK — streptokinase
skatole
skatoxyl
skein cell
skeletal
    s. age
    s. dysplasia
    s. muscle
    s. muscle antibody
skeleton
    appendicular s.
    axial s.
    cardiac s.
    gill arch s.
    s. hand
    "membrane s."
    visceral s.
Skene's glands
skeneitis; skenitis
skew
skewed distribution
skiagraph
skiametry

skin
    alligator s.
    s. biopsy
    congenital localized absence
        of s.
    deciduous s.
    s. dose
    elastic s.
    farmer's s.
    s.-film distance
    fish s.
    s. fungus culture
    glabrous s.
    s. graft
    hyperpigmented s.
    leopard s.
    lizard s.
    loose s.
    s. mycobacteria culture
    parchment s.
    piebald s.
    pig s.
    porcupine s.
    s. puncture
    s.-reactive factor
    sailor's s.
    s.-sensitizing antibody
    shagreen s.
    s. stones
    s. tag
    s. test
    s. test dose
    s. test unit
    s. to tumor distance
    s. tumors
    yellow s.
skinbound disease
skip lesion
SKSD — streptokinase-streptodornase
skull
    natiform s.
SL — sensation level
    Sibley-Lehninger (unit)
    streptolysin
sl — slyke
SLA — sacrolaeva anterior
    slide latex agglutination
slant
    citrate agar s.
    s. culture
    phenylalanine deaminase
        agar s.

slaty anemia
SLD or SLDH — serum lactic
                 dehydrogenase
SLE — St. Louis encephalitis
       systemic lupus erythematosus
sleep
        s. apnea
        s. deprivation
        drug-induced s.
        s. latency
        NREM (non–rapid eye move-
           ment) s.
        REM (rapid eye movement) s.
        s. spindle
sleeping sickness
sleepwalking
SLEV — St. Louis encephalitis virus
          St. Louis encephalitis virus
          serology
SLFIA — substrate-labeled fluores-
          cence immunoassay
SLI — splenic localization index
slide
        s. coagulase test
        s. latex agglutination
        s.-wire potentiometer
sliding
        s. hernia
        s. microtome
slit
        filtration s's
        s.-lamp examination
SLKC — superior limbic
          keratoconjunctivitis
SLN — superior laryngeal nerve
SLO — streptolysin-O
slope culture
slot exhaust
slough
sloughing ulcer
slow
        s. axonal transport
        s. channel
        "s." hemoglobin
        s.-moving protease
        s. neutron
        s.-reacting substance
        s.-reacting substance of anaphy-
           laxis
        s. twitch
        s. viruses
slowly adapting receptor

SLP — sacrolaeva posterior
       sex-limited protein
SLR — *Streptococcus lactis* R
SLS — segment long-spacing
       (collagen)
SLT — sacrolaeva transversa
sludge
sludged blood
SL (Sibley-Lehninger) unit
slurring
slurry
slyke
SM — streptomycin
       submucous
       suction method
       systolic mean
       systolic murmur
Sm — samarium
SMA — sequential multichannel
          autoanalyzer
          superior mesenteric artery
SMA-12 profile test
SMAF — specific macrophage-arming
          factor
small
        s. calorie
        s. cell carcinoma
        s. cell lung cancer
        s. cell sarcoma
        s. cell tumor
        s. cleaved cell lymphoma
        s. intestinal mesentery
        s. intestine
        s. intestine polyp
        s. intestine tumors
        s. lymphocytic lymphoma
        s. noncleaved cell lymphoma
        s. nuclear ribonucleoproteins
        s. nuclear RNA
        s. uncleaved cell
smaller occipital nerve
smallpox
        coherent s.
        confluent s.
        discrete s.
        hemorrhagic s.
        s. immunization
        inoculation s.
        malignant s.
        modified s.
        s. virus
Sm antigen

smart terminal
smear
    alimentary tract s.
    s. background
    blood s.
    Breed s.
    bronchoscopic s.
    buccal s.
    buffy coat s.
    cervical s.
    colonic s.
    cul-de-sac s.
    cytologic s.
    duodenal s.
    ectocervical s.
    endocervical s.
    endometrial s.
    esophageal s.
    fast s.
    FGT (female genital tract) cy-
      tologic s.
    fungal s.
    gastric s.
    lateral vaginal wall s.
    lower respiratory tract s.
    malaria s.
    oral s.
    pancervical s.
    Pap s.; Papanicolaou s.
    peripheral blood s.
    s. preparation and staining for
      blood parasites
    sputum s.
    TB s.
    urinary s.
    vaginal irrigation s.
    VCE s.
smegma
    s. bacillus
    s. clitoridis
    s. embryonum
    s. preputii
smegmalith
Smith (Sm) antigen
smog
    photochemical s.
smoldering leukemia
SMON — subacute myelo-optical neu-
      ropathy
smooth
    s. bacterium
    s. colony

    s. endoplasmic reticulum
    s. leprosy
    s. muscle
    s. muscle antibody
    s.-rough variation
smoothing
SMP — slow-moving protease
SMR — somnolent metabolic rate
      standard mortality ratio
SMRR — submucous resection and
      rhinoplasty
smudge cells
SN — serum-neutralizing
      suprasternal notch
Sn — tin
snakebite
snake venom
snapback DNA
snapping hip
SNB — scalene node biopsy
Snellen chart
Snell's law
"sniff test"
SNM — Society of Nuclear Medicine
SNOP — Systematized Nomenclature
      of Pathology
SNR — signal-to-noise ratio
SNRPs — small nuclear
      ribonucleoproteins
snuff
SO — salpingo-oophorectomy
"soap bubble" lesion
SOB — short(ness) of breath
SOC — sequential-type oral contra-
      ceptive
Society of Computer Medicine
Society of Nuclear Medicine
sodium
    s. acetate formalin
    s. acetrizoate
    s. alginate
    s. aminosalicylate
    s. arsanilate
    s. arsenate
    s. arsenite
    s. ascorbate
    s. bicarbonate test
    s. biphosphate
    s. bitartrate
    s. cacodylate
    s. caprylate
    carbenicillin s.

carbenoxolone s.
carboxymethylcellulose s.
s. caustic alkali
s. chloride
s. chloride and dextrose injection
s. chloride and fructose injection
s. chloride (6.5%) broth
s. chloride (6.5%) culture medium
s. chloride, injection
s. chloride, isotonic
s. chromate
s. chromate Cr-51
s. citrate
cloxacillin s.
colistimethate s.
s. cyanide
s. dehydrocholate
s. desoxycholate
dextrothyroxine s.
s. diatrizoate
s. 2,4-dichlorophenoxyethyl sulfate
s. dihydrogen phosphate
s. dinitro-ortho-cresylate
s. diprotrizoate
s. diuresis
s. dodecyl sulfate
s. endothal
s. escape
s. estrone sulfate
s. ethyl xanthate
etidronate s.
s. fluoride
s. fluoroacetate
s. fluorosilicate
s. glutamate
heparin s.
s. hexafluorosilicate
s. hippurate hydrolysis test
s. hydroxide
s. hyposulfate
s. indigotindisulfonate
s. iodide
s. iodipamide
s. iodohippurate
s. iodomethamate
iodothalamate s.
s. ion
ipodate s.

s. isopropyl xanthate
isotonic s. chloride solution
s. isotope
s. lactate injection
s. levothyroxine
s. liothyronine
s.-lithium counter transport
mercaptomerin s.
s. metaborate
s. N-methyl dithiocarbamate
s. monofluoroacetate
s. morrhuate
s.-β-naphthoquinone-4-sulfonate
s. nitrite
s. nitroprusside
oxacillin s.
s. oxalate
s. pentachlorophenate
s. perborate
s. pertechnetate
s. phosphate
s. phytate
plasma s.
s. polyanethol sulfonate
s. polystyrene sulfonate
potassium s. nitrate
s. propionate
s. psylliate
s. rhodanide
s. ricinoleate
rose bengal s.
s. salicylate
s. selenate
s. silicate
s. silicofluoride
s. succinate
s. sulfate
s. sulfide
s. sulfite
sulfobromophthalein s.
s. sulfocyanate
s. tartrate
s. tetraborate
s. tetradecyl
s. thiocyanate
s. thioglycollate
s. thiosulfate
s. trichloroacetate
s. tungstoborate
tyropanoate s.
s. urate crystals

s. warfarin
s. wasting
Yb-169 pentetate s.
sodoku
Soemmering's ring cataract
soft
s. chancre
s. palate
s. papilloma
s. sore
s. tissue
s. tissue calcification
s. tissue sarcoma
s. tissue tumor
s. tubercle
s. ulcer
s. wart
software
Sol — solution
SOL — space-occupying lesion
sol
metal s.
solid s.
solanine
solanocyte
solanoid cancer
Solanum
solar
s. elastosis
s. keratosis
s. urticaria
soldier's patches
sole
convex s.
solenoid
Solenopsis
soleus muscle
solid
s. ameloblastoma
s. angle
s. carbon dioxide
s. carcinoma
s. cell nests
s. cystic hidradenoma
s.-cystic tumor
s. edema
s.-phase immunoassay
s.-phase radioimmunoassay
s. sol
s. state
s.-state electrode
s.-state radiation detector

s. teratoma
urinary s's
solidistic pathology
solitary
s. bone cyst
s. cell
s. cyst
s. keratoacanthoma
s. myeloma
s. nodule
s. osteocartilaginous exostosis
s. plasmacytoma
solubility
s. coefficient
s. product constant
s. test
solubilize
solubilizer
soluble
s. antigen fluorescent antibody
test
s. immune response suppressor
s. insulin
s. interleukin-2 receptors
s. ribonucleic acid
s. RNA
solute
total body s.
solution
Alsever's s.
ammoniacal silver s's
aqueous s.
azeotropic s.
Balamuth's buffer s.
balanced salt s.
Benedict's s.
buffered saline s.
Burow's s.
Cajal's formol ammonium bromide s.
cetrimide-citrate-saline s.
cobra venom s.
Dakin's s.
Diaphane s.
disclosing s.
Dobell and O'Connor's iodine s.
Dragendorff's s.
Earle's s.
Fehling's s.
Fonio's s.
formaldehyde s.

formol ammonium bromide s.
Fowler's s.
Gallego's differentiating s.
Gram's s.
Hank's s.
Hartmann's s.
Hayem's s.
Hucker-Conn crystal violet s.
s. hybridization
Krebs-Ringer s.
lactated Ringer's s.
Lange's s.
Locke-Ringer s.
Locke's s.
low ionic strength salt s.
Lugol's s.
Lugol's iodine s.
physiological saline s.
Ringer's s.
Ringer's lactate s.
saline s.
saturated s.
standard s.
test s.
Tyrode's s.
volumetric s.
Weigert's iodine s.

solvate
solvation
solvent
    aprotic s.
    s. extraction
    protic s.
solvolysis
SOM — secretory otitis media
        serous otitis media
soma
somasthenia
somatesthesia
somatic
    s. agglutinin
    s. cell
    s. cell genetics
    s. chromosome
    s. death
    s. efferent fibers
    s. fibers
    s. layer
    s. mutation
    s. mutation theory of cancer
    s. pairing
    s. sensations

somatognosis
somatomammotropin
    chorionic s.
    human chorionic s.
    immunoradioassayable human
        chorionic s.
somatomedin A, B, C
somatomedins
somatosensory
    s. area
    s. evoked potential
somatostatin
    s. analog
    s. cell
somatostatinoma
somatotroph adenoma
somatotrophic
somatotropic hormone
somatotropin-releasing factor
somesthesia
somite
somnambulism
somnolence
somnolent metabolic rate
Somogyi
    effect
    method
    unit
sonar
sonicate
sonication
sonification
sonifier
sonify
Sonne-Duval bacillus
Sonne's dysentery
sonogram
sonography
sonolucent
soot wart
S-100 protein
sorbefacient
sorbent
sorbitol
    s. dehydrogenase
    s. phenol-red broth
sore
    canker s.
    fungating s.
    hard s.
    oriental s.
    soft s.

tropical s.
venereal s.
Sörensen's phosphate buffer
Soret's band
sorption
sorter
    fluorescence-activated cell s.
SOS repair system
SOTT — synthetic old tuberculin tri-
        chloroacetic acid
sound
    alteration s., cardiac
    alteration s., heart
    respiratory s., abnormal
    s. waves
source
    s. language
    s. program
    s. statement
South African–type porphyria
South American
    blastomycosis
    hemorrhagic fever
Southern
    blot analysis
    blot technique
    blot test
    blotting
Souttar's tube
soybean
    s.-casein digest
    s.-casein digest blood agar
    s. trypsin inhibitor
SP — shunt procedure
    skin potential
    status post
    steady potential
    summating potential
    suprapubic
    symphysis pubis
    systolic pressure
2-S P —transport medium used for
        mycoplasma isolation
sp. or spp. — species
SPA — suprapubic aspiration
space
    apical s.
    capsular s.
    s. charge
    Disse's s's
    female genital s.
    fetal s.

Fontana's s.
gastrointestinal s.
Held's s.
His's s.
iliocostal s.
intercristal s.
intervillous s.
intracristal s.
intramembranous s.
male genital s.
medullary s.
meningeal s.
s.-occupying lesion
periaxial s.
perinuclear s.
phrenocostal s.
placental s.
Poiseuille's s.
respiratory s.
retrobulbar s.
urinary tract s.
Virchow-Robin s.
spacer
spade
    s. fingers
    s. hand
    s. penis
SPAI — steroid protein activity index
spallation products
Spanish psyllium
Sp antigen
sparganoma
sparganosis
Sparganum proliferum
sparteine
spasm
    cadaveric s.
    torsion s.
spastic
    s. anemia
    s. bladder
    s. bulbar palsy
    s. colitis
    s. gait
    s. ileus
spasticity
spät apoplexy
spatial
    s. distortion
    s. frequency
    s. isomerism

s. resolution
visual-s.
SPBI — serum protein–bound iodine
SPCA — serum prothrombin conver-
        sion accelerator
SPCA
    deficiency
    factor
SPE — serum protein electrophoresis
Spearman's rank correlation coeffi-
    cient
special
    s. pathology
    s. reference method
specialist
specialized transduction
speciation
species
    sibling s.
specific
    s. absorptivity
    s. coagulation factor deficiency
    s. dynamic action
    s. etiologic agent
    s. granule
    s. gravity
    s. heat
    s. heat capacity
    s. ionization
    s. macrophage-arming factor
    s. pathogen–free
    s. rate
    s. rotation
    s. soluble substance
specificity
    diagnostic s.
    neuronal s.
    organ s.
    public s.
    relative s.
    species s.
    spill-over s.
specimen
    anaerobic urine s.
    bacteriologic s's
    blood s.
    brush s's
    clinical bacteriologic s's
    cytologic s.
    random urine s.
speckled leukoplakia
spectinomycin

spectral
    s. color
    s. interference
    s. resolution
    s. response
spectrin
spectrofluorometer
spectrograph
    mass s.
spectrometer
    gamma s.
    mass s.
spectrometry
    clinical s.
    gamma s.
    gas chromatography–mass s.
    infrared s.
    isotope dilution–mass s.
    mass s.
spectrophotometer
    AA s.
    atomic absorption s.
spectrophotometric
spectrophotometry
    atomic absorption s.
    diode array s.
    double beam s.
    flame emission s.
    infrared s.
    ultraviolet/visible s.
spectroscope
    direct vision s.
spectroscopic analysis
spectroscopy
    clinical s.
    emission s.
    flame emission s.
    infrared s.
    magnetic resonance s.
    mass s.
    Raman s.
spectrotype
spectrum (pl., spectra, spectrums)
    absorption s.
    s. analyzer
    atomic s.
    band s.
    clinical s.
    continuous s.
    emission s.
    excitation s.
    fiber s.

fluorescence s.
gamma-ray s.
line s.
specular reflection
speculum (pl., specula)
speech
s. disorder
s. impediment
slurred s.
Spelotrema
Spengler's fragment
sperm
s.-containing cyst
s. count
s. crystal
s. duct ectasia
s. flagellum
s. granuloma
s. maturation
muzzled s.
spermacytic seminoma
spermatic
s. cord
s. fistula
s. vein
spermatid stalk
spermatin
spermatocele
epididymal s.
spermatocyst
spermatocyte
spermatocytic seminoma
spermatogenesis
spermatogenic
s. arrest
s. epithelium
s. granuloma
s. maturation arrest
spermatogonium (pl., spermatogonia)
spermatozoon (pl., spermatozoa)
spermaturia
spermia
spermiation
spermidine
spermin crystal
spermine
spermiogenesis
spermolith
SPF — specific pathogen–free
split products of fibrin
sp. gr. — specific gravity

SPH — secondary pulmonary hemosiderosis
sph — spherical
spherical lens
sphacelate
sphacelation
sphacelism
sphaceloderma
sphacelous
sphacelus
Sphaerophorus necrophorus
S phase
sphenoid
s. bone
s. sinus
s. suture
sphenoiditis
spheno-occipital synchondrosis
sphenopalatine
s. artery
s. ganglion
s. neuralgia
sphenoparietal sinus
sphenopetrosal synchondrosis
sphere
attraction s.
embryonic s.
Morgagni's s's
prelytic s.
segmentation s.
vitelline s.
spherical
s. aberration
s. erythrocyte
s. polar coordinates
spherocyte
spherocytic
s. anemia
s. jaundice
spherocytosis
hereditary s.
spheroid erythrocyte
spherophakia-brachymorphia syndrome
spheroplast
spherule
spherulin
sphincter
s. of ampulla
anal s.
s. ani externus muscle
cardiac s.

cardioesophageal s.
inguinal s.
s. of Oddi
palatopharyngeal s.
s. pupillae muscle
pupillary s.
pyloric s.
rectal s.
s. urethrae muscle
urinary s.
sphincteral achalasia
sphincteritis
sphincterotomy
sphinganine
sphingenine
sphingoin
sphingolipid storage disease
sphingolipidosis (pl., sphingolipidoses)
sphingolipodystrophy
sphingomyelin
s. lipidosis
s. phosphodiesterase
sphingomyelinase deficiency
sphingomyelinosis
sphingophospholipid
sphingosine
sphygmic
SPI — serum precipitable iodine
spiculated
s. bodies
s. erythrocyte
spicule
spider
s. angioma
arterial s.
black widow s.
brown recluse s.
s.-burst
s. cancer
s. cell
s. cell rhabdomyoblast
s. mole
s. nevus
s. pelvis
s. telangiectasia
vascular s.
Spiegler-Fendt
pseudolymphoma
sarcoid
spike
s. and dome complex
H s.

s. and slow-wave complex
s. and slow-wave rhythm
spill
cellular s.
s. control
s. control kit
s. residue
spiloma
spilus
spina (pl., spinae)
s. bifida
s. bifida cystica
s. bifida occulta
open s. bifida
s. ventosa
spinal
s. accessory nerve
s. arachnoid
s. artery
s. cord
s. cord tumors
s. dura mater
s. embolism
s. epidural space
s. fluid
s. fluid culture
s. fluid leukocyte count
s. fluid pressure
s. ganglion
s. hemangioblastoma
s. lemniscus
s. medulla
s. muscle
s. needle
s. nerve
s. pia mater
s. puncture
s. region of subdural space
s. sensory afferent system
s. somatosensory evoked potential
s. subarachnoid space
s. tap
s. tract nucleus
s. tract of trigeminal nerve
spin-cool filter method
spindle
achromatic s.
s. alteration
s. attachment
barbiturate s.
bipolar s.

s. cell
s. cell carcinoma
s. cell lipoma
s. cell melanoma
s. cell nevus
s. cell nodule
s. cell sarcoma
s. cell thymoma
s. cell tumor
Krukenberg's s.
multipolar s.
muscle s.
s. tendon
spindling
spindly squamoid cell
spine
anterior inferior iliac s.
anterior superior iliac s.
ischial s.
posterior inferior iliac s.
posterior superior iliac s.
spinnbarkeit
spinner method
spinocerebellar degeneration
spino-olivary tract
spinorubral
spinotectal
spinothalamic
spiny neuron
spiradenitis
spiradenoma
eccrine s.
spiral
s. canal, cochlea
Curschmann's s's
s. fracture
s. ganglion
Herxheimer's s.
s. lamina
s. membrane
s. plica
s. wound
spiramycin
spirilla
Spirillaceae
spirillar dysentery
spirillosis
Spirillum
S. *minor*
S. *minus*
spirillum
Obermeier's s.

spirit lamp
Spirochaeta
S. *daxensis*
S. *eurystrepta*
S. *marina*
S. *plicatilis*
S. *stenostrepta*
spirochetal
s. infection
s. jaundice
spirochete
nontreponemal s.
spirochetemia
spirochetosis
spirogram
forced expiratory s.
Spirometra
spirometric
spirometry
spironolactone test
Spirurata
Spirurida
Spiruroidea
spiruroid larva migrans
Spitz nevus
SPL — sound pressure level
spontaneous lesion
splanchnic
s. blood flow
s. nerve
splanchnoptosis; splanchnoptosia
splanchnosclerosis
spleen
accessory s.
Banti's s.
diffuse waxy s.
lardaceous s.
sago s.
scrotal s.
sugar-coated s.
waxy s.
splenauxe
Splendore-Hoeppli phenomenon
splenectomy
splenectopia; splenectopy
splenelcosis
splenemphraxis
splenic
s. anemia
s. anemia of infants
s. artery
s. capsule

s. cords
s. corpuscle
s. flexure
s. hilus
s. leukemia
s. lymphatic follicle
s. lymphoma
s. muscle
s. mycosis
s. neutropenia
s. red pulp
s. sinusoids
s. trabeculae
s. tumor
s. vein
s. white pulp
splenitis
    acute s.
    nonspecific acute s.
    spodogenous s.
splenium corporis callosi
splenocele
splenogonadal fusion
splenohepatomegaly; splenohepato-
    megalia
splenoma
splenomalacia
splenomedullary leukemia
splenomegalic
    s. polycythemia
    s. thrombocytopenia
splenomegaly; splenomegalia
    congestive s.
    Egyptian s.
    fibrocongestive s.
    hemolytic s.
splenomyelogenous
splenomyelomalacia
splenoncus
splenoportography
splenosis
spliceosome
splicing
    gene s.
    RNA s.
split
    s. gene
    s. pelvis
    s. renal function
    s. renal function study
    s. renal function test
    s. thickness skin graft

splitting
    beam s.
spodogram
spodography
spondylitis
    ankylosing s.
    rheumatoid s.
    tuberculous s.
spondyloarthropathy
spondyloepiphyseal dysplasia
spondylolisthesis
spondylolisthetic pelvis
spondylosis
    cervical s.
    s. deformans
    lumbar s.
spongiform
    s. encephalitis
    s. pustule of Kogoj
spongioblast
    polar s.
spongioblastoma
    s. multiforme
    s. polare
    s. unipolare
spongioid
spongiosis
    status s.
spongiositis
spongiotic dermatitis
spongy
    s. degenerative-type leukodys-
        trophy
    s. nevus
spontaneous
    s. abortion
    s. agglutination
    s. amputation
    s. delivery
    s. generation
    s. lesion
    s. mutation
    s. pneumothorax
sporadic
    s. diffuse goiter
    s. dysentery
    s. nodular goiter
    s. simple goiter
sporangia
sporangiophore
sporangiospore
sporangium (pl., sporangia)

spore
- bacterial s.
- drumstick s.
- s. form
- s.-forming bacilli
- fungal s.
- s. strips

sporoagglutination
sporoblast
sporocyst
sporogony
Sporothrix schenckii
sporotrichosis
- lymphatic s.
- s. serology

sporotrichositic chancre
Sporotrichum
- *S. beurmanni*
- *S. schenckii*

sporozoan
sporozoea
sporozoid
sporozoite
sporozoon (pl., sporozoa)
spot
- Bitot's s's
- blood s's
- blue s.
- café au lait s's
- cherry red s.
- De Morgan's s's
- electronic focal s.
- s. film
- Fordyce's s's
- Koplik's s's
- milk s's
- mongolian s.
- Roth's s's
- ruby s's
- Tardieu's s's
- tendinous s.
- s. test
- s. test for infectious mononucleosis
- white s.
- yellow s.

spotted
- s. fever
- s. retina

spotting
- leopard s.

Sp (Pr) antigen

spray
- antistatic s.

spreading factor
spread plate
sprue
- celiac s.
- nontropical s.
- tropical s.

spruelike syndrome
SPS — sodium polyanethol sulfonate
          sulfite polymyxin sulfadiazine
Spumavirinae
spur cell
spuria
- placenta s.

spurious
- s. cast
- s. parasite
- s. polycythemia

sputum (pl., sputa)
- s. aeroginosum
- s. coctum
- s. crudum
- s. cruentum
- s. culture
- s. cytology
- s. examination
- s. fungus culture
- globular s.
- green s.
- s. mycobacteria culture
- nummular s.
- prune-juice s.
- rusty s.
- s. smear

SQ — subcutaneous
squalene cyclohydroxylase
squama (pl., squamae)
squamate
squamatization
squame
squamocolumnar junction
squamous
- s. cell
- s. cell breast cancer
- s. cell carcinoma antigen
- s. cell papilloma
- s. epithelial cells
- s. epithelium
- s. hyperplasia
- s. metaplasia
- s. metaplasia of amnion

s. odontogenic tumor
s. papilloma
s. pearl
s. suture
square wave
SQUID — superconducting quantum-interference device
squill
    red s.
SR — sarcoplasmic reticulum
    secretion rate
    sedimentation rate
    sensitization response
    sigma reaction
    sinus rhythm
    skin resistance
    superior rectus
    systemic resistance
Sr — strontium
sr — steradian
SRBC — sheep red blood cells
SRC — sedimented red cells
    sheep red cells
src gene
SRF — skin-reactive factor
    somatotropin-releasing factor
    split renal function
    subretinal fluid
SRFS — split renal function study
SRNA — soluble ribonucleic acid
SRS — slow-reacting substance
SRSA — slow-reacting substance of anaphylaxis
S-R (smooth-rough) variation
SS — *Salmonella* and *Shigella*
    saturated solution
    statistically significant
    subaortic stenosis
    supersaturated
SSA — salicylsalicylic acid
    skin-sensitizing antibody
    sulfosalicylic acid (test)
SSD — source to skin distance
    sum of square deviations
SSKI — saturated solution of potassium iodide
SSN — severely subnormal
SSP — Sanarelli-Shwartzman phenomenon
    subacute sclerosing panencephalitis
SSPE — subacute sclerosing panencephalitis

SSS — scalded skin syndrome
    specific soluble substance
SSU — sterile supply unit
SSV — simian sarcoma virus
ST — esotropia
    sternothyroid
    subtalar
    subtotal
    surface tension
St — stoke
St.
    St. Anthony's fire
    St. Jude's staging system
    St. Louis encephalitis
    St. Louis encephalitis virus
STA — serum thrombotic accelerator
stab — stab cell
    stab neutrophil
stabile
stability
stable
    s. cells
    s. factor
    s. factor deficiency
    s. fly
stachybotryotoxicosis
stachyose
stack
stage
    Arneth s's
    end s.
    Tanner's s.
    tumor s.
staggered
staghorn calculus
staging
    cancer s.
    Jewett-Strong s.
    TNM s.
    tumor s.
stagnant
    s. anoxia
    s. hypoxia
Stagnicola
Stahr's gland
stain (and staining methods)
    Abbott's s. for spores
    aceto-orcein s.
    Achucárro's s.
    acid s.
    acid-fast s.
    acid phosphatase s.

acid-Schiff s.
acridine orange s.
Ag-AS s.
Albert's s.
Alcian blue s.
alkaline phosphatase s.
Altmann's aniline-acid
    fuchsin s.
amyloid s.
antimony s's
arsenic s.
astrocyte s.
ATPase s.
auramine O fluorescent s.
auramine-rhodamine s.
automated slide s.
azan s.
azure A/B/C s's
azure-eosin s.
bacterial s.
basic s.
basic fuchsin–methylene blue s.
Bauer's chromic acid leucofuch-
    sin s.
Becker's s. for spirochetes
Bennhold's Congo red s.
Berg's s.
Best's carmine s.
Bethe's s.
Betke s.
Bielschowsky's s.
Biondi-Heidenhain s.
bipolar s.
Birch-Hirschfeld s.
Bodian's copper-PROTARGOL s.
Borrel's blue s.
Bowie s.
Brown-Brenn s.
Cajal's astrocyte s.
Cajal's s. method
carbol fuchsin s.
carbol-thionin s.
C-banding s.
centromere banding s.
certified s's
chlorazol black E s.
chondroitin sulfate s.
chromate s. for lead
chrome alum hematoxylin-
    phloxine s.
Ciaccio's s.
colloidal iron s.

Congo red s.
contrast s.
cresyl violet s.
Da Fano's s.
Dane's s.
deoxyribonucleic acid s.
diazo s. for argentaffin granules
Dieterle's s.
differential s.
direct fluorescent antibody s.
Dorner s.
double s.
Ehrlich's acid hematoxylin s.
Ehrlich's aniline crystal
    violet s.
Ehrlich's triacid s.
Ehrlich's triple s.
Einarson's s.
elastic fiber s's
enterochromaffin s.
eosin s.
Eranko's fluorescence s.
fat s.
Feulgen's s. method
fibrin s.
Field's rapid s.
Fink-Heimer s.
Flemming's triple s.
fluorescence plus Giemsa s.
fluorescent s.
fluorescent-auramine-
    rhodamine s.
fluorochrome s.
Fontana-Masson silver s.
Fontana's s.
Foot's reticulum impregna-
    tion s.
Fouchet's s.
Fraser-Lendrum s. for fibrin
Friedländer's s. for capsules
fungal s.
G-banding s.
Giemsa s.
Giemsa chromosome
    banding s.
Gimenez s.
Glenner-Lillie s.
glycogen s.
glycolipid s.
glycoprotein s.
Golgi's s.

Gomori-Jones periodic acid–
methenamine-silver s.
Gomori's aldehyde fuchsin s.
Gomori's chrome alum hema-
toxylin-phloxine s.
Gomori's methenamine-
silver s's
Gomori's nonspecific acid phos-
phatase s.
Gomori's nonspecific alkaline
phosphatase s.
Gomori's one-step trichrome s.
Gomori's silver impregnation s.
Gomori's trichrome s.
Goodpasture's s.
Gordon and Sweet s.
Gram's s.
Gram-Weigert s.
Gridley s.
Gridley's s. for fungi
Grimelius' argyrophil s.
method
Grocott-Gomori methenamine-
silver s.
Hale's colloidal iron s.
H and E (hematoxylin and eo-
sin) s.
Hansel's secretion s.
Heidenhain's azan s.
Heidenhain's iron hematox-
ylin s.
hematoxylin-eosin s.
hematoxylin–malachite green–
basic fuchsin s.
hematoxylin-phloxine B s.
hemosiderin s.
Hirsch-Peiffer s.
Hiss' s.
histochemical s.
histologic s.
Holmes' s.
Hortega's neuroglia s.
Hucker-Conn s.
immunofluorescent s.
immunohistochemical s.
immunoperoxidase s.
India ink s.
India ink capsule s.
intravital s.
iodine s.
Jenner-Giemsa s.
Jenner's s.

Kasten's fluorescent Feulgen s.
Kasten's fluorescent PAS s.
keratin s.
Kinyoun s.
Kinyoun carbol fuchsin s.
Kittrich's s.
Kleihauer's s.
Klinger-Ludwig acid-thionin s.
Klüver-Barrera Luxol fast
blue s.
Kossa s.
Kronecker's s.
Laquer's s. for alcoholic hyalin
Lawless' s.
lead hydroxide s.
Leishman's s.
Lendrum's inclusion body s.
Lendrum's phloxine-
tartrazine s.
Lepehne-Pickworth s.
leukocyte acid phosphatase s.
Levaditi s.
Lillie's allochrome connective
tissue s.
Lillie's azure-eosin s.
Lillie's ferrous iron s.
Lillie's sulfuric acid Nile
blue s.
lipid s's
Lison-Dunn s.
Löffler's s.
Löffler's caustic s.
Luna-Ishak s.
Luxol fast blue s.
Macchiavello's s.
MacNeal's tetrachrome
blood s.
malarial pigment s.
Maldonado-San Jose s.
Mallory's s. for actinomyces
Mallory's aniline blue s.
Mallory's collagen s.
Mallory's s. for hemofuchsin
Mallory's iodine s.
Mallory's phloxine s.
Mallory's phosphotungstic acid
hematoxylin s.
Mallory's trichrome s.
Mallory's triple s.
Mann's methyl blue–eosin s.
Marchi's s.
Masson s.

Masson-Fontana ammoniacal silver s.
Masson's argentaffin s.
Masson's trichrome s.
mast cell s.
Maximow's s. for bone marrow
Mayer's acid alum hematoxylin s.
Mayer's hemalum s.
Mayer's mucicarmine s.
Mayer's mucihematein s.
May-Grünwald s.
May-Grünwald-Giemsa s.
metachromatic s.
methenamine silver s.
methylene blue s.
methyl green–pyronin s.
Mowry's colloidal iron s.
MSB trichrome s.
mucicarmine s.
mucopolysaccharide s.
multiple s.
Nakanishi's s.
Nauta's s.
negative s.
Neisser's s.
neutral s.
Nicolle's s. for capsules
Ninhydrin-Schiff s.
Nissl's s.
Noble's s.
nuclear s.
oligodendroglia s.
Orth's s.
oxytalan fiber s.
p21 s.
Padykula-Herman s. for myosin ATPase
Paget-Eccleston s.
Palmgren's silver impregnation s.
pancreatic islet s.
panoptic s.
Papanicolaou's s.
Pappenheim's s.
paracarmine s.
PAS s.
periodic acid–Schiff s.
Perls' Prussian blue s.
peroxidase s.
phloxine-tartrazine s.
phospholipid s.

phosphotungstic acid s.
picrocarmine s.
picro-Mallory trichrome s.
picronigrosin s.
plasma s.
plasmic s.
plastic section s.
polychrome methylene blue s.
port-wine s.
positive s.
progressive s.
Prussian blue s.
PTA (phosphotungstic acid) s.
Puchtler-Sweat s. for basement membranes
Puchtler-Sweat s. for hemoglobin and hemosiderin
Q-banding s.
quinacrine s.
quinacrine chromosome banding s.
Rambourg's chromic acid–phosphotungstic acid s.
Rambourg's periodic acid–chromic methenamine–silver s.
R-banding s.
regressive s.
resorcin-fuchsin s.
reticulin s.
Romanowsky's s.
Romanowsky's blood s.
Roux's s.
Schaeffer-Fulton s.
Schmorl's ferric-ferricyanide reduction s.
Schmorl's picrothionin s.
Schultz' s.
selective s.
silver s.
silver-ammoniacal silver s.
silver protein s.
Stirling's modification of Gram's s.
Sudan black B s.
supravital s.
Taenzer's s.
Taenzer-Unna s.
Takayama's s.
telomeric R-banding s.
thiazine s.
thioflavine T s.
Tizzoni's s.

Toison's s.
toluidine blue s.
trichrome s.
Truant's s.
trypsin G-banding s.
Unna-Pappenheim s.
Unna's s.
Unna-Taenzer s.
uranyl acetate s.
urate crystal s.
van Ermengen's s.
van Gieson's s.
Verhoeff's s.
Verhoeff's elastic tissue s.
Verhoeff–van Gieson s.
vital s.
von Kossa s.
Wachstein-Meissel s. for cal-
   cium-magnesium-ATPase
Wade-Fite-Faraco s.
Warthin-Starry silver s.
Wayson's s.
Weigert-Gram s.
Weigert's s.
Weigert's s. for actinomyces
Weigert's s. for elastin
Weigert's s. for fibrin
Weigert's s. for myelin
Weigert's s. for neuroglia
Weigert's iron hematoxylin s.
Wheatley trichrome s.
Wilder's s. for reticulum
Williams' s.
Wright's s.
Ziehl-Neelsen s.
Ziehl's s.
stained urinary sediment
stalk
abdominal s.
allantoic s.
cerebellar s.
hypophyseal s.
infundibular s.
neural s.
optic s.
pituitary s.
spermatid s.
yolk s.
STA-MCA — superficial temporal ar-
         tery to middle cere-
         bral artery
Stamey test

Stammler's reaction
standard
air-quality s's
s. bicarbonate
certified s's
s. curve
s. deviation
s. electrode potential
s. enthalpy of formation
s. error
s. error of estimate
s. error of the mean
s. free energy
s. hydrogen electrode
internal s.
s. morbidity ratio
s. mortality ratio
primary s.
s. reduction potential
s. score
s. serologic tests for syphilis
s. solution
s. state
s. temperature and pressure
s. test for syphilis
s. urea clearance
standardization
standardize
standardized
s. deviate
s. rate
standing plasma test
standstill
cardiac s.
Stanford protocol
stannic chloride
stannosis
stannous
stanolone
stanozolol
St. Anthony's fire
stapes
Staph — *Staphylococcus*
staph — staphylococcus
staphylocoagulase
staphylococcal
s. bronchopneumonia
s. clumping test
s. colitis
s. endocarditis
s. enteritis
s. folliculitis

s. infection
s. otitis
s. pharyngitis
s. pneumonia
s. protein-A-binding assay
s. scalded skin syndrome
s. septicemia
s. sinusitis
s. tonsillitis
staphylococcemia
staphylococcin
Staphylococcus
    S. *albus*
    S. *aureus*
    S. *citreus*
    S. *epidermidis*
    S. *pyogenes aureus*
    S. *pyogenes* var. *albus*
    S. *saprophyticus*
    S. *septicemia*
    S. *simulans*
staphylococcus (pl., staphylococci)
Staphylococcus aureus nasopharyngeal culture
Staphylococcus aureus neutral proteinase
staphylohemia
staphylokinase
staphylolysin
    α s., alpha s.
    β s., beta s.
    δ s., delta s.
    ε s., epsilon s.
    γ s., gamma s.
staphyloma
staphylomata
staphylo-opsonic index
star
    venous s.
starch
    s. gel electrophoresis
    hydroxyethyl s.
    s. tolerance test
Starling's
    curve
    hypothesis
    law
    mechanism
Starr-Edwards prosthesis
start codon
starvation-induced protein breakdown

stasis (pl., stases)
    bile s.
    s. cirrhosis
    s. dermatitis
    s. ulcer
    venous s.
Stasisia
stat — German unit of radium emanation
    statim (L., "immediately")
state
    absorptive s.
    baseline steady s.
    central excitatory s.
    central inhibitory s.
    complement deficiency s.
    ground s.
    hypercoagulable s.
    immunity deficiency s.
    inotropic s.
    metastable s.
    oxidation s.
    postabsorptive s.
    sample steady s.
    solid s.
    standard s.
    steady s.
    transition s.
statement
    assignment s.
    source s.
static
    s. gangrene
    s. storage allocation
stationary phase
statistic
    Mann-Whitney rank sum s.
    test s.
    Wilcoxon rank sum s.
    Wilcoxon signed rank s.
statistically significant
statistical symbols
statistics
statokinetic labyrinth
stat test
stature
status
    s. asthmaticus
    s. dysraphicus
    s. epilepticus
    s. lymphaticus
    s. marmoratus

secretor s.
s. spongiosis
s. thymicolymphaticus
s. thymicus
Staub-Traugott effect
STC — soft tissue calcification
STD — sexually transmitted disease
    skin test done
    skin to tumor distance
std — saturated
steady-state condition
steam-fitters' asthma
steapsin
stearate
    zinc s.
stearic acid
stearin
stearoyl
steatitis
steatocystoma multiplex
steatolytic enzyme
steatomatosis
steatonecrosis
steatopyga; steatopygia
steatopygous
steatorrhea
steatosis
    alcoholic s.
    s. cordis
    hepatic s.
    macrovesicular s.
    microvesicular s.
Steenbock's unit
Stefan-Boltzmann law
stegnosis
Stegobium
Stegomyia
Steiner's tumor
Steinthol's groupings
Stelangium
Stellantchasmus
stellate
    s. abscess
    s. fracture
    s. ganglion
stem cell
    s.c. leukemia
    s.c. lymphoma
stemline
Stender's dish
Stenoglossa
stenosal

stenosed
stenosis (pl., stenoses)
    aortic s.
    aortic valve s.
    buttonhole s.
    calcific s.
    calcific aortic s.
    calcific nodular s.
    calcific nodular aortic s.
    congenital s.
    congenital pyloric s.
    coronary ostial s.
    discrete subaortic s.
    Dittrich's s.
    fish mouth s.
    hypertrophic pyloric s.
    hypertrophic subaortic s.
    hypopharyngeal s.
    idiopathic hypertrophic subaortic s.
    s. and incompetency
    infundibular s.
    meatal s.
    mitral s.
    muscular subaortic s.
    nodular calcific s.
    nodular calcific aortic s.
    papillary s.
    pulmonary s.
    pulmonary artery s.
    pyloric s.
    renal artery s.
    subaortic s.
    subvalvar s.
    supravalvar s.
    supravalvular aortic s.
    tricuspid s.
    urethral meatal s.
    valvular s.
stenotic
Stensen's duct
step
    s. function
    rate-controlling s.
step-down transformer
step-up transformer
steradian
stercobilin
stercobilinogen
stercolith
stercoraceous ulcer

stercoral
　　s. abscess
　　s. appendicitis
　　s. fistula
　　s. ulcer
stercoroma
Sterculia apetala
sterculia gum
stereocampimeter
stereochemical isomerism
stereochemistry
stereocilia
stereocinefluorography
stereognosis
stereoisomer
stereoisomerism
stereology
stereometer
stereometry
stereoscope
stereoscopic
　　s. microscope
　　s. radiography
stereospecific numbering
stereotactic
stereotaxis
steric hindrance
sterigma (pl., sterigmata)
sterile
　　s. abscess
　　s. cyst
sterility culture
sterilization
　　chemical s.
　　eugenic s.
　　fractional s.
　　intermittent s.
　　mechanical s.
sterilize
sterilizer
　　gas s.
sternal
　　s. notch
　　s. puncture
　　s. synchondrosis
Sternberg-Reed cell
Sternberg's cells
sternoclavicular joint
sternocleidomastoid
　　s. muscle
　　s. musculocutaneous flap

sternocostal
　　s. joint
　　s. triangle
sternohyoid
　　s. flap
　　s. muscle
sternothyroid muscle
sternoxiphoid plane
sternum
steroid
　　11-alpha-hydroxylase s.
　　17-alpha-hydroxylase s.
　　anabolic s's
　　6-beta-hydroxylase s.
　　11-beta-hydroxylase s.
　　s.-binding betaglobulin
　　delta-isomerase s.
　　estrogenic s's
　　s. hormone
　　19-hydroxylase s.
　　s.-21-hydroxylase
　　21-hydroxylase s.
　　ketogenic s's
　　s.-21-monooxygenase
　　s. protein activity index
　　s.-receptor complex
　　s. saponin
steroidogenesis
　　adrenal s.
sterol
　　s. carrier proteins
　　s. glycoside
stetharteritis
stethomyitis; stethomyositis
STH — somatotropic hormone
STI — systolic time interval
stibine
stibophen
stichochrome cell
stiffness
　　chamber s.
stigma (pl., stigmas, stigmata)
　　s. ventriculi
stigmasterol
stilbene dye
stilbestrol
stillbirth
　　macerated s.
still layer
stimulation
　　s. index
　　repetitive s.

stimulator
      long-acting thyroid s.
stimulus (pl., stimuli)
      adequate s.
      maximal s.
      s.-response time
      submaximal s.
      subthreshold s.
      supramaximal s.
      threshold s.
stipple cell
stippled epiphysis
stippling
      basophilic s.
      Schüffner's s.
      Ziemann's s.
Stirling's modification of Gram's stain
stitch abscess
Stix reagent strip test
St. Jude's staging system
STK — streptokinase
St. Louis encephalitis
St. Louis encephalitis virus
St. Louis encephalitis virus serology
STM — streptomycin
stochastic
stock culture
stoichiometry
stoke
Stokes'
      law
      shift
stolon
stoma (pl., stomata)
stomach
      bilocular s.
      drain-trap s.
      dumping s.
      hourglass s.
      "leather-bottle" s.
      sclerotic s.
      thoracic s.
      trifid s.
      s. tumors
      wallet s.
      water-trap s.
stomal ulcer
stomatitis (pl., stomatitides)
      aphthous s.
      gangrenous s.
      herpetic s.

      lead s.
      s. medicamentosa
      Vincent's s.
stomatocyte
stomatocytosis
      hereditary s.
      Mediterranean s.
Stomoxys calcitrans
stone
      kidney s's
      pigment s's
      prostatic s's
      renal s's
      skin s's
      s.-strippers' asthma
      triple s's
      uric acid s's
      urinary s.
      vein s.
stool
      acholic s.
      bilious s.
      s. culture
      s. fungus culture
      s. mycobacteria culture
      tarry s.
stopcock
storage
      s. allocation
      s. capacity
      common s.
      compressed gas s.
      s. disease
      ether s.
      external s.
      internal s.
      s. iron
      s. limits
      s. location
      mass s.
      s. oscilloscope
      transport and s.
storage allocation
      dynamic s.a.
      static s.a.
storiform
      s. neurofibroma
      s.-pleomorphic malignant fibrous histiocytoma
storm
      thyroid s.
Stormer viscosimeter

Stovall-Black method
STP — standard temperature and
      pressure
STPD — standard temperature and
      pressure, dry (0°C,
      760 mm Hg)
strabismus
straddling embolism
strain
    s. birefringence
    cell s.
    s.-gauge plethysmography
    inbred s.
    reference s.
    Taiwan acute respiratory s.
stramonium
strand
    leading s.
    sense s.
strangulated hernia
strangulation
strap cell
Strassburg's test
stratification
stratified
    s. epithelium
    s. random sample
    s. thrombus
stratigraphy
Stratiomyidae
stratum (pl., strata)
    s. basale
    s. cinereum
    s. corneum
    s. granulosum
    s. lucidum
    s. spinosum
    s. zonale
strawberry
    s. birthmark
    s.-cream blood
    s. gallbladder
    s. mark
    s. mucosa
    s. nevus
    s. tongue
    s.-type hemangioma
stray light
streak
    angioid s's
    s. culture
    fatty s's

germinal s.
gonadal s.
s. hyperostosis
medullary s.
meningeal s.
s. ovary
s. plate
primitive s.
streaked gonad
streaming
    cytoplasmic s.
    s. movement
    protoplasmic s.
street virus
Strengeria
strength
    dielectric s.
    s.-duration curve
    ionic s.
    magnetic field s.
strep — streptococcus
streptavidin
strepticemia
Streptobacillus
    S. moniliformis
    S. pseudotuberculosis
Streptococcaceae
streptococcal
    s. antigen test
    s. carditis
    s. cellulitis
    s. endocarditis
    s. erysipelas
    s. fibrinolysin
    s. infection
    s. lymphangitis
    s. nasopharyngitis
    s. pharyngitis
    s. phlegmon
    s. pneumonia
    s. pyoderma
    s. pyrogenic exotoxin
    s. septicemia
    s. tonsillitis
    s. toxin immunization reaction
Streptococceae
streptococcemia
Streptococcus
    S. agalactiae
    S. anaerobius
    S. anginosus-constellatus
    S. bovis

S. *cremoris*
S. *durans*
S. *equi*
S. *equisimilis*
S. *evolutus*
S. *faecalis*
S. *faecium*
S. *hemolyticus*
S. *intermedius*
S. *lactis*
S. *lactis* R
S. *liquefaciens*
S. MG
S. MG-*intermedius*
S. *microaerophilic*
S. *milleri*
S. *mitis*
S. *mutans*
S. *pneumoniae*
S. *pyogenes*
S. *salivarius*
S. *sanguis*
S. *uberis*
S. *viridans*
S. *zooepidemicus*
S. *zymogenes*
streptococcus (pl., streptococci)
   alpha s.
   anaerobic s.
   anhemolytic s.
   Bargen's s.
   beta s.
   Fehleisen's s.
   gamma s.
   group A s.
   group B s.
   group D s.
   group N s.
   hemolytic s.
   β-hemolytic s.
   s. MG
   microaerophilic s.
   nonhemolytic s.
   s. of Ostertag
   s. serum
   viridans s.
streptodornase
streptokinase-streptodornase
streptolysin
   s. O
   s. S

Streptomyces
   S. *ambofaciens*
   S. *antibioticus*
   S. *aureofaciens*
   S. *coeruleorubidus*
   S. *fradiae*
   S. *griseolus*
   S. *griseus*
   S. *hygroscopicus*
   S. *kanamyceticus*
   S. *madurae*
   S. *niveus*
   S. *nodosus*
   S. *nogalater*
   S. *noursei*
   S. *orchidaceus*
   S. *pelletieri*
   S. *peucetius*
   S. *rimosus*
   S. *somaliensis*
   S. *spectabilis*
   S. *tenebrarius*
Streptomycetaceae
streptomycin
streptomycosis
streptosepticemia
Streptothrix
streptotrichosis
streptozocin
streptozotocin
streptozyme agglutinin test
stress
      environmental s.
      s. lymphocyte
      s. polycythemia
      s. protein
      s. reticulocyte
      s. ulcer
stretch
      receptor s.
      s. reflex
stria (pl., striae)
      striae atrophicae
      striae cutis distensae
      striae gravidarum
      s. medullaris
      s. terminalis
      Wickham's striae
      striae of Zahn
striate veins
striation
      basal s.

tabby cat s.
tigroid s.
striatonigral
s. degeneration
s. fibers
stricture
Hunner's s.
ureteral s.
ureteropelvic s.
ureterovesical s.
urethral s.
stridor
laryngeal s.
Strigeata
stringency
stringent response
string sign
strip
BMC test s.
cytochrome oxidase s's
gelatin s's
lactase test s.
Phenistix reagent s.
reagent s.
spore s's
SV s's
test s's
stripped nucleus
stripping
electrolytic s.
Strobane
strobe light
strobila (pl., strobilae)
stroke
apoplectic s.
cerebral s.
heat s.
s. index
sun s.
s. volume
Stroll's dilution egg count technique
stroma (pl., stromata)
s.-free hemoglobin
gonadal s.
Rollet's s.
stromal
s. endometriosis
s.–germ cell tumor
s. hyperplasia
s. luteoma
s. metaplasia
s. myosis

s. nodules
s. sarcoma
s. sex-cord tumor
s. tumor
stromatin
stromatosis
endometrial s.
Strong's bacillus
Strongylata
Strongylidae
Strongyloidea
Strongyloides
S. *fulleborni*
S. *stercoralis*
strongyloidiasis
Strongyloididae
strontium isotope
strontium 90
strophanthin
structural
s. gene
s. isomerism
s. kidney
s. lesion
s. protein
structure
analogous s's
s. collapse
dipolar s.
fine s.
homologous s's
list s.
primary s.
quaternary s.
rudimentary s.
secondary s.
tertiary s.
tuboreticular s.
xanthene s.
struma (pl., strumae)
s. aberranta
s. colloides
Hashimoto's s.
ligneous s.
s. lymphomatosa
s. maligna
s. medicamentosa
s. ovarii
Riedel's s.
strumal carcinoid tumor
strumiform
strumitis

strumous
struvite calculus
strychnine assay
STS — serologic test for syphilis
        standard test for syphilis
S-T segment
STSG — split thickness skin graft
STT — serial thrombin time
STU — skin test unit
Stuart-Prower factor
Stuart's factor
Student's *t*-test
study
      case-control s.
      cohort s.
      double-contrast s.
      dual-contrast s.
      erythrokinetic s's
      fat absorption s's
      ferrokinetic s.
      haplotype association s's
      prospective s.
      renal function s.
      retrospective s.
      split renal function s.
      ultrastructural s.
      water loading s.
stump
      s. cancer
      s. neuralgia
      ureteral s.
stunted
      s. embryo
      s. fetus
stupor
      epileptic s.
      lethargic s.
      postconvulsive s.
"stuttering" infarction
STVA — subtotal villose atrophy
stye
      meibomian s.
      zeisian s.
styloglossus muscle
stylohyoid muscle
styloiditis
styloid process
stylopharyngeus muscle
stylosteophyte
styptic
      chemical s.

      mechanical s.
      vascular s.
Stypven time test
styramate
styrene
styrone
SUA — serum uric acid
        single umbilical artery
subacromial bursa
subacute
      s. abscess
      s. bacterial endocarditis
      s. bronchopneumonia
      s. cerebellar degeneration
      s. combined degeneration
      s. combined sclerosis
      s. glomerulonephritis
      s. granulomatous thyroiditis
      s. hepatitis
      s. infective endocarditis
      s. inflammation
      s. lymphocytic thyroiditis
      s. meningitis
      s. myelomonocytic leukemia
      s. myelo-optical neuropathy
      s. necrotizing encephalomy-
        elopathy
      s. necrotizing encephalomy-
        opathy
      s. necrotizing encephalopathy
      s. nephritis
      s. sclerosing encephalitis
      s. sclerosing panencephalitis
      s. spongiform encephalopathy
      s. thyroiditis
subadventitial fibrosis
subaortic stenosis
      discrete s.s.
      idiopathic hypertrophic s.s.
subaponeurotic
subarachnoid
      s. cistern
      s. hemorrhage
      s. space
subareolar duct papillomatosis
subauricular glands
subbasal projection
subcallosal gyrus
subcapsular cataract
subchorionic
subclass
      immunoglobulin s.

subclavian
    s. artery
    s. lymphatic trunks
    s. vein
subclavicular
subclavius muscle
subcommissural
subcorneal
    s. pustular dermatitis
    s. pustular dermatosis
subcortical aphasia
subcostal
    s. artery
    s. margin
    s. plane
    s. vein
subcu, subcut
    or subq — subcutaneous
subculture
subcutaneous
    s. bursa
    s. emphysema
    s. fat
    s. fat necrosis of newborn
    s. fungus
    s. inguinal ring
    s. mastectomy
    s. nodule
    s. pseudosarcomatous fibro-
       matosis
    s. tissue
    s. trochanteric bursa
    s. zygomycosis
subcutis
subdeltoid bursa
subdiaphragmatic abscess
subdural
    s. empyema
    s. hematoma
    s. hemorrhage
    s. hygroma
    s. space
subendocardial myocardial infarction
subendothelium
subependymal glioma
subependymoma
subepidermal
    s. abscess
    s. fibrosis
suberyl arginine
subfalcine herniation
subfascial bursa

subfornical
subfrontal sulcus
subgranular
subhepatic
    s. abscess
    s. fossa
subicteric
subiculum
subinflammatory
subinguinal lymph node
subinvolution
subjacent
sublabial adhesion
sublenticular posterior limb
sublethal gene
subleukemia
subleukemic
    s. granulocytic leukemia
    s. leukemia
    s. lymphocytic leukemia
    s. monocytic leukemia
    s. myelosis
sublimation
sublingual
    s. caruncle
    s. cyst
    s. duct
    s. gland
    s. tablet
sublobule
    hemispheral s.
subluxation
sublymphemia
submammary mastitis
submandibular
    s. gland
    s. lymph node
submaxillary
    s. duct
    s. ganglion
    s. gland
    s. glycoprotein
submental lymph node
submentovertical
submersion-immersion
submetacentric chromosome
submorphous
submucosa
    adenoid s.
    anal canal s.
    appendiceal s.
    bronchial s.

colonic s.
duodenal s.
esophageal s.
gastric s.
hypopharyngeal s.
ileal s.
jejunal s.
laryngeal s.
nasopharyngeal s.
oropharyngeal s.
pharyngeal s.
rectal s.
small intestinal s.
tonsillar s.
tracheal s.
urinary bladder s.
submucosal leiomyoma
submucous
submuscular bursa
subneural clefts
subnormal
    severely s.
    s. temperature
suboptimal
subpapular
subparietal sulcus
subperiosteal abscess
subperitoneal appendicitis
subphrenic
    s. abscess
    s. fossa
subpleural
subretinal fluid
subroutine
    recursive s.
subscapular
    s. artery
    s. lymph node
    s. muscle
    s. nerve
subsclerotic
subscripted variable
subscription
subseptate uterus
subserosa
    appendiceal s.
    colonic s.
    duodenal s.
    gallbladder s.
    gastric s.
    small intestinal s.
    tubal s.

urinary bladder s.
uterine s.
subserosal leiomyoma
subset
subspecies
substance
    agglutinable s.
    alpha s.
    antidiuretic s.
    autacoid s.
    beta s.
    blood group s.
    blood group–specific s's A
      and B
    cement s.
    chromidial s.
    chromophil s.
    colloid s.
    s. concentration
    controlled s.
    cortical s.
    erythrocyte-sensitizing s.
    exophthalmos-producing s.
    fat-mobilizing s.
    filar s.
    gelatinous s.
    glandular s.
    ground s.
    H s.
    hazardous s's
    hemolytic s.
    immunity s.
    interfibrillar s.
    interspongioplastic s.
    Lewis s.
    medullary s.
    metachromatic s.
    methylene blue active s.
    s. P
    periventricular s.
    pressor s.
    prostaglandin-like s.
    rabbit aorta-contracting s.
    renal pressor s.
    reticular s.
    sarcous s.
    slow-reacting s.
    specific soluble s.
    threshold s.
    thromboplastic s.
    tumor polysaccharide s.

white s. of Schwann
zymoplastic s.
substantia (pl., substantiae)
    s. gelatinosa
    s. metachromaticogranularis
    s. nigra
    s. reticulofilamentosa
substernal goiter
substituent
substitute
    blood s.
    plasma s.
    Scott's tap water s.
    volume s.
substitution
    creeping s. of bone
    s. product
    reaction s.
    s. reaction
substrate
    s. cycle
    defined s.
    hippurate s.
    s.-labeled fluorescence immuno-
      assay
    s. level phosphorylation
subsynchronous
subtelocentric
subtendinous bursa
subthalamic
    s. fasciculus
    s. nucleus
subthalamus
subtotal
    s. amputation
    s. villose atrophy
subungual
    s. abscess
    s. exostosis
    s. fibroma
    s. melanoma
subunit
    hCG-α s.
    hCG-β s.
subvalvar stenosis
subvital mutation
succenturiata
    placenta s.
succimer
succinate
    s. dehydrogenase

s. loxapine
s. semialdehyde
succinchlorimide
succinic acid
Succinivibrio dextrinosolvens
succinylcholine chloride
succinyl-coenzyme A
    s.-c. A hydrolase
    s.-c. A synthetase
succinylsulfathiazole
succus entericus
sucking louse
Sucquet-Hoyer canal
sucrase-isomaltase deficiency
sucrose
    bile salts s.
    s. α-D-glucohydrolase
    s. glucohydrolase
    s. hemolysis test
    s. intolerance
    s. tolerance test
sucrosemia
sucrosuria
suction
    s. method
    post-tussive s.
Suctoria
SUD — sudden unexpected death
        sudden unexplained death
sudamen (pl., sudamina)
Sudan
    black
    black B stain
    brown
    G
    red III
    yellow G
    I, II, III, IV
sudanophil
sudanophilia
sudanophilic leukodystrophy
sudanophobic zone
sudden
    s. cardiac death
    s. coronary death
    s. death syndrome
    s. infant death syndrome
    s. unexpected death
    s. unexpected, unexplained
      death
    s. unexplained death
    s. unexplained infant death

Sudeck's atrophy
sudor
    s. sanguineus
    s. urinosus
sudoriferous
    s. breast cancer
    s. gland
sudorikeratosis
sudoriparous abscess
sufficient
    s. condition
    quantity not s.
suffocation
suffocative goiter
suffusion
sugar
    s. acid
    s. alcohol
    amino s.
    blood s.
    s.-coated spleen
    fasting blood s.
    s.-icing liver
    invert s.
    postprandial blood s.
    reducing s.
    s. tumor
    s. water test screen
suggillation
    postmortem s.
suicidal
suicide
SUID — sudden unexplained infant
      death
sulci cutis
sulcomarginal fasciculus
sulcus (pl., sulci)
    Campbell's cruciate s.
    central s.
    cingulate s.
    circular s.
    collateral s.
    dorsal s.
    fimbriodentate s.
    inferior frontomarginal s.
    inferior temporal s.
    intraparietal s.
    lateral occipital s.
    marginal s.
    middle frontal s.
    middle temporal s.
    occipital s.

    olfactory s.
    orbital s.
    paracentral s.
    parieto-occipital s.
    postcentral s.
    precentral s.
    Reil's limiting s.
    subfrontal s.
    subparietal s.
    superior frontal s.
    superior temporal s.
    s. terminalis
    ventral lateral s.
sulfa
    s. drug
    s. film
sulfabenzamide
sulfacetamide
sulfachloropyridazine
sulfadiazine
sulfadimethoxine
sulfadoxine-pyrimethamine
sulfaethidole
sulfaguanidine
sulfamerazine
sulfameter
sulfamethazine
sulfamethizole
sulfamethoxazole
sulfamethoxypyridazine
sulfanilamide
sulfanilic acid
sulfaphenazole
sulfapyridine
sulfasalazine
sulfatase
    iduronic s.
    phenol s.
    sulfatide s.
    L-sulfoiduronate s.
sulfate
    acid s.
    adenine s.
    adenylyltransferase s.
    ammonium s.
    betamicin s.
    cerebroside s.
    chondroitin s.
    colistin s.
    conjugated s.
    copper s.
    cupric s.

dermatan s.
diethyl s.
dimethyl s.
ferrous s.
heparan s.
hydrazine s.
indoxyl s.
isoproterenol s.
keratan s.
metaproterenol s.
netilmicin s.
neutral s.
Nile blue s.
quinine s.
sodium dodecyl s.
sulfated acid mucopolysaccharide
sulfatemia
sulfathiazole
sulfatidase
sulfatide
cerebroside s.
s. lipidosis
s. sulfatase
sulfation factor
sulfhemoglobin
sulfhemoglobinemia
sulfhemoglobinuria
sulfhydryl group
sulfide
cadmium s.
dichlorodiethyl s.
sulfindigotic acid
sulfinic acid
sulfinpyrazone
sulfinyl
sulfisoxazole
acetyl s.
s. diolamine
sulfite
s. oxidase
s. oxidase deficiency
s. polymyxin sulfadiazine
s. reductase
sulfmethemoglobin
sulfobromophthalein sodium
S-sulfoglutathione
L-sulfoiduronate sulfatase
sulfolipid
sulfolithiocholylglycine
sulfomucin
sulfonamide
s. antagonist
s. assay

sulfonate
alkylbenzene s.
sodium-β-naphthoquinone-4-s.
2,4,6-trinitrobenzene s.
sulfonated bathophenanthroline 2,4,6-
tripyridyl-S-triazene
sulfonation
sulfone
sulfonethylmethane
sulfonic acid
sulfonmethane
sulfonyl
sulfonylurea assay
sulfoprotein
sulforhodamine B
sulfosalicylate
sulfosalicylic acid turbidity test
sulfoxide
dimethyl s.
sulfoxone sodium
sulfur
s. bacterium
s. dioxide
s. dye
s. granules
iron s. protein
s. isotope
s. trioxide
sulfuric
s. acid
s. esterase
s. ester hydrolase
sulfurous acid
sulfurtransferase
Sulkowitch's
reagent
test
sulphenone
sum of square deviations
SUN — serum urea nitrogen
sunstroke
sup — superficial
superior
superacidity
superconducting quantum-interference
device
supercooled
superdistention
superdominance
superficial
"s." bladder
s. burn

s. cervical artery
s. circumflex iliac vein
s. dorsal nucleus
s. epigastric artery
s. implantation
s. lymphatics
s. multicentric basal cell carcinoma
s. palmar artery
s. peroneal nerve
s. petrosal nerve
s. spreading melanoma
s. sylvian vein
s. temporal artery
s. transverse fibers
s. volar artery
s. wound
superheated
superinfection
superior
s. aperture
s. brachium
s. cardiac branch
s. cardiac nerve
s. central nucleus
s. cerebellar artery
s. cerebellar peduncle
s. cerebral vein
s. cervical ganglion
s. colliculus
s. colliculus of corpora quadrigemina
s. commissure
s. deep cervical lymph node
s. displacement
s. division, oculomotor nerve
s. epigastric artery
s. frontal gyrus
s. frontal sulcus
s. fronto-occipital fasciculus
s. ganglion
s. genicular artery
s. gluteal nerve
s. hemorrhoidal artery
s. hemorrhoidal vein
s. intercostal artery
s. laryngeal aperture
s. laryngeal nerve
s. left pulmonary vein
s. limbic keratoconjunctivitis
s. lingular bronchus
s. longitudinal fasciculus

s. mediastinum
s. medullary velum
s. mesenteric artery
s. mesenteric ganglion
s. mesenteric plexus
s. mesenteric vein
s. nasal turbinate
s. oblique muscle
s. oblique nerve
s. occipital gyrus
s. olivary nucleus
s. ophthalmic vein
s. pancreaticoduodenal artery
s. parietal lobe
s. petrosal nerve
s. petrosal sinus
s. phrenic artery
s. phrenic vein
s. posterior fissure
s. principal preoptic nucleus
s. pulmonary sulcus tumor
s. rectal artery
s. rectal vein
s. rectourethral muscle
s. right pulmonary vein
s. sagittal sinus
s. segment
s. sensory nucleus
s. striate vein
s. temporal gyrus
s. temporal sulcus
s. thalamic radiation
s. thoracic artery
s. thyroid artery
s. trunk, brachial plexus
s. vena cava
s. vena caval syndrome
supernatant
postmitochondrial s.
supernumerary
s. kidney
s. nipple
s. organs
s. testis
superoinferior
superonasal
superotemporal
superoxide
s. assay
s. dismutase
superpigmentation
supersaturated

supersecretion
supersonic
Superstitionia
supervoltage
supination
supinator muscle
supine
supplemental
    s. inheritance
    s. tooth
supplementary genes
supply
    power s.
support medium
supporting structure
suppressibility
suppression
    adrenocortical s.
    allotype s.
    immune s.
suppressor
    s. cell
    s. gene
    s. lymphocyte
    s. macrophage
    s. mutation
    soluble immune response s.
    s. T cells
    s. T lymphocyte
    tRNA s.
suppurant
suppurate
suppuration
suppurative
    s. acute appendicitis
    s. acute inflammation
    s. appendicitis
    s. arthritis
    s. cholangitis
    s. chronic inflammation
    s. chronic otitis media
    s. cystitis
    s. granulomatous inflammation
    s. hepatitis
    s. hidradenitis
    s. inflammation
    s. keratitis
    s. mastitis
    s. necrosis
    s. nephritis
    s. pericarditis
    s. pleurisy

    s. pleuritis
    s. pneumonia
    s. sialoadenitis
    s. synovitis
    s. tenosynovitis
    s. thyroiditis
supracallosal gyrus
suprachiasmatic nucleus
supraclavicular
    s. lymph node
    s. nerve
    s. region
suprafetation
suprageniculate nucleus
suprahyoid muscle
supramammillary
    s. decussation
    s. nucleus
supramarginal
    s. artery
    s. gyrus
supranuclear palsy
supraoptic nucleus
supraorbital
    s. artery
    s. nerve
    s. neuralgia
suprapatellar bursa
suprapubic
    s. needle aspiration
    s. puncture
suprarenal
    s. epithelioma
    s. gland
    s. medulla
suprascapular
suprasellar meningioma
supraspinous muscle
suprasternal
supratentorial
supratrochlear
    s. artery
    s. nerve
supratype
supravalvar stenosis
supravalvular aortic stenosis
supravergence
supravital stain
supreme genicular artery
sural
    s. artery
    s. nerve

suramin sodium
surface
    s.-active agent
    s. alteration
    s. area of body
    s.-barrier detector
    s. epithelium
    s. markers
    s. tension
surfactant
    amniotic fluid pulmonary s.
    pulmonary s.
surgery
    exploratory s.
surgical
    s. amputation
    s. defect
    s. dissection
    s. emphysema
    s. incision
    s. instrument
    s. pathology
    s. scar
    s. wound
Surgicutt device
suroplantar
surveillance
    immune s.
    immunologic s.
survey
    cross-sectional s.
    s. meter
    proficiency s.
    s. program
survival
    Kaplan-Meier s. curve
    red blood cell s.
    s. time
SUS — stained urinary sediment
susceptibility
    electric s.
    genetic s.
    magnetic s.
    s. testing
suspended particulates
suspension
suspensory ligament
suspicious cytologic alteration
sustentacular cells
Sutton's
    nevus
    ulcer

suture
    coronal s.
    ethmoidomaxillary s.
    frontal s.
    s. granuloma
    intermaxillary s.
    lacrimal s.
    lambdoid s.
    nasal s.
    palatal s.
    parietomastoid s.
    sagittal s.
    sphenoid s.
    squamous s.
    temporozygomatic s.
    zygomaticomaxillary s.
SUUD — sudden unexpected,
        unexplained death
SV — severe
    simian virus
    snake venom
    stroke volume
    subclavian vein
    supravital
SV strips
SV40 virus
SVAS — supravalvular aortic stenosis
SVC — slow vital capacity
        superior vena cava
SVCG — spatial vectorcardiogram
SVD — spontaneous vaginal delivery
        spontaneous vertex delivery
Svedberg's
    flotation unit
    unit
    unit of sedimentation coeffi-
        cient
SVI — stroke volume index
SVM — syncytiovascular membrane
SVR — systemic vascular resistance
SW — spiral wound
        stroke work
swab
    nasopharyngeal s.
    throat s.
swamp fever
Swan-Ganz catheter
Swann antigen
swan-neck deformity
swarm
S wave

sweat
    s. center
    s. duct adenoma
    s. test
sweat gland
    s.g. adenocarcinoma
    s.g. adenoma
    s.g. carcinoma
    s.g. tumor
sweating
    excessive s.
Sweet's method
swelling
    albuminous s.
    Calabar s.
    cellular s.
    cloudy s.
    fugitive s.
SWI — stroke work index
swimmer's itch
swimming
    s. pool conjunctivitis
    s. pool granuloma
swine
    s. flu
    s. rotlauf bacillus
Swiss
    -type agammaglobulinemia
    -type hypogammaglobulinemia
Swiss cheese
    endometrium
    hyperplasia
    liver
    pattern
switch
    double-pole double-throw s.
    double-pole single-throw s.
    isotype s.
    silicon-controlled s.
Sx — signs
    symptoms
sycoma
sycosis
Sydenham's chorea
sylvatic plague
Sylvius
    aqueduct of S.
    fissure of S.
    iter of S.
sym — symmetrical
    symptom
symbiont

symbiosis
symblepharon
symbol (*see also* Appendix 5,
    Symbols)
    hazard s.
    phallic s.
    statistical s's
Symmers'
    clay pipestem fibrosis
    fibrosis
symmetric
    s. adenolipomatosis
    s. distribution
symmetrical gangrene
symmetry
    bilateral s.
    s. element
    s. group
    icosahedral s.
    s. operation
    s. plane
    radial s.
sympathectomy
sympathetic
    s. chain
    s. fiber
    s. ganglion
    s. imbalance
    s. nervous system
    s. neuroblast
    s. ophthalmia
    s. ophthalmitis
    s. trunk
    s. uveitis
sympathetoblastoma
sympathicoblast
sympathicoblastoma
sympathicogonioma
sympathoblastoma
sympathogonioma
sympathomimetic
sympexis
symphysis (pl., symphyses)
    s. menti
    s. pubis
    s. sacrococcygea
sympodia
symport
symptom
symptomatic
    s. myeloid metaplasia
    s. porphyria

s. ulcer
s. varicocele
symptomatology
symptomatolytic
synanamorph
synapse
    chemical s.
    electrical s.
synapsis
synaptic
    s. bouton
    s. cleft
    s. glomerulus
    s. transmission
    s. vesicles
synaptonemal complex
synaptophysin
synaptosome
synarthrosis
Syncephalastrum
syncephalus
synchondrosis
    costochondral s.
    petroso-occipital s.
    spheno-occipital s.
    sphenopetrosal s.
    sternal s.
synchronism
    developmental s.
synchronized culture
synchronous
    s. counter
    s. data transmission
synchrony
    atrioventricular s.
syncopal
syncope
    cardiac s.
    carotid sinus s.
    exertional s.
    micturition s.
    postural s.
    vasovagal s.
syncyanin
syncytial
    s. alteration
    s. endometritis
    s. giant cells
    s. meningioma
    s. rhabdomyoblast
    s. trophoblast
syncytiotrophoblast

syncytiotrophoblastic
syncytium (pl., syncytia)
    s. formation
syndactyly
syndesis
syndesmitis
syndesmophyte
syndrome (*see also* Eponymic Diseases and Syndromes, Appendix 2)
    abdominal muscle deficiency s.
    acquired immunodeficiency s.
    acrofacial s.
    acute respiratory distress s.
    addisonian s.
    adrenal feminizing s.
    adrenal gland virilizing s.
    adrenogenital s.
    adult hemolytic uremic s.
    adult respiratory distress s.
    amenorrhea-galactorrhea s.
    amniotic infection s. of Blane
    angio-osteohypertrophy s.
    antibody-deficiency s.
    aortic arch s.
    apallic s.
    arthritis-dermatitis s.
    bare lymphocyte s.
    bacterial overgrowth s.
    basal cell nevus s.
    bile salt deficiency s.
    blue diaper s.
    body of Luys s.
    bowel bypass s.
    brachymesomelia-renal s.
    brain death s.
    branchio-oto-renal s.
    carcinoid s.
    carotid sinus s.
    cat-cry s.
    cat's eye s.
    cellular immunity deficiency s.
    cerebrohepatorenal s.
    cervical rib s.
    chancriform s.
    childhood hemolytic uremic s.
    chromosomal breakage s.
    chromosomal malformation s.
    chronic brain s.
    ciliary dyskinesis s.
    cold agglutinin s.
    compartmental s.

cri du chat s.
crush s.
cryopathic hemolytic s.
cryptophthalmus s.
cutaneomucouveal s.
defibrination s.
disappearing bile duct s.
dysmyelopoietic s.
dysplastic nevus s.
dystrophy-dystocia s.
dysuria-pyria s.
ectopic ACTH s.
endocrine polyglandular s.
erythrodysesthesia s.
excited skin s.
"expanded rubella s."
fertile eunuch s.
fetal alcohol s.
fetal face s.
fetal hydantoin s.
fetal trimethadione s.
fibrinogen-fibrin conversion s.
first arch s.
focal dermal hypoplasia s.
folded-lung s.
fragile X s.
gay lymph node s.
glomangiomatous osseous malformation s.
gracilis s.
gray platelet s.
hand-foot s.
heart-hand s.
hemangioma-
   thrombocytopenia s.
hemolytic-uremic s.
hemophagocytic s.
hemorrhagic varicella s.
herniated disk s.
hypereosinophilic s.
hyperimmunoglobulin E s.
hyperimmunoglobulin M s.
hyperviscosity s.
hypophysial s.
hypophysio-sphenoidal s.
idiopathic nephrotic s.
idiopathic respiratory distress s.
ill-defined s.
immotile cilia s.
immunodeficiency s.
inappropriate antidiuretic hormone s.

s. of inappropriate antidiuretic
   hormone secretion
juvenile polyposis s.
lazy leukocyte s.
linear sebaceous nevus s.
lymphadenopathy s.
lymphoproliferative s.
malabsorption s.
malformation s.
malignant carcinoid s.
mandibulofacial dysostosis s.
mandibulo-oculofacial s.
marfanoid hypermobility s.
megacystic s.
megacystis-microcolon intestinal hypoperistalsis s.
menopausal s.
metastatic carcinoid s.
methionine malabsorption s.
milk alkali s.
minimal-change nephrotic s.
mixed cryoglobulin s.
mucocutaneous lymph node s.
mucosal neuroma s.
multiple endocrine neoplasia
   s's, types 1 and 2
multiple hamartoma s.
multiple lentigines s.
multiple mucosal neuroma s.
myelodysplastic s.
myeloproliferative s's
myofascial s.
nail-patella s.
nephritic s.
nephrotic s.
neurocutaneous phacomato-
   sis s.
neuroleptic malignant s.
newborn respiratory s.
null s.
ocular s.
ocular-mucous membrane s.
oculobuccogenital s.
oculocerebrorenal s.
oculodentodigital s.
oculovertebral s.
organic brain s.
orofaciodigital s.
osteomyelofibrotic s.
otomandibular s.
papillary muscle s.
paraneoplastic s.

parkinsonian s.
parotitis s.
periodic s.
pickwickian s.
pituitary Cushing's s.
polycystic ovary s.
polysplenia s.
postpump s.
postrubella s.
premature senility s.
primary fibromyalgia s.
prune belly s.
pseudothalidomide s.
pterygium s.
pulmonary dysmaturity s.
radial aplasia-thrombocyto-
    penia s.
red cell fragmentation s.
respiratory distress s.
respiratory distress s. of
    newborn
right ovarian vein s.
rudimentary testis s.
scalded skin s.
scalenus anticus s.
sicca s.
spherophakia-brachymorphia s.
spruelike s.
staphylococcal scalded skin s.
sudden death s.
sudden infant death s.
superior vena caval s.
testicular feminization s.
testicular regression s.
thrombocytopenia-absent ra-
    dius s.
thrombopathic s.
toxic shock s.
triad s.
trichorhinophalangeal s.
trisomy 8 s.
trisomy 13 s.
trisomy 13-15 s.
trisomy 16-18 s.
trisomy 18 s.
trisomy 20 s.
trisomy 21 s.
trisomy 22 s.
trisomy C s.
trisomy D s.
trisomy E s.
tropical splenomegaly s.

tryptophan malabsorption s.
tumor lysis s.
ulnar tunnel s.
urogenital s.
uveo-encephalitic s.
vasculocardiac s. of hypersero-
    tonemia
vertebral basilar artery s.
vertebral crush-fracture s.
virilizing s.
virus-associated hemophago-
    cytic s.
wasting s.
whistling face s.
X-linked lymphoproliferative s.
XO s.
XXX s.
XXXXX s.
XXXXY s.
XXXY s.
XXY s.
XXYY s.
XYY s.
XYZ s.
synechia (pl., synechiae)
    s. pericardii
syneresis
synergism
synergist
synergistic
synergy
    antimicrobial s.
syn. fl.— synovial fluid
Syngamidae
Syngamus
    S. *laryngeus*
    S. *trachea*
syngamy
syngeneic transplantation
syngenesioplastic transplantation
syngraft
synkaryon
synophthalmia
synorchism
Synosternus pallidus
synostosis
synotus
synovectomy
synovia
synovial
    s. biopsy
    s. chondromatosis

s. chondrosarcoma
s. cyst
s. fluid
s. fluid analysis
s. fluid effect
s. fluid examination
s. histopathology
s. joint
s. layer of articular capsule
s. membrane
s. osteochondromatosis
s. plica
s. sarcoma
s. stromal cells
s. tendon sheath
s. tissue
s. villus
synoviography
synovioma
malignant s.
synovitis
acute serous s.
diffuse pigmented villonodular s.
pigmented villonodular s.
proliferative s.
purulent s.
serous acute s.
suppurative s.
tendinous s.
vaginal s.
villonodular pigmented s.
synovium
syntectic
syntenic genes
synteny
syntexis
synthase
glycogen s.
methionine s.
porphobilinogen s.
uroporphyrinogen I s.
synthesis
abnormal globulin s.
DNA s.
fatty acid s.
glycogen s.
protein s.
testosterone s.
urea s.
synthetase
acetyl-CoA s.

acyl-CoA s.
alanyl RNA s.
argininosuccinate s.
glutathione s.
heme s.
methionyl-RNA s.
polydeoxyribonucleotide s.
thromboxane s.
tyrosyl-RNA s.
valyl-RNA s.
synthetic
s. dyes
s. tuberculin trichloroacetic acid (precipitated)
syntrophism
syntropic
Syphacia obvelata
syphilemia
syphilid
gummatous s.
nodular s.
syphilimetry
syphilis
anorectal s.
cardiovascular s.
congenital s.
genital s.
infantile s.
perinatal s.
primary s.
secondary s.
serologic test for s.
standard test for s.
tertiary s.
venereal disease s.
syphilitic
s. abscess
s. aneurysm
s. aortitis
s. arteritis
s. condyloma latum
s. fever
s. gastritis
s. gumma
s. meningitis
microscopic s.
s. nephritis
s. osteochondritis
s. periarteritis
serodiagnostic s.
s. ulcer
syphiloma of Fournier

syphilomatous
syringadenoma
    papillary s.
    s. papilliferum
syringe
    fountain s.
    hypodermic s.
    Omnistik blood gas s.
    probe s.
    Roughton-Scholander s.
    s. shield
syringitis
syringoacanthoma
syringoadenoma
syringobulbia
syringocarcinoma
syringocystadenoma papilliferum
syringocystoma
syringoencephalomyelia
syringoid
syringoma
    chondroid s.
syringomyelia
syringomyelocele
syrosingopine
Syrphidae
Sysmex multichannel hematology analyzer
system
    10–20 s.
    Abel expert s.
    ABO blood group s.
    absolute s. of units
    antigen blood group s.
    Astler-Coller rectal s.
    Auberger's blood group s.
    Autobac s.
    AutoMicrobic s.
    Auto SCAN s.
    Avantage s.
    avidin-biotin s.
    Bactec s.
    Bergh's staging s.
    bicarbonate buffer s.
    biliary s.
    blood group s's
    Bodin-Gibb staging s.
    body substance isolation s.
    Broders' grading s.
    buffer s.
    Butchart grading s.
    cardiac conduction s.

Cartwright's blood group s.
cell-free s.
centimeter-gram-second s.
cgs s.
coagulation s.
Colton's blood group s.
complement s.
consultation s.
Cost Sterling blood group s.
diffuse neuroendocrine s.
Dombrock's blood group s.
Duffy's blood group s.
Duke's staging s.
Electrion s.
electro-optical s.
endocrine s.
erythrocyte-phosphate buffer s.
Evans' staging s.
fibrinolytic s.
Fisher-Race s.
Fuhrman's grading s.
Gerbich blood group s.
Halon s.
hematopoietic s.
immune s.
isolator s.
Jakobson's malignancy grading s.
Jewett-Strong staging s.
Jones and Campbell staging s.
kallikrein s.
Kell blood s.
Kell blood group s.
Kempson's grading s.
Kidd blood group s.
kinin s.
Landsteiner's blood group s.
Lutheran blood group s.
lymphoreticular s.
lysis centrifugation s.
McLeod blood group s.
meter-kilogram-second s.
metric s.
microbiology identification s.
microsomal enzyme s.
mononuclear phagocyte s.
musculoskeletal s.
myeloperoxidase s.
on-demand s.
operating s.
PALI (Programmed Accelerated Laboratory Investigation) s.

paraganglionic s.
plasmid vector s.
portal s.
properdin s.
renin-angiotensin-
   aldosterone s.
reticuloendothelial s.
Robson's staging s.
Schmidt's blood group s.
Scianna blood group s.
Septi-Chek blood culture s.
Shimoda's blood group s.
SOS repair s.
St. Jude's staging s.
turnkey s.
upper collecting s.
urogenital s.
vascular s.
Whitmore's staging s.
Wiener s.
Wilkerson point s.
Wright's s.
Xga blood group s.
systematic
   s. bacteriology
   s. error
   s. family
systematized nevus
Systematized Nomenclature of Pathology
Système Internationale d'Unités
systemic
   s. anaphylaxis

s. arterial pressure
s. calciphylaxis
s. chondromalacia
s. collagenosis
s. death
s. edema
s. embolism
s. familial primary amyloidosis
s. fungus
s. hemosiderosis
s. histiocytosis
s. hyalinosis
s. hyperfibrinolysis
s. lesion
s. lupus erythematosus
s. mastocytosis
s. necrotizing vasculitis
s. poisoning
s. primary amyloidosis
s. proliferating angioendotheliomatosis
s. resistance
s. reticuloendotheliosis
s. sclerosis
s. vascular resistance
systemoid
systole
systolic
   s. hypertension
   s. murmur
   s. pressure
   s. time interval
Sz — schizophrenia
Szent-Györgyi reaction

T

T — temperature
   tension (intraocular)
   tesla
   thoracic
   thorax
   thymidine
   torque
   tritium
T. — *Taenia*
   Treponema
   Trichophyton
   Trypanosoma

T3RU

T+ — increased tension
T− — decreased tension
T_0 — no evidence of primary tumor
$T^{1/2}$, $T_{1/2}$, or $t^{1/2}$ — half-life
T_3 — triiodothyronine
T_3 uptake test
T_4 — thyroxine
t — temporal
   tertiary
   test of significance
TA — alkaline tuberculin
   therapeutic abortion

titratable acid
toxin-antitoxin
tube agglutination
Ta — tantalum
TA-4 — squamous cell carcinoma antigen
TAA — tumor-associated antigen
TA-AIDS — transfusion-associated AIDS
TAB — typhoid, paratyphoid A and paratyphoid B
tabanid
Tabanidae
Tabanus
tabby cat striation
tabescence
tabescent
tabes dorsalis
tabetic bladder
tabetiform
tabic
tabid
table
    contingency t.
    Gaffky's t.
    life t.
    periodic t.
tablet
    buccal t.
    diazo t.
    hypodermic t.
    ictotest reagent t.
    sublingual t.
tabletop shield
taboparesis
Tac antigen
tache
    t. blanche
    t. laiteuse
tachetic
tachogram
tachometer
tachyarrhythmia
tachycardia
    atrial t.
    junctional t.
    nodal t.
    paroxysmal atrial t.
    paroxysmal ventricular t.
    ventricular t.
tachykinin
tachyphylaxis

tachypnea
tachyzoite
tactile
    t. anesthesia
    t. disc
    t. hypesthesia
    t. receptor
    t. sensation
TAD — thoracic asphyxiant dystrophy
tadpole cell
Taenia
    T. *africana*
    T. *bremneri*
    T. *canina*
    T. *confusa*
    T. *diminuta*
    T. *echinococcus*
    T. *lata*
    T. *murina*
    T. *nana*
    T. *philippina*
    T. *saginata*
    T. *solium*
    T. *taeniaeformis*
taeniasis
Taeniidae
Taeniorhynchus saginatus
Taenzer's stain
Taenzer-Unna stain
TAF — albumose-free tuberculin
    toxoid-antitoxin floccules
    trypsin-aldehyde-fuchsin
    tumor angiogenic factor
tag
    anal t.
    hymenal t.
    sentinel t.
    skin t.
T agglutination
TAGVHD — transfusion-associated graft-versus-host disease
TAH — total abdominal hysterectomy
tail
    t. of caudate nucleus
    t. of epididymis
    t. of pancreas
    t. poikilocyte
    polyA t.
    polyadenylate t.

tailing
Taiwan acute respiratory strain
Takata-Ara test
Takayama's stain
Takayasu's arteritis
TAL — thymic alymphoplasia
talbutal
talc granuloma
talcosis
talipes
  t. calcaneovalgus
  t. calcaneovarus
  t. calcaneus
  t. cavus
  t. equinovalgus
  t. equinovarus
  t. equinus
  t. planovalgus
  t. valgus
T-ALL — T-cell acute lymphoblastic
    anemia
talocalcaneonavicular joint
talocrural joint
talose
talus (pl., tali)
TAM — toxoid-antitoxin mixture
TAME — toluene-sulfo-trypsin argi-
    nine methyl ester
Tamm-Horsfall
  mucoprotein
  protein
tamoxifen
tamponade
  cardiac t.
  pericardial t.
Tamulus
tangent
tangential projection
tangle
  neurofibrillary t's
tannase
tanned
  t. red cell hemagglutination
    inhibition test
  t. red cells
Tanner-Roux procedure
Tanner stage
tannic acid
tantalum isotope
T antigen (tumor antigen)
TAO — thromboangiitis obliterans
    triacetyloleandomycin

tape
  cellulose t.
  t. drive
  magnetic t.
  t. mark
  t. transport
tapetum (pl., tapeta)
tapeworm
  beef t.
  broad fish t.
  t. cyst
  dog t.
  dwarf t.
  fish t.
  pork t.
  rat t.
tapir mouth
TAPVD — total anomalous pulmo-
    nary venous drainage
"tap water bacillus"
TAR — thrombocytopenia with ab-
    sence of radius
tar
  coal t.
  t. keratosis
TARA — tumor-associated rejection
    antigen
Tardieu's
  ecchymoses
  petechiae
  spots
tare
target
  t. cell
  t. cell anemia
  t. lesion
  t. organ
tarry
  t. cyst
  t. stool
tarsal
  t. artery
  t. bone
  t. cyst
  t. gland
  t. joint
  t. plate
  t. tunnel syndrome
tarsitis
tarsoepiphyseal aclasis
tarsomegaly
tarsometatarsal joint

tarsophyma
tarsus
TAR syndrome
TART — tumorectomy, axillary dissection, radiotherapy
tartaric acid
tart cell
tartrate
   ammonium t.
   t.-inhibited acid phosphatase
   t.-resistant leukocyte acid phosphatase
tartrazine
taste
   t. bud
   color t.
   franklinic t.
   t. receiving area
TAT — tetanus antitoxin
   thromboplastin activation test
   total antitryptic activity
   toxin-antitoxin
   transacting transcriptional (regulation)
   turn-around time
   tyrosine aminotransferase
tat gene
Tatlockia micdadei
tattoo
Tatumella ptyseos
tau
   Kendall's t.
taurine
taurochenodeoxycholate
taurochenodeoxycholic acid
taurocholate
taurocholic acid
taurodeoxycholic acid
taurolithocholic acid
Taussig-Bing malformation
tautomer
tautomeral
tautomerase
   phenylpyruvate t.
tautomerism
   enol-keto t.
   proton t.
   ring chain t.
   valence t.
taxis
taxon (pl., taxa)
taxonomy

Taxus
TB — terminal bronchiole
   toluidine blue
   tracheobronchitis
   tubercle bacillus
   tuberculosis
Tb — terbium
TBA — tertiary butylacetate
   testosterone-binding affinity
   thiobarbituric acid
T banding — telomere or terminal banding
TBC — tuberculosis
TBD — total body density
TBE — tuberculin bacillary emulsion
TBF — total body fat
TBG — thyroxine-binding globulin
TBG assay
TBG cap
TBGP — total blood granulocyte pool
TBH — total body hematocrit
TBI — thyroxine-binding index
   total body irradiation
TBII — TSH-binding inhibitory immunoglobulin
TBK — total body potassium
T/B lymphocyte assay
T and B lymphocyte subset assay
TBM — tuberculous meningitis
   tubular basement membrane
TBP — thyroxine-binding protein
TBPA — thyroxine-binding prealbumin
TB-RD — tuberculosis-respiratory disease
TBS — total body solute
   tribromosalicylanilide
   triethanolamine-buffered saline
TB smear
TBT — tolbutamide test
   tracheobronchial toilet
TBV — total blood volume
TBW — total body water
   total body weight
TBX — total body irradiation
TC — taurocholate
   temperature compensation
   tetracycline
   thermal conductivity
   tissue culture

total cholesterol
tubocurarine
$T_4(C)$
Tc — technetium
TCA — tricarboxylic acid
    trichloroacetate
    trichloroacetic acid
    tricyclic antidepressant
TCA (tricarboxylic acid) cycle
TCAP — trimethylcetylammonium
        pentachlorophenate
TCBS — thiosulfate citrate bile salts
        sucrose
TCBS agar
TCC — trichlorocarbanilide
TCD — T cell depletion
    tissue culture dose
TCD_{50} — median tissue culture
        dose
TC detector
TCE — trichloroethylene
T cell
        T-c. antigen receptor
        cytotoxic T c.
        T-c. function
        T-c. growth factor
        T-c. helper cells
        T-c. leukemia
        T-c. lymphocytes
        T-c.–mediated immunity
        T-c. mitogens
        T-c. proliferation
        T-c.–replacing factor
T4 cells
T8 cells
TCF — total coronary flow
TCGF — T-cell growth factor
TCH — total circulating hemoglobin
TCI — transient cerebral ischemia
TCID — tissue culture infective dose
$TCID_{50}$ — median tissue culture infec-
        tive dose
TCIE — transient cerebral ischemic
        episode
TCM — tissue culture medium
TCMI — T-cell–mediated immunity
TCP — tricresyl phosphate
TCR — T-cell receptor
tcRNA — translation control RNA
TCSA — tetrachlorosalicylanilide
TCT — thrombin-clotting time
    thyrocalcitonin

TD — tetanus-diphtheria
    thoracic duct
    thymus-dependent
    torsion dystonia
    transverse diameter
TDA — TSH-displacing antibody
TDF — thoracic duct fistula
    thoracic duct flow
TDI — toluene-diisocyanate
    total-dose infusion
TDL — thoracic duct lymph
TDP — thoracic duct pressure
    thymidine diphosphate
TDT — terminal deoxynucleotidyl
        transferase
TE — threshold energy
    tissue-equivalent
    total estrogen (excretion)
    tracheoesophageal
Te — tellurium
    tetanus
TEA — tetraethylammonium
TEAC — tetraethylammonium
        chloride
teaching hospital
tear
        Mallory-Weiss t.
teardrop
        t. bladder
        t. cell
tear-shaped erythrocyte
TeBG — testosterone-estradiol-
        binding globulin
technetium
        t.-99m aggregated albumin
        t.-99m albumin microspheres
        t.-99m dihydrothiotic acid
        t.-99m dimercaptosuccinic acid
        t.-99m diphosphonate
        t.-99m etidronate sodium
        t.-99m glucoheptonate
        t.-99m iron ascorbate complex
        t.-99m medronate sodium
        t.-99m pentetic acid
        t.-99m pertechnetate
        t.-99m polyphosphate
        t.-99m pyrophosphate
        t.-99m red blood cells
        t.-99m serum albumin
        t.-99m sulfur colloid
        t. Tc 99m pentetic acid

t. Tc 99m red blood cells
t. Tc 99m serum albumin
technical
technician
    histologic t.
    medical laboratory t.
Technicon analyzer
technique; technic
    arterial puncture t.
    Brecher's new methylene
      blue t.
    Brown-Brenn t.
    Carey's Ranvier t.
    Castenada t.
    clamp t.
    Corbin t.
    cough swab t.
    Delves cup t.
    Dennis' t.
    dilution-filtration t.
    direct Coombs' t.
    enzyme-assisted immunoas-
      say t.
    enzyme-multiplied immunoas-
      say t.
    FA (fluorescent antibody) t.
    Ficoll-Hypaque t.
    flotation t's
    fluorescence t.
    fluorescent antibody t.
    glyoxylic acid–induced t.
    Highman's Congo red t.
    Hotchkiss-McManus PAS t.
    immunoblot t.
    immunofluorescence t's
    immunohistochemical t's
    immunoperoxidase t.
    Jerne plaque t.
    Kato's thick smear t.
    Kjeldahl's t.
    Knott's t.
    Kohn's one-step staining t.
    Laurell t.
    Martinez' t.
    McMaster t.
    membrane filter t's
    Mohr's t.
    nephelometric immunopreci-
      pitin t.
    Northern blot t.
    Ouchterlony t.
    Oudin's t.

    PAP (peroxidase-
      antiperoxidase) t.
    peroxidase-antiperoxidase t.
    plaque t.
    program evaluation and re-
      view t.
    Rebuck's skin window t.
    Ritter-Oleson t.
    roll-tube t.
    saline t.
    scintillation t.
    scintillation counting t.
    sealed envelope t.
    section freeze substitution t.
    sedimentation t's
    Seldinger's t.
    Southern blot t.
    Stroll's dilution egg count t.
    time diffusion t.
    titration t.
    transfixion t.
    van den Bergh's t.
    Webster's t.
    Western blot t.
    Westgard multi-rule t.
    zinc sulfate centrifugal flota-
      tion t.
technologic life
technologist
    medical t.
technology
tectobulbar tract
tectorial membrane
tectospinal tract
tectum of mesencephalon
TED — threshold erythema dose
          thromboembolic disease
Tedion
TEE — tyrosine ethyl ester
TEF — tracheoesophageal fistula
Teflon
tegmen (pl., tegmina)
    t. tympani
tegmental
    t. cells
    t. pons
    t. radiation
tegmentum (pl., tegmenta)
Tegretol
TEIB — triethyleneiminobenzo-
         quinone
teichoic acid antibody

TEL — tetraethyl acid
tela (pl., telae)
    t. choroidea
    t. conjunctiva
    t. subcutanea
    t. submucosa
    t. subserosa
telangiectasia
    t. ataxia
    capillary t.
    cephalo-oculocutaneous t.
    essential t.
    hereditary ataxic t.
    hereditary hemorrhagic t.
    t. lymphatica
    t. macularis eruptiva perstans
    spider t.
    t. verrucosa
telangiectasis (pl., telangiectases)
telangiectatic
    t. angioma
    t. cancer
    t. fibroma
    t. glioma
    t. lipoma
    t. osteogenic sarcoma
    t. osteosarcoma
    t. wart
telangiectodes
telangioma (pl., telangiomata)
telecardiography
telecurietherapy
telefluoroscopy
telemetry
telencephalon
teleomorph
teleonomy
telepathology
teleradiography
teleradium treatment
telereceptor
teleroentgenography
teleroentgentherapy
telescoped sediment
tellurate
tellurite medium
tellurium
    t. assay
    t. dioxide
telocentric
telodendron
telogen hair

telomere banding
telomeric R-banding stain
telophase
TEM — transmission electron micro-
        scope
      triethylenemelamine
temperate phage
temperature
    absolute t.
    ambient t.
    body t.
    t. coefficient
    t. compensation
    critical t.
    effective t.
    eutectic t.
    flash-point t.
    ignition t.
    maximal growth t.
    melting t.
    minimal growth t.
    normal body t.
    optimal growth t.
    optimum t.
    t. programming
    t.-sensitive mutation
    subnormal t.
template theory
temporal
    t. arteritis
    t. artery
    t. bone
    t. branch
    t. dispersion
    t. epilepsy
    t. fascia
    t. gyrus
    t. horn
    t. lobe
    t. lobe epilepsy
    t. muscle
    t. operculum
    t. pole
    t. radiation
    t. region
    t. sulcus
temporary parasite
temporomandibular joint
temporomaxillary
temporo-occipital fasciculus
temporopontile
temporopontine

temporozygomatic
TEN — toxic epidermal necrolysis
tenac — tenaculum
tenaculum
tendency
    central t.
tenderness
tendinitis
    hypertrophic infiltrative t.
tendinous
    t. spot
    t. synovitis
    t. xanthoma
tendo (pl., tendines)
    t. Achillis
    t. calcaneus
    t. conjunctivus
    t. cordiformis
    cricoesophageal t.
    t. oculi
tendon
    Achilles t.
    ankle t.
    anterior tibial muscle of t.
    biceps t.
    calcaneal t.
    central t.
    digital t.
    elbow t.
    t. organ
    patellar t.
    posterior tibial muscle of t.
    quadriceps t.
    t. sheath
    shoulder t.
    spindle t.
    superior oblique muscle of t.
    triceps t.
    wrist t.
tendonitis
tendovaginitis
    radial styloid t.
Tenebrio
tenesmus
tenia (pl., teniae)
    t. choroidea
    teniae coli
    t. libera
    t. mesocolica
    t. omentalis
    t. plexus
    t. telae

    t. thalami
    t. ventriculi quarti
    t. ventriculi tertii
teniposide
Tenney changes
tennis thumb
tenonitis
tenontitis
tenontolemmitis
tenontophyma
tenontothecitis
tenophyte
tenositis
tenostosis
tenosynovectomy
tenosynovitis
    t. crepitans
    de Quervain's t.
    gonorrheal t.
    t. granulosa
    nodular t.
    pigmented villonodular t.
    suppurative t.
    traumatic t.
    tuberculous t.
    villonodular pigmented t.
    villous t.
tenovaginitis
TENS —transcutaneous electrical
        nerve stimulator
tension
    carbon dioxide t.
    t. cyst
    t. cyst of breast
    end-tidal CO_2 t.
    oxygen t.
    t. pneumothorax
    premenstrual t.
    surface t.
tensor muscle of velum palatini
tenth cranial nerve
tentorial
    t. branch, ophthalmic nerve
    t. meningioma
tentorium (pl., tentoria)
    t. cerebelli
    t. of hypophysis
TEP — thromboendophlebectomy
TEPP — tetraethyl pyrophosphate
teracurie
terahertz
teratoblastoma

teratocarcinogenesis
teratocarcinoma
    mediastinal t.
teratocarcinosarcoma
teratogen
teratogenesis
teratogenic
teratoid tumor
teratology
teratoma (pl., teratomata)
    adult cystic t.
    benign t.
    cystic dermoid t.
    embryonal t.
    immature t.
    malignant t.
    malignant trophoblastic t.
    mature t.
    monodermal t.
    ovarian t.
    retinoblastic t.
    sacrococcygeal t.
    solid t.
    testicular t.
    triphyllomatous t.
teratomatous cyst
terbium
terbutaline sulfate
terebene
teres major muscle
teres minor muscle
terminal
    t. addition enzyme
    t. airway unit
    amino t.
    t. bar
    t. bar alteration
    t. bronchiole
    carboxyl t.
    t. cisterna
    t. conducting fibers of Purkinje
    CRT t.
    t. deletion
    t. deoxynucleotidyl transferase
    t. deoxyribonucleotidyl trans-
      ferase
    t. duct carcinoma
    t. endocarditis
    graphic t.
    t. half-life
    t. hematuria
    t. ileitis

    t. latency
    t. leukocytosis
    t. respiratory unit
    smart t.
    t. vein
    t. web
terminalization
termination
    t. codon
    t. factor
    t. sequence
terminator
    DNA-chain t.
terminus (pl., termini)
    cohesive t.
ternary acid
terosite
terpenal metabolites
terpene
terpineol
terpin hydrate
terra alba
Terridens diminutus
Terridens diminutus tertiary syphilis
tertian
    t. fever
    t. malaria
tertiary
    t. granule
    t. hyperparathyroidism
    t. sequestrum
    t. structure
    t. syphilis
TES — trimethylaminoethane-
      sulfonic acid
Teschen's virus
tesla
test
    abnormal glucose tolerance t.
    Abrams' t.
    acetic acid t.
    acetic acid and potassium ferro-
      cyanide t.
    acetoacetic acid t.
    acetoin t.
    acetone t.
    acid challenge t.
    acid elution slide t.
    acid hemolysin t.
    acidified serum t.
    acidity reduction t.
    acid-lability t.

acidosis t.
acid perfusion t.
acid phosphatase t.
✳ acid phosphatase t. for semen
ACTH t.
ACTH stimulation t.
activated partial thromboplastin substitution t.
active rosette t.
Adamkiewicz's t.
Adler's t.
adrenal ascorbic acid depletion t.
adrenal function t.
adrenalin t.
adrenocortical inhibition t.
adrenocorticotropic hormone stimulation t.
adrenocorticotropic hormone suppression t.
A/G t.
agglutination t.
A/G (albumin/globulin) ratio t.
albumin t.
albumin suspension t.
aldolase t.
aldosterone stimulation t.
aldosterone suppression t.
alizarin t.
alkali t.
alkali denaturation t.
alkaline phosphatase t.
alkali tolerance t.
alkaloid t.
alkaptonuria t's
Allen-Doisy t.
Allen's t.
Almén's t. for blood
alpha-amino nitrogen t.
Ames t.
p-aminohippurate clearance t.
aminopyrine breath t.
ammoniacal silver nitrate t.
amylase t.
Anderson-Collip t.
antibiotic sensitivity t.
anti–Chlamydia antibody t's
antiglobulin t.
antihuman globulin t.
antistreptolysin-O t's
antithrombin III t.

antitoxoplasma antibody t's
Anton's t.
Apt t.
arginine t.
arginine insulin tolerance t.
arylsulfatase t.
Aschheim-Zondek t.
ascorbate cyanide t.
ascorbic acid t.
Aspergillus antibody t's
Astwood's t.
atropine suppression t.
augmented histamine t.
autohemolysis t.
automated reagin t.
A-Z t.
babesiosis serological t.
Bachman-Pettit t.
Bachman's t.
bacitracin differential disk t.
Baker's acid hematein t.
Baker's pyridine extraction t.
barium t.
Barr body t.
basophil degranulation t.
Beard's t.
BEI (butanol-extractable iodine) t.
Bence Jones protein t.
Benedict's t.
bentiromide t.
bentonite flocculation t.
benzidine t.
Bernstein t.
Berson t.
Betke-Kleihauer t.
Bettendorff's t.
Beutler t.
Bial's t.
bicarbonate titration t.
bicolor guaiac t.
bile acid t.
bile acid tolerance t.
bile-esculin hydrolysis t.
bile pigment t.
bile salt breath t.
bile solubility t.
bilirubin t., direct, indirect
bilirubin tolerance t.
Binz' t.
biuret t.
blind t.

✳ acid-Schiff for fungal infection

Blondheim t.
blood urea nitrogen t.
Bloor's t.
blot t.
Blount's t.
Bloxam's t.
Boas' t.
Bonanno's t.
Bonsignore t.
borderline glucose tolerance t.
Bradshaw's t.
breath analysis t.
bromocriptine suppression t.
bromphenol t.
Bromsulphalein t.
brucella agglutination t.
BSP excretion t.
butanol extractable iodine t.
calcium t.
calcium oxalate t.
CAMP t.
Candida precipitin t.
candidiasis serologic t.
capillary fragility t.
capon-comb-growth t.
carbohydrate fermentation t.
carbohydrate identification t.
carbohydrate utilization t.
carbon dioxide combining
    power t.
Cartwright t.
Casoni's intradermal t.
Castellani's t.
catalase t.
catatorulin t.
catecholamine t.
cellobiose/mannitol sugar per-
    meability t.
cephalin-cholesterol floccula-
    tion t.
cephalin flocculation t.
cetylpyridium chloride t.
CFF (critical flicker fusion) t.
CFT (complement-fixation) t.
Chagas' disease serological t.
Chédiak's t.
chelation t.
chemical inhibition isoamy-
    lase t.
chemiluminescence t.
Chemstrip t.
Chen's t.

Chick-Martin t.
Chido t.
chi-squared t.
chloride plate t.
chlormerodrin accumulation t.
cholesterol t.
cholesterol-lecithin floccula-
    tion t.
cholinesterase t.
chromaffin reaction t.
chromogenic cephalosporin t.
cis-trans t.
citrate t.
Clark's t.
Clauberg's t.
clomiphene t.
clonidine suppression t.
coagulase t.
coagulation t.
coagulation time t.
coccidioidin t.
cold agglutinin t.
cold hemolysin t.
colloidal gold t.
comb-growth t.
compatibility t.
complement-fixation t.
complement lysis sensitivity t.
conglutinating complement ab-
    sorption t.
Congo red t.
Coombs' t., direct, indirect
copper reduction t.
coproporphyrin t.
Corner-Allen t.
cortisone-glucose tolerance t.
cortisone-primed oral glucose
    tolerance t.
cosyntropin t.
C-reactive protein t.
creatine t.
creatinine clearance t.
critical flicker fusion t.
C-stix t.
cyanide-ascorbate t.
cyanide-nitroprusside t.
cystic fibrosis t's
cystinuria t's
cytochrome oxidase t.
cytotoxicity t.
cytotropic antibody t.
Davidsohn's differential t.

Day's t.
deoxyribonuclease t.
deoxyuridine suppression t.
dexamethasone suppression t.
dextrose t.
DFA-TP (direct fluorescent antibody–*Treponema pallidum*) t.
Diagnex blue t.
diazepam breath t.
Dick t.
differential renal function t.
differential ureteral catheterization t.
dilution t.
dinitrophenylhydrazine t.
direct agglutination pregnancy t.
direct antiglobulin t.
direct bilirubin t.
direct Coombs' t.
disaccharide tolerance t.
disk diffusion t.
disk dilution susceptibility t.
dithionite solubility t.
Dixon's t.
DNase (deoxyribonuclease) t.
Dold's t.
Donath-Landsteiner t.
Donné's t.
dot blot t.
double diffusion t.
Dragendorff's t.
Duke's t.
D-xylose absorption t.
D-xylose tolerance t.
dye t.
dye exclusion t.
dye excretion t's
echinococcosis serological t.
edrophonium chloride t.
E (erythrocyte)-rosette t.
Ehrlich's t.
electrophoresis t.
electrotransfer t.
Elek immunodiffusion t.
Ellsworth-Howard t.
Emmens' S/L t.
Envacor t.
enzyme-linked antibody t.
erythrocyte fragility t.
erythrocyte rosette t.

esculin hydrolysis t.
esterase t.
ethanol gelation t.
ethyl hydrocupreine hydrochloride t.
euglobulin clot t.
euglobulin lysis t.
exoantigen t.
factor VIII–related antigen t.
FANA (fluorescent antinuclear antibody) t.
Farr t.
fat absorption t.
febrile agglutination t.
Fehling's t.
fermentation t.
fern t.
ferric chloride t.
ferric ferricyanide reduction t.
fetal hemoglobin t.
Feulgen's t.
Fevold t.
fibrinogen t.
fibrinogen titer t.
fibrin-stabilizing factor t.
fibrin titer t.
FIGLU (formiminoglutamic acid) t.
filariasis serological t.
filter paper microscopic t.
Finn chamber t.
Fishberg's concentration t.
Fisher's exact t.
Fleitmann's t.
flocculation t.
Florence's t.
fluorescent antibody t.
fluorescent antinuclear antibody t.
fluorescent spot t.
fluorescent treponemal antibody absorption t.
fluorocortisone t.
foam stability t.
Folin-Looney t.
Folin's t.
formazan t.
formol-gel t.
Foshay t.
Fouchet's t.
fragility t.
Francis' skin t.

Freda t.
Frei's t.
Friedman's t.
frog t.
fructose intolerance t.
Frye t.
FTA-ABS (fluorescent treponemal antibody absorption) t.
Gaddum and Schild t.
galactose breath t.
galactose tolerance t.
Galli-Mainini toad t.
gastric function t's
gastrin-calcium infusion stimulation t.
gastrin-protein stimulation t.
gastrin-secretin stimulation t.
gastroccult t.
gastrointestinal blood loss t.
gastrointestinal protein loss t.
Geraghty's t.
Gerhardt's ferric chloride t.
Gerhardt's t. for acetoacetic acid
Gerhardt's t. for urobilin in the urine
germ tube t.
Gibson-Cooke sweat t.
glucagon t.
glucocorticoid suppression t.
glucose insulin tolerance t.
glucose oxidase paper strip t.
glucose-6-phosphate dehydrogenase t's
glucose tolerance t.
glutathione stability t.
glycogen storage t.
glycosylated hemoglobin t.
glycyltryptophan t.
Gmelin's t.
Gofman t.
gold-sol t.
Gordon's t.
Graham-Cole t.
Gravindex t.
guaiac t.
Gudmand-Hoyer lactose tolerance t.
Guilford-Zimmerman personality t.
Günzberg's t.
Guthrie t.

Gutzeit's
Haagensen t.
Ham's t.
Hanger's t.
Harris and Ray t.
Harrison spot t.
Harris's t.
Heaf's t.
heat coagulation t.
heat instability t.
heat precipitation t.
Heinz body t.
hemadsorption t.
hemagglutination t.
hemagglutination-inhibition t.
hematein t.
Hemoccult t.
hemolysin t.
Hemo-Quant t.
hemosiderinuria t.
HEMPAS (hereditary erythroblastic multinuclearity with positive acidified serum) t.
Henry fructose t.
hepatitis B surface antigen t's
heterophil antibody t.
heterophile antibody t.
Hicks-Pitney thromboplastin generation t.
Hinton t.
hippurate hydrolysis t.
hippuric acid t.
hippuric acid excretion t.
Histalog t.
histamine release t.
histoplasmin-latex t.
HIVAGEN t.
Hoesch t.
Hogben t.
Hollander t.
homocystinuria t.
homogentisic acid t.
homovanillic acid t.
Hooker-Forbes t.
Howard's t.
Howell's t.
Huhner t.
human chorionic gonadotropin injection t.
human erythrocyte agglutination t.
HVA (homovanillic acid) t.

hydrogen breath t.
17-hydroxycorticosteroid t.
5-hydroxyindoleacetic t.
5-hydroxyindoleacetic acid t.
ICG (indocyanine green) excretion t.
icterus index t.
Ide t.
immunoblot t.
immunofluorescence t.
immunologic pregnancy t.
implantation t.
IMViC (indole, methyl red, Voges-Proskauer, and citrate) t.
indican t.
indigo-carmine t.
indirect bilirubin t.
indirect Coombs' t.
indirect hemagglutination t.
indole t.
indole, methyl red, Voges-Proskauer, and citrate t.
indophenol t.
inhibition t.
insulin clearance t.
insulin hypoglycemia t.
insulin sensitivity t.
insulin tolerance t.
interference t.
intradermal t.
intravenous glucose tolerance t.
intravenous tolbutamide tolerance t.
invasive activity t.
iodine-azide t.
iodine-131 uptake t.
iron-binding capacity t.
isoiodeikon t.
isoniazid phenotype t.
isopropanol precipitation t.
^{131}I (radioactive iodine) uptake t.
Jacquemin's t.
Jaffé's t.
Jolles' t.
Jones-Cantarow t.
Kahn's t.
Katayama's t.
Kerry reducing substance t.
ketogenic corticoids t.

17-ketogenic steroid assay t.
ketone bodies t.
17-ketosteroid assay t.
Kirby-Bauer t.
Kleihauer t.
Kleihauer-Betke t.
Kober's t.
Kobert's t.
Kolmer's t.
Kunkel's t.
Kurzrok-Ratner t.
Kveim t.
Kveim-Siltzbach t.
lactic acid t.
lactic dehydrogenase t.
lactose t's
lactose tolerance t.
lactulose/mannitol t.
Ladendorff's t.
Landsteiner-Donath t.
Lange's t.
Lange's colloidal gold t.
lateral position t.
latex agglutination t.
latex agglutination-inhibition t.
latex fixation t.
latex flocculation t.
latex slide agglutination t.
LE cell t.
Lee-White clotting t.
Legal's t.
leishmaniasis serological t.
lepromin t.
lepromin skin t.
lethal titer t.
leucine aminopeptidase t.
leukocyte adherence assay t.
leukocyte bactericidal assay t.
leukocyte histamine release t.
Levinson's t.
levulose tolerance t.
Liebermann-Burchard t.
Liley's t.
limulus lysate t.
line t.
lipase t.
lipid t.
liver flocculation t.
liver function t.
Lücke's t.
lupus erythematosus cell t.

lymphocyte transfer t.
lymphocyte transformation t.
Machado-Guerreiro t.
magnesium t.
malaria film t.
mallein t.
Malmejde's t.
Mantoux's t.
Mantoux skin t.
Master two-step t.
mastic t.
maximal Histalog t.
Mazzini's t.
Mazzotti t.
McPhail t.
t. meal
melanin t.
melanogen t.
metabisulfite t.
metabolic inhibition t.
methemoglobin elution t.
methemoglobin reduction t.
3-methoxy-4-hydroxymandelic
    acid t.
methylene blue t.
methylmalonic acid screen-
    ing t.
methyl red t.
Metopirone t.
metrotrophic t.
metyrapone stimulation t.
MHA-TP (microhemagglutina-
    tion–*Treponema pallidum*) t.
microimmunofluorescent t.
microlymphocytotoxicity t.
microprecipitation t.
Middlebrook-Dubos hemagglu-
    tination t.
migration ihibition t.
Millon-Nasse t.
Minor's starch-iodine t.
mixed t.
mixed lymphocyte culture t.
mobilization t.
Molisch's t.
monocyte function t.
Monospot t.
Montenegro skin t.
Morner's t.
Mosenthal's t.
Motulsky dye reduction t.
mucin t.

mucin clot t.
mucopolysaccharide t.
mucoprotein t.
Multistix t.
Murphy-Pattee t.
mutagenicity t.
Napier formol-gel t.
NBT (nitroblue tetrazolium) t.
neoprecipitin t.
neutralization t.
neutrophil antibody t.
niacin t.
Nickerson-Kveim t.
Nicklès' t.
nitrate reduction t.
nitrate utilization t.
nitroblue tetrazolium t.
nitroprusside t.
nitrosonaphthol t.
nonprotein nitrogen t.
normal lymphocyte transfer t.
Obermayer's t.
Obermüller's t.
occult blood t.
17-OH-corticoids t.
oleic acid uptake t.
one-tailed t.
ONPG (o-nitrophenyl-β-
    galactoside) t.
Optochin susceptibility t.
oral glucose tolerance t.
oral lactose tolerance t.
orcinol t.
osazone t.
osmotic fragility t.
ovarian ascorbic acid deple-
    tion t.
oxidase t.
oxidation-fermentation t.
oxytocin challenge t.
Paget's t.
Paigen t.
pancreatic islet cell antibody t.
pancreozymin-secretin t.
Pandy's t.
Pap t.; Papanicolaou's t.
paper radioimmunosorbent t.
paracoagulation t.
parainfluenza antibody t's
partial thromboplastin time t.
passive hemagglutination t.
patch t.

Paul-Bunnell t.
Paul-Bunnell-Barrett t.
Paul-Bunnell-Davidsohn t.
PBI t.
pentagastrin t.
perchlorate discharge t.
Perls' iron t.
Petri's t.
phenacetin breath t.
Phenistix t.
phenoloxidase production t.
phenolphthalein t.
phenolsulfonphthalein t.
phentolamine t.
phenylketonuria t.
phenylpyruvic acid t's
phosphatase t.
phospholipid t.
phosphoric acid t.
phthalein t.
Piazza's t.
picrate t.
pituitary function t.
placental and fetoplacental
    function t's
plant protease t.
plasmacrit t.
plasma hemoglobin t.
plasma renin activity t.
platelet adhesiveness t.
platelet aggregation t.
platelet retention t.
platelet survival t.
Porges-Meier t.
Porges-Salomon t.
porphobilinogen t.
porphyrin t.
Porter-Silber chromogens t.
Porteus' maze t.
postcoital t.
potassium t.
potassium hydroxide t.
Prausnitz-Küstner t.
precipitin t.
predictive value of negative t.
predictive value of positive t.
pregnancy t's
presumptive heterophile t.
t. profile
prolactin t.
protamine sulfate t.
protamine titration

protein t.
protein-bound iodine t.
protein-bound iodine-131 t.
prothrombin t.
prothrombin consumption t.
prothrombin-proconvertin t.
prothrombin time t.
provocative t.
provocative chelation t.
provocative Wassermann t.
pulmonary function t.
purine bodies t.
pyrrolidonyl aminopeptidase t.
quantitation t.
Queckenstedt's t.
Quellung t.
Quick's t.
quinine carbacrylic resin t.
Quinlan's t.
rabbit t.
radioactive copper t.
radioactive iodide uptake t.
radioactive iodine t.
radioactive iodine uptake t.
radioallergosorbent t.
radioimmunosorbent t.
radiosensitivity t.
RAI t.
RA latex fixation t.
random plasma glucose t.
rank sum t.
rapid plasma reagin t.
rapid streptococcal antigen t.
Rapoport t.
rat-line t.
rat ovarian hyperemia t.
reactone red t.
reagin t.
red t.
red cell survival t.
Rehfuss' t.
Reiner D-xylose absorption t.
Reinsch's t.
Reiter protein complement-
    fixation t.
resorcinol t.
respiratory syncytial virus anti-
    body t's
respiratory syncytial virus anti-
    gen t.
Reuss' t.
Rh blocking t.

rheumatoid factor t's
riboflavin loading t.
Rimini's t.
Rinne's t.
ristocetin aggregation t.
Rocky Mountain spotted fever
    antibody t's
Rogers t.
Ropes t.
rose bengal t.
rose bengal radioactive (^{131}I) t.
Rosenbach-Gmelin t.
Rosenbach's t.
Rose's t.
Rose-Waaler t.
Ross-Jones t.
Rothera's t.
Rothera's nitroprusside t.
Rotter's t.
Rous' t.
Rowntree and Geraghty's t.
RPR (rapid plasma reagin) t.
rubella antibody t's
rubella HI t.
Rubin's t.
Rubner's lactose t.
Rumpel-Leede t.
Sabin-Feldman dye t.
Sachs-Georgi t.
salicylic acid t.
saline agglutination t.
Sanford's t.
Saundby's t.
Schäffer's t.
Schick t.
Schiller's t.
Schilling t.
Schirmer's t.
schistosomiasis serological t.
Schönbein's t.
Schultz-Dale t.
Schumm's t.
Schwarz's t.
scratch t.
screening t.
secretin stimulation t.
sedimentation t.
Selivanoff's t.
Sereny t.
serial dilution protamine sul-
    fate t.
serologic t. for syphilis (STS)

serology t.
serum alkaline phosphatase t.
serum bacterial t.
serum globulin t.
sex chromatin t.
shake t.
sheep cell agglutination t.
Sia t.
sickle cell t.
sickling t.
signed rank t.
silver nitrate t.
silver nitroprusside t.
Sims-Huhner t.
single-breath nitrogen t.
single diffusion t.
skin t.
slide coagulase t.
SMA-12 profile t.
"sniff" t.
sodium bicarbonate t.
sodium hippurate hydrolysis t.
solubility t.
soluble antigen fluorescent anti-
    body t.
t. solution
Southern blot t.
spironolactone t.
split renal function t.
spot t.
spot t. for infectious mononu-
    cleosis
Stamey t.
standard serologic t's for
    syphilis
standing plasma t.
staphylococcal clumping t.
starch tolerance t.
stat t.
t. statistic
Stix reagent strip t.
Strassburg's t.
streptococcal antigen t.
streptozyme agglutinin t.
t. strips
Student's *t* t.
Stypven time t.
sucrose hemolysis t.
sucrose tolerance t.
sulfosalicylic acid turbidity t.
Sulkowitch's t.
sweat t.

t (statistical hypothesis)-t.
Takata-Ara t.
tanned red cell hemagglutination inhibition t.
tetrazolium t.
Thayer-Martin t.
thermoagglutination t.
Thompson's t.
Thormählen's t.
Thorn t.
three-glass t.
thrombin time t.
thromboplastin activation t.
thromboplastin generation t.
thymol turbidity t.
thyroid-stimulating hormone stimulation t.
thyroid suppression t.
thyroid uptake t's
thyrotropin-releasing hormone stimulation t.
thyroxine-binding index t.
tine t.
tissue thromboplastin inhibition t.
titratable acidity t.
toad t.
tolbutamide t.
tolbutamide tolerance t.
Töpfer's t.
total catecholamine t.
TPI (*Treponema pallidum* immobilization) t.
transaminase t.
transcriptase reverse t.
treponemal immobilization t.
Treponema pallidum hemagglutination t.
Treponema pallidum immobilization t.
TRH (thyrotropin-releasing hormone) stimulation t.
triiodothyronine resin uptake t.
triiodothyronine suppression t.
triiodothyronine uptake t.
trypsin t.
tryptophan load t.
TSH (thyroid-stimulating hormone) t.
T_3U (triiodothyronine uptake) t.

tube coagulase t.
tube dilution t.
tubeless gastric analysis t.
tuberculin t.
tumor skin t.
T_3 uptake t.
two-glass t.
two-tailed t.
typhus antibody t.
tyramine t.
tyrosine t.
Tzanck's t.
Uffelmann's t.
unheated serum reagin t.
urea clearance t.
urea nitrogen t.
urease t.
urinary concentration t.
urine acetone t.
urobilinogen t.
Valentine's t.
van Deen's t.
van de Kamer t.
van den Bergh's t.
van der Velden's t.
vanillylmandelic acid t.
Van Slyke's t.
varicella-zoster antibody t.
VDRL (Venereal Disease Research Laboratories) t.
vitamin A clearance t.
vitamin B_{12} absorption t.
VMA (vanillylmandelic acid) t.
Voges-Proskauer t.
Volhard's t.
Vollmer's t.
Wagner's t.
Waldenström's t.
Wang's t.
Wassén t.
Wassermann's t.
water deprivation t.
Watson-Schwartz t.
Weber's t.
Webster's t.
Weil-Felix t.
Werner's t.
Western blot t.
Westgard quality control t.
Wetzel's t.
wheal-and-erythema skin t's

Wheeler-Johnson t.
Widal's t.
Wilbrand's prism t.
wire loop t.
Woldman's t.
Wormley's t.
Wurster's t.
xylose absorption t.
D-xylose absorption t.
xylose concentration t.
D-xylose tolerance t.
Yvon's t.
Zappacosta's t.
Zimmermann's t.
zinc flocculation t.
zinc-sulfate turbidity t.
zinc turbidity t.
Zondek-Aschheim t.
Zsigmondy's t.

Tes-Tape
testcross
testicle
testicular
t. adenocarcinoma
t. agenesis
t. artery
t. atrophy
t. biopsy
t. cancer
t. compression reflex
t. dysgenesis
t. feminization
t. feminization syndrome
t. germ-cell tumor
t. germinoma
t. hormone
t. interstitium
t. ischemia
t. leukemia
t. maturation
t. purpura
t. regression syndrome
t. teratoma
t. tubular adenoma
t. tumor
t. vasculitis
t. vein
testiculoma ovarii
testing
antibacterial agent susceptibility t.
antimicrobial susceptibility t.

automated reagin t.
avidity t.
bacterial susceptibility t.
calcitonin t.
forensic t.
hypothesis t.
paternity t.
performance t.
susceptibility t.
testis (pl., testes)
appendix of t.
Cooper's irritable t.
cryptorchid t.
ectopic t.
efferent ductule of t.
fetal t.
gubernaculum of t.
interstitial tissue of t.
inverted t.
lobule of t.
lymphatics of t.
mediastinum t.
mesothelioma of t.
movable t.
obstructed t.
prepubertal t.
pulpy t.
t. redux
retained t.
retractile t.
rudimentary t.
supernumerary t.
undescended t.
testitis
testoid hyperthecosis
testolactone
testopathy
testosterone
t.-binding affinity
t. cyclopentylpropionate
t. cypionate
t. enanthate
t.-estradiol-binding globulin
fetal t.
free t.
t. ketolaurate
methyl t.
t. phenylacetate
t. production rate
t. synthesis
t.-to-estradiol ratio

testotoxicosis
    familial t.
Tet — tetanus
    tetralogy of Fallot
tetanic contraction
tetanolysin
tetanospasmin
tetanus
    t. antibody
    t. antitoxin
    t. antitoxin unit
    t. bacillus
    t.-diphtheria
    t. toxin immunization
      reaction
tetany
TETD — tetraethylthiuram disulfide
tetrabromobenzoquinone
tetrabromo-o-cresol
tetrabromophenol blue
tetracaine hydrochloride
tetracarcinoma cells
tetrachlorethane poisoning
tetrachloride
    carbon t.
tetrachlorobenzoquinone
tetrachlorodiphenyl sulfone
tetrachloroethane
tetrachloroethylene
tetrachlorophenol-
    tetrabromosulfophthalein
tetrachloroquinone
n-tetracosanoic acid
tetracyclic
tetracycline
tetrad
tetradecanoyl phorbol acetate
tetraethyl
    t. lead
    t. pyrophosphate
tetrahedron chest
tetrahydrobiopterin
tetrahydrocannabinol
tetrahydro-compound S
tetrahydrocortisol
tetrahydrocortisone
tetrahydrodeoxycorticosterone
tetrahydro-11-deoxycortisol
tetrahydrofolate
    t. dehydrogenase
    methylene t.
tetrahydrofolic acid

tetrahydrofuran
tetrahydronaphthalene
tetrahydropteroylglutamate methyl-
    transferase
tetrahydrozoline hydrochloride
tetralogy
    t. of Eisenmenger
    t. of Fallot
tetramastigote
tetramer
tetramethyl
    t. acridine
    t. lead
tetramethylbenzidine
Tetramitidae
tetranitrate
    pentaerythritol t.
tetranitromethane
tetraphenylporphine sulfonate
tetraplegia
tetraploid
tetraploidy
tetrapyrrole
tetrasodium pyrophosphate
tetrasomic
tetrasomy
Tetratrichomonas
    T. buccalis
    T. hominis
tetravalent
tetra-X chromosomal aberration
tetrazole
tetrazolium
    nitroblue t.
    t. reduction
    t. reduction inhibition
    t. salts
    t. test
tetrazonium salts
tetrodotoxin
tetrohydrodeoxyuridine
tetrose
tetroxide
    dinitrogen t.
    nitrogen t.
    osmium t.
tetrulose
tetryl
TF — tactile fremitus
    tetralogy of Fallot
    thymol flocculation
    tissue-damaging factor

transfer factor
tuberculin filtrate
tubular fluid
TFA — total fatty acids
T factor
TFE — polytetrafluoroethylene
    tetrafluoroethylene
Tfm — testicular feminization syndrome
TF-R — transferrin receptor
TFS — testicular feminization syndrome
TG — thioguanine
    thyroglobulin
    toxic goiter
    triglyceride
TGA — transposition of the great arteries
TGAR — total graft area rejected
TGFA — triglyceride fatty acid
TGL — triglyceride
    triglyceride lipase
TGT — thromboplastin generation test
    thromboplastin generation time
TGV — thoracic gas volume
    transposition of the great vessels
TH — thyrohyoid
Th — thorium
th — thoracic
THA — total hydroxyapatite
thalamencephalon
thalamic
    t. fasciculus
    t. radiation
thalamocortical
thalamogeniculate artery
thalamo-olivary tract
thalamosensory cortical fibers
thalamotemporal radiation
thalamus (pl., thalami)
    external medullary lamina of t.
    inferior peduncular interstitial nucleus of t.
    internal medullary lamina of t.
    interoanterodorsal nucleus of t.
    interoanteromedial nucleus of t.
    interoanteroventral nucleus of t.

    intralaminar nucleus of t.
    lateral ventral nucleus of t.
    medial nucleus of t.
    nucleus circularis of t.
    nucleus dorsointermedius externus of t.
    nucleus limitans of t.
    paracentral nucleus of t.
    parafascicular nucleus of t.
    posterolateral ventral nucleus of t.
    posteroventralis nucleus of t.
    reticular nucleus of t.
    rhomboid nucleus of t.
    superficial dorsal nucleus of t.
    ventral t.
thalassemia; thalassanemia
    A_2 t.
    alpha t.
    α-t.
    beta t.
    β-t.
    β-δ t.
    delta-beta t.
    F t.
    gamma-delta-beta t.
    hemoglobin C–type t.
    hemoglobin E–type t.
    heterozygous t.
    homozygous t.
    t. intermedia
    α-t. intermedia
    Lepore t.
    t. major
    t. minor
    mixed t.
    sickle cell t.
    t. trait
thalassemic hemoglobinopathy
thalidomide
thallitoxicosis
thallium
    t. assay
    t. poisoning
    t. sulfate
thallospore
thallous chloride
thallus
THAM — tris(hydroxymethyl)aminomethane
thanatophoric dwarfism
thanatopsy

thanite
thaumatropy
Thaumetopoea
Thaumetopoeidae
Thayer-Martin
    agar
    medium
    test
THC — tetrahydrocannabinol
THDOC — tetrahydrodeoxycorticos-
    terone
THE — tetrahydrocortisone
thebaine
theca (pl., thecae)
    t. cell
    t. cell–granuloma cell tumor
    t. cell tumor
    t. folliculi
    t. lutein cyst
    t. lutein tumor
thecal
    t. abscess
    t. metaplasia
theca lutein cyst
thecitis
thecoma
thecomatosis
Theiler's virus
Thelazia callipaeda
thelaziasis
theliolymphocyte
thelium (pl., thelia)
theloncus
T helper cells
thenar
thenyldiamine hydrochloride
thenylpyramine
theobromine
theolin
theophylline
    t. assay
    t. poisoning
theorem
    Bayes' t.
    central limit t.
theoretical
    t. plate
    t. science
theory
    Cannon-Bard t.
    Cannon's t.
    Cohnheim's t.
    deletion t.
    emigration t.
    Fisher-Race t.
    "fitter" cell t.
    Frerichs' t.
    gametoid t.
    germ-line t.
    hematogenous t. of endome-
        triosis
    information t.
    Kern's plasma relation t.
    lattice t.
    lymphatic dissemination t. of
        endometriosis
    Metchnikoff's (Mechnikov's)
        cellular immunity t.
    monophyletic t.
    network t.
    polyphyletic t.
    Ribbert's t.
    side-chain t.
    somatic mutation t. of cancer
    template t.
    Warburg's t.
theque
therapeutic
    t. abortion
    t. phlebotomy
    t. pneumothorax
    t. ratio
therapy
    anticoagulant t.
    antiplatelet t.
    Calmette-Guérin bacillus t.
    cancer management t.
    chelation t.
    combined modality t.
    cytoreductive t.
    gold t.
    high-voltage roentgen t.
    hormonal t.
    immunosuppressive t.
    insulin coma t.
    insulin shock t.
    intraosseous t.
    intraperitoneal t.
    intrathecal t.
    intravesical t.
    iron chelation t.
    laser t.
    neoadjuvant t.
    neutron beam t.
    nutritional t.

opsonic t.
oxygen t.
radiation t.
radium t.
thrombolytic t.
thermal
    t. anesthesia
    t. conductivity
    t. conductivity detector
    t. death point
    t. death time
    t. equilibrium
    t. hypesthesia
    t. neutron
    t. receptor
thermelometer
thermionic emission
thermistor
Thermoactinomyces
    T. candidus
    T. sacchari
    T. vulgaris
thermochemistry
thermocoagulation
thermocouple thermometer
thermodilution
thermoduric
thermodynamic equilibrium
thermodynamics
thermogenesis
    nonshivering t.
    shivering t.
thermogenic action
thermogenin
thermogram
thermograph
    continuous scan t.
thermography
    infrared tympanic t.
    tympanic t.
thermolabile
Thermolospora viridis
thermoluminescence
thermoluminescent
    t. detector
    t. dosimeter
Thermolyne Maxi-Mix
thermolysis
thermometer
    air t.
    alcohol t.
    axilla t.

Beckmann's t.
bimetal t.
Celsius t.
centigrade t.
clinical t.
differential t.
Fahrenheit t.
gas t.
Kelvin's t.
liquid-in-glass t.
maximum t.
mercurial t.
metallic t.
metastatic t.
minimum t.
oral t.
Rankine's t.
Réaumur's t.
recording t.
rectal t.
resistance t.
thermocouple t.
thermometry
thermophile
thermophilic
    t. actinomycete
    t. bacterium
thermoprecipitin reaction
thermoresistant
thermostable
    t. alkaline phosphatase
    t. body
thermotaxis
thermotropism
thesaurismosis
thesaurocyte
theta
    t. antigen
    t. band
THF — tetrahydrofolic acid
    tetrahydrofuran
    thymic humoral factor
THFA — tetrahydrofolic acid
THI — transient hypogammaglobuli-
    nemia of infancy
thial
thiamin; thiamine
    t. assay
    t. chloride unit
    t. deficiency
    t. hydrochloride
    t. hydrochloride unit

t. mononitrate
t. nitrate
phosphorylated t.
t. pyrophosphokinase
thiaminase
thiamphenicol assay
thiamylal sodium
Thiara
Thiaridae
thiazide
t. diabetes
t. diuretic
thiazin
thiazinamium chloride
thiazine
t. dye
t. stain
thiazole dye
thiazolsulfone
thickening
hyaline t.
thick-layer autoradiography
thickness
absorption-equivalent t.
Breslow's t.
mean corpuscular t.
thiemia
Thiersch's canaliculi
thiethylperazine maleate
thihexinol methylbromide
thimerosal
thin-layer
t.-l. chromatography
t.-l. electrophoresis
t.-l. immunoassay
"thin line" apolipoprotein
thin-needle biopsy
thin section
thio-acid
thioaldehyde
thiobarbiturate
thiocarbarsone
thiocarbonyl group
thiocholine
propionyl t.
thiochrome
thioctic acid
thiocyanate
potassium t.
Thiodan
thiodiphenylamine
thioester

thioethanolamine acetyl-transferase
thioether
thioflavine; thioflavin
t. S
t. T
t. T stain
thioglycolic acid
thioglycollate
t. broth
fluid t.
t. medium
thioglycollate-135 C broth
thioglycollic acid
thioguanine
thioketone
thiokinase
thiol
thiolaminopropionic acid
thiolase
acetoacetyl-CoA t.
thiolesterase
thiolester hydrolase
thioltransacetylase
thiolysis
thionamide
thione
thioneb
thionin; thionine
thiopental sodium
thiophene
thiophosphate
thiopropazate hydrochloride
thioproperazine mesylate
thioredoxin
thioridazine
t. assay
t. hydrochloride
thiosulfate
t. citrate
t. citrate bile salts sucrose
t. salt
t. sulfurtransferase
thiotepa
thiothixene hydrochloride
thiouracil
thiourea
thioxanthene tranquilizers
thiram
third
t. corpuscle
t. cranial nerve
t.-degree burn

t.-degree frostbite
t.-degree heart block
t.-degree radiation injury
t. trimester pregnancy
thistle seed agar
thixotropic
thixotropy
TH_2O — titrated water
Thoma's
counting chamber
fixative
Thompson's test
Thomsen-Friedenreich antigen
Thoms method
thonzylamine hydrochloride
thoracentesis
thoracic
t. actinomycosis
t. aneurysm
t. aorta
t. artery
t. asphyxiant dystrophy
t. branches, axillary artery
t. cavity
t. duct
t. duct fistula
t. dysplasia
t. esophagus
t. fistula
t. gas volume
t. goiter
t. index
t. kidney
t. limb
t. myotome
t. nerve
t.-pelvic-phalangeal dystrophy
t. portion, sympathetic nervous system
t. spinal cord
t. sympathetic ganglion
t. sympathetic nervous system
t. sympathetic trunk
t. vein
t. vertebra
t. vertebral joint
t. viscera
thoracoabdominal
thoracoacromial artery
thoracoepigastric vein
thoracolaparotomy

thoracolumbar
t. fascia
t. region
thoracopagus parasiticus
thoracopathy
thoracoplasty
thoracopulmonary
thoracostomy
thoracotomy
thorax (pl., thoraces)
Thorazine
thorium isotope
Thormählen's test
thorn apple crystals
Thorn test
Thornwaldt's
abscess
cyst
thoron
Thorotrast
THP — total hydroxyproline
Thr — threonine
thread
mucous t's
threadworm
threatened abortion
three-day test
three-glass test
three-Hertz spike and slow waves
three-part mitosis
three-phase current
three-point cross
threonine; threonin
t. aldolase
t. dehydratase
threonyl
threonyl-RNA synthetase
threose
thresher's lung
threshold
arousal t.
t. body
t. dose
t. erythema dose
t. limit values
mean cell t.
median detection t.
renal t.
t. substance
thrill
aneurysmal t.
aortic t.

diastolic t.
hydatid t.
presystolic t.
systolic t.
throat
    t. culture
    putrid t.
    t. swab
thrombase
thrombasthenia
    Glanzmann-Naegeli t.
    Glanzmann's t.
    hereditary hemorrhagic t.
thrombin
    t. clotting time
    t. time
    t. time test
thrombinogen
thrombinogenesis
thromboagglutinin
thromboangiitis obliterans
thromboarteritis purulenta
thromboasthenia
thromboblast
thromboclasis
thrombocounter whole blood
    lysing kit
thrombocyst; thrombocystis
thrombocytapheresis
thrombocytasthenia
thrombocyte
thrombocythemia
    essential t.
    hemorrhagic t.
    primary t.
thrombocytic
    t. leukemia
    t. series
thrombocytin
thrombocytocrit
thrombocytolysis
thrombocytopathy
thrombocytopenia
    amegakaryocytic t.
    autoimmune t.
    drug-induced t.
    essential t.
    hypersplenic t.
    immune t.
    isoimmune t.
    neonatal t.
    post-transfusion t.

    splenomegalic t.
    thrombotic t.
    t. with absence of radius
thrombocytopenic purpura
    autoimmune t.p.
    idiopathic t.p.
thrombocytopoiesis
thrombocytosis
thromboelastogram
thromboembolic disease
thromboembolism
    pulmonary t.
    venous t.
thromboendarterectomy
thromboendarteritis
thromboendocarditis
thrombogene; Thrombogen
thrombogenesis
    hemodynamic t.
thrombogenic
thrombogenicity
β-thromboglobulin
thromboid
thrombokatilysin
thrombokinase
thrombolic
thrombolus
thrombolymphangitis
thrombolysis
thrombolytic
    t. agents
    t. therapy
thrombometer
thrombomodulin
thrombon
thrombonecrosis
    arteriolar t.
thrombo-occlusive
thrombopathia
thrombopathic syndrome
thrombopathy
    constitutional t.
thrombopenia
thrombopenic anemia
thrombophilia
thrombophlebitis
    t. migrans
    migrating t.
    migratory t.
    t. saltans
thromboplastic
    t. plasma component
    t. substance

thromboplastid
thromboplastin
    t. activation test
    t. antecedent deficiency
    automated activated partial t.
    t. generation test
    t. generation time
    tissue t.
thromboplastinogen
thromboplastinogenase
thromboplastinogenemia
thromboplastin substitution test
thrombopoiesis
thrombopoietin
thrombosed
    t. aneurysm
    t. arteriosclerotic aneurysm
    t. hemorrhoid
thrombosin
thrombosis (pl., thromboses)
    agonal t.
    arterial t.
    atrophic t.
    cardiac t.
    cerebral t.
    coagulative t.
    coronary t.
    dilatation t.
    hemodynamic t.
    marantic t.
    marasmic t.
    mesenteric t.
    microcirculatory t.
    mural t.
    occlusive t.
    placental t.
    plate t.
    platelet t.
    portal vein t.
    propagating t.
    puerperal t.
    renal vein t.
    traumatic t.
    venous t.
thrombospondin
thrombostasis
thrombosthenin
thrombotic
    t. endocarditis
    t. gangrene
    t. infarct
    t. microangiopathy

    t. nonbacterial endocarditis
    t. occlusion
    t. phlegmasia
    t. thrombocytopenic purpura
thrombotonin
thromboxane
    t. A_2
    t. B_2
    t. synthetase
thrombozyme
thrombus (pl., thrombi)
    agglutinative t.
    agonal t.
    antemortem t.
    arterial t.
    ball t.
    ball-valve t.
    bile t.
    blood platelet t.
    canalized t.
    fibrin t.
    globular t.
    hyaline t.
    infective t.
    laminated t.
    marantic t.
    marasmic t.
    mixed t.
    mural t.
    old t.
    organized t.
    pale t.
    parietal t.
    platelet t.
    postmortem t.
    recent t.
    red t.
    secondary t.
    stratified t.
    tumor t.
    valvular t.
    white t.
through-and-through myocardial
    infarction
thrush
    t. culture
THS — tetrahydro-compound S
thulium
thumb
    bifid t.
    hitchhiker t's
    metacarpophalangeal joint of t.

phalanges of t.
tennis t.
Z t.
thumbprinting
Thy-1 antigen
thylacitis
thyme
thymectomy
thymic
    t. abscesses
    t. agenesis
    t. alymphoplasia
    t. aplasia
    t. artery
    t. capsule
    t. carcinoma
    t. cortex
    t. dysplasia
    t. epithelial cells
    t. epithelium
    t. factor
    t. hormone
    t. humoral factor
    t. hypoplasia
    t. leukemia
    t. lobule
    t. lymphocyte
    t. lymphopoietic factor
    t. medulla
    t.-parathyroid aplasia
    t. peptides
    t.-replacing factor
    t. reticulum cell
    t. transplantation
    t. tumors
    t. vein
thymidine
    t. diphosphate
    t. monophosphate
    t.-5'-phosphate
    t. phosphorylase
    t. triphosphate
    tritiated t.
thymidylic acid
thymidylyl
thymin
thymine
    t.-2-deoxyriboside
    t. dimer
    t. ribonucleoside
    t. ribonucleoside phosphate
    t. ribonucleoside-5'-phosphate

thymitis
thymocyte
thymocytotoxic autoantibody
thymol
    t. blue indicator
    t. flocculation
    t. iodide
    t. phthalein
    t. turbidity
    t. turbidity test
Thymolin
thymolipoma
thymolphthalein
    t. indicator
    t. monophosphate
thymoma
    cervical t.
    epithelial t.
    granulomatous t.
    hamartomatous t.
    lymphocytic t.
    perithyroidal t.
    spindle cell t.
thymometastasis
thymonucleic acid
thymopathy
    mitochondrial t.
thymopharyngeal duct
thymopoietin
thymosin alpha-1
thymostimulin
thymulin
thymus
    t. cell
    t.-dependent antigen
    t.-dependent lymphocytes
    t. gland
    t.-independent antigen
    t.-independent lymphocytes
    t.-leukemia antigen
thyristor
thyroadenitis
thyrocalcitonin
thyrocele
thyrocervical trunk
thyrocolloid
thyroglobulin
thyroglossal
    t. duct/cyst
    t. fistula
thyrohyoid muscle

thyroid
- aberrant t.
- t. antimicrosomal antibodies
- t. antithyroglobulin antibodies
- t. artery
- t. cachexia
- t. capsule
- t. carcinoma
- t. cartilage
- t. colloid
- t. crisis
- t. cyst
- ectopic t.
- t. endocrine disorder
- t. extract
- t. follicle
- t. gland
- t. hormone
- t. isthmus
- t. ^{131}I uptake
- lateral t.
- t. leukemia
- lingual t.
- t. lobe
- t. lobule
- medullary carcinoma of t.
- t. microsomal antibodies
- t. nerve
- t. nodule
- ovarian t.
- t. radioiodine uptake
- t. rests
- t. scan
- t.-stimulating hormone assay
- t.-stimulating hormone stimulation
- t.-stimulating immunoglobulin
- t. storm
- t. suppression test
- t.-to-serum ratio
- t. tumor
- t. uptake of radioactive iodine
- t. uptake tests
- t. vein

thyroidal
- t. agenesis
- t. clearance

thyroidea
- t. accessoria
- t. ima
- t. ima artery

thyroidectomize

thyroidectomy

thyroiditis
- acute t.
- amiodarone-associated t.
- autoimmune t.
- chronic t.
- chronic atrophic t.
- de Quervain's t.
- diphenylhydantoin-associated t.
- drug-associated t.
- focal lymphocytic t.
- fungal t.
- giant cell t.
- granulomatous t.
- Hashimoto's t.
- induced t.
- invasive fibrous t.
- iodide-associated t.
- ligneous t.
- lithium-associated t.
- lymphocytic t.
- lymphoma-like t.
- "martial arts" t.
- nonspecific t.
- nonsuppurative t.
- palpation t.
- parasitic t.
- pseudogranulomatous t.
- pseudotuberculous t.
- radiation-related t.
- Riedel's t.
- subacute t.
- subacute granulomatous t.
- subacute lymphocytic t.
- suppurative t.
- tuberculous t.

thyroidization

thyrolingual cyst

thyrolipoma

thyrolytic

thyromegaly

thyropathy

thyroplasia

thyroptosis

thyrosis

thyrotome

thyrotomy

thyrotoxic
- t. cardiomyopathy
- t. crisis/storm

t. myopathy
t. serum
thyrotoxicosis
autoimmune t.
t. factitia
thyrotoxin shock
thyrotrope; thyrotroph
thyrotropic
t. adenoma
t. hormone
t. tumor
thyrotropin
t.-producing adenoma
t.-receptor antibody
t.-releasing factor
t.-releasing hormone
t.-releasing hormone stimulation test
thyroxine; thyroxin
t. assay
t.-binding albumin
t.-binding globulin
t.-binding globulin assay
t.-binding index
t.-binding index test
t.-binding prealbumin
t.-binding protein
free (unbound) t.
t. specific activity
total t.
THz — terahertz
TI — thoracic index
time interval
transverse inlet
tricuspid incompetence
tricuspid insufficiency
Ti — titanium
TIA — transient ischemic attack
TIBC — total iron-binding capacity
tibia (pl., tibiae)
saber t.
t. valga
t. vara
tibial
t. anterior muscle bursa, subtendinous
t. artery
t. astragaloid joint
t. muscle, anterior
t. muscle, posterior
t. nerve
t. tuberosity

t. tuberosity of subcutaneous bursa
t. vein
tibialgia
tibiofibular joint
TIC — trypsin-inhibitory capacity
ticarcillin
tic douloureux
tick
African t.-borne fever
t. bite
t.-borne virus
Colorado t. fever
t. fever
t. paralysis
tic-tac rhythm
TID — titrated initial dose
tide
acid t.
alkaline t.
fat t.
TIE — transient ischemic episode
Tierfellnaevus
Tietz-Fiereck method
tiger heart
tiglium
tigroid striation
time
access t.
activated coagulation t.
activated partial thromboplastin t.
bleeding t.
blood-clot lysis t.
calcium t.
cell cycle t.
circulation t.
clot-lysis t.
clot retraction t.
clotting t.
coagulation t.
conduction t.
dead t.
decimal reduction t.
t. diffusion technique
doubling t.
Duke bleeding t.
Duke's method of bleeding t.
electrode response t.
euglobulin clot lysis t.
euglobulin lysis t.
execution t.

gastric emptying t.
generation t.
grain count halving t.
helium equilibration t.
t. interval
isovolumic relaxation t.
Ivy's method of bleeding t.
kaolin partial thromboplas-
     tin t.
t.-kill rate
lag t.
t. of maximum concentration
mean circulation t.
mean generation t.
occlusion t.
one-stage prothrombin t.
operating t.
partial thromboplastin t.
particle transport t.
plasma clotting t.
plasma-iron disappearance t.
prolonged bleeding t.
prolonged coagulation t.
prothrombin t.
prothrombin consumption t.
reaction t.
recalcification t.
recovery t.
t.-resolved fluoroimmunoassay
resolving t.
retention t.
Russell's viper venom t.
RV (residual volume) t.
serial thrombin t.
t. series analysis
serum prothrombin t.
t.-sharing
shortened bleeding t.
shortened coagulation t.
stimulus-response t.
Stypven t.
survival t.
t.-tension index
thermal death t.
thrombin t.
thrombin-clotting t.
thromboplastin generation t.
turnaround t.
utilization t.
wash t.
wheal reaction t.

whole blood clot lysis t.
whole-blood clotting t.
timer
timolol maleate
timothy bacillus
TIN — tubulointerstitial nephropathy
tin
     t. chloride
     t. oxide
tinctable
tinction
tinctorial
tincture
     belladonna t.
     t. of iodine
tinea
     t. amiantacea
     t. barbae
     t. capitis
     t. ciliorum
     t. circinata
     t. corporis
     t. cruris
     t. favosa
     t. glabrosa
     t. imbricata
     t. kerion
     t. manuum
     t. nigra
     t. pedis
     t. sycosis
     t. unguium
     t. versicolor
Tinel's sign
tine test
tingibility
tingible
tinnitus
tint
TIS — tumor in situ
Tiselius' apparatus
tissue
     aberrant t.
     adipose t.
     areolar t.
     areolar connective t.
     bile pigment demonstration
          in t.
     bilirubin demonstration in t.
     "bursa-equivalent" t.
     cancellous t.
     chondroid t.

cicatricial t.
t.-coding factor
connective t.
t. culture
t. culture dose
t. culture infectious dose
t. culture infective dose
t. culture medium
t.-damaging factor
diffuse lymphatic t.
ectopic thyroid t.
elastic t.
endothelial t.
t.-equivalent
extracellular t.
t. factor
fibroadipose t.
fibrous t.
t. glycogen
granulation t.
gut-associated lymphoid t.
hard t.
hematopoietic t.
hemoglobin demonstration
   in t.
homologous t.
hormone demonstration in t.
inflammation of connective t.
interstitial t.
t. kallikrein
lead demonstration in t.
t. lymph
lymphoid t.
mesenchymal t.
monocytic t.
mucosa-associated lymphoid t.
mucous connective t.
myeloid t.
nephrogenic t.
osteogenic t.
t. plasminogen activator
t. polypeptide antigen
t. processing
soft t.
t.-specific antigen
splenic t.
subcutaneous t.
t. thromboplastin
t. thromboplastin inhibition
   test
t. tolerance dose
tuberculosis granulation t.
t. typing

TIT — triiodothyronine
titanium dioxide
titanium ray
titer
   agglutination t.
   antibody t.
   antihyaluronidase t.
   anti-Rh t.
   ASO (antistreptolysin-O) t.
   CF antibody t.
   coxsackie A virus t.
   fibrin t.
   hemagglutination t.
   mumps antibody t.
   Q fever t.
titian yellow
titrant
titratable
   t. acid
   t. acidity
   t. acidity test
titrated initial dose
titration
   coulometric t.
   potentiometric t.
   t. technique
titrator
   Cotlove t.
titrimetric
titrimetry
Tityus serrulatus
TIVC — thoracic inferior vena cava
Tizzoni's stain
TKA — transketolase activity
TKD — tokodynamometer
TKG — tokodynagraph
Tl — thallium
TL (thymus-leukemia) antigen
TLA — translumbar aortogram
TLC — thin-layer chromatography
   total L-chain concentration
   total lung capacity
   total lung compliance
TLD — thermoluminescent dosimeter
   tumor lethal dose
T/LD_{100} — minimum dose causing
      death or malformation
      of 100% of fetuses
TLE — thin-layer electrophoresis
TLV — threshold limit value
T lymphocyte
   T l. cytotoxicity
   T l. hybridoma

TM — temporomandibular
temporomandibular
transmetatarsal
tympanic membrane
T_m — maximal tubular excretory
capacity of the kidneys
T_{max} — time of maximum concentration
T_{mg} or TmG — maximal tubular reabsorption of glucose
Tm — thulium
TMA — trimethoxyamphetamine
TMJ — temporomandibular joint
TML — tetramethyl lead
T-4 molecule
TMP — thymidine monophosphate
thymine ribonucleoside
phosphate
trimethoprim
TMTD — tetramethylthiuram disulfide
TMV — tobacco mosaic virus
Tn — normal intraocular tension
Tn antigen
T_4 newborn screen
TNF — tumor necrosis factor
TNI — total nodal irradiation
TNM — (primary) tumor, (regional
lymph) nodes, (remote)
metastases—cancer grading system
TNM staging
TNT — trinitrotoluene
TNTC — too numerous to count
TO — original tuberculin
tincture of opium
TOA — tubo-ovarian abscess
toad
t. test
t. toxin
tobacco mosaic virus
Tobie, von Brand, and Mehlman diphasic medium
tobramycin
tocainide
tocol
tocopherol
tocopheryl
tocotrienol
TOCP — triorthocresyl phosphate
Todd
bodies
units

Todd-Hewitt broth
toe
clubbed t's
Hong Kong t.
Morton's t.
webbed t's
togavirus
toggle
Toison's stain
tokodynagraph
tokodynamometer
tolazamide
tolazoline hydrochloride
tolbutamide
t. test
t. tolerance test
tolerance
B-cell t.
drug t.
glucose t.
high-zone t.
immunologic t.
t. interval
low-zone t.
tolerogen
tolerogenic
o-tolidine
tolmetin sodium
tolnaftate
tolonium chloride
toluene
t. diisocyanate
t. 2,4-diisocyanate
p-toluenesulfonic acid reagent
toluic acid
toluidine
alkaline t.
t. blue O
t. blue stain
p-toluidine
toluol
p-toluylenediamine
toluylene red
N-m-tolyl phthalamic acid
tomaculous
tomato tumor
Tomes'
fibers
process
tomogram
tomographic imaging

tomography
>   axial transverse t.
>   computed t.
>   panoramic t.
>   plesiosectional t.
>   positron emission t.
>   rotational t.
>   simultaneous multifilm t.
>   transversal t.
>   ultrasonic t.

tomolaryngography
tone
toner
tongue
>   bifid t.
>   black t.
>   black hairy t.
>   cleft t.
>   raspberry t.
>   strawberry t.
>   t. worms

tonic-clonic attack
tonicity
toning
>   gold t.

tonofibril
tonofilament
tonography
tonometer
tonotopic
tonsil
>   cerebellar t.
>   faucial t.
>   lingual t.
>   pharyngeal t.

tonsillar
>   t. branch, glossopharyngeal
>   nerve
>   t. branch, ninth cranial nerve
>   t. capsule
>   t. cerebellar herniation
>   t. crypts
>   t. fossa
>   t. herniation
>   t. pillar

tonsillectomy
tonsillitis
>   staphylococcal t.
>   streptococcal t.
>   viral t.
>   *Yersinia* t.

tooth
>   deciduous t.
>   developing t.
>   permanent t.
>   t. pulp
>   t. root
>   t. socket
>   supplemental t.

Töpfer's test
tophaceous gout
tophus (pl., tophi)
>   gouty t.

topical
>   t. calciphylaxis
>   t. chemotherapy

topographic breast
topography
topopathogenesis
TOPV — trivalent oral poliovirus
>   vaccine
TORCH — toxoplasmosis, rubella, cy-
>   tomegalovirus, and her-
>   pes simplex
torcular Herophili
Tornwaldt's
>   abscess
>   cyst

torocyte
torose; torous
TORP — total ossicular replacement
>   prosthesis
torque
torr
torsades de pointes
torsion
>   t. injury
>   intrauterine t.
>   neonatal t.
>   t. spasm
>   t. of testis

torticollis
>   congenital t.

tortuosity
Torula
>   *T. capsulatus*
>   *T. histolytica*

torular meningitis
toruli tactiles
toruloma
Torulopsis glabrata
torulopsosis
torulosis

torus (pl., tori)
  mandibular t.
  t. palatinus
tosylate
total
  t. acidity
  t. antitryptic activity
  t. blood granulocyte pool
  t. blood volume
  t. body clearance
  t. body density
  t. body fat
  t. body hematocrit
  t. body potassium
  t. body radiation
  t. body solute
  t. body water
  t. body weight
  t. calcium assay
  t. catecholamine test
  t. cell count
  t. cholesterol
  t. circulating hemoglobin
  t.-dose infusion
  t. electromechanical systole
  t. estriol
  t. estrogen (excretion)
  t. exchangeable potassium measurement
  t. fatty acids
  t. graft area rejected
  t. hematuria
  t. internal reflection
  t. iron-binding capacity
  t. L-chain concentration
  t. lung capacity
  t. necrosis
  t. oxidants
  t. peripheral resistance
  t. protein
  t. pulmonary resistance
  t. pulmonary vascular resistance
  t. resistance
  t. response
  t. ridge count
  t. serum prostatic acid phosphatase
  t. serum protein
  t. thyroxine
  t. urinary gonadotropin
  t. ventilation

totipotency
totipotential cells
touch receptor
tourniquet
Touton giant cells
Towne's projection
toxalbumin
toxanemia
toxaphene
toxemia
  pre-eclamptic t.
  t. of pregnancy
toxemic
  t. jaundice
  t. schistosomiasis
toxic
  t. acute tubular necrosis
  t. adenoma
  t. chemical handling
  t. cirrhosis
  t. cyanosis
  t. dermatitis
  t. epidermal necrolysis
  t. equivalent
  t. erythema
  t. glycosuria
  t. goiter
  t. granulation
  t. granule
  t. hemoglobinuria
  t. hemolytic anemia
  t. idiopathy
  t. leukocytosis
  t. megacolon
  t. methemoglobinemia
  t. multinodular goiter
  t. nephrosis
  t. neuropathy
  t. nodular goiter
  t. oxygen radicals
  t. shock
  t. shock syndrome
  t. unit
  t. waste
toxicant
toxicemia
toxicity
  acetaminophen hepatic t.
  aluminum t.
  aspirin t.
  EP t.
  renal t.

toxicologic
toxicologist
toxicology
     analytical t.
     clinical t.
     environmental t.
     forensic t.
     industrial t.
toxicopathic
toxicosis
toxigenic bacterium
toxigenicity
toxin
     antitetanus t.
     t.-antitoxin
     bee venom t.
     botulinum t.
     Coley's t.
     erythrogenic t.
     fungal t.
     Shiga's t.
     toad t.
Toxocara
     T. canis
     T. cati
     T. mystax
toxocariasis
toxohormone
toxoid
     alum-precipitated t.
     t.-antitoxin floccules
     t.-antitoxin mixture
     t.-antitoxoid
Toxoplasma
     T. gondii
     T. pyrogenes
Toxoplasmea
toxoplasmic encephalitis
toxoplasmin
toxoplasmosis
     acquired t. in adults
     cerebral t.
     congenital t.
     fetal t.
     t., rubella, cytomegalovirus,
       and herpes simplex
     t. serology
TP — temperature and pressure
     thrombocytopenic purpura
     total protein
     tryptophan

tube precipitin
     tuberculin precipitation
TPA — *Treponema pallidum* agglutination
TPBF — total pulmonary blood flow
TPC — thromboplastic plasma component
TPCF — *Treponema pallidum* complement-fixation
TPG — transplacental gradient
TPH — transplacental hemorrhage
TPHA — *Treponema pallidum* hemagglutination assay
TPI — treponemal immobilization test (cardiolipin)
     Treponema pallidum immobilization (test)
     triose phosphate isomerase
TPIA — *Treponema pallidum* immobilization (immune) adherence
TPM — triphenylmethane
TPN — total parenteral nutrition
     triphosphopyridine nucleotide
TPNH — reduced triphosphopyridine nucleotide
TPO — triose phosphate isomerase
     tryptophan peroxidase
TPP — thiamine pyrophosphate
TPPS — tetraphenylporphine sulfonate
TPR — temperature, pulse and respiration
     testosterone production rate
     total peripheral resistance
     total pulmonary resistance
TPS — tumor polysaccharide substance
TPT — typhoid-paratyphoid (vaccine)
TPTZ — tripyridyltriazine
TPVR — total pulmonary vascular resistance
TR — tetrazolium reduction
     total resistance
     total response
     tuberculin R (new tuberculin)
tr — trace
TRA — transaldolase
trabecula (pl., trabeculae)
     arachnoid trabeculae
     trabeculae of bone

trabeculae cranii
trabeculae lienis
septomarginal t.
splenic trabeculae
trabecular
t. adenocarcinoma
t. adenoma
t. bone
t. carcinoma
t.-tubular adenoma
trabeculation
trace
t. element
t. routine
tracer
radioactive t.
trachea (pl., tracheae)
tracheal
t. aspiration
t. bifurcation
t. cartilage
t. gland
t. ligament
t. lumen
t. lymph node
t. mucus
t. muscle
t. submucosa
t. vein
tracheitis
trachelematoma
trachelocystitis
trachelomyitis
trachelopanus
trachelophyma
tracheoaerocele
tracheobiliary fistula
tracheobronchial
t. dyskinesia
t. lymph node
t. secretion
t. tuberculosis
tracheobronchitis
bronchial t.
necrotizing herpetic t.
tracheobronchomegaly
tracheobronchoscopy
tracheoesophageal fistula
tracheomalacia
tracheomegaly
tracheopathia; tracheopathy
t. osteoplastica

tracheoscopy
tracheostoma
tracheostomy
tracheotomy
trachitis
trachoma (pl., trachomata)
t.-inclusion conjunctivitis
t. virus
trachomatis
Trachybdella bistriata
trachychromatic
tracing
tract
biliary t.
Burdach's t.
cerebellar t.
cerebrospinal t.
extrapyramidal t.
Flechsig's t.
gastrointestinal t.
genital t.
genitourinary t.
Goll's t.
Gowers' t.
Lissauer's t.
motor t.
olfactory t.
pyramidal t.
respiratory t.
spinothalamic t.
urinary outflow t.
urogenital t.
traction
t. aneurysm
t. atrophy
t. diverticulum
tractotomy
tractus solitarius nucleus
tragal
tragus (pl., tragi)
TRAIDS — transfusion-related AIDS
trait
alpha-thalassemia t.
beta-thalassemia t.
Cooley's t.
hemoglobin C t.
secretor t.
sickle cell t.
thalassemia t.
tram-track appearance
trance
death t.

tranexamic acid
tranquilizer
 major t.
 minor t.
 phenothiazine t's
 thioxanthene t's
trans-acting factor
transactivating gene
transacylase
transaldolase
transamidinase
transaminase
 aspartate t.
 erythrocyte glutamic-oxaloacetic t.
 glutamate oxaloacetate t.
 glutamate-pyruvate t.
 glutamic-oxaloacetic t.
 glutamic-pyruvic t.
 serum glutamate oxaloacetate t.
 serum glutamate pyruvate t.
 serum glutamic-oxaloacetic t.
 serum glutamic-pyruvic t.
 t. test
 valine t.
transamination
transbronchial biopsy
transcarbamoylase
 ornithine t.
transcarboxylase
transcobalamin I, II, III
transcolonic endoscopy
transconfiguration
transcortical aphasia
transcortin
transcript
 primary t.
transcriptase
 reverse t.
 reverse t. test
transcription
 t. inhibitor
 t. promoter
 reverse t.
 ribonucleic acid t.
 t. unit
transcutaneous
 t. monitoring
 t. needle aspiration
transcytosis

transducer
 electroacoustic t.
 neuroendocrine t.
transducin
transduction
 generalized t.
 t. map
 sensory t.
 specialized t.
 visual t.
transection
transepidermal water loss
transfection
transfectoma
transfer
 t. factor
 t. function
 group t.
 t. host
 linear energy t.
 t. operon
 passive t.
 t. pipet
 replication and t.
 t. RNA
transferability
transferase
 bilirubin glucuronosyl t.
 α-glutamine t.
 γ-glutamine t.
 hypoxanthine guanine phosphoribosyl t.
 terminal deoxynucleotidyl t.
 terminal deoxyribonucleo-
  tidyl t.
 UDP (uridine diphosphate)-
  glucuronyl t.
transferred
 t. antigen-cell-bound antibody
  reaction
 antigen-transferred antibody reaction
transferrin
 t. assay
 t. receptor
 t. saturation
transfixion technique
transformation
 asbestos t.
 bacterial t.
 blast t.
 cell t.

globular-fibrous t.
human lymphocyte t.
logit t.
lymphocytic t.
t. mechanism
nodular t. of liver
probit t.
transformer
high-voltage t.
step-down t.
step-up t.
voltage-regulating t.
transformiminase
transforming
t. agent
t. growth factor
t. virus
transformylase
transfuse
transfusion
autologous t.
blood t.
coagulation factor t.
directed t.
exchange t.
fetal t.
granulocyte t.
hemolytic t.
t. hemosiderosis
t. hepatitis
incompatible t.
intrauterine t.
leukocyte t.
massive t.
neonatal t.
t. nephritis
non-hemolytic t.
platelet t.
t. reaction
t.-related lymphoma
transfusion reaction
acute hemolytic t.r.
allergic t.r.
anaphylactic t.r.
bacterial t.r.
delayed hemolytic t.r.
febrile nonhemolytic t.r.
hemolytic t.r.
transglottic
transglutaminase
transglycosylase
transhepatic

transhiatal
transhydrogenase
transhydroxymethylase
transient
t. agammaglobulinemia
t. albuminuria
t. cerebral ischemia
t. cerebral ischemic episode
t. derepression
t. equilibrium
t. erythroblastopenia of
childhood
t. hypogammaglobulinemia
t. hypogammaglobulinemia of
infancy
t. ischemic attack
t. ischemic episode
t. proteinuria
transillumination
transistor
field effect t.
insulated gate field effect t.
junction t.
junction field effect t.
t.-transistor logic
unijunction t.
transition
isomeric t.
t. mutation
t. state
transitional
t. cell carcinoma
t. cell metaplasia
t. cell neoplasm
t. cell papilloma
t. cell tumors
t. epithelial cells
t. leukocyte
t. meningioma
transketolase assay
translation
t. control RNA
inhibitors of t.
translator
translocase
translocation
autosome t.
balanced t.
chromosome t.
t. factor
insertional t.
reciprocal t.

robertsonian t.
t. trisomy
translucent
transluminal coronary angioplasty
transmandibular projection
transmembrane
    t. glycoprotein
    t. potential
transmethylase
transmethylation
transmissible
transmission
    asynchronous data t.
    t. electron microscope
    t. scan
    serial data t.
    sexual t.
    synchronous data t.
transmittance
    peak t.
transmitted light
transmural
    t. colitis
    t. myocardial infarction
transmutation
transonic
transoral
transorbital
transoximinase
transpalatal
transparent
transparotid
transpeptidase
    glutamyl t.
transperitoneal
transphosphorylase
transplacental hemorrhage
transplant
transplantation
    allogeneic t.
    t. antigen
    autologous bone marrow t.
    bone marrow t.
    heterotopic t.
    homotopic t.
    hyperacute t.
    kidney t.
    organ t.
    orthoptic t.
    t. rejection
    renal t.
    syngeneic t.

syngenesioplastic t.
thymic t.
transport
    active t.
    carrier-mediated t.
    direct t.
    t. disease
    effective oxygen t.
    indirect t.
    lipid t.
    t. medium
    membrane t.
    passive t.
    primary active t.
    t. protein
    reverse cholesterol t.
    secondary active t.
    t. and secretion
    slow axonal t.
    t. and storage
    tape t.
transposable element
transposition
    corrected t.
    gastric t.
    t. of great arteries
    t. of great vessels
    penoscrotal t.
transposon
transpulmonary pressure
transpyloric plane
transsexualism
transsynaptic degeneration
transtentorial herniation
transthoracic aspiration
transthyretin
transtracheal aspiration
transtubercular plane
transudate
    acute inflammatory t.
    peritoneal t.
    pleural t.
transudation
transudative inflammation
transurethral resection
transversalis fascia
transverse
    t. caudate vein
    t. colon
    t. fracture
    t. gyri
    t. mesocolon

t. muscle of abdomen
t. muscle of peritoneum
t. muscle of thorax
t. myelitis
t. myelopathy
t. peduncular tract nucleus
t. presentation
t. scapular artery
t. sinus
transversion mutation
transversospinal muscle
tranylcypromine sulfate
trapezium bone
trapezius
t. muscle
t. musculocutaneous flap
trapezoid
t. body
t. ligament
trapezoidal bone
Trapp-Häser formula
Trapp's formula
Traube-Hering waves
Traube's
corpuscle
plugs
trauma (pl., traumas, traumata)
traumatic
t. abnormality
t. agent
t. anemia
t. aneurysm
t. asphyxial state
t. atrophy
t. bursitis
t. hemolysis
t. myositis ossificans
t. neuroma
t. proctitis
t. shock
t. tenosynovitis
t. thrombosis
t. wet lung
trazodone
TRBF — total renal blood flow
TRC — tanned red cell
total ridge count
treatment
Coffey-Humber t.
Fichera's t.
Koga's t.

Korányi's t.
Minot-Murphy t.
palliative t.
teleradium t.
tree
t. barking
dendritic t.
trehalase
trehalose
Treitz's fossa
Trematoda
trematode
prosostomate t's
t. worm infestation
tremeloid; tremellose
tremor
action t.
intention t.
physiologic t.
static t.
tremulous iris
trench
t. fever
t. foot
t. mouth
Trendelenburg's gait
trephine biopsy
Treponema
T. buccale
T. calligyrum
T. carateum
T. genitalis
T. macrodentium
T. microdentium
T. mucosum
T. orale
T. pallidum
T. pallidum agglutination
T. pallidum complement-fixation
T. pallidum hemagglutination test
T. pallidum immobilization re-action
T. pallidum immobilization test
T. pertenue
T. pintae
T. refringens
T. scoliodontum
T. vincentii
treponemal
t. immobilization test
t. infection

treponematosis
treponeme
trepopnea
treppe
tresis
trestolone acetate
TRF — T-cell-replacing factor
   thymus-replacing factor
   thyrotropin-releasing factor
TRH — thyrotropin-releasing
   hormone
TRH stimulation test
TRI — tetrazolium reduction
   inhibition
triac
triacetin
triacetylglycerol
triacetyloleandomycin
triacylglycerol
  t. acylhydrolase
  t. lipase
triad
  acute compression t.
  adrenomedullary t.
  Andersen's t.
  Beck's
  Carney's t.
  Charcot's t.
  hepatic t's
  Hutchinson's t.
  Osler's t.
  portal t's
  t. of retinal cone
  t. of Schultz
  t. of skeletal muscle
  t. syndrome
  Whipple's t.
triaditis
trial
  clinical t's
  phase I, II, III t's
triamcinolone
triamterene
triangle
  Codman's t.
  Einthoven's t.
  Killan's t.
  sterocostal t.
triangular
  t. bone
  t. ligament
  t. wave

triarylmethane dye
Triatoma
triatomic
triatomid
Triatomidae
triazene
triazinate
tribasic
  t. acid
  t. calcium phosphate
  t. copper sulfate
  t. potassium phosphate
tribe
tribromoethanol
TRIC — trachoma-inclusion conjunctivitis
tricarboxylic
  t. acid
  t. acid cycle
triceps
  t. muscle
  t. tendon
Tricercomonas
trichiasis
trichilemmal cyst
trichilemmoma
Trichina
Trichinella spiralis
trichinosis serology
trichinous embolism
trichitis
trichloracetate
trichloracetic acid
trichlorethylene
trichlorfon
trichloride
  acetylene t.
  vinyl t.
trichlormethiazide
trichloroacetic acid
trichlorobenzene
trichlorobenzoic acid
1,1,1-trichloroethane
1,1,2-trichloroethane
trichloroethanol
trichloroethylene
bis-(trichlorohydroxy ethyl)
  urea
trichloronitromethane
trichlorophenate
  zinc t.
trichlorophenol

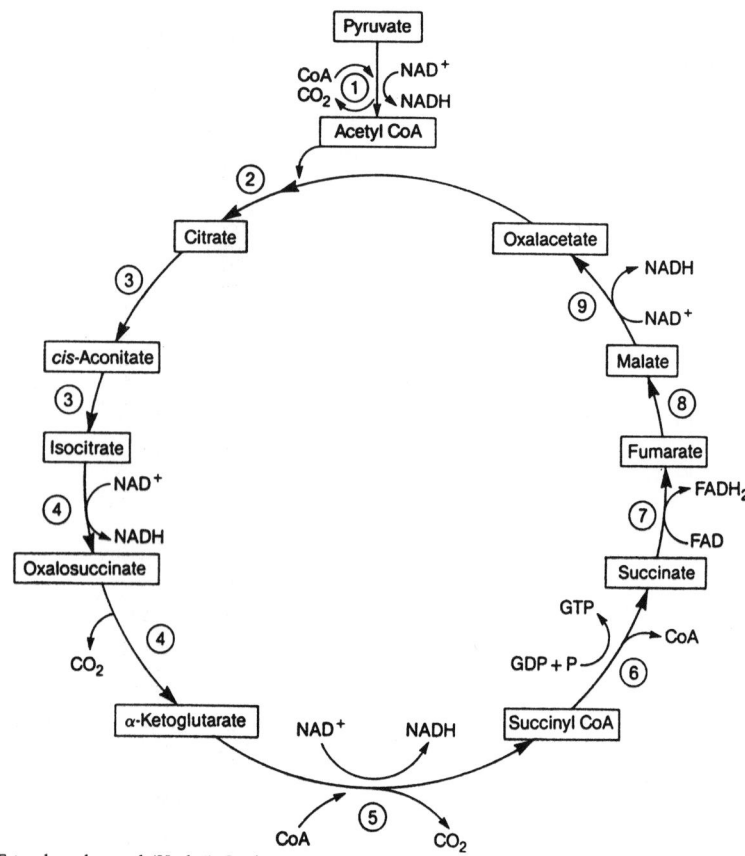

Tricarboxylic acid (Krebs') Cycle. (From Dorland's Illustrated Medical Dictionary. 28th ed. Philadelphia, W.B. Saunders Company, 1994, p.413.)

T. tenax
T. vaginalis
trichomoniasis vaginitis
Trichomycetes
trichomycosis
    t. axillaris
    t. chromatica
    t. favosa
    t. rubra
trichonodosis
trichophytic granuloma
Trichophyton
    T. canis
    T. concentricum
    T. crateriforme
    T. epilans
    T. ferrugineum
    T. gallinae
    T. glabrium
    T. gourvilii
    T. gypseum
    T. megninii
    T. mentagrophytes
    T. purpureum
    T. rosaceum
    T. rubrum
    T. sabouraudi
    T. schoenleini
    T. simii
    T. sulfureum
    T. tonsurans
    T. verrucosum
    T. violaceum
trichophytosis
trichopoliodystrophy
Trichoprosopon
Trichoptera
trichorhinophalangeal syndrome
trichorrhexis nodosa
trichosanthin
Trichosporon
    T. beigelii
    T. cutaneum
    T. giganteum
    T. pedrosianum
trichosporosis
trichostrongyliasis
Trichostrongylidae
Trichostrongyloidae
Trichostrongylus
    T. axei

T. brevis
T. colubriformis
T. instabilis
T. orientalis
T. probolurus
T. vitrinus
Trichothecium roseum
trichotillomania
trichotoxin
trichrome
    Masson t. method
    t. stain
trichuriasis
Trichuris trichiura
Trichuroidea
tricine buffer
triclobisonium chloride
tricresol
tricresyl phosphate
tri-o-cresyl phosphate
tricuspid
    t. atresia
    t. incompetence
    t. insufficiency
    t. orifice
    t. ring
    t. stenosis
    t. valve
tricuspid valve
    anterior leaflet of t.v.
    chordae tendineae of t.v.
    commissure of t.v.
    posterior leaflet of t.v.
    septal leaflet of t.v.
tricyclamol chloride
tricyclic
    t. antidepressant
    t. depressant
trident hand
tridermoma
tridihexethyl
triene
triethanolamine
triethylene
    t. glycol
    t. thiophosphoramide
triethylenemelamine
trifascicular
trifid stomach
trifluoperazine hydrochloride

trifluoride-methanol
    boron t.-m.
triflupromazine hydrochloride
trifluridine
trigeminal
    t. ganglion
    t. lemniscus
    t. nerve
    t. neuralgia
triglyceride
    t. assay
    long-chain t.
    medium-chain t.
    plasma t.
trigonal cystitis
trigone
    olfactory t.
    urinary bladder t.
trigonitis
    pseudomembranous t.
trigonum (pl., trigona)
    t. sternocostale
trihexosidase
    ceramide t.
trihexosylceramide galactosylhydrolase
trihexyphenidyl hydrochloride
trihydroxy
3,4,5-trihydroxybenzoic acid
trihydroxyindole method
triiodothyronine
    t. assay
    free t.
    t. radioimmunoassay
    t. resin uptake test
    reverse t.
    t. suppression test
    t. uptake test
triketohydrindene hydrate
trilobate placenta
trilocular heart
trilostane
trimastigote
trimeprazine tartrate
trimer
trimetaphosphatase
trimethadione
trimethaphan camsylate
trimethidinium
trimethobenzamide hydrochloride
trimethoprim-sulfamethoxazole
trimethoxyamphetamine

trimethyl
    xanthine t.
trimethylamine
trimethylaminuria
bis-trimethylsilyltrifluoroacetamide
trimming resistor
Trinder's reagent
trinitroaniline
2,4,6-trinitrobenzene sulfonate
trinitrophenol
trinitrophenylmethylnitramine
trinitrotoluene
2,4,6-trinitrotoluene
trinocular microscope
Triodontophorus diminutus
triokinase
triol
trioleandomycin
trioleate
    glyceryl t.
triolein I-131
triosephosphate
    t. dehydrogenase
    t. isomerase
    t. isomerase assay
    t. isomerase deficiency
triose-P isomerase
trioxide
    nitrogen t.
trioxymethylene
trioxypurine
2,6,8-trioxypurine
tripalmitate
    glyceryl t.
tripelennamine
    t. citrate
    t. hydrochloride
triphasic wave
triphenylmethane dye
triphenyl phosphate
Triphleps insidiosus
triphosphatase
    adenosine t.
triphosphate
    adenine t.
    adenosine t.
    cytidine t.
    deoxyadenosine t.
    deoxythymidine t.
    guanosine t.
    inosine t.

nucleoside t.
uridine t.
triphosphoric monoester hydrolase
triphthemia
triphyllomatous teratoma
triple
    t.-blind
    t. bond
    t. phosphate crystals
    t. point
    t. stones
    t. sugar iron agar
    t. symptom complex
    t.-X chromosomal aberration
triplegia
triplet
    t. code
    coding t.
triploid
triploidy
triprolidine hydrochloride
triradial
triradiation
tris(2,3-dibromopropyl)phosphate
tris(hydroxymethyl)aminomethane
    buffer
trismus
trisodium
    t. citrate
    t. phosphate
    t. phosphonoformate
trisomic cells
trisomy
    chromosome t.
    t. C syndrome
    double t.
    t. D syndrome
    t. E syndrome
    partial t.
    primary t.
    secondary t.
    t. 8 syndrome
    t. 13 syndrome
    t. 13-15 syndrome
    t. 16-18 syndrome
    t. 18 syndrome
    t. 20 syndrome
    t. 21 syndrome
    t. 22 syndrome
    translocation t.
tristate logic
tristearin

trisulfapyrimidine
trit — triturate
triterpene
triterpenoid saponin
tritiated thymidine
tritium
triton tumor
triturate
trivalent oral poliovirus vaccine
TRK — transketolase
TRMC — tetramethylrhodamino-
        isothiocyanate
tRNA — transfer RNA
tRNA suppressor
TRNG — tetracycline-resistant
        Neisseria gonorrhoeae
trochanter
trochanteric
    t. bursa
    t. bursa of gluteal muscle
    t. bursitis
    subcutaneous t. bursa
troche
trochlea (pl., trochleae)
trochlear
    t. nerve
    t. nucleus
Troglotrema salmincola
Troglotrematidae
Troisier's
    ganglion
    node
Trolard's anastomosing vein
trolley-track sign
trolnitrate phosphate
Trombicula
    T. akamushi
    T. alfreddugèsi
    T. autumnalis
    T. deliensis
    T. irritans
    T. pallida
    T. scutellaris
    T. tsalsahuatl
    T. vandersandi
trombiculiasis
Trombiculidae
trombiculid mite
Trombidoidea
tromethamine
trophedema

trophic
  t. gangrene
  t. lesion
  t. nucleus
  t. ulcer
trophoblast
  syncytial t.
trophoblastic
  t. disease
  gestational t. disease
  t. lacuna
  t. neoplasia
  t. pseudomotor
  t. tumor
trophoblastoma
trophocyte
trophodermatoneurosis
trophoneurosis
  facial t.
  Romberg's t.
trophoneurotic
  t. anemia
  t. leprosy
trophonucleus
trophoplasm
trophoplast
trophoprivic hypothyroidism
trophospongium
trophotaxis
trophozoite
tropical
  t. abscess
  t. bubo
  t. chyluria
  t. diarrhea
  t. macrocytic anemia
  t. mask
  t. pancreatitis
  t. pulmonary eosinophilia
  t. sore
  t. spastic paraparesis
  t. splenomegaly syndrome
  t. sprue
tropicamide
Tropicorbis
tropinesterase
tropism
tropocollagen
tropoelastin
tropomyosin
troponin *C, I, & T*
Trousseau-Lallemand bodies

Trousseau's sign
TRP — tubular reabsorption of
       phosphate
Trp — tryptophan
TRPT — theoretical renal
        phosphorus threshold
TRU — turbidity-reducing unit
T_3RU — triiodothyronine resin
        uptake (test)
Truant's stain
true
  t. aneurysm
  t. cholinesterase
  t. diverticulum
  t. hypertrophy
  t. knot
  t. oxygen
  t. yeast
truncate
truncation
truncus (pl., trunci)
  t. arteriosus
  t. brachiocephalicus
  t. corporis callosi
  t. costocervicalis
  trunci intestinales
  t. jugularis
  t. linguofacialis
  t. lumbosacralis
  t. pulmonalis
  t. subclavius
  t. sympathicus
  t. thyreocervicalis
  t. vagalis
trunk
  t. duplication
  t. ligament
  pulmonary t.
trypan blue
trypanocidal
Trypanosoma
  T. ariari
  T. brucei
  T. brucei brucei
  T. brucei gambiense
  T. brucei rhodesiense
  T. castellani
  T. cruzi
  T. gambiense
  T. hominis
  T. nigeriense
  T. rangeli

troponin I elevatn indicator of acute MI

T. rhodesiense
T. triatomae
T. ugandense
Trypanosomatidae
trypanosome
trypanosomiasis
    African t.
    American t.
    Brazilian t.
    Gambian t.
    Rhodesian t.
trypanosomicidal
trypanosomicide
trypan red
tryparsamide
Trypetidae
trypomastigote
trypsin
    t.-aldehyde-fuchsin
    t. G-banding stain
    immunoreactive t.
    t. inhibitor
    t.-inhibitory capacity
    t. test
trypsinogen
tryptamine
Tryptar
tryptase
tryptic
    t. activity
    t. soy agar
trypticase
    t. soy agar
    t. soy broth
    t. soy with agar broth
    t. soy yeast
tryptone
tryptonemia
tryptophan
    t. 5-hydroxylase
    t. load test
    t. malabsorption syndrome
    t. peroxidase
tryptophanemia
tryptophanuria
tryptophanyl-RNA synthetase
tryptophyl
TS — test solution
    tropical sprue
TSA — thyroid-secreting adenoma
    trypticase soy agar
    tumor-specific antigen

T_4SA — thyroxine-specific activity
TSB — trypticase soy broth
TSC — technetium sulfur colloid
    thiosemicarbazide
TSD — Tay-Sachs disease
TSE — trisodium edetate
tsetse fly
TSF — tissue-coding factor
TSH — thyroid-stimulating hormone
TSH-binding inhibitory immuno-
    globulin
TSH-displacing antibody
TSH-releasing hormone
TSI — thyroid-stimulating
    immunoglobulin
    triple sugar iron
TSI agar
t-s mutation
TSP — total serum protein
TSPAP — total serum prostatic acid
    phosphatase
TSR — thyroid-to-serum ratio
TSS — tropical splenomegaly
    syndrome
TST — tumor skin test
TSTA — tumor-specific
    transplantation antigen
T-strain mycoplasma
T-suppressor cell
tsutsugamushi
    t. disease
    t. fever
TSY — trypticase soy yeast
TT — tetrazol
    thrombin time
    thymol turbidity
    total thyroxine
    transthoracic
T_4:TBG ratio
TTC — triphenyltetrazolium chloride
TTD — tissue tolerance dose
TTH — thyrotropic hormone
    tritiated thymidine
TTI — time-tension index
TTP — thrombotic thrombocyto-
    penic purpura
    thymidine triphosphate
TTS — temporary threshold shift
TTT — tolbutamide tolerance test
T tubule
TU — thiouracil
    Todd unit

toxic unit
tuberculin unit

T₃U — T₃ uptake
tuaminoheptane
tubal
    t. abortion
    t. epithelium
    t. infantilism
    t. insufflation
    t. ostium
    t. plica
    t. pregnancy
    t. serosa
    t. subserosa
    t. tonsil
tube
    t. agglutination
    auditory t.
    Babcock t.
    buccal t.
    t. cast
    cathode-ray t.
    t. coagulase test
    corneal t.
    t. culture
    digestive t.
    t. dilution test
    drainage t.
    Durham's t.
    endobronchial t.
    endotracheal t.
    eustachian t.
    fallopian t.
    germ t.
    glow modulator t.
    granulation t.
    indicator t.
    intubation t.
    Levin t.
    Miller-Abbott t.
    nasogastric t.
    nasolabial t.
    nephrostomy t.
    NIXIE t.
    ovarian t's
    pharyngotympanic t.
    photomultiplier t.
    t. precipitin
    roll t.
    salivary t's
    Sengstaken-Blakemore t.
    Shiner's t.

    Souttar's t.
    test t.
    thoracostomy t.
    Vacutainer t.
    vacuum t.
    voltage-regulator t.
    Wangensteen's t.
    Wintrobe's hematocrit t.
    x-ray t.
tubeless gastric analysis test
tuber (pl., tubera)
    t. cinereum
    t. zygomaticum
tuberal nucleus
tubercle
    t. bacillus
    caseous t.
    darwinian t.
    dissection t.
    fibrous t.
    genital t.
    Ghon's t.
    hard t.
    hyaline t.
    Müller's t.
    orbital t.
    otic t.
    pharyngeal t.
    postmortem t.
    prosector's t.
    sebaceous t.
    soft t.
tubercle bacillus
    avian t.b.
    bovine t.b.
    human t.b.
tubercular; tuberculate; tuberculated
tuberculation
tuberculid
    nodular t.
    papulonecrotic t.
    rosacea-like t.
tuberculin
    albumose-free t.
    alkaline t.
    t. filtrate
    old t.
    original t.
    t. precipitation
    t. R (new tuberculin)
    t. reaction
    t. test

t.-type reaction
t. unit
vacuum t.
t. zymoplastiche
tuberculitis
tuberculization
tuberculofibroid
tuberculoid
t. granuloma
t. leprosy
tuberculoma
tuberculo-opsonic index
tuberculosis
acute t.
acute miliary t.
adrenal t.
adult t.
anthracotic t.
arrested t.
attenuated t.
atypical t.
basal t.
caseous t.
central nervous system t.
childhood type t.
cutaneous t.
t. cutis
t. cutis luposa
t. cutis orificialis
t. cutis verrucosa
dermal t.
disseminated t.
endobronchial t.
endotracheal t.
extrapulmonary t.
fibrocaseous t.
gastrointestinal t.
general t.
genital t.
hematogenous t.
inactive t.
isolated-organ t.
laryngeal t.
miliary t.
open t.
papulonecrotic t.
pericardial t.
pleural t.
postprimary t.
primary t.
progressive pulmonary t.
progressive secondary t.

pulmonary t.
reactivation t.
reinfection t.
renal t.
secondary t.
t. skin test
tracheobronchial t.
ulcerative t.
t. ulcerosa
vertebral t.
tuberculostearic acid
tuberculous
t. abscess
t. arthritis
t. bronchopneumonia
t. cystitis
t. empyema
t. encephalitis
t. endometritis
t. granulation tissue
t. gumma
t. infiltration
t. lymphadenitis
t. lymphadenopathy
t. meningitis
t. nephritis
t. osteomyelitis
t. pericarditis
t. peritonitis
t. pleuritis
t. respiratory disease
t. rheumatism
t. salpingitis
t. scrofuloderma
t. spondylitis
t. tenosynovitis
t. thyroiditis
t. wart
tuberculum (pl., tubercula)
t. arthriticum
tubercula dolorosa
t. sebaceum
t. syphiliticum
tuberhypophyseal
tuberiferous
tuberose
tuberosity
ischial t.
pubic t.
tibial t.
tuberous
t. carcinoma

t. sclerosis
t. xanthoma
Tubifera
tubocurarine chloride
tubo-ovarian
    t.-o. abscess
    t.-o. varicocele
tubo-ovaritis
tuboreticular structure
tubovillous adenoma
tubular
    t. adenoma
    t. adenomatous polyp
    t. aneurysm
    t. basement membrane
    t. breast cancer
    t. cancer
    t. carcinoma
    t. cyst
    t. fluid
    t. immune complex
    t. interstitial nephritis
    t. necrosis
    t. nephritis
    t. nephrosis
    Pick's t. adenoma
    t. proteinuria
    t. vision
tubule
    caroticotympanic t's
    collecting t.
    connecting t's
    galactophorous t's
    lactiferous t's
    mesonephric t's
    proximal t.
    renal t's
    seminiferous t's
    subtracheal t.
    T (transverse) t.
    tracheal t.
    transverse (T) t.
    uriniferous t's
tubulin
tubuloalveolar gland
tubulocyst
tubulodermoid
tubulointerstitial
    t. disease
    t. nephritis
    t. nephropathy
tubulonecrosis

tubulopapillary variant
tubuloreticular particles
tubulorrhectic
tubulorrhexis
tubulovesicle
tubulovesicular
tubulovillous
    t. adenoma
    t. adenomatous polyp
tubulus (pl., tubuli)
    tubuli rectis
tuffstone body
tuft
    glomerular t.
tufted
    t. cell
    t. phalanx
tuftsin deficiency
TUG — total urinary gonadotropin
tularemia
    t. agglutinins
    glandular t.
    oculoglandular t.
    pneumonic t.
    typhoidal (enteric) t.
    ulceroglandular t.
tularemic
    t. chancre
    t. conjunctivitis
tumefacient
tumefaction
tumefy
tumentia
tumescence
tumescent
tumeur
    t. perlée
    t. pileuse
tumid
tumor
    Abrikosov's t. (Abrikos-
      soff's t.)
    acinar cell t.
    acinic cell t.
    acute splenic t.
    adenoid t.
    adenomatoid odontogenic t.
    adipose t.
    adnexal t.
    adrenal rest t.
    adrenocortical rest t.
    aldosterone-producing t.

aldosterone-secreting t.
alveolar cell t.
ameloblastic adenomatoid t.
amyloid t.
t. aneuploidy
t. angiogenesis
t. angiogenic factor
angioinvasive t.
angiomatoid t.
t. anticoagulation
t. antigen (T antigen)
aortic body t.
Askin's t.
t.-associated rejection antigen
Bednar's t.
benign t.
benign epithelial odonto-
   genic t.
bladder t.
blood t.
bone t's
brain t.
breast t's
Brenner's t.
bronchial carcinoid t.
bronchioalveolar intravascular t.
Brooke's t.
brown t.
Brown-Pearce t.
t. burden
Burkitt's t.
Buschke-Löwenstein t.
butyroid t.
calcifying epithelial odontogenic t.
carcinoid t.
carcinoma ex mixed t.
carotid body t.
catecholamine-secreting t.
t. cell kinetics
t. cells
cellular t.
central nervous system t's
chemoreceptor t.
chondromatous giant cell t.
chordoid t.
chromaffin t.
clear cell t.
Codman's t.
collision t.
colloid t.

colon t.
composite t.
composition t.
compound t.
connective t.
t. conversion
dermal duct t.
dermoid t.
desmoid t.
diarrheogenic t.
eccrine t.
t. embolism
t. embolus
embryonal t.
embryonic t.
embryoplastic t.
endobronchial t.
endodermal sinus t.
endometrioid t.
epidermoid t.
epithelial t., benign
Erdheim t.
esophageal t's
estrogen-producing t.
Ewing's t.
extramedullary myeloid t.
eye t's
fallopian tube t's
fatty t.
fecal t.
feminizing t.
fibrohistiocytic t.
fibroid t.
fibromyxoid t.
t. of follicular infundibulum
functional t.
functioning t.
fungating t.
gemistocytic t.
germ cell t.
germ cell–stromal t.
germ cell–stromal–sex cord t.
gestational t.
giant cell t.
t. giant cell
giant cell t. of bone
giant cell t. of tendon sheath
glomus t.
glomus jugulare t.
Godwin t.
gonadal stromal t.
t. grading

granular cell t.
granulosa cell t.
granulosa-theca cell t.
Grawitz's t.
Gubler's t.
heart t's
heterologous t.
hilar cell t. of ovary
histoid t.
homologous t.
hormone-secreting t.
t.-host interaction
Hürthle cell t.
hylic t.
t. immunity
t. infiltrating lymphocytes
innocent t.
interstitial cell t.
juxtaglomerular t.
juxtaglomerular cell t.
Klatskin's t.
Koenen's t.
Krompecher's t.
Krukenberg's t.
Landschutz t.
t. lethal dose
Leydig cell t.
Leydig-Sertoli cell t.
Lindau's t.
lipid cell t.
lung t's
t. lysis syndrome
malignant t.
malignant mixed meso-
    dermal t.
t. marker
mast cell t.
melanotic neuroectodermal t.
Merkel's cell t.
mesenchymal t.
mesodermal mixed t.
mesonephroid t.
metastatic t.
mixed t.
mixed mesodermal t.
mixed t. of salivary gland
mixed t. of skin
monoclonal t.
mucinous t.
mucoepidermoid t.
müllerian mixed t.
t. necrosis

necrosis t.
t. necrosis factor
Nelson's t.
nerve sheath t.
neuroectodermal t.
neuroendocrine t.
neuroendocrine cell t.
no evidence of primary t.
nonfunctional t.
nonfunctioning t.
nonseminomatous germ cell t.
odontogenic t.
oil t.
oncocytic hepatocellular t.
organoid t.
osteoblastic t.
osteoid t.
ovarian t.
ovarian germ cell–stromal–sex
    cord t.
Pancoast's t.
pancreatic t's
papillary t.
papillary cystic t.
paraffin t.
parathyroid t's
pearl t.
Pepper t.
peripheral neuroectodermal t.
Perlmann's t.
phantom t.
phyllodes t.
pilar t. of scalp
Pindborg t.
pituitary t.
plasma cell t.
polyclonal t.
t. polysaccharide substance
potato t. of neck
pregnancy t.
primitive neuroectodermal t.
primitive neuroepithelial t.
prolactin-secreting t.
proliferating trichilemmal t.
t. promoter
prostatic t's
ranine t.
Rathke's pouch t.
Recklinghausen's t.
Regaud's t.
t. registry
renal t's

renomedullary interstitial
cell t.
rete cell t.
retinal anlage t.
rhabdoid t.
Rous t.
salivary gland t's
Schwann cell t.
serous t.
Sertoli cell t.
Sertoli-Leydig cell t.
sex cord–stromal t.
sex cord t., undifferentiated
t. in situ
skin t's
t. skin test
small cell t.
small intestine t's
soft tissue t.
solid cystic t.
t.-specific antigen
t.-specific transplantation antigen
spinal cord t's
spindle cell t.
splenic t.
squamous odontogenic t.
t. stage
t. staging
Steiner's t.
stomach t's
stromal t.
stromal–germ cell t.
stromal–sex cord t.
strumal carcinoid t.
sugar t.
superior pulmonary sulcus t.
t. suppressor genes
sweat gland t.
teratoid t.
testicular t.
testicular germ cell t.
theca cell t.
theca cell–granuloma cell t.
theca lutein t.
thrombus t.
t. thrombus
thymic t's
thyroid t's
thyrotrope t.
thyrotroph t.
tomato t.

transitional cell t's
triton t.
trophoblastic t.
turban t.
ulcerogenic t.
undifferentiated sex cord t.
urethral t.
uterine t's
vaginal t's
villous t.
virilizing t.
vulvar t's
Warthin's t.
Wilms' t.
yolk sac t.
Zollinger-Ellison t.
tumoraffin
tumoral calcinosis
tumorigenesis
    foreign body t.
tumorigenic
tumorlet
tumorlike
tumorous
Tunga penetrans
tungiasis
Tungidae
tungsten
    t. blue
    t. bulb
    t. halogen lamp
    t. lamp
tungstic acid
tunic
    fibrous t.
    mucous t.
    muscular t.
    pharyngeal t.
    serous t.
tunica (pl., tunicae)
    t. adventitia
    t. albuginea
    t. fibrosa
    t. interna
    t. intima
    t. media
    t. mucosa
    t. vaginalis
    t. vasculosa
tunnel anemia
TUPAO — temporary unilateral pulmonary artery occlusion

T₃ uptake test
TUR — transurethral resection
Turbatrix aceti
turbid
turbidimeter
turbidimetric immunoassays
turbidimetry
turbidity
 t.-reducing unit
 thymol t.
turbinal varix
turbinate
 nasal t.
 sphenoid t.
turgescence
turgescent
turgid
turkey red
Türk's
 cell
 irritation leukocyte
 leukocyte
turnaround time
Turnbull's blue
turnkey system
turnover
 t. number
 plasma iron t.
TURP — transurethral resection of
  the prostate gland
turpentine oil
T₃U test
TV — tidal volume
 tuberculin volutin
TVC — timed vital capacity
 total volume capacity
 transvaginal cone
T wave
twelfth cranial nerve
twin
 conjoined t's
 corporea lutea t.
 t. crystal
 dichorionic placenta t's
 dizygotic t's
 fraternal t's
 heterokaryotic t's
 identical t's
 incomplete conjoined t's
 monoamniotic placenta t's
 monochorionic diamniotic placenta t.

 monochorionic placenta t's
 monozygotic t's
 parasitic t.
 placenta t.
 t. placenta
 Siamese t's
twitch
 fast t.
 slow t.
TWL — transepidermal water loss
two-dimensional
 t.-d. chromatography
 t.-d. gel electrophoresis
 t.-d. immunoelectrophoresis
two-emulsion autoradiography
two-glass test
two-sided alternative
two-slide method
two-stage PT (prothrombin-time) test
two-tailed test
Ty — typhoid
Tylenol
tylosis (pl., tyloses)
 t. palmaris et plantaris
tympanic
 t. antrum
 t. canaliculus
 t. cavity
 t. cells
 t. membrane
 t. nerve
 t. thermography
tympanic membrane
 fibrocartilaginous anulus
  of t.m.
 pars flaccida of t.m.
 pars tensa of t.m.
tympanites
tympanography
tympanosclerosis
tympanum
Tymphonotonus
type
 t. A (fundal) gastritis
 t. B (antral) gastritis
 blood t.
 t. I cell
 t. II cell
 t. III cell
 t. culture
 t. 1 dextrocardia
 t. 2 dextrocardia

t. 3 dextrocardia
t. 4 dextrocardia
t. I mucopolysaccharidosis
t. II mucopolysaccharidosis
t. III mucopolysaccharidosis
t. V mucopolysaccharidosis
t. VI mucopolysaccharidosis
t. VII mucopolysaccharidosis
t. IS mucopolysaccharidosis
t. IV mucopolysaccharidosis
Oregon t. hypertyrosinemia
t. I pneumonocyte
t. II pneumonocyte
typhlectasis
typhlenteritis
typhlitis
typhloenteritis
typhlomegaly
typhoid
t. bacillus
t. fever
t. immunization reaction
t. osteomyelitis
paratyphoid A and paraty-
phoid B t.
t.-paratyphoid (vaccine)
t. septicemia
"Typhoid Mary"
typhoidal tularemia
typhosepsis
typhous
typhus
amarillic t.
t. antibody test
endemic t.
t. epidemic
t. fever
louse-borne t.
murine t.
North Asian tick t.
Queensland tick t.

recrudescent t.
scrub t.
typing
ABO t.
ABO-Rh t.
bacteriophage t.
blood t.
phage t.
primed lymphocyte t.
Rh t.
Tyr — tyrosine
tyramine test
Tyrode's solution
Tyroglyphidae
Tyroglyphus siro
tyroid
tyroketonuria
tyroma
tyropanoate sodium
Tyrophagus
tyrosinase deficiency
tyrosine
t. aminotransferase deficiency
t. assay
t. decarboxylase
t. deficiency
t. hydroxylase
t. kinase
t. test
tyrosinemia
tyrosinosis
tyrosinuria
tyrosis
tyrosyl-RNA synthetase
tyrosyluria
tyrothricin
TZ — tuberculin zymoplastiche
Tzanck's
cells
preparation
test

U — unit
    uranium
    urine
UA — umbilical artery
    unaggregated
    uric acid
    urinalysis
    uterine aspiration
U antigen
UB — ultimobranchial body
UBBC — unsaturated vitamin B_{12}–binding capacity
UBF — uterine blood flow
UBG — urobilinogen
UBI — ultraviolet blood irradiation
ubiquinol
    u.-cytochrome reductase
    u. dehydrogenase
ubiquinone reductase
ubiquitin
ubisemiquinone
UC — ulcerative colitis
    ultracentrifugal
    urea clearance
    urethral catheterization
    uterine contractions
U-cell lymphoma
UCG — urinary chorionic gonadotropin
UCP — urinary coproporphyrin
UD — urethral discharge
    uroporphyrinogen decarboxylase
UDP — uridine diphosphate
UDPbilirubin glucuronosyltransferase
UDPgalactose
UDPglucose
UDP glucose-hexose-1-phosphatase
UDPglucuronate
UDPglucuronic acid
UDPglucuronyl transferase
UDPhexose
UDPiduronate
UDPiduronic acid
UDP-N-acetyl-D-galactosamine
UDP-N-acetyl-D-glucosamine
UDPxylose
UDPG — uridine diphosphoglucose
UDPGA — uridine diphosphoglucuronic acid

UDPGT — uridine diphosphoglucuronyl transferase
UF — unknown factor
UFA — unesterified fatty acid
Uffelmann's test
"U" fibers
UG — urogenital
Uganda S virus
UGI — upper gastrointestinal
Uhl's anomaly
UI — uroporphyrin isomerase
UIBC — unsaturated iron-binding capacity
UICC — Union Internationale Contre Cancer
UIF — undegraded insulin factor
UIP — usual interstitial pneumonitis
UIQ upper inner quadrant
UK — urokinase
UL — undifferentiated lymphoma
    upper lobe
ulatrophy
ulcer
    acute u.
    acute hemorrhagic u.
    amebic u.
    amputating u.
    aphthous u.
    Barrett's u.
    Buruli u.
    chancroidal u.
    chiclero u.
    chronic u.
    cockscomb u.
    cold u.
    constitutional u.
    corneal u.
    creeping u.
    Curling's u.
    Cushing's u.
    decubitus u.
    diabetic u.
    diphtheritic u.
    distention u.
    duodenal u.
    elusive u.
    Fenwick-Hunner u.
    focal u.
    follicular u.
    gastric u.

genital u.
groin u.
gummatous u.
hard u.
hemorrhagic u.
Hunner's u.
indolent u.
inflamed u.
Lipschütz' u.
lupoid u.
marginal u.
Marjolin's u.
Meleney's u.
penetrating u.
peptic u.
perambulating u.
perforated u.
perforated gastric u.
perforating u.
phagedenic u.
phlegmonous u.
rodent u.
serpiginous u.
simple u.
sloughing u.
soft u.
stasis u.
stercoraceous u.
stercoral u.
stomal u.
stress u.
Sutton's u.
symptomatic u.
syphilitic u.
trophic u.
varicose u.
venereal u.
warty u.
ulcera
ulcerate
ulcerated
ulceration
aphthous u.
ulcerative
u. colitis
u. cystitis
u. esophagitis
u. inflammation
u. scrofuloderma
u. tuberculosis
ulcerogenic tumor
ulceroglandular tularemia

ulcerogranuloma
ulceromembranous
ulcerosa
blepharitis u.
ulcerous
ulcus (pl., ulcera)
u. ambulans
u. terebrans
u. venereum
u. vulvae acutum
ulegyria
ulerythema ophryogenes
Ulex europaeus lectin
Ullmann's line
ULN — upper limits of normal
ulna (pl., ulnae)
ulnar
u. artery
u. drift
u. nerve
u. tunnel syndrome
u. vein
ulodermatitis
uloid
ULQ — upper left quadrant
ultimobranchial
u. bodies
u. cells
ultimum moriens
ultrabrachycephalic
ultracentrifugal
ultracentrifugation
ultracentrifuge
analytic u.
ultradolichocephalic
ultrafilter
ultrafiltrate
ultrafiltration hemodialyzer
ultrafreezing
ultramicroanalysis
ultramicrotome
ultrasonic
u. nebulizer
u. tomography
ultrasonication
ultrasonogram
ultrasonography
ultrasound
ultrastructural study
ultrastructure
ultrathin section

ultraviolet
>   u. blood irradiation
>   u. burn
>   u. fluorescent dosimeter
>   u. light
>   u. light-induced mutation
>   u. microscope
>   u. radiation
>   u. ray
>   u./visible spectrophotometry

ultropaque method

UM — uracil mustard

umb — umbilicus

umbilical
>   u. artery
>   u. cord
>   u. cyst
>   u. fistula
>   u. hernia
>   u. ligament
>   u. mucous connective tissue
>   u. polyp
>   u. vein

umbilicus

umbrella
>   u. cell
>   u. iris

UMP — uridine monophosphate

UN — urea nitrogen

unaggregated

unbound thyroxine-binding globulin

uncal

Uncinaria
>   U. americana
>   U. duodenalis

uncinariasis

uncinate
>   u. epilepsy
>   u. fasciculus
>   u. process of pancreas

unclassified
>   arborvirus group u.

uncompensated
>   u. acidosis
>   u. alkalosis

unconjugated
>   u. bilirubin
>   u. estriol

unconsciousness

uncouplers
>   oxidative phosphorylation u.

uncoupling protein

uncrossed pyramidal tract

uncus (pl., unci)
>   u. gyri

undecaprenol
>   u. phosphate
>   undecylenate calcium u.

undecoylium chloride-iodine

undecylenate
>   zinc u.

undecylenic acid

undegraded insulin factor

underflow

undernutrition

undescended testis

undifferentiated
>   u. adenocarcinoma
>   u. carcinoma
>   u. cell adenoma
>   u. epidermoid carcinoma
>   u. leukemia
>   u. lymphoma
>   u. neuroepithelium
>   u. sarcoma
>   u. sex cord tumor
>   u. squamous cell carcinoma

undifferentiation

Undritz anomaly

undulant fever

undulating membrane

undulation
>   jugular u.
>   respiratory u.

unesterified fatty acid

ung — unguentum (ointment)

unheated serum reagin (test)

Uniblue A

unicameral
>   u. bone cyst
>   u. cyst

unicellular sclerosis

unicentral

unicentric blastoma

unicystic ameloblastoma

unidirectional

uniflagellate

unifocal eosinophilic granuloma

unigravida

unilocular
>   u. cyst
>   u. echinococcosis
>   u. hydatid
>   u. hydatid cyst

unimodal
union
  faulty u.
  primary u.
  secondary u.
  vicious u.
Union Internationale Contre Cancer
un-ionized hemoglobin
uniovular
unipara
unipolar neuron
uniport
unipotential stem cells
unit
  absolute u.
  activation u.
  alexin u.
  Allen-Doisy u.
  alpha u.
  amboceptor u.
  A-mode u.
  androgen u.
  Angström u.
  Ansbacher u.
  antigen u.
  antitoxin u.
  antivenin u.
  atomic mass u.
  atomic weight u.
  base u.
  Behnken's u.
  Bessey-Lowry u.
  Bessey-Lowry-Brock u.
  Bethesda u.
  biological standard u.
  B-mode u.
  Bodansky's u.
  Bowers-McComb u.
  British thermal u.
  u. cell
  centimeter-gram-second u.
  central processing u.
  chlorophyll u.
  chorionic gonadotropin u.
  Clauberg's u.
  colony-forming u.
  complement u.
  Corner-Allen u.
  corpus luteum hormone u.
  Dam u.
  digitalis u.
  diphtheria antitoxin u.

Doppler u.
Ehrlich's u.
electromagnetic u.
electrostatic u.
endoscopic u.
enzyme u.
equine gonadotropin u.
estradiol benzoate u.
estrone u.
Fishman-Lerner u.
Florey u.
Gutman u.
heat u.
hemagglutinating u.
hemolysin u.
hemolytic u.
heparin u.
Holzknecht's u.
homology u.
Hounsfield u.
Howell's u.
immunizing u.
u. inheritance
insulin u.
u. of intermedin
international u.
international benzoate u.
International System of u's
Jenner-Kay u.
kallikrein-inhibiting u.
Karmen u.
ketal u.
Kienböck's u.
King's u.
King-Armstrong u.
u. of luteinizing activity
Mache u.
u. of mass
meter-kilogram-second u.
Montevideo's u's
mouse u.
mouse uterine u's
u. of neutron dosage
Oxford u.
u. of oxytocin
pantothenic acid u.
u. of penicillin
peripheral resistance u.
phosphatase u.
physiologic u.
plaque-forming u's
u. of progestational activity

progesterone u.
prolactin u.
protein nitrogen u.
radiation-absorbed u.
radiation measuring u's
rat u.
resistance u.
riboflavin u.
Russell's u.
Sherman's u.
Sherman-Bourquin u. of vitamin B_2
Sherman-Munsell u.
Shinowara-Jones-Reinhard u.
SI (Système International d'Unites) u.
Sibley-Lehninger u.
skin test u.
SL (Sibley-Lehninger) u.
Somogyi u.
Steenbock's u.
Svedberg's u.
Svedberg's flotation u.
terminal respiratory u.
tetanus antitoxin u.
thiamine chloride u.
thiamine hydrochloride u.
u. of thyrotrophic activity
Todd u's
toxic u.
transcription u.
tuberculin u.
turbidity-reducing u.
u. of vasopressin
vitamin A u.
u. of vitamin B_1
vitamin D u.
vitamin G u.
u. of wavelength
u. of weight
Wohlgemuth u.
x-ray u.
United States Food and Drug Administration
United States Public Health Service
unit-erythroid
colony-forming u.-e.
unit membrane
asymmetric u. m.
unit of neutron dosage
univalent antibody
univariant analysis

universal donor
univitelline
unknown
u. etiology
u. function
u. morphology
u. topographic site
unmedullated
unmyelinated
Unna-Pappenheim stain
Unna's
alkaline methylene blue
mark
nevus
stain
Unna-Taenzer stain
unopette dilutor
unorganized virus
unresectable
unresolved
u. hepatitis
u. lobar pneumonia
u. pneumonia
unresponsiveness
immunologic u.
unsaturated
u. fatty acids
u. hydrocarbon
u. iron-binding capacity
u. vitamin B_{12} binding capacity
Unschuld's sign
unstable hemoglobin
ununited fracture
unwinding protein
UOQ — upper outer quadrant
UP—ureteropelvic
uroporphyrin
U/P — urine-plasma ratio
UPG — uroporphyrinogen
UPI — uteroplacental insufficiency
UPJ — ureteropelvic junction
upper
u. collecting system
u. extremity
u. limits of normal
u. respiratory disease
u. respiratory infection
u. respiratory tract infection
uptake
absolute iodine u.
oxygen u.

radioactive iodine u.
resin u.
thyroid ^{131}I u.
UR — upper respiratory
ur — urine
urachal
u. adenoma
u. carcinoma
u. cyst
u. fistula
u. neoplasm
u. sinus
u.-umbilical sinus
u.-vesical fistula
u.-vesical sinus
urachus
fetal u.
patent u.
persistent u.
uracil
u. dehydrogenase
u. mustard
u. phosphoribosyltransferase
uracrasia
uragogue
uranin
uranium
u. isotope
u. nephritis
u. nitrate
uranoplasty
uranyl acetate stain
uraroma
urarthritis
urate
u. calculus
u. crystal
u. crystal stain
De Galantha's method for u's
magnesium u.
u. monosodium
u. nephropathy
u. oxidase
uratemia
uratohistechia
uratoma
uratosis
uraturia
URD — upper respiratory disease
urea
u. agar
u. clearance

u. clearance test
u. cycle
u. nitrogen
u. nitrogen test
u. synthesis
Ureaplasma urealyticum
ureapoiesis
urease test
urecchysis
uredema
3-ureidopropionase
urelcosis
uremia
hemolytic u.
hypercalcemic u.
uremic
u. cachexia
u. colitis
u. coma
u. eclampsia
u. encephalopathy
u. esophagitis
u. gastroenteritis
u. inflammation
u. lung
u. medullary cystic disease
u. pericarditis
u. pneumonia
u. pneumonitis
uremigenic
ureotelic
ureter
adynamic u.
atonic u.
bifid u.
double u.
lamina propria of u.
mucous membrane of u.
u. muscularis
retrocaval u.
ureteral
u. achalasia
u. adventitia
u. atresia
u. catheterization
u. ectopy
u. hyperperistalsis
u. ileus
u. lumen
u. orifice
u. peristalsis
u. plaque

u. redundancy
u. stricture
u. stump
u. valve
u. vasocutaneous fistula
ureteralgia
ureterectasia
ureteritis
u. cystica
u. follicularis
glandular u.
u. glandularis
ureterocele
ureterocelectomy
ureterocervical
ureterocutaneous fistula
ureterocystoscope
ureterocystostomy
ureteroduodenal
ureteroenterostomy
ureterogram
ureterography
ureterohydronephrosis
ureteroileostomy
ureterolith
ureterolithiasis
ureterolysis
ureteropelvic stricture
ureteropyelitis
ureteropyelography
ureteropyelonephritis
ureteropyelostomy
ureteropyosis
ureterosigmoidostomy
ureterostenosis
ureterostoma
ureterostomy
ureterotrigonosigmoidostomy
ureterovaginal
ureterovesical
u. obstruction
u. stricture
ureterovesicoplasty
urethan
urethane
urethra
bulb of u.
corpus cavernosum of u.
membranous u.
mucous membrane of u.
penile u.
prostatic u.

urethral
u. artery
u. caruncle
u. catheterization
u. crista
u. discharge
u. diverticulitis
u. diverticulum
u. endometriosis
u. fold
u. gland
u. hematuria
u. lacuna
u. lumen
u. meatal stenosis
u. meatus
u. membrane
u. metaplasia
u. obstruction
u. orifice
u. outlet
u. polyp
u. stricture
u. tumor
u. valve
u. verruca
u. washing
urethratresia
urethrectomy
urethremphraxis
urethrism
urethritis
chlamydial u.
follicular u.
gonococcal u.
gonorrheal u.
granular u.
nongonococcal u.
nonspecific u.
u. petrificans
posterior u.
simple u.
urethrocele
urethrocystitis
urethrocystogram
urethrography
urethrophraxis
urethrophyma
urethroscopy
urethrostenosis
urethrovaginal
urethrovesical

urginin
urhidrosis
URI — upper respiratory infection
uric acid
    u.a. calculus
    u.a. crystals
    u.a. infarct
    u.a. nephropathy
    u.a. stones
uricacidemia
uricase
uricemia
uric monosodium
uricolytic index
uricosuria
uricosuric
uridine
    u. diphosphate galactose-4-
      epimerase
    u. diphosphate glucose-4-
      epimerase
    u. diphosphoglucose
    u. diphosphoglucuronyl-
      transferase
    u. monophosphate
    u. monophosphate pyrophos-
      phorylase
    u.-5'-phosphate
    u. phosphorylase
    u. triphosphate
uridrosis
uridylic acid
uridyltransferase
    hexose-1-phosphate u.
uridylyl
uridyltransferase
    UDP-glucose-hexose-1-
      phosphate u.
urinal
urinalysis
    cytodiagnostic u.
urinary
    u. amylase
    u. bladder
    u. calculus
    u. cast
    u. chorionic gonadotropin
    u. concentration test
    u. conduit
    u. coproporphyrin
    u. cortisol
    u. cyst

    u. cytology
    u. diversion
    u. estriol
    u. fistula
    u. fungus culture
    u. glucose
    u. gonadotropin fragment
    u. incompetence
    u. incontinence
    u. nitrogen
    u. obstruction
    u. outflow
    u. outflow tract
    u. pole, glomerular
    u. retention
    u. sand
    u. sediment
    u. smear
    u. solids
    u. sphincter
    u. stone
    u. tract disease
    u. tract infection
urination
urine
    u. acetone test
    acid u.
    alkaline u.
    ammoniacal u.
    u. bilirubin
    chylous u.
    cloudy u.
    crude u.
    u. culture
    u. cytology
    diabetic u.
    febrile u.
    fetal u.
    feverish u.
    gouty u.
    green u.
    honey u.
    hyposthenuric u.
    isosthenuric u.
    maple syrup u.
    u. mycobacterial culture
    milky u.
    nebulous u.
    u. osmolality
    pale u.
    u.-plasma ratio
    pregnancy u.

red u.
residual u.
u. sediment crystals
u./serum osmolality ratio
u. specimen collection
u. urea nitrogen
u. urobilinogen
urinemia
urinoma
     perirenal u.
urinometer
urinometry
urinophilous
urinoscopy
urinothorax
urinous
UriSystem
uroammoniac
urobenzoic acid
urobilin
urobilinemia
urobilinogen
     u. assay
     fecal u.
     u. test
     urine u.
urobilinogenemia
urobilinogenuria
urobilinuria
urocanic acid
urocele
urocheras
urochrome
urocortisol
urocrisia
urocyanin
urocyanogen
urocyanosis
urocystitis
urodynia
uroedema
uroepithelial cancer
uroerythrin
urofuscohematin
urogastrone
urogenital
     u. anlagen
     u. diaphragmatic fascia
     u. disease
     u. fistula
     u. folds
     u. mesenchyme

u. ridge
u. sinus
u. syndrome
u. system
u. tract
uroglaucin
urogram
     excretory u.
urography
urogravimeter
urohematonephrosis
urohemolytic coefficient
urokinase-like plasminogen activator
urokymography
urolith
urolithiasis
urolithic
urological
urology
urometer
uromucoid assay
uroncus
Uronema caudatum
uronephrosis
uronic acid
uronolactonase
uronoscopy
uropathy
     obstructive u.
uropepsin
uropepsinogen assay
urophanic
urophein
uroporphyria
     erythropoietic u.
uroporphyrin
     u. assay
     u. isomerase
uroporphyrinogen
     u. decarboxylase
     u. I synthase
     u. III synthase
uroporphyrinuria
uropsammus
uroreaction
urorosein
urorubin
urorubrohematin
uroschesis
uroscopic
uroscopy
urosemiology

urosepsin
uroseptic
urothelial
    u. aplasia/dysplasia
    u. atypia
    u. cells
    u. dysplasia
    u. hyperplasia
    u. leukoplakia
    u. metaplasia
    u. papilloma
urothelium
urotoxic coefficient
uroureter
uroxanthin
URQ — upper right quadrant
ursodeoxycholic acid
URTI — upper respiratory tract infection
urticant
urticaria
    aquagenic u.
    cholinergic u.
    factitious u.
    giant u.
    u. gigans
    u. gigantea
    u. perstans
    u. pigmentosa
    solar u.
    u. tuberosa
urticate
Uruma virus
U/S osmol ratio
US — ultrasonic
USN — ultrasonic nebulizer
USO — unilateral salpingo-oophorectomy
USPHS — United States Public Health Service
USR — unheated serum reagin (test)
Ustilaginaceae
ustilaginism
Ustilago maydis
usual interstitial pneumonitis
uta
UTBG — unbound thyroxine-binding globulin
uteri hernia inguinale
uterine
    u. artery
    u. aspiration

    u. bleeding
    u. blood flow
    u. calculus
    u. cancer
    u. cervix
    u. colic
    u. corpus carcinoma
    u. inertia
    u. leiomyoma
    u. ligament
    u. myoma
    u. segment
    u. serosa
    u. subserosa
    u. tube
    u. tumor
    u. vein
uteritis
utero
    in u.
uteroabdominal
uterolith
utero-ovarian varicocele
uteropelvic junction
uteroperitoneal fistula
uteroplacental insufficiency
uteroplasty
uterorectal
uterosacral ligament
uterosalpingography
uterus
    u. arcuatus
    u. bicornis bicollis
    u. bicornis unicollis
    bifid u.
    u. didelphys
    double u.
    duplex u.
    u. masculinus
    rudimentary u., male
    septate u.
    u. unicornis
UTI — urinary tract infection
utilization
    ketone body u.
    net protein u.
    u. time
UTP — uridine triphosphate
utricle
    prostatic u.
    urethral u.
utriculitis

utriculosaccular
UU — urine urobilinogen
UUN — urine urea nitrogen
UV — ultraviolet
    umbilical vein
    urinary volume
UVA — ultraviolet radiation
uvea
uveal melanoma
uveitis
    granulomatous u.
    nongranulomatous u.
    sympathetic u.
uveo-encephalitic syndrome

uveomeningitis
uveoparotid fever
UVJ — ureterovesical junction
UVL — ultraviolet light
uvula
    bifid u.
    u. of bladder
    palatine u.
    u. vermis
    u. vesicae
uvular
uvulitis
uvulotomy
U wave

V

V — factor V
    vanadium
    vein
    vision
    volume
V_{co} — carbon monoxide (endogenous production)
V_{CO_2} — carbon dioxide output
V_d — apparent volume of distribution (V area)
V_γ — tidal volume
V' — velocity
    Vibrio
    voltage
v — vein
volt
VA — vacuum aspiration
    ventriculoatrial
    vertebral artery
    visual acuity
    volt-ampere
Va — alveolar ventilation
vaccenic acid
vaccinate
vaccination
    roseola v.
vaccinatum
    eczema v.
vaccine
    attenuated v.
    autogenous v.
    bacille Calmette-Guérin v.

    Cox v.
    diphtheria, pertussis, and tetanus v.
    duck embryo v.
    Haemophilus pertussis v.
    hepatitis B v.
    influenza v.
    killed v.
    killed measles virus v.
    v. lymph
    pertussis v.
    pneumococcal v.
    polyvalent pneumococcal v.
    RhoGAM v.
    Sabin v.
    Salk v.
    smallpox v.
    trivalent oral poliovirus v.
    typhoid v.
    viral v.
vaccinia
    v. gangrenosa
    v. immune globulin
    v. virus
vaccinoid
VACTERL — vertebral, anal, cardiac, tracheal, esophageal, renal, and limb
vacuolar
    v. degeneration

v. myelopathy
v. nephrosis
vacuolated cell
vacuolating agent
vacuolation
vacuole
    v. alteration phagocytosis
    autophagic v.
    condensing v.
    contractile v.
    digestion v.
    heterophagic v.
    plasmocrine v.
    rhagiocrine v.
vacuolization
    cytoplasmic v.
    nuclear v.
vacuome
Vacutainer tube
VACURG — Veterans Administration Cooperative Urological Research Group
vacuum
    v. aspiration
    v. breaker
    v. distillation
    v. flask
    v. gauge
    high v.
    permeability of v.
    permittivity of v.
    v. phenomenon
    v. tube
    v. tuberculin
    v. tube voltmeter
    ultrahigh v.
VAD — venous admixture
VA factor
vagabond's
    v. disease
    v. melanosis
vagal paraganglioma
vagina (pl., vaginas, vaginae)
    blind-ended v.
    congenital absence of v.
    cyclic v.
    double v.
    fornix of v.
    menstrual v.
    pregnancy v.
    proliferative v.

    secretory v.
    septate v.
    vestibule of v.
vaginal
    v. adenosine
    v. adenosis
    v. apex
    v. artery
    v. atresia
    v. canal
    v. discharge
    v. epithelium
    v. hematocele
    v. irrigation smear
    v. metaplasia
    v. mucous membrane
    v. pool
    v. rhabdomyosarcoma
    v. secretion
    v. synovitis
    v. tumor
    v. vault
vaginalitis
vaginectomy
vaginismus
vaginitis (pl., vaginitides)
    v. adhaesiva
    adhesive v.
    candidal v.
    v. cystica
    desquamative inflammatory v.
    v. emphysematosa
    emphysematous v.
    gonococcal v.
    granular v.
    herpes simplex v.
    trichomonal v.
vaginogram
vaginography
vaginomycosis
vaginoperineal
vaginoperineoplasty
vaginoperineorrhaphy
vaginoperineotomy
vaginoperitoneal
vaginoplasty
vaginoscope
vaginosis
    bacterial v.
vaginotomy
vaginovesical
vaginovulvar

vagotomy
vagotonia
vagus nerve
Vahlkampfia
VAHS — virus-associated hemophago-
　　　　cytic syndrome
Val — valine
valence
　　　v. electron
　　　v. tautomer
Valentine's test
valeric acid
valethamate bromide
VALG — Veterans Administration
　　　　　Lung Cancer Study
　　　　　Group
valgus deformity
validation
valine
　　　v. aminotransferase
　　　v. transaminase
valinemia
valinuria
Valium
vallate
vallecula
　　　v. cerebelli
　　　v. epiglottica
　　　v. ovata
　　　v. for petrosal ganglion
　　　v. sylvii
　　　v. unguis
valley fever
villous adenomatous polyp
valproic acid
Valsalva's
　　　maneuver
　　　posterior sinus
value. (*See* Laboratory Reference Inter-
　　val Values, Appendix 1.)
　　　absolute v.
　　　acetyl v.
　　　acid v.
　　　buffer v.
　　　cot v.
　　　crot v.
　　　D v.
　　　GC v.
　　　globular v.
　　　iodine v.
　　　normal v's
　　　P v.

　　　predictive v.
　　　reference v's
　　　referent v.
　　　rot v.
　　　threshold limit v's
valve
　　　anal v's
　　　aortic v's
　　　atrioventricular v.
　　　cardiac v's
　　　cleft leaflet, mitral v.
　　　cleft leaflet, tricuspid v.
　　　congenital v.
　　　v. of coronary sinus
　　　v. of foramen ovale
　　　Heister's v.
　　　ileocecal v.
　　　v. of inferior vena cava
　　　Kerckring's v's
　　　mitral v.
　　　pulmonary v.
　　　pulmonic v. of commissure
　　　Singer-Blom stoma v.
　　　sinus v.
　　　spiral v.
　　　tricuspid v.
　　　ureteral v.
　　　urethral v.
　　　v. of veins
　　　venous v.
valvular
　　　v. atresia
　　　v. disease of heart
　　　v. endocarditis
　　　v. incompetence
　　　v. malformation
　　　v. stenosis
　　　v. thrombus
　　　v. tissue embolus
　　　v. vegetation
valvulitis
　　　rheumatic v.
valvulotomy
valyl
valylene
valyl-RNA synthetase
VAMP — vincristine, amethopterin,
　　　　　6-mercaptopurine, and
　　　　　prednisone
vanadium
vancomycin
van Deen's test

van de Kamer test
van den Bergh's
    test
    technique
van der Velden's test
van der Waals
    equation
    force
van Gieson's stain
vanillactic acid
vanillic acid
vanillin
vanillylmandelic acid: homovanillic
    acid ratio
vanishing testis syndrome
Van Slyke's
    amino acid procedure
    test
Van Slyke and Cullen's method
V antigen
vapor (pl., vapores, vapors)
    burning v.
    combustible v.
    v.-phase chromatography
    v. pressure
    v. pressure depression osmom-
        eter
vaporization
vaporize
vapor-phase chromatography
var — variant
variability
    random analytical v.
variable
    v. autotransformer
    v. capacitor
    continuous v.
    dependent v.
    dichotomous v.
    discrete v.
    double-precision v.
    endogenous v.
    exogenous v.
    fixed-point v.
    floating-point v.
    independent v.
    label v.
    v. number tandem repeats
    ordinal v.
    pointer v.
    random v.
    v. resistor

variance
    analysis of v.
    multivariate analysis of v.
    phenotypic v.
variant
    v. hemoglobin
    inherited albumin v's
    L-phase v.
    v. osteosarcoma
    sarcomatoid v.
    storiform-pleomorphic v.
    tubulopapillary v.
variate
    binary v.
variation
    antigenic v.
    coefficient of v.
    contingent negative v.
    interindividual v.
    intraindividual v.
    meristic v.
    microbial v.
    negative v.
    rough-smooth v.
    smooth-rough v.
varication
variceal
varicella
    v. gangrenosa
    v. pneumonia
    v. virus
    v. zoster
varicella-zoster
    v.-z. antibody test
    v.-z. immune globulin
    v.-z. infection
    v.-z. virus
    v.-z. virus culture
    v.-z. virus serology
varicelliform eruption
    Kaposi's v.e.
varices
variciform
varicocele
    ovarian v.
    symptomatic v.
    tubo-ovarian v.
    utero-ovarian v.
varicoid
varicole
varicophlebitis

varicose
    v. aneurysm
    v. ulcer
    v. vein
varicosis (pl., varicoses)
varicosity
varicule
variegate
    v. porphyria
variola
    v. minor
    v. virus
variolation
varix (pl., varices)
    v. anastomoticus
    aneurysmal v.
    cirsoid v.
    esophageal v.
    lymph v.
    orbital v.
    turbinal v.
varus deformity
vas (pl., vasa)
    v. deferens
    vasa efferentia
    v. lymphaticum
    v. lymphocapillare
    vasa recta
    vasa vasorum
vascormone
vascular
    v. anomaly
    v. arcade
    v. birthmark
    v. breast
    v. ectasis
    v. endothelium
    v. hemophilia
    v. keratitis
    v. leiomyoma
    v. malformation
    v. myxoma
    v. nephritis
    v. nevus
    v. permeability
    v. pole
    v. polyp
    v. resistance
    v. ring
    v. sclerosis
    v. sinusoid
    v. spider

    v. styptic
    v. system
vascularization
    corneal v.
vascularized
vasculature
vasculitis
    allergic v.
    classic v.
    cutaneous v.
    fungal v.
    granulomatous v.
    hypersensitivity v.
    leukocytoclastic v.
    livedo v.
    necrotizing v.
    nodular v.
    noninfectious v.
    Pseudomonas v.
    rejection v.
    rheumatoid v.
    rickettsial v.
    segmented hyalinizing v.
    systemic necrotizing v.
    testicular v.
vasculocardiac syndrome
vasculolymphatic
vasculomyelinopathy
vasculotoxic
vas deferens
    v.d. adventitia
    v.d. agenesis
    v.d. ampulla
    v.d. lumen
    v.d. mucosa
    v.d. muscularis
vasectomy
vasitis nodosa
vasoactive
    v. intestinal polypeptide
    v. peptide
    v. spasmogenic mediator
vasoactivity
vasoconstriction
vasocutaneous fistula
vasodepressor
vasodilatation
vasodilation
vasodilator
vasoexcitor
vasoformative cells

VASOG — Veterans Administration Surgical Oncology Group
vasogenic
 v. edema
 v. shock
vasomotor
 v. apparatus
 v. dysfunction
 v. hypotonia
 v. paralysis
 v. rhinitis
vaso-occlusive crisis
vasoparalysis
vasoparesis
vasopermeability
vasopressin
 arginine v.
vasopressor
vasospasm
vasospastic
vasotonin
vasovagal
vasovasostomy
vaspar
vastus
 v. intermedius muscle
 v. lateralis muscle
 v. medialis muscle
VATER — vertebral defects, imperforate anus, tracheoesophageal fistula, and radial and renal dysplasia
Vater-Pacini corpuscles
Vater's
 ampulla
 corpuscle
 papilla
VB — vinblastine
VBP — vinblastine, bleomycin, and Platinol
VBS — veronal-buffered saline
VBS : FBS — veronal-buffered saline : fetal bovine serum
VC — vena cava
 ventilatory capacity
 vincristine
 vital capacity
VCA — viral capsid antigen
VCG — vectorcardiogram
VCR — vincristine

VCU — voiding cystourethrogram
VD — vapor density
 venereal disease
VDA — visual discriminatory acuity
VDBR — volume of distribution of bilirubin
VDEL — Veneral Disease Experimental Laboratory
VDG — venereal disease—gonorrhea
VDH — valvular disease of heart
VDM — vasodepressor material
VDP — vincristine, daunorubicin, prednisone
VDRL — Venereal Disease Research Laboratory (test)
VDS — venereal disease—syphilis
VE — visual efficiency
 volumic ejection
V & E — Vinethene and ether
 vector
vector
 cloning v.
 dendritic v.
 v. diagram
 electric field v.
 expression v.
VEE virus — Venezuelan equine encephalomyelitis virus
vegetation
 bacterial v.
 dendritic v.
 valvular v.
 verrucous v.
vegetative endocarditis
veil
 aqueduct v.
Veillonella
 V. *alcalescens*
 V. *discoides*
 V. *orbiculus*
 V. *parvula*
 V. *reniformis*
 V. *vulvovaginitidis*
Veillonellaceae
vein
 azygos v.
 Galen's great cerebral v.
 Galen's lesser v.
 hepatic v.
 iliac v.
 innominate v.
 jugular v.

Labbé's anastomosing v.
mesenteric v.
omphalomesenteric v.
ophthalmic v.
ovarian v.
penile v.
pericardial v.
pulmonary v.
radial v.
Rosenthal's v.
saphenous v.
v. stone
striate v.
testicular v.
Trolard's anastomosing v.
ulnar v.
umbilical v.
uterine v.
varicose v's
velamen (pl., velamina)
v. vulvae
velamentous insertion
Velban
velocity
v. coefficient
v. constant
v. diffusion
nerve conduction v.
wave v.
velopharyngeal insufficiency
velum (pl., vela)
medullary v.
VEM — vasoexcitor material
vena (pl., venae)
v. cava
v. cava inferior
venae cordis
venacavogram
veneniferous
venenous
venereal
v. disease
v. disease — gonorrhea
v. disease — syphilis
v. lymphogranuloma
v. sore
v. ulcer
v. wart
Venereal Disease Experimental Laboratory
Venereal Disease Research Laboratory
venereology

venereum
lymphogranuloma v.
lymphopathia v.
Venezuelan
equine A encephalomyelitis virus
equine encephalitis
equine encephalomyelitis virus
venin
venipuncture
Venn diagram
venofibrosis
venogram
venography
peripheral v.
portal v.
splenic v.
splenoportal v.
venom
antisnake v.
cobra v.
Kokoi v.
v. leukocytolysis
Malayan pit viper v.
Russell's viper v.
snake v.
viper v.
veno-occlusive disease
venosclerosis
venostasis
venous
v. admixture
v. anastomosis
v. angioma
v. blood
v. cannulation
v. capillaries
v. claudication
v. congestion
v. embolism
v. gangrene
v. hematocrit
v. hum
v. infarction
v. insufficiency
v. murmur
v. obstruction
v. occlusion plethysmography
v. plexus
v. pressure

v. puncture
v. return curve
v. sclerosis
v. sinus
v. star
v. stasis
v. thromboembolism
v. thrombosis

vent
 pulmonic alveolar v's

ventilation
 alveolar v.
 v./perfusion ratio
 pulmonary v.
 total v.

ventral
 v. cervical nerve
 v. column
 v. corticospinal tract
 v. displacement
 v. external arcuate fibers
 v. hernia
 v. horn
 v. lateral sulcus
 v. lumbar nerve
 v. medial fissure
 v. median fissure
 v. paraflocculus
 v. pontine syndrome
 v. proper fasciculus
 v. respiratory group
 v. reticulospinal tract
 v. sacral nerve
 v. spinal nerve root
 v. spinocerebellar tract
 v. spinothalamic tract
 v. tegmental decussation
 v. thalamus
 v. thoracic nerve

ventricle
 aortic v.
 auxiliary v.
 cerebral v.
 double-outlet right v.
 fifth v.
 first v. of cerebrum
 fourth v.
 Galen's v.
 lateral v.
 left v.
 pineal v.
 right v.

second v. of cerebrum
sixth v.
terminal v.
third v. of cerebrum
Verga's v.

ventricose
ventricular
 v. aneurysm
 v. bigeminum
 v. contraction
 v. diverticulum
 v. escape
 v. fibrillation
 v. filling phase
 v. fold
 v. function curve
 v. gradient
 v. hypertrophy
 v. murmur
 v. performance
 period of v. filling
 v. premature beat
 v. premature contraction
 v. premature depolarization
 v. septal defect
 v. septum
 v. system
 v. tachycardia
 v. vein

ventriculoatrial
ventriculography
ventriculojugular shunt
ventriculoradial dysplasia
ventriculosubarachnoid
ventromedial nucleus
ventroptosia
ventroptosis
Venturi mask
venula (pl., venulae)
venule
 postcapillary v.
VEP — visual evoked potential
VePesid
VER — visual evoked response
vera
 polycythemia v.
verapamil
verdoglobin
verdohemochrome
verdohemoglobin
verdoperoxidase
Verga's ventricle

vergeture
Verhoeff's elastic tissue stain
Verhoeff–van Gieson stain
vermian
    v. lobule
    v. sublobule
vermicular
vermiform granules
vermifuge
vermilion
vermilionectomy
verminous
    v. abscess
    v. colic
vermis
    cerebellar v.
    uvula v.
vernal conjunctivitis
Vernier dial
vernix caseosa
Verocay bodies
veronal
    v. buffer
    v.-buffered saline: fetal bovine
        serum
verotoxins
Verril's sign
verruca (pl., verrucae)
    v. acuminata
    v. digitata
    v. filiformis
    v. glabra
    v. mollusciformis
    v. necrogenica
    v. peruana
    v. plana
    v. plana juvenilis
    v. plana senilis
    v. plantaris
    seborrheic v.
    v. seborrheica
    v. senilis
    v. simplex
    urethral v.
    v. virus
    v. vulgaris
verrucal
    v. atypical endocarditis
    v. nonbacterial endocar-
        ditis
verruciform xanthoma

verruciformis
    acrokeratosis v.
verrucose
verrucosis
    lymphostatic v.
verrucous
    v. carcinoma
    v. carditis
    v. endocarditis
    v. hyperplasia
    v. nevus
    v. papilloma
    v. scrofuloderma
    v. vegetation
    v. xanthoma
verruga peruana
versicolor
vertebra (pl., vertebrae)
    cervical v.
    dorsal v.
    lumbar v.
    sacral v.
    thoracic v.
vertebral
    v. artery
    v. arthritis
    v. basilar artery syndrome
    v. column
    v. compression fracture
    v. crush-fracture syndrome
    v. hemangioendothelioma
    v. joint
    v. nerve
    v. osteomyelitis
    v. polyarthritis
    v. tuberculosis
    v. vein
vertebrate
vertex (pl., vertices)
vertical occipital fasciculus
Verticillium graphii
vertigo
verumontanitis
verumontanum
very-low-density lipoprotein
very-high-density lipoprotein
very late activation anticoagulation
vesica (pl., vesicae)
vesical
    v. artery
    v. blood fluke
    v. calculus

v. diverticulum
v. dysplasia
v. endometriosis
v. fistula
v. hematuria
vesicle
  acoustic v.
  acrosomal v.
  germinal v.
  lens v.
  micropinocytotic v's
  optical v.
  phospholipid v.
vesicoabdominal
vesicobullous
vesicocervical
vesicocolic fistula
vesicocutaneous fistula
vesicointestinal fistula
vesicolithiasis
vesicoperineal
vesicopustular
vesicopustule
vesicosigmoid
vesicostomy
vesicoumbilical fistula
vesicoureteral reflux
vesicourethral
vesicouterine fistula
vesicouterovaginal
vesicovaginal fistula
vesicovaginorectal fistula
vesicula (pl., vesiculae)
vesicular
  v. acute inflammation
  v. emphysema
  v. eruption
  v. granulomatous inflammation
  v. inflammation
  v. keratitis
  v. lesion
  v. mole
  v. murmur
  v. nucleus
  v. pharyngitis
  v. stomatitis
vesiculate
vesiculation
vesiculiform
vesiculin
vesiculitis
vesiculocavernous

vesiculopapular
vesiculoprostatitis
vesiculopustular
vesiculose
vessel
  blood v.
  aberrant renal v's
  transposition of great v's
vestibular
  v. anus
  v. apparatus
  v. ganglion
  v. gland
  v. membrane
  v. nerve
  v. nucleus
  v. root
  v. sensation
  v. window
vestibule
  Gibson's v.
  labyrinth v.
  nasal v.
  oral v.
vestibulocochlear
  v. nerve
  v. organ
vestibulospinal
vestigial
vesuvine
VF — ventricular fibrillation
  ventricular fluid
  visual field
  vocal fremitus
v.f. — field of vision
V factor
VFP — ventricular fluid pressure
VG — ventricular gallop
VH — vaginal hysterectomy
  venous hematocrit
  viral hepatitis
VHD — viral hematodepressive
  disease
VHDL — very high density lipoprotein
VI — volume index
VIA — virus-inactivating agent
viability
viable cell count
Vi agglutination
Vi antigen
vib — vibration

vibration
    v. receptor
    v. second
    v. sensation
vibrator
    Bart's v.
vibratory
    v. sense
    v. sense loss
Vibrio
    V. *alginolyticus*
    V. *bubulus*
    V. *cholerae*
    V. *cholerae-asiaticae*
    V. *coli*
    V. *comma*
    V. *danubicus*
    V. *eltor*
    V. *fecalis*
    V. *fetus*
    V. *finkleri*
    V. *ghinda*
    V. group EF6
    V. *jejuni*
    V. *massauah*
    V. *metschnikovii*
    V. *niger*
    V. *parahaemolyticus*
    V. *phosphorescens*
    V. *proteus*
    V. *septicus*
    V. *sputorum*
    V. *tyrogenus*
    V. *vulnificus*
vibrio
    Celebes v.
    cholera v.
    El Tor v.
    nonagglutinating v.
    paracholera v.
vibrion septique
Vibrionaceae
vibriosis
vicarious
    v. hemoptysis
    v. hypertrophy
    v. menstruation
Vicia faba (fava)
vicinal
vicine
vicious union
Victoria blue

Victoria orange
vidarabine
videognosis
vidian neuralgia
Vierra's sign
VIG — vaccinia-immune globulin
villiform
villin
villitis
villoma
villonodular
    v. pigmented synovitis
    v. pigmented tenosynovitis
villositis
villous
    v. adenoma
    v. adenomatous polyp
    v. carcinoma
    v. papilloma
    v. polyp
    v. tenosynovitis
    v. tumor
villus (pl., villi)
    abnormal chorionic v.
    arachnoid v.
    chorionic v.
    intestinal v.
    mature abnormal chorionic v.
    synovial v.
viloma
vimentin
vinbarbital
vinblastine sulfate
vinca alkaloid
Vincent's
    angina
    organism
    stomatitis
vincristine
    v. neuropathy
    v. sulfate
vinculin
vindesine
vinegar acid
vinyl
    v. chloride
    v. cyanide
    v. ether
    v. polymer
    v. trichloride
vinzolidine
violaceous

violet
    amethyst v.
    aniline gentian v.
    Bensley's safranin acid v.
    Bernthesen's methylene v.
    chrome v.
    cresyl v. acetate
    crystal v.
    gentian v.
    hexamethyl v.
    methylene v.
    pentamethyl v.
viomycin
viosterol
VIP — vasoactive intestinal poly-
      peptide
    voluntary interruption of
      pregnancy
viper venom
VIPoma — vasoactive intestinal poly-
      peptide + -oma
Vira A
viral
    v. bronchiolitis
    v. bronchopneumonia
    v. capsid antigen
    v. conjunctivitis
    v. culture
    v. cystitis
    v. diarrhea
    v. dysentery
    v. encephalitis
    v. enteritis
    v. enterocolitis
    v. gastroenteritis
    v. hemagglutination
    v. hematodepressive disease
    v. hepatitis (type A and
      type B)
    v. inclusion cells
    v. infection
    v. meningitis
    v. myocarditis
    v. oncogenesis
    v. otitis
    v. particles
    v. pharyngitis
    v. pleuritis
    v. pneumonia
    v. probe
    v. respiratory infection
    v. rhinitis
    v. sinusitis

    v. tonsillitis
    v. wart
viral disease
    abortive v.d.
    arboviral v.d.
    arthropod borne v.d.
    herpetic v.d.
    persistent v.d.
    respiratory v.d.
    retroviral v.d.
Virazole
Virchow-Robin space
Virchow's
    crystals
    gland
    hydatid
    law
    nociceptor
    node
    viremia
virginity
viridans streptococcus (streptococci)
virilism
    adrenal v.
    congenital adrenal v.
virility
virilization
    adrenal v.
virilizing
    v. adenoma
    v. carcinoma
    v. syndrome
    v. tumor
virion
virogene
virology
virostatic
virucidal
virucopria
virulence
virulent
viruria
virus (pl., viruses)
    Abelson's murine leukemia v.
    acute laryngotracheobronchi-
      tis v.
    v. A hepatitis
    AIDS-related v.
    animal v's
    v. animatum
    Apeú v.

arbor v's, groups A, B, C, un-
    classified
Argentine hemorrhagic
    fever v.
v.-associated hemophagocytic
    syndrome
attenuated v.
Australian X disease v.
Australian X encephalitis v.
avian erythroblastosis v.
avian leukosis v.
avian myeloblastosis v.
avian myelocytomatosis v.
bacterial v.
v. B hepatitis
biundulant milk fever v.
BK v.
v. blockade
bovine leukemia v.
bovine papilloma v.
Brunhilde v.
Bunyamwera v.
Bwamba fever v.
C v. (Coxsackie virus)
CA v. (croup-associated parain-
    fluenza virus)
Cache Valley v.
California encephalitis v.
Central European encephali-
    tis v.
chickenpox v.
chikungunya fever v.
Coe v.
Colorado tick fever v.
Columbia SK v.
common cold v.
coryza v.
cowpox v.
Coxsackie v., A, type 1; B,
    type 1
Crimean hemorrhagic
    fever v.
croup-associated v.
cytomegalic inclusion dis-
    ease v.
cytopathic v.
defective v
dengue v., types 1, 2, 3, 4
diphasic meningoencephali-
    tis v.
diphasic milk fever v.
distemper v.

eastern equine encephalomyeli-
    tis v.
EB v. (Epstein-Barr virus)
Ebola v.
ECBO v. (ecbovirus)
ECDO v. (ecdovirus)
ECHO v. (echovirus)
ECMO v. (ecmovirus)
ECSO v. (ecsovirus)
ecthyma infectiosum v.
EEE v. (eastern equine enceph-
    alomyelitis virus)
EMC v. (encephalomyocarditis
    virus)
encephalomyocarditis v.
enteric cytopathogenic bovine
    orphan v.
enteric cytopathogenic human
    orphan v.
enteric cytopathogenic monkey
    orphan v.
enteric cytopathogenic swine
    orphan v.
entomopox v.
epidemic keratoconjunctivi-
    tis v.
epidemic parotitis v.
Epstein-Barr v.
equine encephalomyelitis v.
erythema infectiosum v.
exanthem subitum v.
feline leukemia v.
fifth disease v.
filterable v.
fixed v.
foot-and-mouth disease v.,
    types A, B, C
Guama v.
Guaroa v.
Hantaan v.
hemadsorption v., types 1, 2
hemagglutinating v.
hepatitis v.
herpangina v.
herpes v.
herpes-like v.
herpes simplex v., I, II
herpes-type v.
herpes zoster v.
human immunodeficiency v.
human T-cell leukemia-
    lymphoma v.

human T-cell lymphotropic v.
Ilheus v.
v.-inactivating agent
inclusion conjunctivitis v.
infectious hepatitis v.
influenza v., types A, B, C
Itaqui v.
Japanese B encephalitis v.
JC v.
JCV v.
JH v.
Junin v.
Kumba v.
Kyasanur Forest disease v.
LaCrosse v.
lactic dehydrogenase v.
Lansing v.
Lassa v.
latent v.
LCM (lymphocytic choriomeningitis) v.
Leon v.
lepori pox v.
louping ill v.
Lunyo v.
lymphadenopathy-associated v.
lymphocytic choriomeningitis v.
lymphogranuloma venereum v.
Machupo v.
mammary tumor v.
Marburg v.
Marituba v.
masked v.
Mason Pfizer monkey v.
Mayaro v.
measles v.
Mengo v.
MM v.
molluscum contagiosum v.
molluscum sebaceum v.
Moloney's leukemogenic v.
Moloney's sarcoma v.
monkey B v.
mouse leukemia v.
mouse mammary tumor v.
mumps v.
murine leukemia v.
murine sarcoma v.
Murray Valley encephalitis v.
neurotropic v.
v.-neutralizing

Newcastle disease v.
nonbacterial gastroenteritis v.
Norwalk v.
Ntaya v.
Omsk hemorrhagic fever v.
oncogenic v.
O'nyong-nyong fever v.
orf v.
Oriboca v.
ornithosis v.
Oropouche v.
orphan v's
panleukopenia v.
pappataci fever v.
parainfluenza v., types 1,
 2, 3, 4
parapox v.
parrot v.
pharyngoconjunctival
 fever v.
phlebotomus fever v.
pneumonitis v.
poliomyelitis v.
polyoma v.
Powassan v.
pox v.
psittacosis v.
rabies v.
rat v.
reservoir of v.
respiratory exanthematous v.
respiratory infection v.
respiratory syncytial v.
Rift Valley fever v.
RNA v.
roseola infantum v.
Rous' sarcoma v.
RS (respiratory synctial) v.
rubella v.
rubeola v.
Russian spring-summer encephalitis v.
Salisbury common cold v.
salivary gland v.
sand-fly fever v.
Schwartz leukemia v.
Semliki Forest v.
Sendai v.
serum hepatitis v.
v. shedding
Simbu v.
simian v.

simian immunodeficiency v.
simian sarcoma v.
simian T-cell leukemia
 v. — III
Sindbis v.
slow v's
smallpox v.
St. Louis encephalitis v.
street v.
SV 40 v.
T-cell lymphotropic v.
Teschen's v.
Theiler's v.
tickborne v's
tobacco mosaic v.
trachoma v.
transforming v.
v. transport medium
Uganda S v.
unorganized v.
Uruma v.
vaccinia v.
vacuolating v.
varicella v.
varicella-zoster v.
variola v.
VEE (Venezuelan equine encephalomyelitis) v.
Venezuelan equine A encephalomyelitis v.
verruca v.
vesicular stomatitis v.
WEE (western equine encephalomyelitis) v.
Wesselsbron v.
western equine enncephalomye-
 litis v.
West Nile v.
Willowbrook v.
yellow fever v.
Zika v.
zoster-varicella v.
2060 v.

VIS — vaginal irrigation smear
viscera
 abdominal v.
 thoracic v.
visceral
 v. edema
 v. fibers, afferent, efferent
 v. inversion
 v. larva migrans

 v. layer
 v. leishmaniasis
 v. membrane
 v. metastasis
 v. neuralgia
 v. pericardium
 v. peritoneum
 v. pleurisy
visceromegaly
visceroptosia
visceroptosis
viscerotomy
viscerotrophic reflex
viscid
viscidosis
viscometer
viscoplastic
viscosimeter
 Ostwald's v.
 Stormer's v.
viscosimetry
viscosity
 absolute v.
 dynamic v.
 kinematic v.
viscous metamorphosis
viscus (pl., viscera)
visor flap
visual
 v. association areas
 v. cortex
 v. cycle
 v. disorder
 v. evoked cortical potential
 v. field defect
 v. pathway
 v. pigments
 v. receiving area
 v.-spatial
 v. transduction
 v. yellow
 v. zone
visuomotor
visuospatial
vital
 v. capacity
 v. dye
 v. red
 v. signs
 v. staining
vitamin
 v. A

v. A and carotene assay
v. A clearance test
v. A unit
v. A_1 (retinol) (aldehyde)
v. A_2 (dehydroretinol)
v. B
v. B complex
v. B_1 (thiamine) (hydrochloride unit)
v. B_2 (riboflavin)
v. B_3
v. B_6
v. B_7
v. B_{12} (cyanocobalamin)
v. B_{12} absorption test
v. B_{12b} (hydroxocobalamin)
v. B_c conjugate (folic acid)
v. C (ascorbic acid)
v. D (calciferol)
v. D–dependent types I, II rickets
v. D_2 (ergosterol)
v. D_3 (cholecalciferol)
v. D hormone
v. D poisoning
v. E (alpha-tocopherol)
fat soluble v's
v. G (riboflavin)
v. H (biotin)
v. K
v. K deficiency
v. K_1 (phytonadione)
v. K_2 (menaquinone)
v. K_3 (menadione)
v. L
v. L_1
v. L_2
v. M (folic acid)
water soluble v's
vitaminoid
vitellin
vitelline
v. duct
v. sphere
vitellointestinal
v. cyst
v. duct
vitiation
vitiliginous
vitiligo (pl., vitiligines)
circumnevic v.
vitiligoidea

vitreous
v. body
v. humor
vitriol oil
vitronectin
vivax
v. fever
v. malaria
Viviparidae
Viviparus
vivum contagium
VLA — very late appearing antigen
VLB — vinblastine
VLDL — very low density lipoprotein
VLSI — very large scale integration
VM — viomycin
voltmeter
VMA — vanillylmandelic acid (test)
V max — total enzyme activity
VMR — vasomotor rhinitis
VN — virus-neutralizing
VNS — villonodular synovitis
VNTRs — variable number tandem repeats
vocal
v. cord
v. fold
Voges-Proskauer
broth
reaction
reagent
test
volar
v. artery
v. digital vein
v. metacarpal artery
v. metacarpal vein
volatile
v. oil
v. organic substances
v. screen
volatility
volatilization
vole bacillus
Volhard's test
Volkmann's
canal
contracture
paralysis
Vollmer's test
volt
v.-ampere

electron v.
giga electron v.
kilo electron v.
megaelectron v.
million electron v.
v.-ohm-milliammeter
v.-ohm-millimeter

voltage
anode v.
v. divider
v.-gated channel
v.-regulating transformer
v. regulator
v.-regulator tube
ripple v.
v.-to-frequency converter

voltammetry
voltmeter
digital v.
vacuum tube v.

volt-ohm-milliammeter
volt-ohm-millimeter
volume
atomic v.
blood v.
cell v.
central blood v.
circulating blood v.
v. coefficient
v. conduction
conductivity cell v.
corrected blood v.
v. of distribution of bilirubin
effective circulating blood v.
end-diastolic v.
end-systolic v.
expiratory reserve v.
extracellular v.
extracellular fluid v.
fluid v.
forced expiratory v.
v. index
inspiratory reserve v.
intracellular fluid v.
intrathoracic gas v.
mean cell v.
mean corpuscular v.
mean platelet v.
minute v.
v. overload
packed cell v.
v. of packed red cells

v. per cent
placental residual blood v.
plasma v.
pulmonary capillary blood v.
red blood cell v.
red cell v.
regional cerebral blood v.
residual v.
retention v.
stroke v.
v. substitute
thoracic gas v.
tidal v.
total blood v.
weight per v.

volumetric
v. analysis
v. flask
v. pipet
v. solution

voluntary
v. activity
v. interruption of pregnancy
v. muscle

Volutella cinerescens
volutin
volvulus
gastric v.

VOM — volt-ohm-millimeter
vomer
vomeronasal
v. cartilage
v. organ

vomica
vomicose
vomit
vomitus
colonic v.

v-onc
von Haberer's gastroenterostomy
von Hansemann cells
von Jaksch's anemia
von Kossa's method
von Kupffer's cells
von Meyenburg's complex
von Recklinghausen's neurofibromatosis
von Willebrand's
antigen
factor

vortex (pl., vortices)
voxel — volume element

VP — vasopressin
    venipuncture
    venous pressure
    Voges-Proskauer (reaction)
    volume-pressure
VP-16-epidophyllotoxin
VPB — ventricular premature beat
VPC — vapor-phase chromatography
    ventricular premature con-
      traction
    volume per cent
VPD — ventricular premature depolar-
      ization
VPRC — volume of packed red cells
V/Q — ventilation-perfusion ratio
VR — valve replacement
    vascular resistance
    venous return
    ventilation ratio
    vocal resonance
VRBC — red blood cell volume
VRD — von Recklinghausen's disease
VRI — viral respiratory infection
VS — venesection
    vital signs
    volumetric solution
v.s. — vibration seconds
VSD — ventricular septal defect
VSS — vital signs stable
V strips
VSV — vesicular stomatitis virus
VSW — ventricular stroke work
VT — vacuum tuberculin
    ventricular tachycardia

VTE — venous thromboembolism
V & T — volume and tension
V-Tech urinalysis system
vulgaris
    acne v.
    psoriasis v.
vulva
vulvar
    v. connective tissue
    v. dystrophy
    v. hyperplasia
    v. mucous membrane
    v. tumor
vulvectomy
vulvitis
    chronic atrophic v.
    chronic hypertrophic v.
    leukoplakic v.
vulvorectal
vulvouterine
vulvovaginal
    v. anus
    v. gland
vulvovaginitis
VUR — vesicoureteral reflux
VV — viper venom
vv — veins
v/v — volume for volume
VW — vessel wall
VWD — von Willebrand's disease
VZ — varicella-zoster
VZIG — varicella-zoster immune
      globulin
VZV — varicella-zoster virus
VZV culture

W

W — tungsten
    Weber's (test)
    wehnelt (unit of roentgen
      ray penetrating
      ability)
W+ — weakly positive
w — water
    watt
Wachstein-Meissel stain
Wade-Fite-Faraco stain
Wagner's test

Waldenström's
    macroglobulinemia
    purpura
    test
Waldeyer's
    gland
    tonsillar ring
Walker's
    carcinoma
    carcinosarcoma
"walking pneumonia"

wall
    anterior w.
    cell w.
    cross w.
    ureteral w.
wallerian degeneration
wallet stomach
Wallhauser and Whitehead's method
Walsh's average
Walthard's
    cell rests
    islets
wandering
    w. abscess
    w. goiter
    w. liver
    w. organ
    w. pacemaker
    w. pneumonia
Wangensteen's tube
Wangiella dermatitidis
Wang's test
warble fly
warbles
Warburg's theory
warfarin
    w. assay
    w. potassium
    sodium w.
warm
    w. agglutinin
    w. antibody
    w. auto antibodies
    w. hemagglutinin
warmth receptor
Warren's incision
wart
    anatomical w.
    common w.
    digitate w.
    fig w.
    filiform w.
    flat w.
    genital w.
    infectious w.
    moist w.
    mosaic w.
    necrogenic w.
    pitch w.
    plane w.
    plantar w.
    pointed w.

    postmortem w.
    prosector's w.
    seborrheic w.
    senile w.
    soft w.
    soot w.
    telangiectatic w.
    tuberculous w.
    venereal w.
    viral w.
Warthin-Finkeldey
    cell
    giant cell
Warthin-Starry silver stain
Warthin's tumor
warty
    w. carcinoma
    w. dyskeratoma
    w. dyskeratosis
    w. horn
    w. ulcer
WAS — Wiskott-Aldrich syndrome
wash
    Gravlee jet w.
washed
    w. red blood cells
    w. red cells
washing
    bronchial w.
    w. cytology
    gastric w.
    renal pelvic w.
    renal salt w.
    salt-w.
    urethral w.
WASP — World Association of
            Societies of Pathology
Wassén test
wasserhelle
    w. cell
    w. hyperplasia
Wassermann's
    antigen
    reaction
    test
Wassermann-fast
waste
    chemical w.
    infectious w.
    w. product
    radioactive w.
    toxic w.

wasting
    sodium w.
    syndrome
Watanabe heritable hyperlipidemic
    rabbetting
water
    w. aspirator
    w. bacterium
    w. bath
    w. brash
    w.-clear cell
    w.-clear-cell hyperplasia
    w. conductivity
    w.-deprivation test
    extracellular w.
    w. gas
    gentian aniline w.
    w. immersion
    interstitial w.
    w. intoxication
    intracellular w.
    w. loading study
    w.-soluble scarlet
    w.-soluble vitamins
    total body w.
    w.-trap stomach
watering-can
    w.c. perineum
    w.c. scrotum
watershed
    abdominal w's
    w. infarct
    w. infarction
Watson-Crick helix
Watsonius watsoni
Watson-Schwartz test
watt
watts-second
wave
    acid w.
    alkaline w.
    alpha w's
    w. amplitude
    w. analyzer
    beta w's
    brain w's
    C w.
    cannon a w's
    contraction w.
    delta w's
    dicrotic w.
    diphasic w.
    E w.

    Erb's w's
    F w's
    giant a w's
    H w.
    M w.
    Mayer's w's
    monophasic w.
    w. number
    P w.
    periodic w.
    polyphasic w.
    Q w.
    R w.
    S w.
    sawtooth w.
    sine w.
    square w.
    T w.
    theta w's
    three-hertz spike and slow w's
    Traube-Hering w's
    triangular w.
    tricrotic w.
    triphasic w.
    U w.
    v w.
    w. velocity
    ventricular w.
    x w.
    y w.
waveform
waveguide
wavelength
    w. accuracy
    nominal w.
    w. repeatability
wavy fibers
wax
    bone w.
    w. gland
    grave w.
waxy
    w. cast
    w. degeneration
    w. fingers
    w. kidney
    w. liver
    w. spleen
    w. urinary cast
Wayson stain
WB — weight bearing
    whole blood

whole body
Willowbrook (virus)
Wb — Weber
WBC — white blood cell
white blood count
WBC/hpf — white blood cells per
high power field
WBCT — whole blood clotting time
WBF — whole-blood folate
WBH — whole-blood hematocrit
whole body hyperthermia
WBR — whole body radiation
WC — white cell
white cell casts
whooping cough
WC′ — whole complement
WCC — white cell count
WD — wallerian degeneration
WDHA — watery diarrhea,
hypokalemia, and
achlorhydria
WDLL — well-differentiated
lymphocytic lymphoma
WE — western encephalitis
western encephalomyelitis
weakly
w. positive
w. reactive
wear-and-tear pigmentation
web
cell w.
esophageal w.
laryngeal w.
subsynaptic w.
terminal w.
webbed
w. fingers
w. neck
w. penis
w. toes
webbing
Weber-Christian panniculitis
Weber-Ferguson incision
Weber's
gland
test
Webster's
technique
test
weddellite calculus
wedge
w. method
w. resection

wedged hepatic vein pressure
WEE — western equine encephalomyelitis
WEE virus — western equine encephalomyelitis virus
Weeks' bacillus
Wegener's granulomatosis
Wegner's line
wehnelt (unit of penetration of roentgen rays)
Weibel-Palade bodies
Weichselbaum's diplococcus
Weidel's reaction
Weigert-Gram stain
Weigert's
iodine solution
iron hematoxylin
iron hematoxylin stain
weight
apothecaries' w.
atomic w.
avoirdupois w.
equivalent w.
fat-free dry w.
fat-free wet w.
gram-molecular w.
high birth w.
high molecular w.
ideal body w.
low birth w.
low molecular w.
molar w.
molecular w.
w. per volume
total body w.
Weil-Felix
agglutinins
reaction
test
Weinberg's reaction
Weinman's medium
Welch's bacillus
Welcker's method
welders'
w. conjunctivitis
w. lung
well-differentiated
w.d. lymphocytic lymphoma
w.d. liposarcoma
welt
wen
Wenckebach's block

Werdnig-Hoffmann paralysis
Werner's test
Wernicke's encephalopathy
Wesenberg-Hamazaki body
Wesselsbron's virus
West Nile
    fever
    virus
Westergren's
    method
    sedimentation rate
Western
    blot analysis
    blot technique
    blot test
    blotting
western
    w. encephalitis
    w. encephalomyelitis
    w. equine encephalitis
    w. equine encephalomyelitis
    w. equine encephalomyelitis
        virus
Westgard
    multi-rule technique
    quality control test
Westphal-Strümpell pseudosclerosis
wet
    w. beriberi
    w. gangrene
    w. lung
    w. pleurisy
Wetzel's test
WFR — Weil-Felix reaction
WGA — wheat germ agglutinin
Wharton's duct
wheal
    w.-and-erythema skin test
    w. reaction time
wheat germ agglutinin
Wheatley trichrome stain
Wheatstone's bridge
Wheeler-Johnson test
wheel rotation
wheeze
whetstone crystals
whewellite calculus
whey
    litmus w.
WHHL — Watanabe heritable hyper-
        lipidemic rabbetting
whiplash

Whipple's
    method
    resection
    triad
whipworm
whistling face syndrome
white
    w. bile
    w. blood cell
    w. blood cell count
    w. blood cells per high power
        field
    w. blood cell urinary cast
    w. cell
    w. cell casts
    w. cell count
    w. corpuscle
    w. gangrene
    w. infarct
    w. (anemic) infarction
    w. lead
    w. leg
    w. line
    w. matter
    w. muscle
    w. patch
    w. piedra
    w. pulp
    w. ramus
    w. spot
    w. spot disease
    w. substance (Schwann's)
    w. thrombus
whitehead
whitlow
    herpetic w.
    melanotic w.
Whitmore's
    bacillus
    staging system
Whitnall's ligament
Whitten effect
WHO — World Health Organization
WHO histological classification of
        ovarian tumors
whole
    w.-arm fusion
    w. blood
    w. blood cells
    w. blood clot lysis time
    w. body irradiation
    w.-body titration curve

w. complement
w. ragweed extract
whole-blood
w.b. folate
w.b. hematocrit
whooping cough
Wickham's striae
Widal's
reaction
test
width
red-cell distribution w.
Wiener system
Wilbrand's prism test
Wilcoxon
rank sum statistic
signed rank statistic
Wilder's stain
wild-type gene
Wilkerson point system
Wilkins-Chilgren agar
Williams' stain
Willis'
circle
pancreas
Willowbrook virus
Wills' factor
Wilms' tumor
wind contusion
window
cochlear w.
skin w.
vestibular w.
Winslow's
epiploic foramen
pancreas
Wintrobe's
hematocrit
macromethod
method
sedimentation rate
tube
Wintrobe and Landsberg's method
wire-loop
w.-l. lesion
w.-l. test
wire-wound resistor
Wirsung's duct
Wisconsin medium
within normal limits
WK — Wernicke-Korsakoff
(syndrome)

WMA — World Medical Association
WMR — work metabolic rate
WNL — within normal limits
W/O — water in oil
Wohlfahrtia
W. *magnifica*
W. *opaca*
W. *vigil*
Wohlgemuth unit
Woldman's test
Wolff-Chaikoff effect
wolffian
w. body
w. cyst
w. duct
w. duct carcinoma
w. rest
Wolf-Orton body
Wolhynian fever
Wood's
glass
lamp
light
Wookey skin flap
woolsorters' disease
work metabolic rate
Working Formulation of National
Cancer Institute
Working Formulation of non-
Hodgkin's lymphoma for clinical
usage
workload recording system
World Association of Societies of Pathology
World Health Organization
WHO histologic classification
of ovarian tumors
World Medical Association
worm
w. abscess
Bancroft's filarial w.
dragon w.
eye w.
serpent w.
tongue w's
Wormley's test
wound
abraded w.
avulsed w.
contused w.
w. culture
first intention w.

gunshot w.
incised w.
lacerated w.
missile w.
mutilating w.
penetrating w.
perforating w.
second intention w.
spiral w.
stab w.
superficial w.
surgical w.
WP — weakly positive
WPW — Wolff-Parkinson-White (syndrome)
WR — Wassermann reaction
    weakly reactive
Wratten filter
W rays
WRC — washed red cells

WRE — whole ragweed extract
Wright
    blood group system
    respirometer
Wright's
    antigen
    stain
wrinkled nucleus
Wrisberg's nerve
wryneck
ws — watts-second
wt — weight
Wuchereria
    W. bancrofti
    W. malayi
    W. pacifica
wuchereriasis
Wu-Kabat plot
Wurster's test
w/v — weight per volume
Wyeomyia

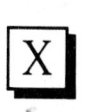

X — homeopathic symbol for the decimal scale of potencies
    Kienböck's unit of x-ray dosage
    magnification
    respirations (anesthesia chart)
Xa — antifactor X
xanthate
xanthelasma
    generalized x.
    x. palpebrarum
xanthelasmoidea
xanthematin
xanthemia
xanthene
    x. dye
    x. structure
xanthic calculus
xanthine
    x. dimethyl
    x. oxidase
    x. ribonucleoside
    x. trimethyl
xanthinuria
xanthinuric
xanthiuria

xanthochromatic
xanthochromia
xanthochromic
xanthocyte
xanthoderma
xanthoerythrodermia perstans
xanthogranuloma
    juvenile x.
    necrobiotic x.
xanthogranulomatous
    x. cholecystitis
    x. pyelonephritis
xanthoma
    x. cell
    cerebrotendinous x.
    x. diabeticorum
    x. disseminatum
    fibrous x.
    juvenile x.
    normolipemic x.
    x. palpebrarum
    plane x.
    x. planum
    x. striatum palmare
    x. tendinosum

tendinous x.
x. tuberosum simplex
tuberous x.
verruciform x.
verrucous x.
xanthomatosis
    biliary x.
    cerebrotendinous x.
    normal cholesteremic x.
xanthomatous
    x. deposition
    x. granuloma
Xanthomonas
xanthopsia
xanthopsydracia
xanthopterin
xanthosarcoma
xanthosine
    x. monophosphate
    x. phosphate
xanthosis
xanthous
xanthoxanthomatosis
xanthurenic
    x. acid
    x. aciduria
xanthuria
xanthylic acid
x-axis
X body
XC — excretory cystogram
X chromatin bodies
X chromosome
XDP — xeroderma pigmentosum
Xe — xenon
xenoantigen
xenobiotic
xenodiagnosis
xenogeneic antigen
xenogenetic
xenograft
xenology
xenon
xenon-127
xenon-133
xenoparasite
Xenopsylla
    X. *astia*
    X. *brasiliensis*
    X. *cheopis*
Xenopus laevis
xenylamine

xeransis
xerantic
xerocytosis
xeroderma pigmentosum
xeromammography
xeronosus
xerophthalmia
xeroradiography
xerosialography
xerosis
xerostomia
xerotic
xerotomography
X factor
Xg antigen
Xga antigen
Xga blood group system
X histiocytosis
X-inactivation
xiphisternum
xiphoiditis
xiphoid process
Xk^a antigen
X karyotype
XLA — X-linked agammaglobuli-
    nemia
XLD — xylose-lysine-deoxycholate
    (agar)
X-linked
    X-l. agammaglobulinemia
    X-l. character
    X-l. dominant inheritance
    X-l. familial hypophosphatemia
    X-l. gene
    X-l. genetic disorder
    X-l. heredity
    X-l. hyper-IgM immunodefi-
        ciency
    X-l. hypogammaglobulinemia
        with growth hormone defi-
        ciency
    X-l. hypophosphatemic rickets
    X-l. ichthyosis
    X-l. infantile agammaglobuli-
        nemia
    X-l. infantile hypogammaglob-
        ulinemia
    X-l. lymphoproliferative syn-
        drome
    X-l. recessive inheritance
    X-l. sideroblastic anemia

XLP — X-linked lymphoproliferative
    disease
XM — crossmatch
XMP — xanthosine monophosphate
XO syndrome
XP — xanthogranulomatous pyelone-
    phritis
    xeroderma pigmentosum
XR — x-ray
x-ray
    x-r. crystallography
    x-r. microscope
XS — excess
    xiphisternum
XT — exotropia
XU — excretory urogram
Xu — x-unit
XV strips
XX gonadal dysgenesis
XX karyotype
XX male syndrome
XXX karyotype
XXX syndrome
XXXXX syndrome
XXXXY syndrome
XX/XY sex chromosome pattern
XXXY syndrome
XXY karyotype
XXY syndrome
XXYY syndrome
XY gonadal dysgenesis
XY karyotype
xylan

xylanase
xylene cyanol FF
xylenol
xylidine
xylitol
    x. dehydrogenase (NADP-
    linked)
    x. oxidoreductase
Xylocaine
Xylohypha bantiana
xyloketose
xylol
xylometazoline hydrochloride
xylose
    x. absorption test
    x. concentration test
    x.-lysine-deoxycholate medium
D-xylose
    D-x. absorption test
    D-x. tolerance test
xylosuria
xylulokinase
xylulose
L-xylulose
    L-x. dehydrogenase
    L-x. reductase
xylulose 5-phosphate
xylulosuria
L-xylulosuria
xylyl
xysma
XYY karyotype
XYY syndrome
XYZ syndrome

Y — yttrium
Y
    Y body
    Y chromatin
    Y chromosome
    fragment Y
    Y protein
Yakima hemoglobin
yaws
    crab y.
    forest y.
y-axis

Yb — ytterbium
Yb-169 pentetate sodium
Y body
Y chromatin
Y chromosome
yeast
    y. fungus
    trypticase soy y.
yellow
    alizarin y.
    y. atrophy of liver
    y. body

y. corallin
fast y.
y. fat
y. fever
y. fever virus
y. hepatization
metaniline y.
y. phosphorus
titian y.
y. urine
visual y.
yellowish eosin
yerbine
Yergason's sign
Yersinia (pl., *Yersinieae*)
    Y. *enterocolitica*
    Y. *pestis*
    Y. *pseudotuberculosis*
Yersinia tonsillitis
yersiniosis
YF — yellow fever
yield
    quantum y.
Yk[a] antigen

Y-linked
    Y-l. character
    Y-l. gene
yohimbine
Yokogawa's fluke
yolk
    accessory y.
    formative y.
    y. sac carcinoma
    y. sac tumor
    y. stalk
Yorke's autolytic reaction
Youdon plot
yperite
Y protein
ypsiliform
YS
    yellow spot
    yolk sac
Yt[a] antigen
Yt[b] antigen
ytterbium
yttrium
Yvon's test

Z

Z — atomic number
    zero
Zahn's
    infarct
    lines
Z antigen
Zappacosta's test
Zappert counting chamber
Zarontin
z-axis
Z/D — zero defects
zebra bodies
Zebrina
Zeeman's
    correction method
    effect
zeisian stye
Zellballen pattern
Zener's
    breakdown
    diode

Zenker's
    degeneration
    diverticulum
    dysplasia
    fixative
    fluid
    formol fixative
    necrosis
    pulsation diverticulum
zenoplated tumor cells
zeolite
zephiran-trisodium phosphate
zero
    absolute z.
    z. defects
    z.-order reaction
zeta
    z. potential
    z. sedimentation rate
    z. sedimentation ratio
    z. sedimentation ratio method

zetacrit
zeta sedimentation ratio method
zidovudine
Ziehl-Neelsen stain
Ziehl's stain
Ziemann's
    dots
    stippling
ZIG — zoster immune globulin
Zika virus
Zimmermann's
    corpuscle
    elementary particle
    granule
    pericyte
    reaction
    test
zinc
    z. arsenate
    z. arsenite
    z. assay
    z. bacitracin
    z. caprylate
    z. chloride
    z. cyanide
    z. deficiency
    z. dimethyldithiocarbamate
    z. finger protein
    z. flocculation test
    z. gelatin
    z. isotope
    z. oxide
    z. pelargonate
    z. peroxide
    z. phenolsulfonate
    z. phosphide
    z. poisoning
    z. propionate
    z. protoporphyrin
    z. stearate
    z. sulfate centrifugal flotation
      technique
    z. sulfate turbidity test
    z. trichlorophenate
    z. turbidity test
    z. undecylenate
zincalism
Zinn's
    annulus
    artery
    zonule
zinterol hydrochloride

zipper
    leucine z.
ziram
zirconium
    z. dioxide
    z. granuloma
    z. oxide
Z line
Zn — zinc
Zollinger-Ellison tumor
zona (pl., zonae)
    z. fasciculata
    z. glomerulosa
    z. incerta
    z. pellucida
    z. reticularis
zonal
    z. electrophoresis
    z. necrosis
zonate
Zondek-Aschheim test
zone
    active z.
    antibody excess z.
    epileptogenic z.
    equivalence z.
    fetal z.
    flame intensity z's
    focal z.
    hemorrhoidal z.
    hyperesthetic z.
    interpalpebral z.
    Looser's transformation z's
    motor z.
    nephrogenic z.
    placental z.
    sudanophobic z.
    visual z.
zoning
zonula (pl., zonulae)
    z. adherens
    z. ciliaris
    z. occludens
zonular keratitis
zonule
    ciliary z.
    lens z.
    Zinn's z.
zooanthroponosis
zoofulvin
Zoogloea
Zoomastigophorea

zoomylus
zoonosis
zoonotic
> z. filariasis
> z. infection

Zoon's balanitis
zoophilic
zooprophylaxis
zoster
> dermatomal herpes z.
> disseminated z.
> herpes z.
> z. immune globulin
> varicella-z.
> z. varicella virus

Zovirax
Zr — zirconium
Zsigmondy's test
ZSR — zeta sedimentation rate
> zeta sedimentation ratio

Z thumb
Zuberella
zuckergussleber
Zuckerkandl's organs
Zurich hemoglobin
Zwischenferment
zwitterions
zygoma
zygomatic
> z. arch

z. bone
z. branch of facial nerve
z. nerve
z. process

zygomaticomaxillary
Zygomycetes
zygomycosis
> rhinofacial z.
> subcutaneous z.

zygomycota
zycomycotina
zygonema
zygote
zygotene
Zymobacterium
zymodeme
zymogen granules
zymogenic
zymogram
zymohexase
zymolysis
Zymomonas
zymophore
zymoplastic substance
zymosan
zymosis
zymosthenic
zytase
Zz — zingiber (ginger)
Z. Z.' Z." — increasing degrees of contraction

PART II

APPENDICES

APPENDIX 1
Laboratory Reference Interval Values of Clinical Importance*

Reference intervals are valuable guidelines for the assessment of health and disease by the clinician, but they should not be used as absolute indicators of health and disease. For essentially every test, there is a significant overlap between the normal and diseased populations. Many factors may influence the determination of the reference interval. The method and mode of standardization are variables for the reference interval, particularly for immunologic and enzymatic tests. The selection of the "normal" population is also important, since factors such as age, sex, race, diet, personal habits (e.g., alcohol consumption, smoking), and exercise may influence the reference interval for a given analyte. Last, the statistics chosen to define the reference interval are also a factor. These multiple variables for the determination of the reference interval indicate why there are differences among institutions for the same analyte.

The values in this chapter are primarily for adults in the fasting state. Values for other groups, when included, are clearly identified. For convenience, this chapter is divided into the following three sections: clinical chemistry, toxicology, and serology; hematology and coagulation; and drugs—therapeutic and toxic. The list includes reference intervals for the most common tests used in the practice of internal medicine. For more information about the reference interval for a given test or a test not included in the list, see *Clinical Guide to Laboratory Tests*, second edition, edited by Dr. Norbert W. Tietz. This book contains literature citations for most of the tests listed in this chapter.

All laboratory values are given in conventional and international units. If the value and units for a reference interval are the same for conventional and international units, the interval is listed only in the column for international units. The temperature for all enzyme assays listed in the chapter is 37°C. The pertinent prefixes denoting the decimal factors are listed.

---

* From Elin RJ: Laboratory reference interval values of clinical importance. In Wyngaarden JB, Smith LH, Bennett JC: Cecil Textbook of Medicine, 19th ed. Philadelphia, W.B. Saunders Company, 1992. The material in this appendix was partially extracted from Tietz NW (ed.): Clinical Guide to Laboratory Tests. Philadelphia, W.B. Saunders Company, 1990. The material for the section on Therapeutic Drug Concentrations was partially extracted from Tietz NW: Textbook of Clinical Chemistry. Philadelphia, W.B. Saunders Company, 1986. The main contributors to this section of the book are NW Tietz and NM Logan. Other sources are listed under References.

PREFIXES DENOTING DECIMAL FACTORS

Prefix	Symbol	Factor
mega	M	10^6
kilo	k	10^3
hecto	h	10^2
deka	da	10^1
deci	d	10^{-1}
centi	c	10^{-2}
milli	m	10^{-3}
micro	μ	10^{-6}
nano	n	10^{-9}
pico	p	10^{-12}
femto	f	10^{-15}

ABBREVIATIONS

AU   Arbitrary units
EU   Ehrlich unit
GD   General diagnostics
IFA   Immunofluorescent assay
IU   International unit (of hormone activity)
RIA   Radioimmunoassay
RID   Radial immunodiffusion
S   Substrate
U   International unit (of enzyme activity)

REFERENCES

Beutler E: Hemolytic Anemia in Disorders of Red Cell Metabolism. New York, Plenum Publishing Company, 1978.

Brown SS, Mitchell FL, Young DS (eds.): Chemical Diagnosis of Disease. Amsterdam, Elsevier/North-Holland Biomedical Press, 1979.

Conn RB (ed.): Current Diagnosis. 7th ed. Philadelphia, W.B. Saunders Company, 1985.

Gilman AG, Rall TW, Nies AS, Taylor P (eds.): Goodman and Gilman's The Pharmacological Basis of Therapeutics. 8th ed. New York, Pergamon Press, 1990.

Henry JB (ed.): Clinical Diagnosis and Management by Laboratory Methods. 18th ed. Philadelphia, W.B. Saunders Company, 1991.

Hoeg JM, Gregg RE, Brewer HB: An approach to the management of hyperlipoproteinemia. JAMA 255:512, 1986.

Mabry C, Tietz NW: Tables of normal laboratory values. In Nelson WE, Vaughan VC, McKay JR, et al. (eds.): Nelson Textbook of Pediatrics. 23rd ed. Philadelphia, W.B. Saunders Company, 1983.

Miale JB: Laboratory Medicine: Hematology. 6th ed. St. Louis, The C.V. Mosby Company, 1982.

Tietz NW (ed.): Textbook of Clinical Chemistry. Philadelphia, W.B. Saunders Company, 1986.

Tietz NW, Blackburn RH (eds.): Reference Ranges and General Information. Clinical Laboratories, A.B. Chandler Medical Center, University of Kentucky, Lexington, Kentucky, 1984.

Tietz NW (ed.): Clinical Guide to Laboratory Tests. Philadelphia, W.B. Saunders Company, 1990.

Williams WJ, Beutler E, Erslev AJ, et al.: Hematology. 3rd ed. New York, McGraw-Hill Book Company, 1983.

CLINICAL CHEMISTRY, TOXICOLOGY, SEROLOGY

Test	Specimen	Reference Interval (Conventional Units)	Reference Interval (International Units)
Acetoacetate	Serum or plasma	Negative (<1 mg/dL)	Negative (<0.1 mmol/L)
Semiquantitative	(fluoride/oxalate)		
Acetone	Urine	Negative	Negative
Semiquantitative	Serum or plasma		
	(fluoride or oxalate)	Negative (<1.0 mg/dL)	Negative (<0.17 mmol/L)
Semiquantitative	Urine	Negative	Negative
Acid phosphatase	Serum		M: 2.5–11.7 U/L
(S:p-nitrophenylphosphate)			F: 0.3–9.2 U/L
Adrenocorticotropic	Plasma (heparin)	0800 h: 8–79 pg/mL	8–79 ng/L
hormone (ACTH)		1600 h: 7–30 pg/mL	7–30 ng/L
Alanine aminotransferase	Serum		8–20 U/L
(ALT, SGPT)			
Albumin			
Nephelometric, colorimetric	Serum	3.5–5.0 g/dL	35–50 g/L
Turbidimetric	CSF	15–45 mg/dL	150–450 mg/L
	Urine	<80 mg/d at rest	<80 mg/d
		<150 mg/d ambulatory	<150 mg/d
Aldolase	Serum		1.0–7.5 U/L
Aldosterone	Plasma (heparin EDTA)	Adult, average sodium diet	
	or serum	supine: 3–10 ng/dL	0.08–0.28 nmol/L
		upright: 5–30 ng/dL	0.14–0.83 nmol/L
Alkaline phosphatase	Serum		Adult (>18 y)
(S:4–NPP)			F: 42–98 U/L
			M: 53–128 U/L
δ-Aminolevulinic acid			
(δ-ALA)	Serum	15–23 µg/dL	1.1–8 µmol/L
	Urine	1.5–7.5 mg/d	11.4–57.2 µmol/d
Ammonia nitrogen	Serum or plasma		
Resin or enzymatic	(Na-heparin)	Adult 15–45 µg N/dL	11–32 µmol/L
	Urine, 24-h	140–1500 mg/d	10–107 mmol/d
Amylase	Serum		25–125 U/L
(S:Beckman, defined substrate)			
	Urine, timed specimen		1–17 U/h
Angiotensin I	Peripheral venous	11–88 pg/mL	11–88 ng/L
	plasma (EDTA)		
Angiotensin II	Plasma (EDTA)	10–60 pg/mL	10–60 ng/L
	Arterial blood		
α₁-Antitrypsin	Serum	78–200 mg/dL	0.78–2.00 g/L
(nephelometry)			
Anion gap	Plasma (heparin) or	7–14 mEq/L	7–14 mmol/L
[Na − (Cl⁻ + HCO₃⁻)]	serum		
Arsenic	Whole blood (heparin)	0.2–2.3 µg/dL	0.03–0.31 µmol/L
		Chronic poisoning: 10–50 µg/dL	1.33–6.65 µmol/L
		Acute poisoning: 60–93 µg/dL	7.98–12.37 µmol/L
	Urine, 24-h	5–50 µg/d	0.067–0.665 µmol/d
Ascorbic acid (see Vitamin C)			
Aspartate aminotransferase			
(AST, SGOT)	Serum		10–30 U/L
Base excess	Whole blood (heparin)	− 2 to 3 mEq/L	− 2 to 3 mmol/L
Bicarbonate	Serum	18–23 mEq/L	18–23 mmol/L
Bile acids, total	Serum, fasting	0.3–2.3 µg/mL	0.74–5.64 µmol/L
	Serum, 1-h postprandial	1.8–3.2 µg/mL	4.41–7.84 µmol/L
	Feces	120–225 mg/d	294–551 µmol/d
Bilirubin			
Total	Serum	0.2–1.0 mg/dL	3.4–17.1 µmol/L
	Urine	Negative	Negative
Conjugated (direct)	Serum	0–0.2 mg/dL	0–3.4 µmol/L
Calcium, ionized (iCa)	Serum	4.65–5.28 mg/dL	1.16–1.32 mmol/L
Calcium, total	Serum	8.4–10.2 mg/dL	2.10–2.55 mmol/L
	Urine, 24-h	100–300 mg/d	2.5–7.5 mmol/d
	CSF	4.2–5.4 mg/dL	1.05–1.35 mmol/L
Carbon dioxide,	Serum or plasma	23–29 mEq/L	23–29 mmol/L
total (TCO₂)	(heparin)		
Carcinoembryonic	Serum	Nonsmokers: <2.5 ng/mL	<2.5 µg/L
antigen (CEA)			
β-Carotene	Serum	10–85 µg/dL	0.19–1.58 µmol/L
Catecholamines, total	Urine, 24-h	<100 µg/d	<5.91 nmol/d
Ceruloplasmin (RID)	Serum	18–45 mg/dL	180–450 mg/L
Chloride	Serum or plasma	98–106 mEq/L	98–106 mmol/L
	(heparin)		
	CSF	118–132 mEq/L	118–132 mmol/L
	Urine, 24-h	110–250 mEq/d	110–250 mmol/d

CLINICAL CHEMISTRY, TOXICOLOGY, SEROLOGY *Continued*

Test	Specimen	Reference Interval (Conventional Units)	Reference Interval (International Units)
Cholesterol, total	Serum or plasma (EDTA)	Recommended: <200 mg/dL	<5.18 mmol/L
		Moderate risk: 200–239 mg/dL	5.18–6.19 mmol/L
		High risk: ≥240 mg/dL	≥6.22 mmol/L
Chorionic gonadotropin, β-subunit (β-HCG)	Serum or plasma (EDTA)	M and nonpregnant F: <5.0 mU/mL	<5.0 IU/L
Complement			
Total hemolytic Complement activity	Plasma (EDTA)	75–160 U/mL	75–160 kU/L
Copper	Serum	M: 70–140 μg/dL	10.99–21.98 μmol/L
		F: 80–155 μg/dL	12.56–24.34 μmol/L
	Erythrocyte (heparin)	90–150 μg/dL	14.13–23.55 μmol/L
	Urine, 24-h	3–35 μg/d	0.047–0.55 μmol/d
Coproporphyrin	Urine, 24-h	34–234 μg/d	51–351 nmol/d
	Feces, 24-h	<30 μg/g dry wt	<45 nmol/g dry wt
Corticosteroid-binding globulin (CBG) (see Transcortin)		400–1200 μg/d	600–1800 nmol/d
Corticosterone	Serum	0800 h: 130–820 ng/dL	4–24 nmol/L
		1600 h: 60–220 ng/dL	2–6 nmol/L
Cortisol	Serum or plasma (heparin)	0800 h: 5–23 μg/dL	138–635 nmol/L
		1600 h: 3–15 μg/dL	82–413 nmol/L
		2000 h: ≤50% of 0800 h	Fraction of 0800 h: ≤0.50
Cortisol, free	Urine, 24-h	10–100 μg/d	27–276 nmol/d
C-Peptide	Serum	0.78–1.89 ng/mL	0.26–0.62 nmol/L
C-Reactive protein	Serum	68–8200 ng/mL	68–8200 μg/L
Creatine kinase (CK)	Serum		M: 38–174 U/L
			F: 26–140 U/L
Isoenzymes	Serum	Fraction 2 (MB) <4–6% of total (method-dependent)	Fraction of total: <0.04–0.06
Creatinine Jaffe, kinetic or enzymatic	Serum or plasma	M: 0.7–1.3 mg/dL	62–115 μmol/L
		F: 0.6–1.1 mg/dL	53–97 μmol/L
	Urine, 24-h	M: 14–26 mg/kg/d	124–230 μmol/kg/d
		F: 11–20 mg/kg/d	97–177 μmol/kg/d
Creatinine clearance (endogenous)	Serum or plasma, and urine	M: 90–139 mL/min/1.73 m²	0.87–1.34 mL/s/m²
		F: 80–125 mL/min/1.73 m²	0.77–1.20 mL/s/m²
Dehydroepiandrosterone serum (DHEA)	Serum	M: 1.8–12.5 ng/mL	6.2–43.3 nmol/L
		F: 1.3–9.8 ng/mL	4.5–34.0 nmol/L
Dehydroepiandrosterone sulfate (DHEA-S)	Serum	M: 1.7–6.7 μg/mL	4.6–18.2 μmol/L
		F: Premenopausal: 0.5–5.4 μg/mL	1.4–14.7 μmol/L
		Postmenopausal: 0.3–2.6 μg/mL	0.8–7.1 μmol/L
11-Deoxycortisol (compound S)	Serum	12–158 ng/dL	0.3–4.6 nmol/L
Estrogens, total	Serum	M: 20–80 pg/mL	20–80 ng/L
		F, cycle:	
		Follicular phase: 60–200 pg/mL	60–200 ng/L
		Luteal phase: 160–400 pg/mL	160–400 ng/L
		Postmenopausal: ≤130 pg/mL	≤130 ng/L
	Urine, 24-h		M: 15–40 μg/d
			F: Preovulation: 4–25 μg/d
			Ovulation: 28–100 μg/d
			Luteal peak: 22–80 μg/d
			Pregnancy, term: <45,000 μg/d
			Postmenopausal: <20 μg/d
Fat, fecal	Feces, 72-h		<7 g/d
			fat-free diet: <4 g/d
Fatty acids, nonesterified (free)	Serum or plasma (heparin)	8–25 mg/dL	0.28–0.89 mmol/L
Ferritin	Serum	M: 20–250 ng/mL	20–250 μg/L
		F: 10–120 ng/mL	10–120 μg/L
α₁-Fetoprotein	Serum	<10 ng/mL	<10 μg/L
Fibrinogen (see Hematology and Coagulation section)			
Folate	Serum	3–16 ng/mL	7–36 nmol/L
	Erythrocytes (EDTA)	130–628 ng/mL packed cells	294–1422 nmol/L packed cells
Follitropin (FSH)	Serum or plasma (heparin)	M: 4–25 mIU/mL	4–25 IU/L
		F: Follicular phase: 1–9 mU/mL	1–9 U/L
		Ovulatory peak: 6–26 mU/mL	6–26 U/L
		Luteal phase: 1–9 mU/mL	1–9 U/L
		Postmenopausal: 30–118 mU/mL	30–118 U/L
	Urine, 24-h		4–18 U/d
			3–12 U/d
Free thyroxine index (FT₄I)	Serum		4.2–13.0
Gastrin	Serum	<100 pg/mL	<100 ng/L

CLINICAL CHEMISTRY, TOXICOLOGY, SEROLOGY *Continued*

Test	Specimen	Reference Interval (Conventional Units)			Reference Interval (International Units)		
Glucose	Serum	Adult: 70–105 mg/dL			3.9–5.8 mmol/L		
		>60 y: 80–115 mg/dL			4.4–6.4 mmol/L		
	Whole blood (heparin)	65–95 mg/dL			3.6–5.3 mmol/L		
	CSF	40–70 mg/dL			2.2–3.9 mmol/L		
Quantitative, enzymatic	Urine	<0.5 g/d			<2.8 mmol/d		
Qualitative	Urine				Negative		
Glucose, 2-h postprandial	Serum	<120 mg/dL			<6.7 mmol/L		
Glucose tolerance test (GTT), oral	Serum		mg/dL			mmol/L	
			Normal	Diabetic		Normal	Diabetic
		Fasting:	70–105	>140		3.9–5.8	>7.8
		60 min:	120–170	≥200		6.7–9.4	≥11
		90 min:	100–140	≥200		5.6–7.8	≥11
		120 min:	70–120	≥140		3.9–6.7	≥7.8
γ-Glutamyltransferase (GGT)	Serum				M: 9–50 U/L		
					F: 8–40 U/L		
Glycerol, free	Plasma	0.29–1.72 mg/dL			0.032—0.187 mmol/L		
Growth hormone (HGH, somatotropin)	Serum or plasma (EDTA, heparin)	Adult, M: <2 ng/mL			<2 μg/L		
		F: <10 ng/mL			<10 μg/L		
		>60 y, M: 0.4–10 ng/mL			0.4–10 μg/L		
		F: 1–14 ng/mL			1–14 μg/L		
Haptoglobin (see Hematology and Coagulation section)							
HDL-cholesterol (HDLC) (5th percentile from Lipid Research Clinics)	Serum or plasma (EDTA)	M: >29 mg/dL			>0.75 mmol/L		
		F: >35 mg/dL			>0.91 mmol/L		
Hemoglobin A₁c (electrophoresis)	Whole blood (heparin, EDTA, or oxalate)	5.6–7.5% of total Hb			Fraction of Hb: 0.056–0.075		
Homovanillic acid (HVA)	Urine, 24-h	1.4–8.8 mg/d			8–48 μmol/d		
17-Hydroxycorticosteroids (17-OHCS)	Urine, 24-h	M: 3.0–10.0 mg/d			8.3–27.6 μmol/d		
		F: 2.0–8.0 mg/d			5.5–22.1 μmol/d		
5-Hydroxyindole acetic acid (5-HIAA)							
Qualitative	Fresh random urine				Negative		
Quantitative	Urine, 24-h	2–6 mg/d			10.4–31.2 μmol/d		
17-Hydroxyprogesterone (17-OHP)	Serum	M: 0.5–2.5 ng/mL			1.5–7.5 nmol/L		
		F: Follicular: 0.2–1.0 ng/mL			0.6–3.0 nmol/L		
		Luteal: 1.0–5.0 ng/mL			3.0–15.5 nmol/L		
		Postmenopausal: ≤0.7 ng/mL			≤2.1 nmol/L		
Immunoglobulin A (IgA)	Serum	40–350 mg/dL			400–3500 mg/L		
Immunoglobulin D (IgD)	Serum	0–8 mg/dL			0–80 mg/L		
Immunoglobulin E (IgE)	Serum	0–380 IU/mL			0–380 kIU/L		
Immunoglobulin G (IgG)	Serum	650–1600 mg/dL			6.5–16 g/L		
	CSF	0.5–5 mg/dL			5–50 mg/L		
Immunoglobulin M (IgM)	Serum	55–300 mg/dL			550–3000 mg/L		
Insulin (12-h fasting)	Serum	6–24 μIU/mL			42–167 pmol/L		
Intrinsic factor (see Vitamin B₁₂)							
Iron	Serum	M: 65–175 μg/dL			11.6–31.3 μmol/L		
		F: 50–170 μg/dL			9.0–30.4 μmol/L		
Iron-binding capacity, total (TIBC)	Serum	250–450 μg/dL			44.8–80.6 μmol/L		
Iron saturation	Serum	M: 20–50			Fraction of iron saturation: 0.20–0.5 (M)		
		F: 15–50			0.15–0.5 (F)		
17-Ketogenic steroids (17-KGS)	Urine, 24-h	M: 5–23 mg/d			17–80 μmol/d		
		F: 3–15 mg/d			10–52 μmol/d		
Ketone bodies							
Qualitative	Serum	Negative (0.5–3.0 mg/dL)			Negative (5–30 mg/L)		
	Urine, random				Negative		
17-Ketosteroids, total (17-KS)	Urine, 24-h	M: 18–30 y 9–22 mg/d			31–76 μmol/d		
		>30 y 8–20 mg/d			28–70 μmol/d		
		F: 6–15 mg/d			21–52 μmol/d		
L-Lactate	Whole blood (heparin)	Venous: 4.5–19.8 mg/dL			0.5–2.2 mmol/L		
		Arterial: 4.5–14.4 mg/dL			0.5–1.6 mmol/L		
Lactate dehydrogenase (LDH)	Serum				208–378 U/L		
LDH isoenzymes (Electrophoresis, agarose)	Serum	%			Fraction of total:		
		Fraction 1: 18–33			0.18–0.33		
		Fraction 2: 28–40			0.28–0.40		
		Fraction 3: 18–30			0.18–0.30		
		Fraction 4: 6–16			0.06–0.16		
		Fraction 5: 2–13			0.02–0.13		
Lead	Whole blood (heparin)	<40 μg/dL			<1.93 μmol/L		
		Toxic: ≥100 μg/dL			≥4.83 μmol/L		
	Urine, 24-h	<80 μg/L			<0.39 μmol/L		

CLINICAL CHEMISTRY, TOXICOLOGY, SEROLOGY Continued

Test	Specimen	Reference Interval (Conventional Units)	Reference Interval (International Units)
Lipase (turbidimetric)	Serum		Adult: 10–140 U/L
			>60 y: 18–180 U/L
LDL-Cholesterol (LDLC)	Serum or plasma (EDTA)	Recommended: <130 mg/dL	<3.37 mmol/L
		Moderate risk: 130–159 mg/dL	3.37–4.12 mmol/L
		High risk: ≥160 mg/dL	≥4.14 mmol/L
Lutropin (LH)	Serum or plasma (heparin)	M: 1–8 mU/mL	1–8 U/L
		F: Follicular phase: 1–12 mU/mL	1–12 U/L
		Midcycle: 16–104 mU/mL	16–104 U/L
		Luteal: 1–12 mU/mL	1–12 U/L
		Postmenopausal: 16–66 mU/mL	16–66 U/L
	Urine		M: 9–23 U/d
			F: non-midcycle, 4–30 U/d
Lysozyme	Serum, plasma	0.4–1.3 mg/dL	4–13 mg/L
Magnesium	Serum	1.3–2.1 mEq/L	0.65–1.05 mmol/L
	Urine, 24-h	6.0–10.0 mEq/d	3.00–5.00 mmol/d
Mercury	Whole blood (EDTA)	<5.0 μg/dL	<0.25 μmol/L
	Urine, 24-h	<20 μg/L	<0.1 μmol/L
		Toxic: >150 μg/L	<0.75 μmol/L
Metanephrine, total	Urine, 24-h	0.05–1.20 μg/mg creatinine	0.03–0.69 mmol/mol creatinine
Myelin basic protein	CSF		<2.5 ng/mL
Myoglobin	Serum		M: 19–92 μg/L
			F: 12–76 μg/L
	Urine, random		Negative
Osmolality	Serum		275–295 mOsmol/kg
	Urine, random		50–1400 mOsmol/kg, depending on fluid intake
			After 12-h fluid restriction: >850 mOsmol/kg
	Urine, 24-h		~390–900 mOsmol/kg
Oxalate	Serum	1–2.4 μg/mL	11–27 μmol/L
		Ethylene glycol poisoning: >20 μg/mL	Ethylene glycol poisoning: >228 μmol/L
Oxygen (Po₂)	Whole blood, arterial (heparin)	83–100 mm Hg	11–14.4 kPa
Oxygen saturation	Whole blood, arterial (heparin)	95–98%	Fraction saturated: 0.95–0.98
pH (37°C)	Whole blood, arterial (heparin)		7.35–7.45
Phosphorus, inorganic	Serum	2.7–4.5 mg/dL	0.87–1.45 nmol/L
		>60 y, M: 2.3–3.7 mg/dL	0.74–1.2 nmol/L
		F: 2.8–4.1 mg/dL	0.90–1.3 nmol/L
	Urine, 24-h	0.4–1.3 g/d	13–42 mmol/d
Porphobilinogen (PBG)			
Quantitative	Urine, 24-h	0–2.0 mg/d	0–8.8 μmol/d
Qualitative	Urine, fresh random		Negative
Potassium	Serum	3.5–5.1 mEq/L	3.5–5.1 mmol/L
	Plasma (heparin)	3.5–4.5 mEq/L	3.5–4.5 mmol/L
	Urine, 24-h	25–125 mEq/d	25–125 mmol/d
Pregnanediol	Urine, 24-h	M: 0–1.9 mg/d	0–5.9 μmol/d
		F: Follicular: <2.6 mg/d	<8 μmol/d
		Luteal: 2.6–10.6 mg/d	8–33 μmol/d
		Postmenopausal: 0.2–1.0 mg/d	0.6–3.1 μmol/d
Progesterone	Serum	M: 0.13–0.97 ng/mL	0.4–3.1 nmol/L
		F: Follicular: 0.15–0.70 ng/mL	0.5–2.2 nmol/L
		Luteal: 2.0–25 ng/mL	6.4–79.5 nmol/L
Prolactin (hPRL)	Serum	0–20 ng/mL	0–20 μg/L
Protein			
Total	Serum	6.4–8.3 g/dL	64.0–83.0 g/L
Electrophoresis	Serum	Albumin: 3.5–5.0 g/dL	35–50 g/L
		α₁-Globulin: 0.1–0.3 g/dL	1–3 g/L
		α₂-Globulin: 0.6–1.0 g/dL	6–10 g/L
		β-Globulin: 0.7–1.1 g/dL	7–11 g/L
		γ-Globulin: 0.8–1.6 g/dL	8–16 g/L
Total	Urine, 24-h		50–80 mg/d at rest
Total	CSF	Lumbar: 15–45 mg/dL	150–450 mg/L
Protoporphyrin	Whole blood (heparin or EDTA)	17–77 μg/dL RBC	0.30–1.37 μmol/L RBC
	Feces, 24-h	≤60 μg/g dry wt or <1500 μg/d	≤0.11 mmol/kg dry wt or <2.67 μmol/d
Pyruvic acid	Whole blood (heparin)	0.3–0.9 mg/dL	0.03–0.10 mmol/L
Renin (normal diet)	Plasma (EDTA)	ng/mL/h ± 1 SE	μg/L/h ± 1 SE
		Supine: 1.6 ± 1.5	1.6 ± 1.5
		Standing: (4-h): 4.5 ± 2.9	4.5 ± 2.9

CLINICAL CHEMISTRY, TOXICOLOGY, SEROLOGY Continued

Test	Specimen	Reference Interval (Conventional Units)	Reference Interval (International Units)
Riboflavin (see Vitamin B$_2$)			
Sediment	Urine, fresh, random		
Casts			Hyaline: occasional (0–1) casts/hpf
			RBC: not seen
			WBC: not seen
			Tubular epithelial: not seen
			Transitional and squamous epithelial: not seen
Cells			RBC: 0–2/hpf
			WBC: M: 0–3/hpf
			F: 0–5/hpf
			Epithelial: few
			Bacteria:
			Unspun: no organisms/oil immersion field
			Spun: <20 organisms/hpf
Sodium	Serum or plasma (heparin)	136–146 mEq/L	136–146 mmol/L
	Urine, 24-h	40–220 mEq/d	40–220 mmol/d
Specific gravity	Urine, random		1.002–1.030
	Urine, 24-h		1.015–1.025
		% of total	Fraction of total
Testosterone, free	Serum	M: 52–280 pg/mL 1.5–3.2	180.4–971.6 pmol/L 0.015–0.032
		F: 1.6–6.3 pg/mL 0.8–1.4	5.6–21.9 pmol/L 0.008–0.014
Testosterone, total	Serum	M: 300–1000 ng/dL	10.4–34.7 nmol/L
		F: 20–75 ng/dL	0.69–2.6 nmol/L
	Urine	20–50 y,	
		M: 50–135 µg/d	173–470 nmol/d
		F: 2–12 µg/d	7–42 nmol/d
		>50 y,	
		M: 40–60 µg/d	139–210 nmol/d
		F: 2–8 µg/d	7–28 nmol/d
Thiamine (see Vitamin B$_1$)	Serum		
Thyroglobulin (Tg)	Serum	3–42 ng/mL	3–42 µg/L
Thyroglobulin antibodies	Serum		<1:10
Thyroid microsomal antibodies	Serum		Nondetectable (hemagglutination) or <1:10 (IFA)
Thyrotropin (hTSH)	Serum or plasma	2–10 µU/mL	2–10 mU/L
Thyrotropin-releasing hormone	Plasma	5–60 pg/mL	5–60 ng/L
Thyroxine, free (FT$_4$)	Serum	0.8–2.4 ng/dL	10–31 pmol/L
Thyroxine (T$_4$), total	Serum	5–12 µg/dL	65–155 nmol/L
		>60 y, M: 5.0–10.0 µg/dL	65–129 nmol/L
		F: 5.5–10.5 µg/dL	71–135 nmol/L
Thyroxine-binding globulin (TBG)	Serum	15.0–34.0 µg/mL	15.0–34.0 mg/L
Thyroxine index, free (see Free thyroxine index)			
Transcortin	Serum	M: 18.8–25.2 mg/L	323–433 nmol/L
		F: 14.9–22.9 mg/L	256–393 nmol/L
Transferrin	Serum	200–400 mg/dL	2.0–4.0 g/L
		>60 y: 180–380 mg/dL	1.80–3.80 g/L
Triglycerides (TG)	Serum, after ≥12-hr fast	Recommended:	
		M: 40–160 mg/dL	0.45–1.81 mmol/L
		F: 35–135 mg/dL	0.40–1.52 mmol/L
Tri-iodothyronine, free	Serum	260–480 pg/dL	4.0–7.4 pmol/L
Tri-iodothyronine, total (T$_3$)	Serum	100–200 ng/dL	1.54–3.08 mmol/L
Tri-iodothyronine resin uptake test (T$_3$RU)	Serum	24–34%	24–34 AU (arbitrary units)
Urea nitrogen	Serum or plasma	7–18 mg/dL	2.5–6.4 mmol/L
	Urine	12–20 g/d	0.43–0.71 mol/d
Urea nitrogen/creatinine ratio	Serum		12/1–20/1
Uric acid (uricase)	Serum	M: 3.5–7.2 mg/dL	0.21–0.42 mmol/L
		F: 2.6–6.0 mg/dL	0.15–0.35 mmol/L
	Urine, 24-h	250–750 mg/d	1.48–4.43 mmol/d
Urinary sediment (see Sediment)			
Urobilinogen	Urine, 2-h	0.1–0.8 EU	0.1–0.8 U
	Urine, 24-h	0.5–4.0 EU	0.5–4.0 U
	Feces	75–275 EU/100 g	750–2750 U/kg
		75–400 EU/d	75–400 U/d
		40–280 mg/d	67–473 µmol/d
Uroporphyrin	Urine, 24-h	<50 µg/d	<60 nmol/d
	Feces, 24-h specimen	10–40 µg/d	12–48 nmol/d
	Erythrocytes (heparin or EDTA)		Negative

CLINICAL CHEMISTRY, TOXICOLOGY, SEROLOGY *Continued*

Test	Specimen	Reference Interval (Conventional Units)	Reference Interval (International Units)
Vanillylmandelic acid (VMA)	Urine, 24-h	2–7 mg/d	10.1–35.4 μmol/d
Viscosity	Serum		1.10–1.22 centipoise
Vitamin A	Serum	30–80 μg/dL	1.05–2.8 μmol/L
Vitamin B₁ (Thiamine)	Serum	0–2 μg/dL	0–75 nmol/L
Vitamin B₂ (Riboflavin)	Serum	4–24 μg/dL	106–638 nmol/L
Vitamin B₆	Plasma (EDTA)	5–30 ng/mL	20–121 nmol/L
Vitamin B₁₂	Serum	100–700 pg/mL	74–516 pmol/L
Vitamin C	Plasma (oxalate, heparin, or EDTA)	0.5–1.5 mg/dL	28–85 μmol/L
Vitamin D₃, 1,25-dihydroxy	Serum	25–45 pg/mL	60–108 pmol/L
Vitamin D₃, 25-hydroxy	Plasma (heparin)	Summer: 15–80 ng/mL	37.4–200 nmol/L
		Winter: 14–42 ng/mL	34.9–105 nmol/L
Vitamin E	Serum	5.0–18.0 μg/mL	12–42 μmol/L
Zinc	Serum	70–150 μg/dL	10.7–22.9 μmol/L

HEMATOLOGY AND COAGULATION

Test	Specimen	Reference Interval (Conventional Units)	Reference Interval (International Units)
Activated partial thromboplastin time (APTT)	Whole blood (Na citrate)		25–35 sec
Bleeding time (BT)			
Ivy	Blood from skin		Normal: 2–7 min
			Borderline: 7–11 min
Simplate (G-D)			2.75–8 min
Blood volume	Whole blood (heparin)		M: 52–83 mL/kg
			F: 50–75 mL/kg
Bone marrow	Bone marrow aspirate	% (mean)	Number fraction (mean)
Differential count			
Myeloblasts		0.3–5.0 (2.0)	0.003–0.05 (0.02)
Promyelocytes		1.0–8.0 (5.0)	0.01–0.08 (0.05)
Myelocytes:			
Neutrophilic		5.0–19.0 (12.0)	0.05–0.19 (0.12)
Eosinophilic		0.5–3.0 (1.5)	0.005–0.03 (0.015)
Basophilic		0.0–0.5 (0.3)	0.00–0.005 (0.003)
Metamyelocytes		13.0–32.0 (22.0)	0.13–0.32 (0.22)
Polymorphonuclear neutrophils		7.0–3.0 (2.0)	0.07–0.30 (0.20)
Polymorphonuclear eosinophils		0.5–4.0 (2.0)	0.005–0.04 (0.02)
Polymorphonuclear basophils		0.0–0.7 (0.2)	0.0–0.007 (0.002)
Lymphocytes		3.0–17.0 (10.0)	0.03–0.17 (0.10)
Plasma cells		0.0–2.0 (0.4)	0.00–0.02 (0.004)
Monocytes		0.5–5.0 (2.0)	0.005–0.05 (0.02)
Reticulum cells		0.1–2.0 (0.2)	0.001–0.02 (0.002)
Megakaryocytes		0.03–3.0 (0.1)	0.0003–0.03 (0.001)
Pronormoblasts		1.0–8.0 (4.0)	0.01–0.08 (0.04)
Normoblasts		7.0–32.0 (18.0)	0.07–0.32 (0.18)
Clot lysis, 37°C	Whole clotted blood		48–72 h
Clot retraction screen	Whole blood (no anticoagulant)		Retraction begins at 1 h, maximum at 24 h
Clotting time, Lee-White, 37°C	Whole blood (no anticoagulant)		5–8 min
Differential count (see Bone marrow differential count or Leukocyte differential count)			
Eosinophil count	Whole blood (EDTA); capillary blood	50–400 cells/μL (mm³)	50–400 × 10⁶ cells/L
Erythrocyte count (RBC count)	Whole blood (EDTA)	millions of cells/μL (mm³)	× 10¹² cells/L
		M: 4.3–5.7	4.3–5.7
		F: 3.8–5.1	3.8–5.1
Erythrocyte sedimentation rate (ESR), Wintrobe			M: 0–15 mm/h
			F: 0–20 mm/h
Ferritin (see Chemistry section)			
Fibrin degradation products (Agglutination, Thrombo-Wellco test)	Whole blood: special tube containing thrombin and proteolytic inhibitor	<10 μg/mL	<10 mg/L
	Urine: 2 mL in special tube (see above)	<0.25 μg/mL	<0.25 mg/L
Fibrinogen	Plasma (Na citrate)	200–400 mg/dL	2.00–4.00 g/L
Glucose-6-phosphate dehydrogenase (G6PD) in erythrocytes	Whole blood (ACD, EDTA, or heparin)	12.1 ± 2.09 U/g Hb (1 SD)	0.78 ± 0.13 MU/mol Hb (1 SD)
Haptoglobin (Hp) RID	Serum; avoid hemolysis	26–185 mg/dL	260–1850 mg/L
Hematocrit (HCT, Hct)	Whole blood (EDTA)		
Calculated from MCV and RBC (electronic displacement or laser)		M: 39–49%	0.39–0.49 volume fraction
		F: 35–45%	0.35–0.45 volume fraction

HEMATOLOGY AND COAGULATION *Continued*

Test	Specimen	Reference Interval (Conventional Units)		Reference Interval (International Units)	
Hemoglobin (Hb)	Whole blood (EDTA)	M: 13.5–17.5 g/dL		2.09–2.71 mmol/L	
		F: 12.0–16.0 g/dL		1.86–2.48 mmol/L	
	Plasma (heparin, ACD)	<3 mg/dL		<0.47 µmol/L	
	Urine, fresh, random			Negative	
Hemoglobin electrophoresis	Whole blood (EDTA, citrate, or heparin)			Mass fraction	
		HbA >95%		HbA >0.95	
		HbA₂ 1.5–3.5%		HbA₂ 0.015–0.035	
		HbF <2%		HbF <0.02	
Leukocyte count (WBC count)	Whole blood (EDTA)	4.5–11.0 × 10³ cells/µL (mm³)		4.5–11.0 × 10⁹ cells/L	
	CSF	0.5 mononuclear cells/µL		0.5 × 10⁶ cells/L	
Leukocyte	Whole blood (EDTA)	%	Cells/µL (mm³)	Number fraction	Cells × 10⁹/L
Differential count					
Myelocytes		0	0	0	0
Neutrophils—bands		3–5	150–400	0.03–0.05	150–400
Neutrophils—segmented		54–62	3000–5800	0.54–0.62	3000–5800
Lymphocytes		23–33	1500–3000	0.25–0.33	1500–3000
Monocytes		3–7	285–500	0.03–0.07	285–500
Eosinophils		1–3	50–250	0.01–0.03	50–250
Basophils		0–0.75	15–50	0–0.0075	15–50
Leukocyte					
Differential count	CSF	%		Number fraction	
Lymphocytes		62 ± 34		0.62 ± 0.324	
Monocytes (includes pia-arachnoid mesothelial cells)		36 ± 20		0.36 ± 0.20	
Neutrophils		2 ± 5		0.02 ± 0.05	
Histocytes				Rare	
Ependymal cells				Rare	
Eosinophils				Rare	
Mean corpuscular hemoglobin (MCH)	Whole blood (EDTA)	26–34 pg/cell		0.40–0.53 fmol/cell	
Mean corpuscular hemoglobin concentration (MCHC)	Whole blood (EDTA)	31–37% Hb/cell or gHb/dL RBC		4.81–5.74 mmol Hb/L RBC	
Mean corpuscular volume (MCV)	Whole blood (EDTA)	80–100 fL		80–100 fL	
Methemoglobin (MetHb)	Whole blood (EDTA, heparin, or ACD)	0.06–0.24 g/dL		9.3–37.2 µmol/L	
Partial thromboplastin time (PTT)	Whole blood (Na citrate)	60–85 sec		60–85 sec	
Plasma volume	Plasma (heparin)	M: 25–43 mL/kg		0.025–0.043 L/kg	
		F: 28–45 mL/kg		0.028–0.045 L/kg	
Platelet count (thrombocyte count)	Whole blood (EDTA)	150–450 × 10³/µL (mm³)		150–450 × 10⁹/L	
Prothrombin consumption	Whole blood (no anticoagulant)	>30 sec		>30 sec	
Prothrombin time, two-stage modified	Whole blood (Na citrate)	18–22 sec		18–22 sec	
RBC count (see Erythrocyte count)					
Red cell volume	Whole blood (heparin)	M: 20–36 mL/kg		M: 0.020–0.036 L/kg	
		F: 19–31 mL/kg		F: 0.019–0.031 L/kg	
Reticulocyte count	Whole blood (EDTA, heparin, or oxalate)	0.5–1.5% of erythrocytes		0.005–0.015 (number fraction)	
Sulfhemoglobin	Whole blood (EDTA, heparin, or ACD)	≤1.0% of total Hb		<0.010 of total Hb (mass fraction)	
Thrombin time	Whole blood (Na citrate)			Time of control ± 2S when control is 9–13 sec	
Thromboplastin time, activated (see Activated partial thromboplastin time [APTT])					

DRUGS—THERAPEUTIC AND TOXIC

Drug	Specimen	Reference Interval (Conventional Units)		Reference Interval (International Units)
Acetaminophen	Serum or plasma (hep or EDTA)	Therap:	10–30 µg/mL	66–199 µmol/L
		Toxic:	>200 µg/mL	>1324 µmol/L
Amikacin	Serum or plasma (EDTA)	Therap:		
		Peak	25–35 µg/mL	43–60 µmol/L
		Trough (severe infection):	4–8 µg/mL	6.8–13.7 µmol/L
		Toxic:		
		Peak	>35 µg/mL	>60 µmol/L
		Trough	>10 µg/mL	>17 µmol/L
ε-Aminocaproic acid	Serum or plasma (hep or EDTA); trough	Therap:	100–400 µg/mL	0.76–3.05 mmol/L
Amitriptyline	Serum or plasma (hep or EDTA); trough (>12 h after dose)	Therap:	120–250 ng/mL	433–903 nmol/L
		Toxic:	>500 ng/mL	>1805 nmol/L
Amobarbital	Serum	Therap:	1–5 µg/mL	4–22 µmol/L
		Toxic:	>10 µg/mL	>44 µmol/L
Amphetamine	Serum or plasma (hep or EDTA)	Therap:	20–30 ng/mL	148–222 nmol/L
		Toxic:	>200 ng/mL	>1480 nmol/L
Bromide	Serum	Therap:	750–1500 µg/mL	9.4–18.7 mmol/L
		Toxic:	>1250 µg/mL	>15.6 mmol/L

DRUGS—THERAPEUTIC AND TOXIC Continued

Drug	Specimen		Reference Interval (Conventional Units)	Reference Interval (International Units)
Caffeine	Serum or plasma (hep or EDTA)	Therap:	3–15 µg/mL	15–77 µmol/L
		Toxic:	>50 µg/mL	>258 µmol/L
Carbamazepine	Serum or plasma (hep or EDTA); trough	Therap:	4–12 µg/mL	17–51 µmol/L
		Toxic:	>15 µg/mL	>63 µmol/L
Carbenicillin	Serum or plasma	Therap:		Dependent on minimum inhibition concentration of specific organism
		Toxic:	>250 µg/mL	>660 µmol/L
Chloramphenicol	Serum or plasma (hep or EDTA); trough	Therap:	10–25 µg/L	31–77 µmol/L
		Toxic:	>25 µg/mL	>77 µmol/L
Chlordiazepoxide	Serum or plasma (hep or EDTA); trough	Therap:	700–1000 ng/mL	2.34–3.34 µmol/L
		Toxic:	>5000 ng/mL	>16.7 µmol/L
Chlorpromazine	Serum or plasma (hep or EDTA); trough	Therap:	50–300 ng/mL	157–942 nmol/L
		Toxic:	>750 ng/mL	>2355 nmol/L
Cimetidine	Serum or plasma (hep or EDTA); trough	Therap:	0.5–1.2 µg/mL	2–5 µmol/L
Clonazepam	Serum or plasma (hep or EDTA. trough	Therap:	15–60 ng/mL	48–190 nmol/L
		Toxic:	>80 ng/mL	>254 nmol/L
Clonidine	Serum or plasma (hep or EDTA)	Therap:	1.0–2.0 ng/mL	4.4–8.7 nmol/L
Clorazepate	Serum or plasma (hep or EDTA)	As desmethyldiazepam:		
		Therap:	0.12–1.0 µg/mL	0.36–3.01 µmol/L
Cocaine	Serum or plasma (hep or EDTA); on ice	Therap:	100–500 ng/mL	330–1650 nmol/L
		Toxic:	>1000 ng/mL	>3300 nmol/L
Cyclosporine	Serum (12 h after dose)	Therap:	100–400 ng/mL	83–333 nmol/L
		Toxic:	>400 ng/mL	>333 nmol/L
Desipramine	Serum or plasma (hep or EDTA); trough (≥12 h after dose)	Therap:	75–300 ng/mL	281–1125 nmol/L
		Toxic:	>400 ng/mL	>1500 nmol/L
Diazepam	Serum or plasma (hep or EDTA); trough	Therap:	100–1000 ng/mL	0.35–3.51 µmol/L
		Toxic:	>5000 ng/mL	>17.55 µmol/L
Digitoxin	Serum or plasma (hep or EDTA) ≥6 h after dose	Therap:	20–35 ng/mL	24–46 nmol/L
		Toxic:	>45 ng/mL	>59 nmol/L
Digoxin	Serum or plasma (hep or EDTA); trough (≥12 h after dose)	Therap:	0.8–1.5 ng/mL	1.1–1.9 nmol/L
		CHF: Arrhythmias:	1.5–2.0 ng/mL	1.9–2.6 nmol/L
		Toxic:	>2.5 ng/mL	>3.2 nmol/L
Diphenylhydantoin (see Phenytoin)				
Disopyramide	Serum or plasma (hep or EDTA); trough	Therap: Arrhythmias:		
		Atrial	2.8–3.2 µg/mL	8.3–9.4 µmol/L
		Ventricular	3.3–7.5 µg/mL	9.7–22 µmol/L
		Toxic:	>7 µg/mL	>20.7 µmol/L
Doxepin	Serum or plasma (hep or EDTA); trough (≥ 12 h after dose)	Therap:	30–150 ng/mL	107–537 nmol/L
		Toxic:	>500 ng/mL	>1790 nmol/L
Ethchlorvynol	Serum or plasma (hep or EDTA)	Therap:	2–8 µg/mL	14–55 µmol/L
		Toxic:	>20 µg/mL	>138 µmol/L
Ethosuximide	Serum or plasma (hep or EDTA); trough	Therap:	40–100 µg/mL	283–708 µmol/L
		Toxic:	>150 µg/mL	>1062 µmol/L
Fenoprofen	Plasma (EDTA)	Therap:	20–65 µg/mL	82–268 µmol/L
Flecainide	Serum or plasma (hep or EDTA); trough	Therap:	0.2–1.0 µg/mL	0.5–2.4 µmol/L
		Toxic:	>1.0 µg/mL	>2.4 µmol/L
Furosemide	Serum (30 min after dose)	Therap:	1–2 µg/mL	3–6 µmol/L
Gentamicin	Serum or plasma (EDTA)	Therap:		
		Peak (severe infection)	8–10 µg/mL	16.7–20.9 µmol/L
		Trough (severe infection)	2–4 µg/mL	4.2–8.4 µmol/L
		Toxic:		
		Peak	>10 µg/mL	>21 µmol/L
		Trough	>4 µg/mL	>8.4 µmol/L
Glutethimide	Serum	Therap:	2–6 µg/mL	9–28 µmol/L
		Toxic:	>5 µg/mL	>23 µmol/L
Imipramine	Serum or plasma (hep or EDTA); trough (≥12 h after dose)	Therap:	125–250 ng/mL	446–893 nmol/L
		Toxic:	>500 ng/mL	>1784 nmol/L
Isoniazid	Serum or plasma (hep or EDTA)	Therap:	1–7 µg/mL	7–51 µmol/L
		Toxic:	20–710 µg/mL	146–5176 µmol/L
Kanamycin	Serum or plasma (EDTA)	Therap:		
		Peak	25–35 µg/mL	52–72 µmol/L
		Trough (severe infection)	4–8 µg/mL	8–16 µmol/L
		Toxic:		
		Peak	>35 µg/mL	>72 µmol/L
		Trough	>10 µg/mL	>21 µmol/L
Lidocaine	Serum or plasma (hep or EDTA); ≥45 min following bolus dose	Therap:	1.5–6.0 µg/mL	6.4–26 µmol/L
		Toxic:		
		CNS or cardiovascular depression	6–8 µg/mL	26–34.2 µmol/L
		Seizures, obtundation, decreased cardiac output	>8 µg/mL	>34.2 µmol/L
Lithium	Serum or plasma (hep or EDTA); (>12 h after last dose)	Therap:	0.6–1.2 mEq/L	0.6–1.2 mmol/L
		Toxic:	>2 mEq/L	>2 mmol/L
Lorazepam	Serum or plasma (hep or EDTA)	Therap:	50–240 ng/mL	156–746 nmol/L
Meperidine	Serum or plasma (hep or EDTA)	Therap:	400–700 ng/mL	1620–2830 nmol/L
		Toxic:	>1 µg/mL	>4043 nmol/L
Meprobamate	Serum	Therap:	6–12 µg/mL	28–55 µmol/L
		Toxic:	>60 µg/mL	>275 µmol/L

DRUGS—THERAPEUTIC AND TOXIC Continued

Drug	Specimen	Reference Interval (Conventional Units)		Reference Interval (International Units)
Methadone	Serum or plasma (hep or EDTA)	Therap:	100–400 ng/mL	0.32–1.29 μmol/L
		Toxic:	>2000 ng/mL	>6.46 μmol/L
Methaqualone	Serum or plasma (hep or EDTA)	Therap:	2–3 μg/mL	8–12 μmol/L
		Toxic:	>10 μg/mL	>40 μmol/L
Methotrexate	Serum or plasma (hep or EDTA)	Therap:	variable	variable
		Toxic:		
		Low-dose therapy (1–2 wk)	>9.1 ng/mL	>20 nmol/L
		High-dose therapy (48 h)	>454 ng/mL	>1000 nmol/L
Methsuximide (N-desmethyl methsuximide)	Serum	Therap:	10–40 μg/mL	53–212 μmol/L
		Toxic:	>40 μg/mL	>212 μmol/L
Methyldopa	Plasma (EDTA)	Therap:	1–5 μg/mL	4.7–23.7 μmol/L
		Toxic:	>7 μg/mL	>33 μmol/L
Methyprylon	Serum	Therap:	8–10 μg/mL	43–55 μmol/L
		Toxic:	>50 μg/mL	>273 μmol/L
Mexiletine	Serum or plasma (hep or EDTA)	Therap:	0.7–2.0 μg/mL	3.9–11.2 μmol/L
		Toxic:	>2.0 μg/mL	>11.2 μmol/L
Morphine	Serum or plasma (hep or EDTA)	Therap:	10–80 ng/mL	35–280 nmol/L
		Toxic:	>200 ng/mL	>700 nmol/L
N-Acetylprocainamide	Serum or plasma (hep or EDTA); trough	Therap:	5–30 μg/mL	18–108 μmol/L
		Toxic:	>40 μg/mL	>144 μmol/L
Nitroprusside	Serum or plasma (EDTA)	As thiocyanate:		
		Therap:	6–29 μg/mL	103–499 μmol/L
Normethsuximide	Serum	Therap:	10–40 μg/mL	53–212 μmol/L
		Toxic:	>40 μg/mL	>212 μmol/L
Nortriptyline	Serum or plasma (hep or EDTA); trough (≥12 h after dose)	Therap:	50–150 ng/mL	190–570 nmol/L
		Toxic:	>500 ng/mL	>1900 nmol/L
Oxazepam	Serum or plasma (hep or EDTA)	Therap:	0.2–1.4 μg/mL	0.70–4.9 μmol/L
Paraquat	Whole blood (EDTA)	Toxic:	0.1–1.6 μg/mL	0.39–6.2 μmol/L
	Urine	Occup exp:	0.3 μg/mL	1.17 μmol/L
		Toxic:	0.9–64 μg/mL	3.50–249 μmol/L
Pentobarbital	Serum or plasma (hep or EDTA); trough	Therap:		
		Hypnotic	1–5 μg/mL	4–22 μmol/L
		Therap coma	20–50 μg/mL	88–221 μmol/L
		Toxic:	>10 μg/mL	>44 μmol/L
Phenacetin	Plasma (EDTA)	Therap:	1–30 μg/mL	6–167 μmol/L
		Toxic:	50–250 μg/mL	279–1395 μmol/L
Phencyclidine	Serum or plasma (hep or EDTA)	Toxic:	90–800 ng/mL	370–3288 nmol/L
Phenobarbital	Serum or plasma (hep or EDTA); trough	Therap:	15–40 μg/mL	65–170 μmol/L
		Toxic:		
		Slowness, ataxia, nystagmus	35–80 μg/mL	151–345 μmol/L
		Coma with reflexes	65–117 μg/mL	280–504 μmol/L
		Coma without reflexes	>100 μg/mL	>430 μmol/L
Phensuximide (both parent and N-desmethyl metabolites)	Serum or plasma (hep or EDTA)	Therap:	40–60μg/mL	228–324 μmol/L
Phenylbutazone	Plasma (EDTA)	Therap:	50–100 μg/mL	162–324 μmol/L
		(not well defined)		
		Toxic:	>100 μg/mL	>324 μmol/L
Phenytoin	Serum or plasma (hep or EDTA); trough	Therap:	10–20 μg/mL	40–79 μmol/L
		Toxic:	>20 μg/mL	>79 μmol/L
Primidone	Serum or plasma (hep or EDTA); trough	Therap:	5–12 μg/mL	23–55 μmol/L
		Toxic:	>15 μg/mL	>69 μmol/L
Procainamide	Serum or plasma (hep or EDTA); trough	Therap:	4–10 μg/mL	17–42 μmol/L
		Toxic:	>10 μg/mL	>42 μmol/L
		Also consider effect of metabolite, N-acetylprocainamide		
Propoxyphene	Plasma (EDTA)	Therap:	0.1–0.4 μg/mL	0.3–1.2 μmol/L
		Toxic:	>0.5 μg/mL	>1.5 μmol/L
Propranolol	Serum or plasma (hep or EDTA); trough	Therap:	50–100 ng/mL	193–386 nmol/L
Protriptyline	Serum or plasma (hep or EDTA); trough (≥12 h after dose)	Therap:	70–250 ng/mL	266–950 nmol/L
		Toxic:	>500 ng/mL	>1900 nmol/L
Quinidine	Serum or plasma (hep or EDTA); trough	Therap:	2–5 μg/mL	6–15 μmol/L
		Toxic:	>6 μg/mL	>18 μmol/L
Salicylates	Serum or plasma (hep or EDTA); trough	Therap:	150–300 μg/mL	1086–2172 μmol/L
		Toxic:	>300 μg/mL	>2172 μmol/L
Secobarbital	Serum	Therap:	1–2 μg/mL	4.2–8.4 μmol/L
		Toxic:	>5 μg/mL	>21.0 μmol/L
Theophylline	Serum or plasma (hep or EDTA)	Therap:	8–20 μg/mL	44–111 μmol/L
		Toxic:	>20 μg/mL	>110 μmol/L
Thiocyanate	Serum or plasma (EDTA)			
		Nonsmoker:	1–4 μg/mL	17–69 μmol/L
		Smoker:	3–12 μg/mL	52–206 μmol/L
		Therap, after nitroprusside infusion:	6–29 μg/mL	103–499 μmol/L
	Urine	Nonsmoker:	1–4 mg/d	17–69 μmol/d
		Smoker:	7–17 mg/d	120–292 μmol/d
Thiopental	Serum or plasma (hep or EDTA); trough	Hypnotic:	1.0–5.0 μg/mL	4.1–20.7 μmol/L
		Coma:	30–100 μg/mL	124–413 μmol/L
		Anesthesia:	7–130 μg/mL	29–536 μmol/L
		Toxic conc:	>10 μg/mL	>41 μmol/L
Thioridazine	Serum or plasma (hep or EDTA)	Therap:	1.0–1.5 μg/mL	2.7–4.1 μmol/L
		Toxic:	>10 μg/mL	>27 μmol/L
Tobramycin	Serum or plasma (hep or EDTA)	Therap:		
		Peak (severe infection)	8–10 μg/mL	17–21 μmol/L
		Trough (severe infection)	<4 μg/mL	<9 μmol/L
		Toxic:		
		Peak	>10 μg/mL	>21 μmol/L
		Trough	>4 μg/mL	>9 μmol/L
Tocainide	Serum or plasma (hep or EDTA)	Therap:	4–10 μg/mL	21–52 μmol/L
Valproic acid	Serum or plasma (hep or EDTA); trough	Therap:	50–100 μg/mL	347–693 μmol/L
		Toxic:	>100 μg/mL	>693 μmol/L
Vancomycin	Serum or plasma (hep or EDTA); trough	Therap:	5–10 μg/mL	3–7 μmol/L
		Toxic:	>80–100 μg/mL	>55–69 μmol/L
		(not well established)		
Verapamil	Serum or plasma (hep or EDTA)	Therap:	100–500 ng/mL	220–1100 nmol/L
Warfarin	Serum or plasma (hep or EDTA)	Therap:	1–10 μg/mL	3–32 μmol/L

Eponymic Diseases and Syndromes

Aarskog-Scott s.

Aarskog's s.

Abercrombie's s.

Abrami's d.

Achard s.

Achard-Thiers s.

Achenboch's s.

Acosta's d.

Adair-Dighton s.

Adams' d.

Adams-Stokes d.

Addison's d.

Addison-Biermer d.

addisonian s.

Adie's s.

Ahumada–del Castillo s.

Aicardi's s.

Akureyri d.

Albarrán's d.

Albers-Schönberg d.

Albert's d.

Albright's s.

Albright-McCune-Sternberg s.

Aldrich's s.

Alexander's d.

Alezzandrini's s.

Alibert's d.

Allen-Masters s.

Almeida's d.

Alper's d.

Alport's s.

Alström's s.

Alzheimer's d.

amniotic infection s. of Blane

Anders' d.

Andersen's d., s.

Andes d.

Andrews' d.

Angelucci's s.

Anton's s.

Apert-Crouzon d.

Apert's d., s.

Aran-Duchenne d.

Argonz–Del Castillo s.

Arias' s.

Armstrong's d.

Arndt-Gottron s.

Arnold-Chiari s.

Arnold's nerve reflex cough s.

Ascher's s.

Asherman's s.

Aufrecht's d.

Aujeszky's d.

Avellis' s.

Axenfeld's s.

Ayerza's d., s.

Baastrup's d.

Babinski-Fröhlich s.

s. of Babinski-Nageotte

Babinski's s.

Babinski-Vaquez s.

Baelz's d.

Bäfverstedt's s.

Balfour's d.

Balint's s.

Baller-Gerold s.

Ballet's d.

Ballingall's d.

Baló's d.	Bekhterev's d.
Bamberger-Marie d.	Bell's d.
Bamberger's d.	s. of Benedikt
Bamle d.	Bennett's d.
Bang's d.	Benson's d.
Bannister's d.	Berardinelli's s.
Banti's d., s.	Bergeron's d.
Barclay-Baron d.	Berger's d.
Barcoo d.	Berlin's d.
Bardet-Biedl s.	Bernard's s.
Barlow's d., s.	Bernard-Horner s.
Barraquer's d.	Bernard-Sergent s.
Barré-Guillain s.	Bernard-Soulier s.
Barrett's s.	Bernhardt-Roth s.
Barthélemy's d.	Bernhardt's d.
Bart's s.	Bernheim's s.
Bartter's s.	Bertolotti's s.
Basedow's d.	Besnier-Boeck d.
Basel d.	Besnier-Boeck-Schaumann d., s.
Bassen-Kornzweig s.	Best's d.
Bateman's d., s.	Bianchi's s.
Batten-Mayou d.	Biedl's d.
Batten's d.	Bielschowsky-Jansky d.
Batten-Spielmeyer-Vogt d.	Bielschowsky's d.
Bayle's d.	Biemond's s.
Bazex's s.	Biermer's d.
Bazin's d.	Biett's d.
Beard's d.	Bilderbeck's d.
Beau's d., s.	Billroth's d.
Beauvais' d.	Binswanger's d.
Bechterew's (Bekhterev's) d.	Bird's d.
Becker's d.	Björnstad's s.
Beck's d.	Blackfan-Diamond s.
Beckwith's s.	Blatin's s.
Beckwith-Wiedemann s.	Bloch-Sulzberger s.
Begbie's d.	Blocq's d.
Béguez César d.	Bloodgood's d.
Behçet's s.	Bloom's s.
Behr's d.	Blount-Barber d.
Beigel's d.	Blount's d.

Blumenthal's d.

Blum's s.

body of Luys s.

Boeck's d.

Boerhaave's s.

Bogaert's d.

Bonnet-Dechaume-Blanc s.

Bonnevie-Ullrich s.

Bonnier's s.

Böök's s.

Börjeson-Forssman-Lehmann s.

Börjeson's s.

Bornholm d.

Bostock's d.

Bouchard's d.

Bouchet-Gsell d.

Bouillaud's d., s.

Bourneville-Pringle d.

Bourneville's d.

Bouveret's d., s.

Bowen's d.

Brachmann–de Lange s.

Bradley's d.

Brailsford-Morquio d.

Breda's d.

Breisky's d.

Brennemann's s.

Bretonneau's d.

Bright's d.

Brill's d.

Brill-Symmers d.

Brill-Zinsser d.

Brinton's d.

Brion-Kayser d.

Briquet's s.

Brissaud-Marie s.

Brissaud's d.

Brissaud-Sicard s.

Bristowe's s.

Brock s.

Brocq's d.

Brodie's d.

Brooke's d.

Brown-Séquard d., s.

Brown's vertical retraction s.

Brown-Symmers d.

Bruck's d.

Brugsch's s.

Bruns' s.

Brunsting's s.

Brushfield-Wyatt d., s.

Bruton's d.

Buckley's s.

Budd-Chiari s.

Budd's d., s.

Buerger-Grütz d.

Buerger's d.

Buhl's d.

Bürger-Grütz s.

Burnett's s.

Bury's d.

Buschke-Ollendorff s.

Buschke's d.

Busquet's d.

Buss d.

Busse-Buschke d.

Byler's d.

Bywaters' s.

Cacchi-Ricci d.

Caffey's d., s.

Caffey-Silverman s.

California d.

Calvé-Perthes d.

Camurati-Engelmann d.

Canada-Cronkhite s.

Canavan's d.

Caner-Decker s.

Capdepont's d.

Capgras' s.

Caplan's s.

Caroli's d.

Carpenter's s.

Carrión's d.

Castellani's d.

Castleman's d.

Cavare's d.

Cazenave's d.

Ceelen-Gellerstedt s.

Céstan-Chenais s.

Céstan-Raymond s.

Céstan's s.

Chabert's d.

Chagas-Cruz d.

Chagas' d.

Championniére's d.

Charcot-Marie-Tooth d.

Charcot's d., s.

Charcot-Weiss-Barker s.

Charlin's s.

Charlouis' d.

Charrin's d.

Chauffard's s.

Chauffard-Still s.

Cheadle's d.

Chédiak-Higashi s.

Chédiak-Steinbrinck-Higashi s.

Cheney s.

Cherchevski's (Cherchewski's) d.

Chester's d.

Chiari-Arnold s.

Chiari-Budd s.

Chiari-Frommel s.

Chiari II s.

Chiari's s.

Chilaiditi's s.

Chotzen's s.

Christensen-Krabbe d.

Christian's d., s.

Christian-Weber d.

Christmas d.

Christ-Siemens s.

Christ-Siemens-Touraine s.

Churg-Strauss s.

Ciarrocchi's d.

Cistelli's s.

Citelli's s.

Civatte's d.

Clarke-Hadfield s.

Claude Bernard–Horner s.

Claude's s.

Clérambault-Kandinsky s.

Clough and Richter's s.

Clouston's s.

Coats' d.

Cockayne's s.

Coffin-Lowry s.

Coffin-Siris s.

Cogan's s.

Collet-Sicard s.

Collet's s.

Concato's d.

Conn's s.

Conor and Bruch's d.

Conradi's d., s.

Cooley's d.

Cooper's d.

Corbus' d.

Core-Forbes d.

Cori's d.

Cornelia de Lange's s.

Corrigan's d.

Corvisart's d.

Costen's s.

Cotard's s.

Cottunius' d.

Cotugno's d.

Courvoisier-Terrier s.

Cowden's d.

Crandall's s.

Creutzfeldt-Jakob d., s.

Crigler-Najjar s.	Dercum's d.
Crocq's d.	De Sanctis-Cacchione s.
Crohn's d.	de Toni-Fanconi s.
Cronkhite-Canada s.	Deutschländer's d.
Cronkhite's s.	Devergie's d.
Crouzon's d.	Devic's d.
Crow-Fukase s.	DiGeorge's s.
Cruveilhier-Baumgarten s.	Dighton-Adair s.
Cruveilhier's d.	Di Guglielmo d., s.
Cruz-Chagas d.	Dimitri's d.
Csillag's d.	Döhle d.
Curschmann's d.	Donohue's s.
Curtius' s.	Down's s.
Cushing's d., s.	Dresbach's s.
Cyriax's s.	Dressler's s.
Czerny's d.	Duane's s.
Daae-Finsen d.	Dubini's d.
Daae's d.	Dubin-Johnson s.
DaCosta's d., s.	Dubin-Sprinz d., s.
Dalrymple's d.	Dubois' d.
Danbolt-Closs s.	Dubreuil-Chambardel s.
Dandy-Walker s.	Duchenne-Aran d.
Danielssen-Boeck d.	Duchenne-Erb s.
Danielssen's d.	Duchenne-Griesinger d.
Danlos' s.	Duchenne's d., s.
Darier's d.	Duhring's d.
Darling's d.	Dukes' d.
David's d.	Duncan's d.
Davies' d.	Duplay's s.
Debré-Sémélaigne s.	Dupré's s.
de Clerambault s.	Dupuytren's d.
Degos' d., s.	Durand-Nicolas-Favre d.
Déjérine-Klumpke s.	Durand's d.
s. of Déjérine-Roussy	Durante's d.
Déjérine's d., s.	Duroziez's d.
Déjérine-Sottas d., s.	Dutton's d.
de Lange's s.	Dyggve-Melchior-Clausen s.
Del Castillo s.	Dyke-Davidoff-Masson s.
Dennie-Marfan s.	Eagle s.
de Quervain's d.	Eales's d.

Eaton-Lambert s.

Ebstein's d.

Economo's d.

Eddowes' s.

Edsall's d.

Edwards' s.

Edwards-Patau s.

Ehlers-Danlos s.

Eichstedt's d.

Eisenlohr's s.

Eisenmenger's s.

Ekbom s.

Ellis–van Creveld s.

Engelmann's d.

Engel-Recklinghausen d.

English d.

Engman's d.

Epstein's d., s.

Erb-Charcot d.

Erb-Goldflam d.

Erb-Landouzy d.

Erb's d., s.

Erdheim d.

Eulenburg's d.

Evans' s.

Faber's s.

Fabry's d.

Fahr's d.

Fahr-Volhard d.

Fallot's s.

Fanconi's s.

Fanconi-Zinsser s.

Farber's d., s.

Farber-Uzman s.

Fauchard's d.

Favre-Durand-Nicholas d.

Favre-Racouchot s.

Fede's d.

Feer's d.

Felty's s.

Fenwick's d.

Feuerstein-Mims s.

Fiedler's d.

Fiessinger-Leroy-Reiter s.

Fiessinger's s.

Figueira's s.

Filatov-Dukes d.

Filatov's d.

Fisher's s.

Fitz-Hugh-Curtis s.

Fitz's s.

Flajani's d.

Flatau-Schilder d.

Flegel's d.

Fleischner's d.

Flynn-Aird s.

Foix's s.

Fölling's d.

Forbes' d.

Forbes-Albright s.

Fordyce's d.

Forestier's d.

Forney's s.

Forssman's carotid s.

Förster's d.

Foster Kennedy s.

Fothergill's d.

Fournier's d.

Foville's s.

Fox-Fordyce d.

Fraley s.

Franceschetti s.

Franceschetti-Jadassohn s.

Francis' d.

François' s.

Frankl-Hochwart's d.

Franklin's d.

Fraser's s.

Freeman-Sheldon s.

Frei's d.

Freiberg's d.

Frenkel's anterior ocular traumatic s.

Frey's s.

Friderichsen-Waterhouse s.

Friedländer's d.

Friedmann's d.

Friedmann's vasomotor s.

Friedreich's d.

Friend d.

Fröhlich's s.

Froin's s.

Frommel-Chiari s.

Frommel's d.

Fuchs's s.

Furst-Ostrum s.

Fürstner's d.

Gailliard's s.

Gairdner's d.

Gaisböck's d.

Gamma's d.

Gamstorp's d.

Gandy-Nanta d.

Ganser's s.

Gard-Girnoux s.

Gardner-Diamond s.

Gardner's s.

Garré's d.

Gasser's s.

Gaucher's d.

Gee-Herter d.

Gee-Herter-Heubner d.

Gee's d.

Gee-Thaysen d.

Gélineau's s.

Gensoul's d.

Gerhardt's d., s.

Gerlier's d.

Gerstmann's s.

Gerstmann-Straussler-Schenker s.

Gianotti-Crosti s.

Gibert's d.

Gibney's d.

Gierke's d.

Gilbert's d., s.

Gilchrist's d.

Gilles de la Tourette's s.

Glanzmann-Riniker s.

Glanzmann's d.

Glasser's d.

Glénard's d.

Glisson's d.

Goldberg-Maxwell s.

Goldenhar's s.

Goldflam-Erb d.

Goldflam's d.

Goldscheider's d.

Goldstein's d.

Goldston s.

Goltz-Gorlin s.

Goltz's s.

Goodpasture's d., s.

Good's s.

Gopalan's s.

Gorham's d.

Gorlin-Chaudhry-Moss s.

Gorlin-Goltz s.

Gorlin-Psaume s.

Gorlin's s.

Gorman's s.

Gougerot and Blum d.

Gougerot-Carteaud s.

Gougerot-Nulock-Houwer s.

Gougerot-Ruiter d.

Gougerot-Sjögren d.

Gowers' s.

Gradenigo's s.

Graefe's d.

Graham Little s.

Graves' d.

Greenfield's d.

Greenhow's d.

Gregg's s.

Greig's s.

Griesinger's d.

Griscelli s.

Grönblad-Strandberg s.

Gross's d.

Grover's d.

Gruber's s.

Gubler's s.

di Guglielmo's d.

Guillain-Barré s.

Guinon's d.

Gull's d.

Gull-Sutton d.

Gunn's s.

Günther's d.

Habermann's d.

Haber's s.

Hadfield-Clarke s.

Haff d.

Haglund's d.

Hagner's d.

Hailey-Hailey d.

Hakim's s.

Hallermann-Streiff s.

Hallermann-Streiff-Francois s.

Hallervorden s.

Hallervorden-Spatz d., s.

Hallgren's s.

Hallopeau's d.

Hallopeau-Siemens s.

Hall's d.

Haltia-Santavuori s.

Hamman-Rich s.

Hamman's d.

Hammond's d.

Hand's d.

Hand-Schüller-Christian d.

Hanhart's s.

Hanot-Chauffard s.

Hanot's d.

Hansen's d.

d. of the Hapsburgs

Harada's s.

Hare's s.

Harley's d.

Harris' s.

Hartnup d., s.

Hashimoto's d.

Hassin's s.

Hayem-Widal s.

Heberden's d.

Hebra's d.

Heerfordt's d., s.

Hegglin's s.

Heidenhaim's s.

Heine-Medin d.

Heller-Döhle d.

Helweg-Larssen s.

Hench-Rosenberg s.

Henderson-Jones d.

Henoch-Schönlein s.

Herlitz s.

Hermansky-Pudlak s.

Herrmann's s.

Hers' d.

Herter-Heubner d.

Herter's d.

Heubner's d.

Hildenbrand's d.

Hines-Bannick s.

Hippel-Lindau d.

Hippel's d.

Hirschfeld's d.

Hirschowitz s.

Hirschsprung's d.

His's d.

His-Werner d.

Hjärre's d.

Hodara's d.

Hodgkin's d.

   lymphocyte depletion type

   lymphocyte predominance type

   mixed cellularity type

   nodular sclerosis type

Hodgson's d.

Hoffa's d.

Hoffmann-Werdnig s.

Holmes-Adie s.

Holt-Oram s.

Homén's s.

Hoppe-Goldflam d.

Horner-Bernard s.

Horner's s.

Horton's d., s.

Houssay s.

Huchard's d.

Hünermann's d.

Hunter-Hurler s.

Hunter's s.

Huntington's d.

Hunt's d., s.

Hurler-Pfaundler s.

Hurler's d., s.

Hurler-Scheie s.

Hutchinson-Boeck d.

Hutchinson-Gilford d.

Hutchinson's d.

Hutchison s.

Hutinel's d.

Hyde's d.

Imerslund-Gräsbeck s.

Irvine's s.

Isambert's d.

Itai-Itai d.

Ivemark's s.

Jaccoud's s.

Jackson's s.

Jacod's s.

Jadassohn-Lewandowsky s.

Jaffe-Lichtenstein d., s.

Jahnke's s.

Jakob-Creutzfeldt d.

Jakob's d.

Jaksch's d.

Janet's d.

Jansen's d.

Jansky-Bielschowsky d.

Jensen's d.

Jervell and Lange-Nielsen s.

Jeune's s.

Job-Buckley s.

Job's s.

Johne's d.

Johnson-Stevens d.

Joseph d.

Jourdain's d.

Jüngling's d.

juvenile Paget's d.

Kahlbaum's d.

Kahler's d.

Kaiserstuhl d.

Kalischer's d.

Kallmann's s.

Kanner's s.

Kartagener's s.

Kasabach-Merritt s.

Kashin-Beck d.

Kast's s.

Kawasaki's d.

Kayser's d.

Kearns' s.

Kearns-Sayre s.

Kedani d.

Kellgren's d.

Kennedy's s.

Keshan d.

Kienböck's d.

Kiloh-Nevin s.

Kimmelstiel-Wilson s.

Kimura's d.

Kinnier Wilson d.

Kinsbourne s.

Kirkland's d.

Klauder's s.

Klebs' d.

Kleine-Levin s.

Klemperer's d.

Klinefelter's s.

Klippel-Feil s.

Klippel's d.

Klippel-Trenaunay s.

Klippel-Trenaunay-Weber s.

Klumpke-Déjerine s.

Klüver-Bucy s.

Kneist s.

Kocher-Debré-Sémélaigne s.

Kocher's s.

Koenig's s.

Koenig-Wichman d.

Koerber-Salus-Elschnig s.

Köhler-Pellegrini-Stieda d.

Köhler's bone d.

Köhlmeier-Degos d.

Kokka d.

König's s.

Korsakoff's d., s.

Koshevnikoff's d.

Kostmann's s.

Krabbe's d., s.

Krause's s.

Krishaber's d.

Kufs' d.

Kugelberg-Welander d.

Kuhnt-Junius d.

Kümmell's d.

Kümmel-Verneuil d.

Kunkel's s.

Kuskokwim s.

Kussmaul-Maier d.

Kussmaul's d.

Kyrle's d.

Laband's s.

Labbé's d.

Labbé's neurocirculatory s.

Ladd's s.

Laënnec's d.

Lafora's d.

Lambert-Eaton s.

Lancereaux-Mathieu d.

Landouzy's d.

Landry's d., s.

Landry-Guillain Barré s.

Lane's d.

Langdon-Down's d.

Larrey-Weil d.

Larsen-Johansson d.

Larsen's d., s.

Laségue's d.

Lauber's d.

Laubry-Soulle s.

Launois' s.

Launois-Bensaude s.

Launois-Cléret s.

Laurence-Biedl s.

Laurence-Moon s.

Laurence-Moon-Bardet-Biedl s.

Laurence-Moon-Biedl s.

Läwen-Roth s.

Lawford's s.

Lawrence-Seip s.

Leber's d.

Legal's d.

Legg-Calvé d.

Legg-Calvé-Perthes d.

Legg-Calvé-Waldenström d.

Legg-Perthes d.

Legg's d.

Leigh's d.

Leiner's d.

Leloir's d.

Lenegre's d.

Lennox s.

Lenz's s.

Leredde's s.

Leriche's d., s.

Leri-Weill d., s.

Lermoyez's s.

Leroy's d.

Lesch-Nyhan s.

Letterer-Siwe d.

Lévi's d., s.

Lev's d.

Lévy-Roussy s.

Lewandowsky-Lutz d.

Leyden-Moebius s.

Leyden's d.

Lhermitte-McAlpine s.

Libman-Sacks d., s.

Lichtheim's d., s.

Liddle's s.

Li-Fraumeni cancer s.

Lightwood's s.

Lignac-Fanconi d., s.

Liganc's d., s.

Lindau's d.

Lindau-von Hippel d.

Lipschütz's d.

Little's d.

Lobo's d.

Lobstein's d., s.

Löffler's s.

Looser-Milkman s.

Lorain-Lévi s.

Lorain's d.

Louis-Bar s.

Lowe's d., s.

Lowe-Terrey-MacLachlan s.

Lown-Ganong-Levine s.

Lucas-Championniére d.

Lucey-Driscoll s.

Luft's d.

Lutembacher's s.

Lutz-Splendore-Almeida d.

Luys' body s.

Lyell's d., s.

Lyme d.

Mackenzie's d., s.

MacLean-Maxwell d.

Macleod's s.

Madelung's d.

Maffucci's s.

Magitot's d.

Maher's d.

Majocchi's d.

Malassez's d.

Malherbe's d.

Malibu d.

Malin's s.

Mallory-Weiss s.

Manson's d.

Marañón's s.

Marburg virus d.

Marchesani's s.

Marchiafava-Bignami d.

Marchiafava-Micheli d.

March's d.

Marcus Gunn's s.

Marek's d.

Marfan's d., s.

Margolis's s.

Marie-Bamberger d., s.

Marie-Robinson s.

Marie's d., s.

Marie-Strümpell d.

Marie-Tooth d.

Marinesco-Garland s.

Marinesco-Sjögren's s.

Marion's d.

Maroteaux-Lamy s.

Marshall's s.

Marsh's d.

Martin's d.

Martorell's s.

Mathieu's d.

Maunier-Kuhn d.

Mauriac s.

Maxcy's d.

Mayer-Rokitansky-Küster s.

McArdle's d.

McArdle-Schmid-Pearson d.

McCune-Albright s.

McLean-Maxwell d.

Meckel-Gruber s.

Meckel's s.

Medin's d.

Meige's d.

Meigs' s.

Meleda d.

Melkersson-Rosenthal s.

Melkersson's s.

Melnick-Needles s.

Ménétrier's d., s.

Mengert's shock s.

Meniere's d., s.

Menkes' kinky hair s.

Merzbacher-Pelizaeus d.

Meyenburg-Altherr-Uehlinger s.

Meyenburg's d.

Meyer-Betz d.

Meyer-Schwickerath and Weyers s.

Meyer's d.

Mibelli's d.

Miescher's d.

Mikulicz's d., s.

Milkman's s.

Millard-Gubler s.

Mills' d.

Milroy's d.

Milton's d.

Milwaukee shoulder s.

Minamata d.

Minkowski-Chauffard s.

Minor's d.

Minot-von Willebrand s.

Miranda s.

Mirrizzi's s.

Mitchell's d.

Miyasoto's d.

Möbius' d., s.

Moeller-Barlow d.

Molten's d.

Monakow's s.

Mondor's d.

Monge's d.

Montreal platelet d.

Moore's s.

Morel-Kraepelin d.

Morel's s.

Morgagni-Adams-Stokes s.

Morgagni's d., s.

Morgagni-Stewart-Morel s.

Morquio-Brailsford d.

Morquio's s.

Morquio-Ullrich s.

Morris s.

Morton's d., s.

Morvan's d., s.

Moschcowitz's d.

Mosse's s.

Mounier-Kuhn s.

Mozer's d.

Mucha-Habermann d., s.

Mucha's d.

Muckle-Wells s.

Muir-Torre s.

Munchausen's s.

Munchmeyer's d.

Murchison-Sanderson s.

Murri's d.	Owren's d.
Myá's d.	Paas's d.
Nadia d.	Paget's d.
Naegeli's s.	Paget's d., extramammary
Naffziger's s.	Pancoast's s.
Neftel's d.	Panner's d.
Nelson's s.	Papillon-Léage and Psaume s.
Netherton's s.	Papillon-Lefèvre s.
Neumann's d.	Parinaud's oculoglandular s.
Newcastle d.	Parinaud's s.
Nezelof's s.	parkinsonian s.
Nicolas-Favre d.	Parkinson's d.
Nidoko d.	Parrot's d.
Nieden's s.	Parry-Romberg s.
Niemann-Pick d.	Parry's d.
Niemann's d.	Parsons' d.
Noack's s.	Patau's s.
Nonne-Milroy d.	Patella's d.
Nonne-Milroy-Meige s.	Paterson-Brown-Kelly s.
Nonne's s.	Paterson-Kelly s.
Noonan's s.	Paterson's s.
Nordau's d.	Pauzat's d.
Norrie's d.	Pavy's d.
Norum's d.	Payr's d.
Nothnagel's s.	Pel-Ebstein d.
Novy's rat d.	Pelizaeus-Merzbacher d.
Ogilvie's s.	Pellegrini's d.
Oguchi's d.	Pellegrini-Stieda d.
Ohara's d.	Pellizzi's s.
Ollier's d.	Pendred's s.
Olmer's d.	Pepper s.
Opitz's d.	Perlman's s.
Oppenheim's d., s.	Perrin-Ferraton d.
Ormond's d.	Perthes' d.
Osgood-Schlatter d.	Pette-Döring d.
Osler's d.	Peutz' s.
Osler-Vaquez d.	Peutz-Jeghers s.
Osler-Weber-Rendu d.	Peyronie's d.
Ostrum-Furst s.	Pfaundler-Hurler s.
Otto's d.	Pfeiffer's d., s.

Phocas' d.

Picchini's s.

Pick's d.

pickwickian s.

Pictou d.

Pierre Robin s.

Pinkus' d.

Plummer's d.

Plummer-Vinson s.

POEMS s.

Poland's s.

Polhemus-Schafer-Ivemark s.

Pompe's d.

Poncet's d.

Posada's d.

Posada-Wernicke d.

Potter's s.

Pott's d.

Poulet's d.

Prader-Willi s.

Preiser's d.

Pringle's d.

Profichet's s.

pseudo-Hurler's d.

pseudo-Turner's s.

Purtscher's d.

Putnam-Dana s.

Pyle's d.

Quervain's d.

Quincke's d.

Quinquaud's d.

Raeder's paratrigeminal s.

Ramsay Hunt s.

Ranikhet d.

Rayer's d.

Raymond-Céstan s.

Raynaud's d.

Recklinghausen-Applebaum d.

Recklinghausen's d.

Recklinghausen's d. of bone

Reclus' d.

Reed-Hodgkin d.

Refetoff s.

Refsum's d.

Reichmann's d., s.

Reifenstein's s.

Reiter's d., s.

Rendu-Osler d.

Rendu-Osler-Weber d.

Renpenning's s.

Rett s.

Reye's s.

Ribas-Torres d.

Richards-Rundle s.

Richter's s.

Riedel's d.

Rieger's s.

Riga-Fede d.

Riga's d.

Riggs' d.

Riley-Day s.

Riley-Smith s.

Ritter's d.

Roaf's s.

Robert's s.

Robinow's s.

Robin's s.

Robinson's d.

Robles' d.

Roger's d., s.

Rokitansky-Küster-Hauser s.

Rokitansky's d.

Romano-Ward s.

Romberg's d., s.

Rose d.

Rosenbach's s.

Rosenthal-Kloepfer s.

Rosenthal's s.

Rosewater's s.

Rossbach's d.

Rot-Bernhardt d., s.

Roth-Bernhardt d., s.

Rothmann-Makai s.

Rothmund-Thomson s.

Roth's d., s.

Rotor's s.

Rot's d., s.

Rotter's s.

Rougnon-Heberden d.

Roussy-Déjérine s.

Roussy-Lévy's d., s.

Rovsing s.

Rubarth's d.

Rubinstein's s.

Rubinstein-Taybi s.

Rud's s.

Rummo's d.

Rundles-Falls s.

Russell's s.

Russell-Silver s.

Rust's d., s.

Ruysch's d.

Sabin-Feldman s.

Sachs' d.

Saethre-Chotzen s.

St. Agatha's d.

St. Aignon's d.

St. Anthony's d.

St. Appolonia's d.

St. Avertin's d.

St. Avidus' d.

St. Blasius' d.

St. Dymphna's d.

St. Erasmus' d.

St. Fiacre's d.

St. Gervasius' d.

St. Gotthard's tunnel d.

St. Hubert's d.

St. Job's d.

St. Mathurin's d.

St. Modestus' d.

St. Roch's d.

St. Sement's d.

St. Valentine's d.

St. Zachary's d.

Sanchez Salorio s.

Sander's d.

Sanders' d.

Sandhoff's d.

Sanfilippo's s.

Saunders' d.

Savill's d.

Schafer's s.

Schamberg's d.

Schanz' d., s.

Schaumann's d., s.

Scheie's s.

Schenck's d.

Scheuermann's d.

Schilder's d.

Schimmelbusch's d.

Schirmer's s.

Schlatter-Osgood d.

Schlatter's d.

Schmid-Fraccaro s.

Schmidt's s.

Schmorl's d.

Scholz's d.

Schönlein-Henoch d., s.

Schönlein's d.

Schottmüller's d.

Schridde's d.

Schroeder's d., s.

Schüller-Christian d., s.

Schüller's d., s.

Schultz' d., s.

Schwartz s.

Schwediauer's d.

Schweninger-Buzzi d.

Seabright bantam s.

Seckel's s.

Secretan's s.

Seitelberger's d.

Selter's d.

Selye s.

Senear-Usher s.

Sertoli-cell–only s.

Sever's d.

Sézary reticulosis s.

Sézary s.

Shaver's d.

Sheehan's s.

Shichito d.

Shwachman-Diamond s.

Shwachman's s.

Shy-Drager s.

Sicard's s.

Silver-Russell s.

Silverskiöld's s.

Silver's s.

Silvestrini-Corda s.

Simmonds' d.

Simons' d.

Simopoulos s.

Sipple's s.

Sjögren-Larsson s.

Sjögren's d., s.

Skevas-Zerfus d.

Sluder's s.

Sly d., s.

Smith-Lemli-Opitz s.

Smith-Riley s.

Smith's d.

Smith-Strang d.

Sneddon-Wilkinson d.

Sohval-Soffer s.

Sorsby's s.

Sotos' s.

Sotos' s. of cerebral gigantism

Spencer's d.

Spens's s.

Speransky-Richen-Siegmund s.

Spielmeyer-Stock d.

Spielmeyer-Vogt d.

Sprinz-Dubin s.

Sprinz-Nelson s.

Spurway s.

Stanton's d.

Stargardt's d.

Steele-Richardson-Olszewski s.

Steinbrocker's s.

Steiner's s.

Steinert's d.

Stein-Leventhal s.

Sterbe d.

Sternberg's d.

Stevens-Johnson s.

Stewart-Morel s.

Stewart-Treves s.

Sticker's d.

Stickler's s.

Stieda's d.

Still-Chauffard s.

Stilling s.

Stilling-Turk-Duane s.

Still's d.

Stokes' d.

Stokes-Adams d.

Stokvis' d.

Stokvis-Talma s.

Strachan's s.

Strümpell-Leichtenstern d.

Strümpell-Lorrain d.

Strümpell's d.

Strümpell-Marie d.

Strümpell-Westphal d.

Stryker-Halbeisen s.

Stühmer's d.

Sturge-Kalischer-Weber s.

Sturge's s.

Sturge-Weber d., s.	Tommaselli's d.
Sudeck-Leriche s.	Tooth d.
Sudeck's d.	Tornwaldt's d.
Sulzberger-Garbe s.	Torre's s.
Sutton and Gull's d.	Torsten-Sjögren's s.
Sutton's d.	Touraine-Solente-Golé s.
Swediaur's d.	Tourette's d.
Sweet's d., s.	Treacher Collins s.
Swift-Feer d.	Trevor's d.
Swift's d.	Troisier's s.
Sydenham's d.	Trousseau's s.
Sylvest's d.	Turcot s.
Symmers' d.	Turner's s.
Takahara's d.	Tyzzer's d.
Takayasu's d., s.	Uehlinger's s.
Talfan d.	Ullrich-Feichtiger s.
Talma's d.	Ullrich-Turner s.
Tangier d.	Ulysses s.
Tapia's s.	Underwood's d.
Tarui d.	Unna's d.
Taussig-Bing s.	Unna-Thost s.
Taylor's d.	Unverricht's d.
Tay-Sachs d.	Urbach-Oppenheim d.
Tay's d.	Urbach-Wiethe d.
Terry's s.	Usher's s.
Teschen d.	van Bogaert's d.
Thaysen's d.	van Buchem's s.
Theiler's d.	van Buren's d.
Thibierge-Weissenbach s.	van der Hoeve's s.
Thiele s.	Van der Woude's s.
Thiemann's d.	Vaquez-Osler d.
Thomsen's d.	Vaquez's d.
Thomson's d.	Verner-Morrison s.
Thorn's s.	Vernet's s.
Thornwaldt's d., s.	Verneuil's d.
Thygeson's d.	Verse's d.
Tietze's s.	Vidal's d.
Tillaux's d.	Villaret's s.
Timme's s.	Vincent's d.
Tolosa-Hunt s.	Vinson-Plummer s.

Vinson's s.

Virchow's d.

Vogt-Koyanagi s.

Vogt-Spielmeyer d.

Vogt's s.

Vohwinkel's s.

Volkmann's d., s.

Voltolini's d.

von Bechterew's (Bekhterev's) d.

von Economo's d.

von Gierke's d.

von Hippel–Lindau d.

von Hippel's d.

von Jaksch's d.

von Meyenburg's d.

von Recklinghausen's d.

von Willebrand's d., s.

Voorhoeve's d.

Vrolik's d.

Waardenburg's s.

Wagner's d.

Waldenström's d.

Wallenberg's s.

Ward-Romano s.

Wardrop's d.

Wartenberg's d.

Wassilieff's d.

Waterhouse-Friderichsen s.

s. of Weber

Weber-Christian d.

Weber-Cockayne s.

Weber-Dimitri d.

Weber-Dubler s.

Weber's d.

Wegener's s.

Wegner's d.

Weill-Marchesani s.

Weil's d., s.

Weir Mitchell's d.

Wells' s.

Wenckebach's d.

Werdnig-Hoffmann d., s.

Werlhof's d.

Wermer's s.

Werner-His d.

Werner-Schultz d.

Werner's s.

Wernicke-Korsakoff s.

Wernicke's d., s.

Wesselsbron d.

Westphal's d.

Westphal-Strümpell d.

West's s.

Weyers' oligodactyly s.

Weyers-Thier s.

Whipple's d.

White's d.

Whitmore's d.

Whytt's d.

Widal s.

Widal-Abrami d.

Wildervanck s.

Wilkie's d.

Willebrand's s.

Williams-Campbell s.

Williams s.

Willis' d.

Wilson-Mikity s.

Wilson's d., s.

Winckel's d.

Windscheid's d.

Winiwarter-Buerger d.

Winkler's d.

Winter's s.

Winton d.

Wiskott-Aldrich s.

Witkop's d.

Witkop–Von Sallmann d.

Wohlfart-Kugelberg-Welander d.

Wolff-Parkinson-White s.

Wolf-Hirschhorn s.	Zahorsky's d.
Wolfram s.	Zellweger s.
Wolman's d.	Ziehen-Oppenheim d.
Woringer-Kolopp d.	Zieve's s.
Wright's s.	Zinsser-Cole-Engman s.
Young's s.	Zollinger-Ellison s.

Culture Media*

(a. = agar; b. = broth; c. = culture medium; m. = medium)

acetate differential a.
agar c.
albumin b. (Dubos)
Anderson's m.
antibiotic c.
Aronson's c.
asparagin c.
Avery's c.
azide violet blood a.
bacteriostasis a.
Balamuth's c.
Barile-Yaguchi-Eveland (BYE) a.
basal c.
beef infusion c.
beer wort c.
bile c., bile salt c.
bismuth sulfite a.
blood c. (Kracke)
Boeck and Drbohlav's c.
Bordet-Gengou a.
boric acid b.
brain-heart infusion m.
Braun's c.
brilliant green a.
brilliant green-bile a.
bromcresol purple desoxycholate (BCP-D) a.
Brucella a.
buffered desoxycholate glucose (BDG) b.
carbohydrate b.
Cary-Blair transport m.
Casman's b.
cell c.
Chapman-Stone a.
charcoal a.
chlamydospore a.

chocolate c.
Clark and Lubs c.
Clauberg's a.
clearing m.
clostrisel a.
coagulase-mannitol a.
corn meal a.
Corper's c.
Craig's c.
cystine-heart a.
Czapek-Dox a.
decarboxylase c.
deoxycholate-citrate m.
deoxycholate citrate lactose saccharose (DCLS) a.
dextrose a.
dextrose starch a.
Dieudonné's c.
differential c.
Dorset's egg c.
Dubos' c.
Durham's c.
Eagle's basal m.
egg c.
egg albumin c.
egg-meat c.
Eijkman lactose b.
Eisenberg's milk-rice c.
EMB a.
Emerson a.
Endo a.
enriched c.
eosin-methylene blue (EMB) a.
eosin-methylthionine chloride c.
esculin c.
ethyl violet azide b.
extract a.

* Adapted from Dorland's Illustrated Medical Dictionary, 26th ed. Philadelphia, W.B. Saunders Company, 1981.

FDA m.
Fildes' c.
fish b.
Fletcher's m.
Forget-Fredette a.
formate ricinoleate m.
Fränkel and Voges' asparagin c.
fuchsin a., fuchsin sulfite a.
gelatin a., c.
glucose-formate b.
glycerin b.
glycerinated potato c.
glycerin-potato b.
hanging block m.
haricot b.
Hershell's c.
hormone c.
Hoyle's m.
indicator c.
infusion m.
inosite-free b.
iron b.
Jordan's tartrate c.
Kendall's c.
KF streptococcal m.
Kitasato's b.
Kligler iron a.
Koser citrate b.
Krumwiede triple sugar a.
Kulp's c.
lactose-litmus b.
lauryl sulfate b.
lead b.
Les' c.
Levine's EMB a., Levine's eosin-
    methylene blue a.
Li-Rivers c.
litmus-milk c.
litmus-whey c.
Littman a.
Löffler's m.
Löwenstein-Jensen c.
Löwenstein's c.
L.S.U. m.
MacConkey a., b.
malachite green b.
malt a.
malt extract a., b.
mannitol salt a.
Martin's b.
meat extract m.
meat infusion m.

membrane filter m.
milk c.
milk-rice c.
mineral salts a.
Monsur's a.
motility test m.
MR-VP b.
Mueller-Hinton a.
Mycoplasma a.
Naegeli's c.
Neill's m.
neomycin assay a.
neutral red c.
NIH agar m.
nitrate b.
N.N.N. c.
Noguchi's c.
nutrient c.
nystatin assay a.
oleic a. (Dubos)
Omeliansky's nutritive c.
Pai's c.
Parietti's b.
Park and Williams' chocolate c.
Pasteur's c.
peptone water c.
Petragnani c.
Petroff's synthetic c.
Petruschky's c.
phenol red m.
phenylalanine a.
Pike's streptococcal b.
polymyxin test a's
potato blood a.
potato dextrose a.
proof a.
Proskauer-Beck m.
protein-free c.
rice extract a.
Robertson's c.
Rogosa SL m.
Rosenow's veal-brain b.
rosolic acid-peptone c.
Russell's double sugar a.
Sabouraud's a.
saccharose-mannitol a.
Salmonella-Shigella (SS) a.
seed a.
selective c.
selenite b.
selenite-cystine b.
semisolid c.

serum b.
silicate jelly c.
Simmons' citrate a.
Snyder's a.
Soyka's milk-rice c.
spirit blue a.
Spirolate b.
standard methods a.
sterility test b., c.
streptomycin assay a. with yeast
    extract
Stuart b.
sugar b.
sulfite a.
sulfite polymyxin sulfadiazine
    (SPS) a.
tartrate c.
TB charcoal a.
TCBS a.
tellurite a.
tellurite glycine a.

tetrathionate b.
tetrathionate enrichment b.
Thayer-Martin m.
thiosulfate citrate bile salts sucrose
    (TCBS) a.
Tindale's m.
Todd-Hewitt b.
tomato juice a.
triple sugar iron a.
Trudeau's m.
urea a.
urease test b.
Uschinsky's c.
veal infusion c.
Venkatraman-Ramikrishnan m.
wheat b.
Wilson-Blair c.
Winogradsky's c.
wort a., b.
yeast autolysate c.
zein a.

APPENDIX 4
Table of Elements

TABLE OF ELEMENTS

NAME	SYMBOL	AT. NO.	AT. WT.*	NAME	SYMBOL	AT. NO.	AT. WT.*
Actinium	Ac	89	227.028	Mendelevium	Md	101	(258)
Aluminum	Al	13	26.982	Mercury	Hg	80	200.59
Americium	Am	95	(243)	Molybdenum	Mo	42	95.94
Antimony	Sb	51	121.75	Neodymium	Nd	60	144.24
Argon	Ar	18	39.948	Neon	Ne	10	20.179
Arsenic	As	33	74.922	Neptunium	Np	93	237.0482
Astatine	At	85	(210)	Nickel	Ni	28	58.69
Barium	Ba	56	137.33	Niobium	Nb	41	92.906
Berkelium	Bk	97	(247)	Nitrogen	N	7	14.007
Beryllium	Be	4	9.012	Nobelium	No	102	259
Bismuth	Bi	83	208.980	Osmium	Os	76	190.2
Boron	B	5	10.811	Oxygen	O	8	15.999
Bromine	Br	35	79.904	Palladium	Pd	46	106.42
Cadmium	Cd	48	112.41	Phosphorus	P	15	30.974
Calcium	Ca	20	40.08	Platinum	Pt	78	195.08
Californium	Cf	98	(251)	Plutonium	Pu	94	(244)
Carbon	C	6	12.011	Polonium	Po	84	(209)
Cerium	Ce	58	140.12	Potassium	K	19	39.098
Cesium	Cs	55	132.905	Praseodymium	Pr	59	140.908
Chlorine	Cl	17	35.453	Promethium	Pm	61	(145)
Chromium	Cr	24	51.996	Protactinium	Pa	91	231.036
Cobalt	Co	27	58.933	Radium	Ra	88	226.025
Copper	Cu	29	63.546	Radon	Rn	86	(222)
Curium	Cm	96	(247)	Rhenium	Re	75	186.207
Dysprosium	Dy	66	162.50	Rhodium	Rh	45	102.906
Einsteinium	Es	99	(252)	Rubidium	Rb	37	85.468
Element 106		106	(263)	Ruthenium	Ru	44	101.07
Erbium	Er	68	167.26	Rutherfordium	Rf	104	(261)
Europium	Eu	63	151.96	Samarium	Sm	62	150.36
Fermium	Fm	100	(257)	Scandium	Sc	21	44.956
Fluorine	F	9	18.998	Selenium	Se	34	78.96
Francium	Fr	87	(223)	Silicon	Si	14	28.086
Gadolinium	Gd	64	157.25	Silver	Ag	47	107.868
Gallium	Ga	31	69.72	Sodium	Na	11	22.990
Germanium	Ge	32	72.59	Strontium	Sr	38	87.62
Gold	Au	79	196.967	Sulfur	S	16	32.064
Hafnium	Hf	72	178.49	Tantalum	Ta	73	180.948
Hahnium	Ha	105	(261)	Technetium	Tc	43	(98)

Element	Symbol	No.	Atomic Weight	Element	Symbol	No.	Atomic Weight
Helium	He	2	4.003	Tellurium	Te	52	127.60
Holmium	Ho	67	164.930	Terbium	Tb	65	158.925
Hydrogen	H	1	1.008	Thallium	Tl	81	204.383
Indium	In	49	114.82	Thorium	Th	90	232.038
Iodine	I	53	126.905	Thulium	Tm	69	168.934
Iridium	Ir	77	192.22	Tin	Sn	50	118.69
Iron	Fe	26	55.847	Titanium	Ti	22	47.88
Krypton	Kr	36	83.80	Tungsten	W	74	183.85
Lanthanum	La	57	138.906	Uranium	U	92	238.029
Lawrencium	Lw	103	(260)	Vanadium	V	23	50.942
Lead	Pb	82	207.2	Xenon	Xe	54	131.29
Lithium	Li	3	6.941	Ytterbium	Yb	70	173.04
Lutetium	Lu	71	174.967	Yttrium	Y	39	88.906
Magnesium	Mg	12	24.312	Zinc	Zn	30	65.38
Manganese	Mn	25	54.938	Zirconium	Zr	40	91.22

*Atomic weights are corrected to conform with the 1979 values of the International Union of Pure and Applied Chemistry, expressed to the fourth decimal point, rounded off to the nearest thousandth. The numbers in parentheses are the mass numbers of the most stable or most common isotope.

(From Dorland's Illustrated Medical Dictionary, 28th ed., p. 539. Philadelphia, W. B. Saunders Company, 1994).

Symbols*

Ⓛ	left	↑V	increase due to in vivo effect
Ⓜ	murmur	↓V	decrease due to in vivo effect
®	right trademark	↑C	increase due to chemical
⊙	start of operation		interference during the
⊗	end of operation		assay
□	male	↓C	decrease due to chemical
○	female		interference during the
♂	male		assay
♀	female	→	causes, no change,
*	birth		transfer to
†	death	←	is due to
τ	life (time)	⊖	normal
τ½	half-life (time)	√c̄	check with
p̄	after	φ	none
ā	before	∨	systolic blood pressure
c̄	with	∧	diastolic blood pressure
s̄	without	#	gauge, number, weight
?	question of, questionable,	24°	24 hours
	possible	Δt	time interval
>	greater than	ΔA	change in absorbance
≥	greater than or equal to	ΔpH	change in pH
<	less than	Δ	prism diopter
≤	less than or equal to	3 = D	delayed double diffusion
~	approximate		(test)
≃	approximately equal to	606	arsphenamine
±	not definite, plus/minus	914	neoarsphenamine
(+)	significant	℞	take
(−)	insignificant	6-MP	6-mercaptopurine
(±)	possibly significant	³HT	H₃T, tritiated thymidine
↓	decreased, depression	1°	primary
↑	elevation, increased	2d	second
♠	up	2°	secondary

---

*Decimal prefixes are given in Appendix 1.

2ndry	secondary	μc	microcurie
2×	twice	μEq	microequivalent
×2	twice	μf	microfarad
1×	once	μg	microgram
°	degree	μl	microliter
′	foot	μμc	micromicrocurie (picocurie)
″	inch	μμg	micromicrogram (picogram)
ⅲ̈	two	μM	micromolar
/	of, per	μr	microroentgen
:	ratio (is to)	μsec	microsecond
+	positive, present	μu	microunit
−	absent, negative	μv	microvolt
$\overline{X}$	average of all X's	μw	microwatt
α	alpha particle, is	μγ	milligamma (nanogram)
	proportional to	mμ	millimicron
≠	does not equal	mμc	millimicrocurie (nanocurie)
X²	chi square (test)	mμg	millimicrogram (nanogram)
σ	1/100 of a second, standard	Ω	ohm
	deviation	℈	drachm, dram
℈	scruple	f℈	fluidrachm, fluidram
℥	ounce	∞	infinity
f℥	fluid ounce	☌	combined with
μ	micron	X	crossed with, as in
μμ	micromicron		hybridization

Greek Alphabet

Name of letter	Capital	Lower case	Transliteration
alpha	A	α	a
beta	B	ь or β	b
gamma	Γ	γ	g
delta	Δ	δ	d
epsilon	E	ϵ	e short
zeta	Z	ζ	z
eta	H	η	e long
theta	Θ	θ	th
iota	I	ι	i
kappa	K	κ	k, c
lambda	Λ	λ	l
mu	M	μ	m
nu	N	ν	n
xi	Ξ	ξ	x
omicron	O	o	o short
pi	Π	π	p
rho	P	ρ	r
sigma	Σ	σ or ς	s
tau	T	τ	t
upsilon	Υ	υ	y
phi	Φ	ϕ or φ	f
chi	X	χ	ch, kh
psi	Ψ	ψ	ps
omega	Ω	ω	o long